Dietary Pattern and Health
Volume 2

Special Issue Editor
Zumin Shi

MDPI • Basel • Beijing • Wuhan • Barcelona • Belgrade

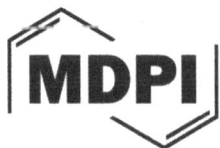

MDPI

Special Issue Editor
Zumin Shi
University of Adelaide
Australia

Editorial Office
MDPI AG
St. Alban-Anlage 66
Basel, Switzerland

This edition is a reprint of the Special Issue published online in the open access journal *Nutrients* (ISSN 2072-6643) from 2015–2016 (available at: http://www.mdpi.com/journal/nutrients/special_issues/dietary-pattern-health).

For citation purposes, cite each article independently as indicated on the article page online and as indicated below:

Author 1; Author 2. Article title. *Journal Name* **Year**, *Article number*, page range.

First Edition 2017

Volume 1
ISBN 978-3-03842-587-8 (Pbk)
ISBN 978-3-03842-588-5 (PDF)

Volume 2
ISBN 978-3-03842-595-3 (Pbk)
ISBN 978-3-03842-596-0 (PDF)

Volume I – Volume II
ISBN 978-3-03842-597-7 (Pbk)
ISBN 978-3-03842-610-3 (PDF)

Table of Contents

About the Special Issue Editor

Zumin Shi is an associate professor at the University of Adelaide. He got his medical degree in Beijing Medical University in 1988. From 1988 to 2001, he worked at Jiangsu Provincial Center for Disease Control and Prevention, China. Having 13 years' experience in nutrition and foodborne disease prevention, he started his master in international community health in University of Oslo in 2001. He was conferred a PhD in the area of epidemiology from University of Oslo in Feb 2007. After his PhD he had his postdoc in University of Newcastle, and University of Oslo. In 2009, he joined SA Health and University of Adelaide. Dr. Shi's main research interest is the relationship between food intake, lifestyles and chronic diseases. He also has interests in food safety and foodborne disease prevention. He has published over 150 journal articles and authored a number of books.

Preface to "Dietary Pattern and Health"

This special issue is divided into two volumes based on how dietary patterns were constructed for use in dietary studies: Volume 1 contains studies considering the relationship between posteriori dietary patterns and health outcome (18 papers) while Volume 2 includes studies considering: a priori dietary patterns and health outcome (20 papers).

In Volume 1, a posteriori dietary patterns based on factor analysis/principal component analysis (PCA, 15 papers), cluster analysis (2 papers), reduced rank regression (RRR, 2 papers) and various health outcomes are covered. Seven papers from China, Spain, the Netherlands and South Africa focus on dietary patterns and obesity. Six papers have assessed the association between dietary patterns and metabolic diseases in Ghana, Australia, China, Qatar, and USA. Studies on the associations between dietary patterns and cognitive function, atopic dermatitis and general health are also included. Most of the studies use a comprehensive food frequency questionnaire (FFQ) to assess food intake. A small number of studies use a short version of FFQ.

Three papers use data from national representative studies including the National Health and Nutrition Examination Survey (NHANES) in the USA, China Kadoorie Biobank survey, and Australian Health Survey 2011.

There are three pioneering papers in terms of methodology in the volume. Using principal component analysis, Pisa et al. construct nutrient patterns and find a positive association between animal-based nutrient pattern and obesity among rural South African adolescents. Thani et al. construct lifestyle patterns by incorporating dietary habits and lifestyle factors among Qatari women of childbearing age. Similarly, Perez-Rodrigo et al. combine factor analysis and cluster analysis to assess the association between lifestyle patterns and obesity among Spanish children and adolescents. This novel data-driven approach highlighted the synergistic effect of the clustering of dietary habits and other lifestyles. It can be used as an alternative to the priori healthy lifestyle scores.

In Volume 2, there are four sections. In the review and perspective section, four papers focus on Mediterranean diet. Davis et al. systematically review the definition of Mediterranean diet used in population based research. Hoffman et al discuss the influence of food processing techniques on nutritional values (e.g. phytochemicals) in the Mediterranean diet. This is an important area but often neglected in the research or promotion of Mediterranean diet. It may help to understand the association between diet and health in populations with different cooking practices. D'Alessandro et al review population studies on the association between Mediterranean diet and cardiovascular diseases. The review by Fito discusses the role of nutritional genomics in the association between Mediterranean diet and cardiovascular disease.

In section 2, seven original research papers describe the association between priori dietary pattern scores (e.g. Mediterranean diet score, Nordic Food Index, diet quality score) and health outcomes (bone mineral density, polycystic ovary syndrome, diabetes, cardiovascular disease, nasopharyngeal carcinoma, and general health).

Three papers are included in the clinical trial section focusing on 1) the effect of weight loss on leptin and adiponectin; 2) sex difference in the effect of Mediterranean diet on LDL, and 3) feasibility of recruiting families in intervention program based on dietary patterns.

The last section of Volume 2 focuses on the food and nutrients intake as well as the associations with health outcomes. Some of the papers may help to understand the association between dietary patterns and health outcomes. For example, a study by Cao et al. assesses the association between macronutrient intake and obstructive sleep apnea among Australian men and found high fat intake is associated with daytime sleepiness. Using data from the 2008/2009 New Zealand Adult Nutrition Survey, Brow et al. find that nut consumption was associated with more favorable body composition and cardiometabolic profiles.

The collection of papers suggest that dietary pattern analysis is an area of growing interest. Findings from the papers show the importance of overall dietary patterns. The dietary pattern analysis approach takes into account the synergetic effects of food and nutrients. Factor analysis/PCA is the most commonly used method in the posteriori dietary pattern research. Currently, all the studies using RRR method were conducted using SAS software. As the free RRR packages became available in R (e.g. rrr package, rrpack), more studies in this area will be expected.

Zumin Shi
Special Issue Editor

![nutrients]

Review

MDPI

Definition of the Mediterranean Diet: A Literature Review

Courtney Davis [1,†], Janet Bryan [2,†], Jonathan Hodgson [3,†] and Karen Murphy [1,†,*]

1   Alliance for Research in Exercise, Nutrition and Activity, University of South Australia, Adelaide 5001, Australia; courtney.davis@mymail.unisa.edu.au
2   School of Psychology, Social Work and Social Policy, University of South Australia, Adelaide 5001, Australia; janet.bryan@unisa.edu.au
3   School of Medicine and Pharmacology, University of Western Australia, Crawley 6009, Australia; jonathan.hodgson@uwa.edu.au
*   Correspondence: karen.murphy@unisa.edu.au; Tel.: +61 00 0002 1000
†   These authors contributed equally to this work.

Received: 14 October 2015 ; Accepted: 30 October 2015 ; Published: 5 November 2015

Abstract: Numerous studies over several decades suggest that following the Mediterranean diet (MedDiet) can reduce the risk of cardiovascular disease and cancer, and improve cognitive health. However, there are inconsistencies among methods used for evaluating and defining the MedDiet. Through a review of the literature, we aimed to quantitatively define the MedDiet by food groups and nutrients. Databases PubMed, MEDLINE, Science Direct, Academic Search Premier and the University of South Australia Library Catalogue were searched. Articles were included if they defined the MedDiet in at least two of the following ways: (1) general descriptive definitions; (2) diet pyramids/numbers of servings of key foods; (3) grams of key foods/food groups; and (4) nutrient and flavonoid content. Quantity of key foods and nutrient content was recorded and the mean was calculated. The MedDiet contained three to nine serves of vegetables, half to two serves of fruit, one to 13 serves of cereals and up to eight serves of olive oil daily. It contained approximately 9300 kJ, 37% as total fat, 18% as monounsaturated and 9% as saturated, and 33 g of fibre per day. Our results provide a defined nutrient content and range of servings for the MedDiet based on past and current literature. More detailed reporting amongst studies could refine the definition further.

Keywords: Mediterranean diet; definition; quantity; foods and nutrients

---

1. Introduction

The Mediterranean diet (MedDiet) was first defined by Ancel Keys as being low in saturated fat and high in vegetable oils, observed in Greece and Southern Italy during the 1960s [1]. In the Seven Countries Study this dietary pattern was associated with reduced risk of coronary heart disease (CHD) compared to northern European countries and the United States after 25 years follow-up [2,3]. Over the past several decades the study of the MedDiet has advanced, and the definition originally introduced by Keys has evolved and varied. There are a number of ways to define a dietary pattern, including general descriptions, dietary pyramids, *a priori* scoring systems, *a posteriori* dietary pattern formation, or by food and nutrient content [4–9].

Of these, *a priori* scoring systems have gained most popularity in the past two decades as they simplify analysis of adherence to the diet in relation to primary outcomes [10]. Dietary intake is separated into selected food groups related to health outcomes and points are awarded for higher intakes of health-promoting foods and lower intakes of health-harming foods, to calculate a single adherence score. However there are several *a priori* Mediterranean diet scores (MDS) with different scoring criteria [11–14]. Sofi *et al.* [10] recently compared data from 26 cohort studies utilising some form of MDS, and noted the large range of cut-offs for major food groups such as cereals, even amongst similar populations. When compared on the same nutritional data, 10 different *a priori* MDS resulted in a mean adherence ranging from 22.7% to 87.7%, with poor correlation between most indices [14]. This implies the defining aspects of the MedDiet used to calculate these scores are widely different. Similarly, there are large differences between studies using gram intakes of foods and nutrient content as descriptions/adherence scores. For example, the Greeks in the Seven Countries study consumed an average of 191 g/day of vegetables, in the Prevención con Dieta Mediterránea (PREDIMED) study participants in the intervention group consumed approximately 350 g/day, and the Greeks enrolled in EPIC consumed over 500 g/day [11,15,16].

Marinez-Gonzalez *et al.* [1] suggest that "the very definition of the MedDiet is not a minor issue" (p 10), and point out that two prominent randomised trials investigating health effects of the MedDiet used interventions not fully in line with traditional ideas of the diet, such as the high oil content. A systematic review of intervention trials investigated the relationship between the MedDiet and health outcomes; the authors concluded that there is good evidence the diet improves the lipid profile, endothelial function and blood pressure, but that one of the most limiting factors to drawing conclusions was discrepancies in how the MedDiet had been defined and formulated [17].

Differences in definitions could be limiting our understanding of the mechanisms by which the MedDiet confers its health benefits. The biological actions of key nutritional components of the MedDiet, such as specific fatty acids, have been studied with promising, although somewhat inconsistent results [18]. One reason for this may be differences in dose of foods and nutrients between studies. Additionally it is difficult to formulate new MedDiets for intervention studies which are consistent with previous studies, as there is little consistency on which to base these new diets. One potential approach to address such problems is to form a more universal definition by calculating an average quantity of foods and nutrients from previous MedDiets, which would combine traditional and modern examples from relevant studies and provide a benchmark profile of the MedDiet. This definition could be used in future to design intervention MedDiets or MDS which are comparable to other studies. Our objective was to collate information from a range of studies to form a more comprehensive and quantitative definition of the MedDiet than presently exists, by summarising existing definitions and calculating the mean amounts of foods and nutrients.

2. Results

2.1. Mediterranean Diet: General Descriptions and Pyramids

General descriptions of the MedDiet are similar amongst publications, emphasising the same key components. The definitions include guidelines for high intake of extra virgin (cold pressed) olive oil, vegetables including leafy green vegetables, fruits, cereals, nuts and pulses/legumes, moderate intakes of fish and other meat, dairy products and red wine, and low intakes of eggs and sweets. Each description provides an indication of the frequency these foods should be consumed, for example often, daily, biweekly and the amounts in the diet, described using subjective terms such as abundance, high, moderate, low, some, and vast. Most lack specific suggestions for numbers of servings or serving size, and do not specify amounts of additives to the diet, such as sauces, condiments, tea, coffee, salt, sugar, or honey. Some definitions specify that cereals should be mostly wholegrain. The definitions from Willett *et al.* [6] Panagiotakos *et al.* [19] and Dilis *et al.* [20] add some description of traditional practices; olive oil was added to vegetables and legumes to make them palatable, fruits were eaten as desserts or snacks, cheeses accompanied salads and stews, and red meat was eaten only on special occasions.

Most commonly, recommended numbers of servings for these food groups are represented as a diet pyramid. Diet pyramids are considered a useful way to display the general principles of a diet including approximate recommendations for quantities of food groups (*i.e.*, those consumed in greatest quantities appear in the largest section of the pyramid). Three MedDiet pyramids were chosen as a representative sample for this review, although several others exist. In 1993, the first MedDiet pyramid was produced by Oldway's Preservation and Exchange Trust [6]. This was updated in 2009 [21]. The 1999 Greek Dietary guidelines are based on a traditional MedDiet and are also expressed in pyramid form [22]. A third pyramid model of the diet was released in 2010 by the Mediterranean Diet Foundation (MDF), intended as a flexible, general representation of the MedDiet [5]. The pyramid of the Greek dietary guidelines is semi-quantitative, providing serving number and size. The recommendations of these three pyramids are compared in Table 1.

Table 1. Comparison of dietary recommendations for three Mediterranean diet pyramids.

Foods	Oldway's Preservation and Trust (2009) [21]	Mediterranean Diet Foundation (2011) [5]	1999 Greek Dietary Guidelines (1999) [22] [1]
Olive oil	Every meal	Every meal	Main added lipid
Vegetables	Every meal	≥2 serves every meal	6 serves daily
Fruits	Every meal	1–2 serves every meal	3 serves daily
Breads and cereals	Every meal	1–2 serves every meal	8 serves daily
Legumes	Every meal	≥2 serves weekly	3–4 serves weekly
Nuts	Every meal	1–2 serves daily	3–4 serves weekly
Fish/Seafood	Often, at least two times per week	≥2 serves weekly	5–6 servings weekly
Eggs	Moderate portions, daily to weekly	2–4 serves weekly	3 servings weekly
Poultry	Moderate portions, daily to weekly	2 serves weekly	4 servings weekly
Dairy foods	Moderate portions, daily to weekly	2 serves daily	2 serves daily
Red meat	Less often	<2 serves/week	4 servings monthly
Sweets	Less often	<2 serves/week	3 servings weekly
Red wine	In moderation	In moderation and respecting social beliefs	Daily in moderation

[1] Serving sizes specified as: 25 g bread, 100 g potato, 50–60 g cooked pasta, 100 g vegetables, 80 g apple, 60 g banana, 100 g orange, 200 g melon, 30 g grapes, 1 cup milk or yoghurt, 1 egg, 60 g meat, 100 g cooked dry beans.

The general structure and placement of key food groups in the pyramids is similar however the pyramids differ in their recommendations for vegetables and fruits, nuts and legumes, fish/seafood and poultry. Recommendations for legume intake range from every meal to at least twice a week. The MDF suggests daily nuts, while the Greek guidelines are less specific and recommend fewer servings.

2.2. Mediterranean Diet: Quantity of Food in Grams

The gram quantity for foods or food groups was reported for 15 separate populations in 11 papers, spanning a timeline of 46 years of data collection (1960–2006) [8,11,16,23–30]. Twelve of the 15 reports were based on observations of dietary intake, most commonly collected by food frequency questionnaire or food recalls [8,11,16,23,24,26–28]. All of these observations were of local Mediterranean populations excepting one, which observed Greek-Australian migrants living in Melbourne, Australia [26]. Of the three interventions, two were in a local French Mediterranean population, the third in an Australian population [25,29,30]. All reports included gram values for the groups all cereals, all vegetables, fruits/nuts and meat/meat products. All dairy and legumes were reported for all but one population and fish in all but two. Reporting of bread, potato, cheese, eggs and oil was less consistent; olive oil was reported in 11 data sets, eggs in nine, cheese and potato in seven and bread intake recorded in five. Table 2 shows the amount of foods in grams in the MedDiet by study, and the average and standard deviation for each food group. Table 3 shows the conversion of grams of foods to standard Australian serving sizes, compared to recommendations according to the Australian Dietary Guidelines [19]. According to the lowest and highest intakes reported, the MedDiet contained between three and nine serves of vegetables, half to two serves of fruits, one to 13 serves of cereals and 1.5 to eight serves of olive oil daily. The recommended number of servings according to the Greek Dietary Guidelines and the MDF pyramid differ considerably from the average numbers of servings derived here, based on Australian serving sizes. Fruits, nuts and fish servings are considerably less than recommended.

2.3. Mediterranean Diet: Nutrient Content

Eight papers reported the nutrient content of the MedDiet in sufficient detail to be included in this review [4,15,27–29,31–33]. Table 4 shows the mean nutrient content of the MedDiet. Four of the eight included papers were intervention studies, two were descriptive papers and two were observational studies. The interventions took place in France, Australia, Spain and Sweden [15,25,29,33]. The observations were of Spanish adults recruited for the European Prospective Investigation into Cancer and Nutrition (EPIC) study [27,28]. The two descriptive papers analysed the nutrient content of Mediterranean menus designed specifically for the study, both based on the traditional Cretan diet [4,32]. Two others reported only on specific fatty acid content of the diet (Table 5) [3,11].

All papers reported the energy and fibre content, and all but one reported the per cent energy contribution from saturated fat (SFA). It was possible to derive the monounsaturated fat (MUFA) to SFA ratio for all papers. According to these eight papers, the MedDiet contains approximately 9.3 MJ/day, and provides close to 37% energy from total fat, 19% from MUFA, 5% from PUFA, 9% from SFA, 15% from protein and 43% energy from carbohydrate. The specific fatty acids intakes observed from the Seven Countries Study and amongst the Greek cohort of the EPIC study are shown in Table 5 [3]. The addition of this data did not greatly alter the average total fat and energy contents, although they did result in slightly higher intakes. Two papers included long chain omega-3 PUFA content expressed as % of total energy, with an average of 1.4%, and three papers as grams/day, with an average of 1.1 [4,15,25,27,33].

2.4. Mediterranean Diet: Flavonoid Content

Bioactive compounds include a range of non-nutritive substances thought to confer health benefits, including polyphenolic compounds and phytosterols [34]. The most notable of the polyphenols are flavonoids, water soluble plant components which are known to have antioxidant properties *in vitro* [34]. There are six classes of flavonoids including flavones, flavonols, flavanols (flavan-3ols), flavanones, anthocyanidins and isoflavones [35]. These are sourced primarily from red wine, olive oil, coffee, tea, nuts, fruits, vegetables, herbs and spices. Four papers reported specifically on the flavonoid content of the diet [21,36–38]. The mean daily flavonoid content presented in the four papers is compared in Table 6. Vasilopoulou *et al.* [38] developed a theoretical seven-day traditional Mediterranean menu based on the 1999 Greek dietary guidelines [39]. The 2003 United States Department of Agriculture (USDA) flavonoid tables were used to estimate flavone, flavonol, flavanol, flavanone and anthocyanidin content, and isoflavone content was estimated from the VENUS phytoestrogen database [38]. Dilis *et al.* [21] analysed this same menu chemically for the luteolin, apigenin (flavones), quercetin, kaempferol, myricetin, isorhamnetin (flavonols) and catechin, epicatechin, epigallocatechin, epicatechin gallate and epigallocatechin (flavanols) content and determined the total daily content as 79.01 mg. Vasilopoulou *et al.* [38] found the combined total of flavones, flavonols and flavanols was 67.8 mg/day, as calculated from the 2003 USDA tables (Table 6). Zamora-Ros *et al.* [36] using an updated USDA flavonoid database (2007) estimated the total daily flavonoid intake of the Spanish cohort recruited for the EPIC study. Dietary intake was assessed by a computerised diet history questionnaire administered by a dietitian in a personal interview. Tresserra-Rimbau *et al.* [37] conducted the only analysis of polyphenol intake based partially on an intervention MedDiet. Over 7000 high-risk Spanish adult participants with complete dietary data were included from the PREDIMED study. Polyphenol intake, including flavonoids, was calculated using the Phenol-Explorer database which provides information on polyphenol content for 456 foods. Dietary data was collected from a 137-item FFQ, administered in person by a dietitian.

Table 2. Grams per day of key foods and food groups in the Mediterranean diet, in order of date data was collected, including mean ± SD.

Reference	Study Type/Notes	Years of Data Collection	Bread	All Cereals [1]	Legumes	Potato	All Vegetables [2]	Fruits/Nuts	Meat/Meat Products [3]	Cheese	All Dairy [4]	Eggs	Olive Oil	Fish [5]
							Food Groups							
Alberti-Fidanza and Fidanza (2004) [39][6]	Observational study, Italian cohort, 1960s. Based on WFRs. Male adults only	1960	NR	488	49	NR	344	101	55	15	48	20	NR	42
Alberti-Fidanza and Fidanza (2004) [39]	Observational study, Italian cohort, 1960s. Based on WFRs. Female adults only	1960	NR	348	36	NR	274	76	25	12	49	11	NR	30
Kromhout et al., (1989) [16]	Observational study, Greek cohort 1960s. Based on 7-d WFRs	1960–1965	415	452.5	30	170	361	463	35	13.5	165.5	15	80	39
Kromhout et al., (1989) [16]	Observational study, Italian cohort, 1960s. Based on 7-d WFRs	1960–1969	353	513	5.5	43	210	109.5	119.5	28.5	223.5	46.5	60.5	28.5
Varela-Moreiras et al., (2010) [23][6,7]	Observational study, Spanish cohort, based on FFQ	1964	368	434	20.2	300	451	155	77	NR	~229	NR	~68	63
Trichopoulou et al., (1995) [8][8]	Observational study, Greek cohort. Based on FFQs	1988–1990	NR	288	60.5	NR	296	264	112	NR	246	NR	NR	NR
de Logeril et al., (1994) [24]	Intervention study. MedDiet vs. advice from hospital dietitians. Based on 24-h recalls	1988–1992	167	261	19.9	NR	316	251	105	32.2	NR	NR	15.7	46.5
Kouris-Blazos et al., (1999) [25]	Observational study, Greek-Australians. Based on FFQs	1990–1992	NR	353	86	NR	252	246	190	NR	246	NR	NR	NR
Guallar-Castillon et al., (2012) [26]	Observational study, Spanish middle-age adults. Based on FFQs	1992–1996	NR	230	52	79	334	325	126	27	297	26	NR	63
Buckland et al., (2009) [27][9]	Observational study, Spanish adults. Based on FFQs	1992–1996	NR	198.2	52.2	NR	269.3	353.3	128	NR	323.8	NR	20.7	61.1
Trichopoulou et al., (2003) [11]	Observational study, Greek cohort. Based on FFQs. Males only	1994–1999	NR	191.0	10.4	98.9	682.5	393.0	129	NR	222.6	19.0	46.2	26.4
Trichopoulou et al., (2003) [11]	Observational study, Greek cohort. Based on FFQs. Females only	1994–1999	NR	145.7	7.9	73.5	609.6	385.7	94.5	NR	216.2	15.7	38.9	21.7

Table 2. *Cont.*

Reference	Study Type/Notes	Years of Data Collection	Bread	All Cereals [1]	Legumes	Potato	All Vegetables [2]	Fruits/Nuts	Meat/Meat Products [3]	Cheese	All Dairy [4]	Eggs	Olive Oil	Fish [5]
Itsiopoulos et al., (2011) [28]	Intervention study MedDiet vs. HabDiet. Based on 7-day diet records	1998–2001	190	263	56	116	582	307	45	25	126	19	65	37
Vincent-Baudry et al., (2005) [29]	Intervention study. MedDiet vs. low fat diet. Based on 3-d WFR	1998–2002	NR	200	NR	NR	350	303	150	NR	200	NR	20	100
Varela-Moreiras et al., (2010) [23] [6]	Observational study, Spanish cohort. Based on FFQs	2000–2006	NR	221.1	12.6	NR	302.1	298.6	82.0	NR	398.1	34.7	49.5	98.4
	Mean		298.6	305.8	35.6	125.8	374.9	268.7	05.1	21.9	213.6	23.0	44.0	50.5
	SD		112.3	118.5	24.3	86.5	142.0	115.0	49.9	8.2	96.2	11.2	22.7	25.5

[1] All cereals group includes all refined and whole grain products reported, including bread; [2] All vegetables including potatoes; [3] Meat, Meat products group includes all unprocessed and processed red meat, white meat and delicatessen meats unless otherwise specified; [4] All dairy includes cheese, milk and milk products, and yoghurt as reported; [5] Fish includes oily fish, non-oily fish and shellfish; [6] Fruit and nuts group includes fruit only; [7] Meat/meat products includes chicken only; [8] Original data presented as mean daily consumption in grams adjusted for energy, separated into survivors and dead. Average presented; [9] Intakes divided into tertiles of MedDiet score, average of three tertiles used. Mean of both genders reported. Originally reported as g/1000 Calories, converted to total by (grams*(total Calories/1000)). WFR, weighed food record; NR, not reported; FFQ, food frequency questionnaire.

Table 3. Servings of food groups in the Mediterranean diet, calculated as standard Australian serving sizes, compared to Australian Dietary Guidelines [30], Greek Dietary Guidelines [22] and Mediterranean Diet Foundation [5] recommendations.

	Food Groups												
	Bread	All Cereals	Legumes[1]	Potato	All Vegetables	Fruits[2]	Nuts[1,2]	Meat/Meat Products[1]	Cheese	Other Dairy	Eggs[1]	Olive Oil	Fish[1]
Average content of the MedDiet, g/day[3]	300	305	35	125	375	225	4	105	21	215	23	45	50
Australian standard serving size, g or mL [30]	40	40–120	75–150	75	75	150	30	65–80	40	200–250 g	120	10 mL	100
Number of standard serves	7.5/day	2.5–7.5/day (average 4)	0.25–0.5/day, 1.6–3/week	1.5/day, 11.5/week	5/day	1.5/day	1/week	0.5–0.75/day	0.5/day, 3.5/week	1/day	0.25/day, 1.75/week	4.5/day, 31.5/week	0.5/day, 3.5/week
ADG recommended serves/day, adult men	NS	6	3	NS	6	2	3	3	NS	2.5	3	NS	3
ADG recommended serves/day, adult women	NS	6	2.5	NS	5	2	2.5	2.5	NS	2.5	2.5	NS	2.5
GDG recommended serves	NS	8/day	3–4/week	NS	6/day	3/day	3–4/week	Red meat 4/month, Poultry 4/week	NS	2/day	3/week	Daily, NFS	5–6/week
MDF recommended serves	NS	1–2/meal	>2/week	<3/week	>2/meal	1–2/meal	1–2/day	Red meat <2/week, White meat 2/week	NS	2/day	2–4/week	Every meal, NFS	>2/week

[1] Lean meat/poultry/fish/eggs/nuts and seeds/legumes grouped together in dietary guidelines, no recommendation for number of serves for individual foods such as nuts, legumes, fish or seeds; [2] Fruits and nut intakes based on papers provided this information (8 papers reported fruit, 2 papers reported nuts). Mean combined fruits/nuts was 270 g calculated in Table 2; [3] rounded to nearest 5 g. ADG, Australian Dietary Guidelines; GDG, Greek Dietary Guidelines; NS, not specified NFS, not further specified; MDF, Mediterranean diet foundation.

Table 4. Daily energy and nutrient content of the Mediterranean diet, in order of date of data collection, including mean ± SD.

Reference	Study Type/Notes	Years of Data Collection	Energy [1] (kJ/kCal)	Total Fat (g)	PRO (g)	MUFA (g)	PUFA (g)	SFA (g)	% E from Total Fat	% E from MUFA	% E from PUFA	% E from SFA	MUFA:SFA Ratio [2]	% E from CHO	% E from Protein	Fibre (g)	Vit C (mg)	Folate (ug)	Pot (mg)
Katatos et al., (2000) [4].	Descriptive study. Based on WFR	1960–1965	11016/2633	77	NR	67	18	25	41.3	23	6.0	9	2.68	45	12	47	258	559	4504
de Lorgeril et al., (1994) [31].[3]	Intervention study. Based on 24-h food recall and FFQ	1988–1992	8146/1947	NR	NR	NR	NR	NR	30.4	12.9	4.6	8	1.6	NR	15.2	18.6	115.8	NR	NR
Buckland et al., (2009) [27].[4]	Observational cohort study. Based on FFQs	1992–1996	8669/2072	82.5	90.75	37.5	11.8	22.6	35.2	16	5.1	9.6	1.66	40.8	17.8	27.4	172.7	NR	NR
Guallar-Castillon et al., (2012) [26].[5]	Observational cohort study. Based on FFQs	1992–1996	10021/2395	NR	110.2	NR	NR	NR	NR	NR	NR	NR	2.00	NR	NR	25.3	279.9	512.5	NR
Trichopoulou et al., (2006) [32].	Descriptive study. Based on menu designed from GDG[6]	1999 [6]	2473/10347	110.7	74.5	63.8	9.9	29.8	39.6	22.8	3.5	10.7	2.14	39.6	12.2	29.8	NR	NR	1774
Itsiopoulos et al., (2011) [28].	Intervention study. Based on 7-day diet records	1998–2001	9300/2223	NR	NR	NR	NR	NR	NR	21.3	NR	8.2	2.60	43.5	13.5	36.2	191.1	453	4565
Ambring et al., (2004) [33].	Cross over intervention. Based on 24-h recalls.	NR	7820/1869	NR	NR	NR	NR	NR	NR	14	NR	8	1.75	48	16	40	NR	NR	NR
Estruch et al., (2013) [15].[7]	Intervention study. Based on FFQs	2003–2010	9205/2200	NR	NR	NR	NR	NR	NR	21.5	NR	9.4	2.04	40	15.3	26.2	NR	NR	NR
		Mean	9316/2226	89.9	91.8	56.3	13.3	25.9	36.6	18.8	4.8	9.0	2.1	42.8	14.9	31.3	203.5	508.2	3614.3
		SD	1101/236	18.2	17.9	15.9	4.2	3.5	4.9	4.3	1.0	1.0	0.4	3.3	2.3	9.2	66.3	53.1	1594.1

[1] Where energy reported in kilojoules, converted to Calories (kilojoules/4.184). To convert from Calories to kilojoules, multiply by 4.184; [2] If not provided, calculated from grams fat. If grams not provided, calculated from percentage energy from MUFA and SFA.; [3] Dietary intake from experimental group presented, at an average of 4 years follow-up. Vitamin C presented as ascorbic acid from original publication (June 1994), de Lorgeril et al. [24]. Percent energy from MUFA presented as oleic acid only (18:1 omega-9); [4] Reported mean intakes of highest tertile for MedDiet adherence. Reported as g/1000 Calories. Converted to total grams by formula (grams × (Calories/1000)). Calculated energy contributions (%) from grams of macronutrients; [5] Highest quintile reported for MedDiet adherence score. PRO and total fat reported as g/1000 Calories. Converted to total grams by formula (grams × (Calories/1000)); [6] Based on 1999 Greek dietary guidelines; [7] Average of walnut and olive oil intervention groups presented. PRO, protein; MUFA, monounsaturated fat; PUFA, polyunsaturated fat; SFA, saturated fat; CHO, carbohydrate; Vit, vitamin; mg, milligrams; µg, micrograms; POT, potassium; WFR, weighed food record; NR, Not reported; FFQ, food frequency questionnaire; GDG, Greek dietary guidelines; SD, standard deviation.

Table 5. Mean nutrient intake (grams per day) reported in the Seven Countries Study (Greek and Italian cohorts) and EPIC study (Greek cohort).

	Nutrients and Energy, Mean ± SD				
	Energy (kJ/kCal)	SFA (g)	MUFA (g)	PUFA (g)	MUFA:SFA
Kromhout *et al.*, (1995) [3]. (Greeks)	2749 ± 100	24.9 ± 4.4	73.7 ± 14.7	14.4 ± 1.3	3.0 ± 0.1
Kromhout *et al.*, (1995) [3]. (Italians)	3043 ± 523	38.0 ± 14.1	58.9 ± 12.3	15.3 ± 5.5	1.6 ± 0.3
Trichopoulou *et al.*, (2003) [11]. (Greek Males)	2438 ± 705	34.6 ± 13.2	58.4 ± 20.0	17.5 ± 9.2	1.8 ± 0.5
Trichopoulou *et al.*, (2003) [11]. (Greek Females)	1931 ± 572	28.6 ± 11.6	48.7 ± 17.8	15 ± 8.2	1.7 ± 0.5
Mean ± SD (Table 5 only)	10628.5 ± 1989.2/2540 ± 475	31.5 ± 5.9	59.9 ± 10.3	15.6 ± 1.4	2.0 ± 0.7
Mean ± SD (Tables 4 and 5)	9753.2 ± 1506.2/2331 ± 360	29.1 ± 5.5	58.4 ± 11.9	14.6 ± 2.9	2.0 ± 0.5

EPIC, European Prospective Investigation into Cancer and Nutrition; SFA, saturated fat; MUFA, monounsaturated fat; PUFA, polyunsaturated fat; MUFA:SFA, monounsaturated to saturated fat ratio.

Table 6. Comparison of mean daily flavonoid intakes of the Mediterranean diet.

	Study Type	Years Data Collected	Participant Characteristics	Total Daily Flavonoid Intake (Mean) mg/Day
Zamora-Ros *et al.*, (2010) [34]	Observational study	1992–1996	Spanish adults aged 35–64	313.3
Tresserra-Rimbau *et al.*, (2014) [35]	Intervention study. MedDiet administered to half study sample	2003–2010	Spanish adults aged 55–80	Quintiles from lowest to highest: 273 362 431 512 670
Vasilopoulou *et al.*, (2005) [36]	Descriptive	NA	NA	118.6
Dilis *et al.*, (2007) [20] [1]	Descriptive	NA	NA	79.1
	Average flavonoid content			344.9

[1] Dilis *et al.* [20] included only flavones, flavonols, and flavan-3ols (flavanols) in their analysis; NA = not applicable.

3. Discussion

The MedDiet has been described similarly for the past five decades, and several pyramids represent the general principles. However, this review found that studies vary considerably when defining the amounts of foods in grams and/or nutrients constituting the MedDiet, although less so when the nutrient profiles are compared.

Dietary constituents of the MedDiet may reduce the risk of CVD and cancer in a dose dependent manner, highlighting the need for greater consistency between studies in the amount of foods and nutrients administered as part of a MedDiet. Sofi *et al.* [37] reviewed the dietary data of the Greek component of the EPIC study, and using segmented logistic regression models evaluated the dose-response relationship between intakes of the nine components of the MDS and overall mortality. There appeared to be an increased risk reduction at two threshold levels for intakes of fruits and nuts, meat and meat products, ethanol, vegetables, cereals and dairy [37].

Evidence from the present study shows considerable variation in quantity of MedDiet components. The intake of olive oil ranged from 15.7 to 80 mL/day, legumes from 5.5 to 60.5 g/day, vegetables from 210 to 682 g/day and fruits and nuts from 109 to 463 g/day amongst studies. A 5-fold difference in olive oil intake and 10-fold difference in legume intake could have significant implications for specific and all-cause mortality risk. Menotti *et al.* [2] used Seven Countries Study data to examine whether modest variations in food intake predicted changes in CHD death rate. The daily increase for oils (30 g), legumes (30 g), all vegetables (+ 20%, 189 g) and all vegetable food (+ 25%, 237 g) all predicted decreased death from CHD (by 18%, 28%, 28%, and 32%, respectively). Amongst the Spanish population of the EPIC study, for each 10 g increase in olive oil, the hazard ratio was 0.93 for risk of all-cause mortality (95% CI 0.90–0.97) [38]. Furthermore, sub-analyses from the PREDIMED study showed after 3 months on the intervention, C-reactive protein was significantly decreased in the extra virgin olive oil-enriched arm, but not the nut-enriched arm [40]. After 12 months, a 24 g/day increase in extra virgin olive oil resulted in a 0.3 μg/L decrease in TNF-α receptor 60 concentration, and a 62.7 g/day increase in vegetable intake resulted in a 0.2 μg/L decrease ($p < 0.05$) [41]. The variety of olive oil intake alone seen across different studies could affect whether the study finds significant effects of the MedDiet.

Quantity of foods appears to impact health outcomes, and forms the basis for most *a priori* MDS scoring criteria [11]. Meta-analytic evidence has shown those consuming more vegetables, fruits/nuts, legumes, cereals and fish, less dairy and meat/poultry and who have a higher MUFA:SFA and consume moderate amounts of ethanol have better cardiovascular and cognitive health than those consuming less [42,43]. However, the quantity used to define cut-offs varies between studies; when the 9-point MDS score was first used in 1995 the cut-off for vegetable intake was 303 g/day for men, and when used again in 2003 this increased to 550 g/day [8,11]. Differences of such magnitude are likely to substantially alter intakes of bioactive nutrients. Furthermore any subtle improvements in health with increasing intakes may be lost when only one cut-off point is used. There have been recent attempts to improve these scores—Sofi *et al.* [10,37] in their work have proposed scores with multiple cut-offs and using weighted mean cut-offs from a number of studies. While these newer scores are probably improvements on existing MDS's, they are still limited by a number of factors, such as failing to recognise major foods like nuts, and differences between studies as to foods are included into each food group. An average nutrient content may be more useful as a basis for forming *a priori* scoring systems.

In this review, nutrient content was found to be more consistent across different studies than food quantity. Different foods can provide similar nutrients which allows for preservation of unique foods and dishes observed amongst the different Mediterranean countries while retaining the mechanistic effects of the nutrients and bioactive compounds. Thus there is a distinct advantage to defining the diet by nutrients rather than foods. There are currently no *a priori* based scores which use nutrient content exclusively [11,19]. Consumption of fatty acids as a percentage of total energy intake, protein, the MUFA to SFA ratio and fibre, vitamins C and E, minerals including selenium and potassium, folate, β-carotene, antioxidant or phytosterol content may be useful nutrients to consider in defining the diet, as these nutrients are consistently implicated as combining for anti-CVD, anti-cancer, anti-aging effects and preventing cognitive decline [36,42,44–46]. According to this review, on average PUFA intake contributed 4.9% total energy, MUFA 18.4%, SFA 9.0%, the MUFA:SFA was 2.0, fibre intake was 33 g/day, vitamin C 225 mg/day and folate 508.2 μg/day. Notably, it was not possible to derive detailed information on the content of nutrients such as selenium, vitamin E, beta-carotene, long chain omega-3 PUFA or other bioactives such as plant sterols. Expressing nutrient intake as a percentage of total energy is recommended, as those consuming more energy will usually consume more nutrients [47].

Previously, Sauro-Calixto *et al.*, formed a definition of the MedDiet based on nutrient intakes of the Spanish population in 1964 [9]. This definition focused only on four biologically active components of the diet; fibre, total daily antioxidant capacity, MUFA:SFA and phytosterol content. The MUFA:SFA suggested to define the diet was 1.6–2.0, compared to 2.0 in the present study. This appears to be a consistent element of the MedDiet. A defining dietary fibre intake of 41–62 g/day compares to an average intake of 33 g/day found in the present study, with a large variation amongst both interventions and observations [15,16]. It is possible that fibre intake has been too low in recent interventions. The other two components of this definition are rarely considered in studies, total daily antioxidant capacity and phytosterol intake. From the four studies included in the review investigating the total flavonoid content, intake is likely to be at least 79 mg/day with an average of approximately 350 mg. Estimates for flavonoid intakes ranged from 79 to 670 mg/day, depending on population studied and whether chemical analysis or databases were used. Indeed there are so many methods for determination of flavonoids that it is not possible to compare studies.

Standardization of practices for determination of flavonoids is necessary before we can accurately compare different MedDiets and calculate an approximate range or average [15,24].

Because servings of foods tend to be better received than nutrients or grams in public health, we calculated the number of standard Australian serves provided on average by the MedDiet [30]. Based on the average gram content, the MedDiet provides approximately seven serves of bread, four serves of cereals, five serves of vegetables, 1.5 serves of potato, 1.5 serves of fruit, 0.5–0.75 serves of meat, 0.5 a serve of cheese, and one serve of dairy per day, as well as one serve nuts and three serves of legumes and fish per week. Popular Mediterranean pyramids recommend at least 3–4 weekly serves of nuts, and at least three daily serves of fruit, and usually fewer serves of potato. Considering the averages were based primarily on observation studies these difference are understandable—there appears to be a mismatch between the reality of what Mediterranean populations are eating and pyramid definitions of the MedDiet. This is one limitation of this review, which did not attempt to distinguish between definitions of the MedDiet based on whether they came from observations of diet, or intervention diets.

This review was limited by several other factors. Limited reporting of key nutrient or bioactive molecules has already been mentioned. Only four of 12 food groups had gram values from all 15 data sets. Only energy and fibre was provided by all eight studies, and seven provided the per cent contribution to total energy intake from the macronutrients. Three reported amounts of fats, protein and carbohydrates in grams, and only four reported on other key nutrients including calcium, potassium, phosphate, magnesium, sodium, folate and vitamins A, E and C. There was rarely information provided on sugar, sources of sugar (e.g., desserts or sweets) or wild greens and other herbs, known sources of antioxidants. The average values must be interpreted with some caution.

There were inconsistencies in classification of food groups. For example, the fruit and nuts group consisted only of fruits for intakes reported by Varela-Moreiras *et al.* [23] and Alberti-Fidanza *et al.* [39]. Potentially, separation of fruits and nuts would be worthwhile, as nuts appear to have an independent role in health [48]. Little information was given on the diet formation when administered as an intervention. It was often unclear whether there was consideration for origin of the diet, which (if any) previous research it had been modelled on, and where and how foods were sourced.

It may be becoming increasingly important to distinguish between observed modern MedDiets and the traditional model based primarily on the Cretan, Greek and Southern Italian diets of 1960 and prior, as countries move towards a more Westernised eating pattern. Most pyramids and general descriptions are still based on traditional practices. However the intervention diets included in the review were in some cases "inspired" by the MedDiet but had distinct differences to typical traditional diets. Ambring *et al.* [33] formulated an intervention diet with less calories and total fat than the control diet, despite the traditional MedDiet typically being high in energy and moderate to high in total fat. Several of the observations were of modern MedDiets, for example Spain in the early 2000s [23]. If the uniqueness of the traditional diet is lost, the longevity and protection against CHD observed in the Seven Countries Study may also be lost. However, arguably it is prudent to include modernised MedDiets in the definition, which incorporate new health research and allow for changes in food supply and habits, such as was done in the formation of the MDF pyramid [5]. It may no longer be possible to follow a traditional diet for most populations, especially outside of Mediterranean countries.

4. Materials and Methods

To define the MedDiet a literature review was performed. Databases PubMed [49], MEDLINE [50], Science Direct [51], Academic Search Premier [52] and the University of South Australia Library Catalogue [53] were searched using the following search terms; "Mediterranean diet", "Mediterranean dietary pattern", Mediterranean, and content, nutrient *, "nutrient content", definition, define *, pyramid, and "number of serve *", flavonoid *. Definitions were classified into one of four categories for the purpose of this review: (1) general descriptive definitions; (2) diet pyramids/numbers of servings of key foods and serving size; (3) grams of key foods/food

Nutrients **2015**, *7*, 9139–9153

groups; and (4) nutrient and flavonoid content. Total intakes of other phytochemicals, including total polyphenols, phytosterols and carotenoids, were reported by $n < 2$ papers which was deemed insufficient information to draw conclusions from. Papers were included in the review if they defined the MedDiet in at least two of the above four ways. This included studies reporting the dietary intake of a Mediterranean population in an observational capacity, presenting a Mediterranean menu designed based on evidence, or studies using a Mediterranean diet as an intervention where the grams of foods and/or nutrient content was reported. All studies were published in English. There was no restriction on study design, date of publication or sample characteristics. MedDiets used for weight loss purpose were excluded due to caloric and food restrictions. Studies reporting less than five nutrients or food group quantities were excluded. Where the same MDS had been applied using identical cut-off values in separate articles, only the original paper was included.

To define the diet by quantity of foods in grams or milllitres, the mean intake was recorded for major foods or food groups. Twelve groups were included (bread, all cereals, legumes, potatoes, all vegetables, fruits/nuts, meat/meat products, cheese, all dairy, eggs, olive oil and fish), based on available data. For the all cereals, all vegetables and all dairy groups, if not originally reported the sum of individual components was used; for all cereals, bread and cereals were combined, for all vegetables, potatoes and other vegetables were combined and for all dairy, cheese, yoghurt and milk were combined. Using standard Australian serving sizes [30] the gram value was converted to numbers of serves to provide a defining range or number of servings for key food groups. To define the diet by nutrient intake, the mean of all studies reporting at least five of the following was calculated; energy, total fat, SFA, MUFA, protein, percentage energy contributions from total fat, SFA, MUFA, PUFA, protein, carbohydrate, MUFA:SFA, fibre, vitamin C, folate and potassium. The percentage energy contributions of macronutrients and the MUFA to SFA ratio were calculated based on total gram value where not originally reported.

5. Conclusions

High level evidence from the PREDIMED [15] study shows the MedDiet can improve cardiovascular and cognitive health, which will help guide dietary guideline development for prevention of chronic disease. To help understand the mechanisms of benefit of the MedDiet, we require a definition of the MedDiet which is consistent and describes not only the principles generally, but the nutrient and bioactive content. This is the first review to collate information from across a wide range of different studies, to summarise the general descriptions, servings of foods, grams of key food groups and nutrient and flavonoid content of the MedDiet. The average nutrient content of the diet resulting from this review was relatively consistent amongst different studies. This may be a useful working definition, and could improve *a priori* scoring systems which currently rely on grams of foods rather than nutrient content. Consideration for the geographical location of data collection, sample size, and methodological aspects was beyond the scope of this review, but may be necessary to improve the definition. Examining additional foods, nutrients and bioactive compounds and including an assessment of methodological quality of studies could improve this definition further.

Supplementary Materials: Supplementary materials can be accessed at: http://www.mdpi.com/2072-6643/7/11/5459/s1, Table S1: Study design, objectives, methods, outcomes and details of the MedDiet for each paper included in the review, Table S2: Full list of nutrient content presented by studies defining the MedDiet, intakes presented as total per day.

Acknowledgments: The work for this review was funded by a University of South Australia Post-graduate Award (CRD).

Author Contributions: Courtney Davis, Janet Bryan and Karen Murphy conceived and designed the study; Courtney Davis performed the literature search, analysed the evidence and wrote the manuscript; Janet Bryan, Jonathan Hodgson and Karen Murphy assisted in analysing the evidence and revised the manuscript. All authors read and approved the final submitted manuscript.

Conflicts of Interest: The authors declare no conflict of interest.

References

1. Martínez-González, M.Á.; Sánchez-Villegas, A. The emerging role of mediterranean diets in cardiovascular epidemiology: Monounsaturated fats, olive oil, red wine or the whole pattern? *Eur. J. Epidemiol.* **2004**, *19*, 9–13. [PubMed]

2. Menotti, A.; Kromhout, D.; Blackburn, H.; Fidanza, F.; Buzina, R.; Nissinen, A. Food intake patterns and 25-year mortality from coronary heart diseas: Cross-cultural correlations in the seven countries study. *Eur. J. Epidemiol.* **1999**, *15*, 507–515. [CrossRef] [PubMed]

3. Kromhout, D.; Menotti, A.; Bloemberg, B.; Aravanis, C.; Blackburn, H.; Buzina, R.; Dontas, A.S.; Fidanza, F.; Giampaoli, S.; Jansen, A.; *et al.* Dietary saturated and trans fatty acids and cholesterol and 25-year mortality from coronary heart disease: The seven countries study. *Prev. Med.* **1995**, *24*, 308–315. [CrossRef] [PubMed]

4. Kafatos, A.; Verhagen, H.; Moschandreas, J.; Apostolaki, I.; van Westerop, J.J.M. Mediterranean diet of crete: Foods and nutrient content. *J. Am. Diet. Assoc.* **2000**, *100*, 1487–1493. [CrossRef]

5. Bach-Faig, A.; Berry, E.M.; Lairon, D.; Reguant, J.; Trichopoulou, A.; Dernini, S.; Medina, F.X.; Battino, M.; Belahsen, R.; Miranda, G.; *et al.* Mediterranean diet pyramid today. Science and cultural updates. *Public Health Nutr.* **2011**, *14*, 2274–2284. [CrossRef] [PubMed]

6. Willett, W.C.; Sacks, F.; Trichopoulou, A.; Drescher, G.; Ferro-Luzzi, A.; Helsing, E.; Trichopoulos, D. Mediterranean diet pyramid: A cultural model for healthy eating. *Am. J. Clin. Nutr.* **1995**, *61*, 1402S–1406S. [PubMed]

7. Bamia, C.; Trichopoulos, D.; Ferrari, P.; Overvad, K.; Bjerregaard, L.; Tjønneland, A.; Halkjær, J.; Clavel-Chapelon, F.; Kesse, E.; Boutron-Ruault, M.-C.; *et al.* Dietary patterns and survival of older Europeans: The EPIC-Eldely Study (European Prospective Investigation into Cancer and Nutrition). *Public Health Nutr.* **2007**, *10*, 590–598. [CrossRef] [PubMed]

8. Trichopoulou, A.; Kouris-Blazos, A.; Wahlqvist, M.L.; Gnardellis, C.; Lagiou, P.; Polychronopoulos, E.; Vassilakou, T.; Lipworth, L.; Trichopoulos, D. Diet and overall survival in elderly people. *BMJ* **1995**, *311*, 1457–1460. [CrossRef] [PubMed]

9. Saura-Calixto, F.; Goñi, I. Definition of the mediterranean diet based on bioactive compounds. *Crit. Rev. Food Sci. Nutr.* **2009**, *49*, 145–152. [CrossRef] [PubMed]

10. Sofi, F.; Macchi, C.; Abbate, R.; Gensini, G.F.; Casini, A. Mediterranean diet and health status: An updated meta-analysis and a proposal for a literature-based adherence score. *Public Health Nutr.* **2014**, *17*, 2769–2782. [CrossRef] [PubMed]

11. Trichopoulou, A.; Costacou, T.; Bamia, C.; Trichopoulos, D. Adherence to a Mediterranean diet and surviival in a Greek population. *N. Engl. J. Med.* **2003**, *348*, 2599–2608. [CrossRef] [PubMed]

12. Panagiotakos, D.B.; Chrysohoou, C.; Pitsavos, C.; Stefanadis, C. Association between the prevalence of obesity and adherence to the Mediterranean diet: The ATTICA study. *Nutrition* **2006**, *22*, 449–456. [CrossRef] [PubMed]

13. Gerber, M.J.; Scali, J.D.; Michaud, A.; Durand, M.D.; Astre, C.M.; Dallongeville, J.; Romon, M.M. Profiles of a healthful diet and its relationship to biomarkers in a population sample from mediterranean southern France. *J. Am. Diet. Assoc.* **2000**, *100*, 1164–1171. [CrossRef]

14. Milá-Villarroel, R.; Bach-Faig, A.; Puig, J.; Puchal, A.; Farran, A.; Serra-Majem, L.; Carrasco, J.L. Comparison and evaluation of the reliability of indexes of adherence to the mediterranean diet. *Public Health Nutr.* **2011**, *14*, 2338–2345. [CrossRef] [PubMed]

15. Estruch, R.; Ros, E.; Salas-Salvadó, J.; Covas, M.-I.; Corella, D.; Arós, F.; Gómez-Gracia, E.; Ruiz-Gutiérrez, V.; Fiol, M.; Lapetra, J.; *et al.* Primary prevention of cardiovascualr disease with a mediterranean diet. *N. Engl. J. Med.* **2013**, *368*, 1279–1290. [CrossRef] [PubMed]

16. Kromhout, D.; Keys, A.; Aravanis, C.; Buzina, R.; Fidanza, F.; Giampaoli, S.; Jansen, A.; Menotti, A.; Nedeljkovic, S.; Pekkarinen, M.; *et al.* Food consumption patterns in the 1960s in seven countries. *Am. J. Clin. Nutr.* **1989**, *49*, 889–894. [PubMed]

17. Serra-Majem, L.; Roman, B.; Estruch, R. Scientific evidence of interventions using the mediterranean diet: A systematic review. *Nutr. Rev.* **2006**, *64*, S27–S47. [CrossRef] [PubMed]

18. Hu, F.B.; Manson, J.E.; Willett, W.C. Types of dietary fat and risk of coronary heart disease: A critical review. *J. Am. Coll. Nutr.* **2001**, *20*, 5–19. [CrossRef] [PubMed]

19. Panagiotakos, D.B.; Pitsavos, C.; Stefanadis, C. Dietary patterns: A mediterranean diet score and its relation to clinical and biological markers of cardiovacsular disease risk. *Nutr. Metab. Cardiovasc. Dis.* **2006**, *16*, 559–568. [CrossRef] [PubMed]
20. Dilis, V.; Vasilopoulou, E.; Trichopoulou, A. The flavone, flavonol and flavan-3-ol content of the greek traditional diet. *Food Chem.* **2007**, *105*, 812–821. [CrossRef]
21. Mediterranean Diet Pyramid. Available online: http://oldwayspt.org/resources/heritage-pyramids/mediterranean-pyramid/overview (accessed on 27 February 2013).
22. Ministry of health and welfare, supreme scientific health council: Dietary guidelines for adults in greece. *Arch. Hell. Med.* **1999**, *16*, 516–524.
23. Varela-Moreiras, G.; Ávila, J.; Cuadrado, C.; del Pozo, S.; Ruiz, E.; Moreiras, O. Evaluation of food consumption and dietary patterns in spain by the food consumption survey: Updated information. *Eur. J. Clin. Nutr.* **2010**, *64*, S37–S43. [CrossRef] [PubMed]
24. de Lorgeril, M.; Renaud, S.; Mamelle, N.; Salen, P.; Martin, J.-L.; Monjaud, I.; Guidollet, J.; Touboul, P.; Delaye, J. Mediterranean alpha-linolenic acid-rich diet in secondary prevention of coronary heart disease. *Lancet* **1994**, *343*, 1454–1459. [CrossRef]
25. Kouris-Blazos, A.; Gnardellis, C.; Wahlqvist, M.L.; Trichopoulos, D.; Lukito, W.; Trichopoulou, A. Are the advantages of the mediterranean diet transferable to other populations? A cohort study in melbourne, australia. *Br. J. Nutr.* **1999**, *82*, 57–61. [PubMed]
26. Guallar-Castillon, P.; Rodriguez-Artalejo, F.; Tormo, M.; Sanchez, M.; Rodriguez, L.; Quiros, J.R.; Navarro, C.; Molina, E.; Martinez, C.; Marin, P.; *et al.* Major dietary patterns and risk of coronary heart disease in middle-aged persons from a mediterranean country: The epic-spain cohort study. *Nutr. Metab. Cardiovasc. Dis.* **2012**, *22*, 192–199. [CrossRef] [PubMed]
27. Buckland, G.; González, C.A.; Agudo, A.; Vilardell, M.; Berenguer, A.; Amiano, P.; Ardanaz, E.; Arriola, L.; Barricarte, A.; Basterretxea, M.; *et al.* Adherence to the Mediterranean diet and risk of coronary heart disease in the Spanish EPIC Cohort Study. *Am. J. Epidemiol.* **2009**, *170*, 1518–1529. [CrossRef] [PubMed]
28. Itsiopoulos, C.; Brazionis, L.; Kaimakamis, M.; Cameron, M.; Best, J.; O'Dea, K.; Rowley, K. Can the mediterranean diet lower hba1c in type 2 diabetes? Results from a randomized cross-over study. *Nutr. Metab. Cardiovasc. Dis.* **2011**, *21*, 740–747. [CrossRef] [PubMed]
29. Vincent-Baudry, S.; Defoort, C.; Gerber, M.; Bernard, M.-C.; Verger, P.; Helal, O.; Portugal, H.; Planells, R.; Grolier, P.; Amiot-Carlin, M.-J.; *et al.* The medi-rivage study: Reduction of cardiovascular disease risk factors after a 3-mo intervention with a mediterranean-type diet or a low-fat diet. *Am. J. Clin. Nutr.* **2005**, *82*, 964–971. [PubMed]
30. Australian Dietary Guidelines: Summary. Available online: https://www.eatforhealth.gov.au/sites/default/files/files/the_guidelines/n55a_australian_dietary_guidelines_summary_book.pdf (accessed on 23 February 2015).
31. De Lorgeril, M.; Salen, P.; Martin, J.-L.; Monjaud, I.; Delaye, J.; Mamelle, N. Mediterranean diet, traditional risk factors, and the rate of cardiovascular complications after myocardial infarction: Final report of the lyon diet heart study. *Circulation* **1999**, *99*, 779–785. [CrossRef] [PubMed]
32. Trichopoulou, A.; Vasilopoulou, E.; Georga, K.; Soukara, S.; Dilis, V. Traditional foods: Why and how to sustain them. *Trends Food Sci. Technol.* **2006**, *17*, 498–504. [CrossRef]
33. Ambring, A.; Friberg, P.; Axelsen, M.; Laffrenzen, M.; Taskinen, M.-R.; Basus, S.; Johansson, M. Effects of a mediterranean-inspired diet on blood lipids, vascular function and oxidative stress in healthy subjects. *Clin. Sci.* **2004**, *106*, 519–525. [CrossRef] [PubMed]
34. Zamora-Ros, R.; Andres-Lacueva, C.; Lameula-Raventós, R.M.; Berenguer, T.; Jakszyne, P.; Barricarte, A.; Ardanaz, E.; Amiano, P.; Dorronsoro, M.; Larranaga, N.; *et al.* Estimation of dietary sources and flavonoid intake in a spanish adult population (Epic-Spain). *J. Am. Diet. Assoc.* **2010**, *110*, 390–398. [CrossRef] [PubMed]
35. Tresserra-Rimbau, A.; Rimm, E.B.; Medina-Remón, A.; Martínez-González, M.Á.; López-Sabater, C.M.; Arós, F.; Fiol, M.; Ros, E.; Serra-Majem, L.; Pintó, X.; *et al.* Polyphenol intake and mortality risk: A re-analysis of the predimed trial. *BMC Med.* **2014**, *12*, 77.
36. Vasilopoulou, E.; Georga, K.; Joergensen, B.M.; Naska, A.; Trichopoulou, A. The antioxidant properties of greek foods and the flavonoid content of the mediterranean menu. *Curr. Med. Chem.* **2005**, *5*, 33–45.

37. Sofi, F.; Abbate, R.; Gensini, G.F.; Casini, A.; Trichopoulou, A.; Bamia, C. Identification of change-points in the relationship between food groups in the mediterranean diet and overall mortality: An "a posteriori" approach. *Eur. J. Nutr.* **2012**, *51*, 167–172. [CrossRef] [PubMed]

38. Buckland, G.; Mayén, A.L.; Agudo, A.; Travier, N.; Navarro, C.; Huerta, J.M.; Chirlaque, M.D.; Barricarte, A.; Ardanaz, E.; Moreno-Iribas, C.; *et al.* Olive oil intake and mortality within the spanish population (Epic-Spain). *Am. J. Clin. Nutr.* **2012**, *96*, 142–149. [CrossRef] [PubMed]

39. Alberti-Fidanza, A.; Fidanza, F. Mediterranean adequacy index of italian diets. *Public Health Nutr.* **2004**, *7*, 937–941. [CrossRef] [PubMed]

40. Urpi-Sarda, M.; Casas, R.; Chiva-Blanch, G.; Romero-Mamani, E.S.; Valderas-Martinez, P.; Arranza, S.; Andres-Lacueva, C.; Llorach, R.; Medina-Remón, A.; Lamuela-Raventos, R.M.; *et al.* Virgin olive oil and nuts as key foods of the mediterranean diet effects on inflammatory biomarkers related to atherosclerosis. *Pharmacol. Res.* **2012**, *65*, 577–583. [CrossRef] [PubMed]

41. Urpi-Sarda, M.; Casas, R.; Chiva-Blanch, G.; Romero-Mamani, E.S.; Valderas-Martínez, P.; Salas-Salvadó, J.; Covas, M.I.; Toledo, E.; Andres-Lacueva, C.; Llorach, R., *et al.* The mediterranean diet pattern and its main components are associated with lower plasma concentrations of tumor necrosis factor receptor 60 in patients at high risk for cardiovascular disease. *J. Nutr.* **2012**, *142*, 1019–1025. [CrossRef] [PubMed]

42. Sofi, F.; Abbate, R.; Gensini, G.F.; Casini, A. Accruing evidence on benefits of adherence to the mediterranean diet on health: An updated systematic review and meta-analysis. *Am. J. Clin. Nutr.* **2010**, *92*, 1189–1196. [CrossRef] [PubMed]

43. Fung, T.T.; Rexrode, K.M.; Mantzoros, C.S.; Manson, J.E.; Willett, W.C.; Hu, F.B. Mediterranean diet and incidence of and mortality from coronary heart disease and stroke in women. *Circulation* **2009**, *119*, 1093–1100. [CrossRef] [PubMed]

44. Breslow, J.L. N-3 fatty acids and cardiovascular disease. *Am. J. Clin. Nutr.* **2006**, *83*, 1477S–1482S. [PubMed]

45. Rafnsson, S.B.; Dilis, V.; Trichopoulou, A. Antioxidant nutrients and age-related cognitive decline: A systematic review of population-based cohort studies. *Eur. J. Nutr.* **2013**, *52*, 1553–1567. [CrossRef] [PubMed]

46. Pérez-López, F.R.; Fernández-Alonso, A.; Chedraui, P.; Simoncini, T. Mediterranean lifestyle and diet: Deconstructing mechanisms of health benefits. In *Bioactive Food as Dietary Intervention for the Aging Population*, 1st ed.; Watson, R., Preedy, V.R., Eds.; Academic Press: Waltham, MA, USA, 2013; pp. 129–138.

47. Willett, W.C.; Howe, G.R.; Kushi, L.H. Adjustment for total energy intake in epidemiologic studies. *Am. J. Clin. Nutr.* **1997**, *65*, 1220S–1228S. [PubMed]

48. Souza, R.G.; Gomes, A.C.; Naves, M.M.; Mota, J.F. Nuts and legume seeds for cardiovascular risk reduction: Scientific evidence and mechanisms of action. *Nutr. Rev.* **2015**, *73*, 335–347. [CrossRef] [PubMed]

49. PubMed. Available online: http://www.ncbi.nlm.nih.gov/pubmed (accessed on 19 March 2013).

50. Ovid: Search. Available online: http://ovidsp.tx.ovid.com.access.library.unisa.edu.au/ (accessed on 20 March 2013).

51. Science Direct. Available online: http://www.sciencedirect.com.access.library.unisa.edu.au/ (accessed on 21 March 2013).

52. Academic Search Premier. Available online: http://web.b.ebscohost.com.access.library.unisa.edu.au/ ehost/search/advanced?sid=3f4e9ae3-2b23-4d50-bdc6-fbf330114be5%40sessionmgr114&vid=0&hid=115 (accessed on 22 March 2013).

53. UniSA Library. Available online: http://www.library.unisa.edu.au/ (accessed on 18 March 2013).

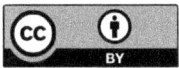

nutrients

MDPI

Review

Nutritional Genomics and the Mediterranean Diet's Effects on Human Cardiovascular Health

Montserrat Fitó [1,*,†] and Valentini Konstantinidou [2,*,†]

1   Cardiovascular Risk and Nutrition Research Group (CARIN), CIBER de Fisiopatología de la Obesidad y Nutrición (CIBEROBN), Institut Hospital del Mar d'Investigació Mèdica (IMIM), Dr. Aiguader, 88, Barcelona 08003, Spain

2   MEDOLIALI S.L. (DNANUTRICOACH®), Calle Diputación, 279, 1, 7, Barcelona 08007, Spain

*   Correspondence: mfito@imim.es (M.F.); valentini@dnanutricoach.com (V.K.); Tel.: +34-933-16-07-20 (M.F.); +34-931-71-88-59 (V.K.)

†   These authors contributed equally to this work.

Received: 11 October 2015; Accepted: 7 April 2016; Published: 13 April 2016

Abstract: The synergies and cumulative effects among different foods and nutrients are what produce the benefits of a healthy dietary pattern. Diets and dietary patterns are a major environmental factor that we are exposed to several times a day. People can learn how to control this behavior in order to promote healthy living and aging, and to prevent diet-related diseases. To date, the traditional Mediterranean diet has been the only well-studied pattern. Stroke incidence, a number of classical risk factors including lipid profile and glycaemia, emergent risk factors such as the length of telomeres, and emotional eating behavior can be affected by genetic predisposition. Adherence to the Mediterranean diet could exert beneficial effects on these risk factors. Our individual genetic make-up should be taken into account to better prevent these traits and their subsequent consequences in cardiovascular disease development. In the present work, we review the results of nutritional genomics explaining the role of the Mediterranean diet in human cardiovascular disease. A multidisciplinary approach is necessary to extract knowledge from large-scale data.

Keywords: nutrigenetics; dietary pattern; prevention

---

1. Introduction

1.1. Dietary Patterns

Food patterns refer to the consumption of differing amounts, proportions, and combinations of diverse foods and beverages, and the variations in the frequency of their intake. The relevance of overall high-quality food patterns should be taken into consideration as the synergies and cumulative effects among different foods and nutrients are behind their health benefits [1]. A single-variable approach has been traditionally followed in nutritional studies. One consequence of this has been to promote debate among proponents of single-nutrient causes and solutions to diet-related health problems [2]. Diets are more than the sum of their components, and this has been a fundamental concern with the one-variable-at-a-time (OVAT) approach due to the fact that the multidimensional essence of nutrition is not captured. Moreover, diets form only part of a healthy lifestyle recommended for the treatment of numerous complex and multifactorial diseases such as cardiovascular ones. Dietary patterns are a major environmental factor that people are exposed to numerous times a day during their lives. Diet is also the environmental factor that people can learn to control from early on to prevent diet-related diseases and promote healthy living and aging.

A healthy dietary pattern, such as the Mediterranean diet, can be a useful and complementary tool to better control classic cardiovascular risk factors within the frame of lifestyle recommendations.

In this regard, the first step in hypertension and other cardiovascular risk factors management is to follow a healthy diet, such as the traditional Mediterranean diet [3] or the DASH (Dietary-Approaches-to-Stop-Hypertension) diets [4]. Both diets are characterised by foods rich in phytochemicals, such as fruit and vegetables, which have been inversely associated with high blood pressure and hypercholesterolemia, among other cardiovascular risk factors.

However, the specific characterization of a dietary pattern remains a challenge because it is hampered by the complexity of interpreting multidimensional dietary data. Interactions between diet and the human genome have led to intense research and debate regarding the effectiveness of personalized nutrition as a more adequate tool to prevent chronic diseases than the traditional one-size-fits all recommendations [5]. The nutritional genomics field, although still in its early stages, offers encouraging results for its widespread incorporation into clinical practice.

1.2. The Mediterranean Dietary Pattern

The traditional Mediterranean diet refers to dietary patterns found in olive-growing areas of the Mediterranean region since the 1960s [6]. It is considered a single entity consisting of diet-variants from each region in the Mediterranean basin. It is based on an abundant and daily consumption of olive oil, which is the main source of fat, and is characterized by: (a) high intake of vegetables, fruit, legumes, whole grains, nuts, and seeds; (b) frequent (and moderate) intake of red wine with meals; (c) moderate consumption of seafood, fermented dairy products (cheese and yogurt), poultry, and eggs; and (d) low consumption of red meat, meat products, and sweets. Moreover, the Mediterranean dietary pattern also encompasses daily physical activity, proper hydration (approximately 2 L of water a day) and social eating habits [7]. Olive oil is considered a hallmark of this dietary pattern, resulting in high intakes of monounsaturated fatty acids (MUFA) and lower intakes of saturated fatty acids (SFA).

The Mediterranean diet may not be markedly different from other recommended diets worldwide but its basic element, olive oil, makes it unique and contributes an additional value to its health benefits [8]. To the best of our knowledge, the Mediterranean diet is the only dietary pattern that, to date, has been investigated in depth and that is why the present review is based on this dietary pattern. Current knowledge from observational studies supports its instrumental role in the context of cardiovascular disease (CVD) prevention. As yet, few randomized, dietary intervention trials have been performed assessing long-term effects of a diet intervention, with a solid design, in primary and secondary prevention. The Lyon Diet Heart Study reported the benefits of a Mediterranean-type dietary pattern on the secondary prevention of CVD with 605 volunteers who had suffered a first myocardial infraction [9]. The protective effect of the diet was maintained up to 4 years after the first infarction. The most relevant impact of the traditional Mediterranean diet (TMD) as a primary protection against cardiovascular endpoints has only recently been described in the PREDIMED (PREvencion con DIeta MEDiterranea) study [10,11]. The PREDIMED study was a randomized, controlled and large-scale (*n* = 7447) intervention trial which tested the long-term effects (5-year follow up) of the TMD on incident cardiovascular diseases. The PREDIMED study reported, for the first time, high-level evidence of the primary prevention for cardiovascular events such as a hard composite endpoint (myocardial infarction, stroke, and cardiovascular mortality) [10,12], stroke [10], atrial fibrillation [13], type-2 diabetes [14], and peripheral vascular disease [15]. In addition, an improvement of the classic cardiovascular risk factors, at the medium and long term, in high-risk individuals was described after adherence to the traditional Mediterranean diet.

Traditionally the healthy benefits of the Mediterranean diet have been attributed to its richness in antioxidants. Antioxidant compounds can exert their beneficial effects through chemical reactions, once incorporated into the organism, but also during the digestion of the diet components. The anti-inflammatory effects in addition to the antioxidant ones, the formation of nitrolipid compounds, the viability of the cell-membranes and monolayers, and the modification of the microbiota can be other remarkable mechanisms. Furthermore, the mechanism of action of antioxidants, and other nutrients, is very much related to their capacity to modulate gene and protein expression.

1.3. Methods

Our aim is to present evidence concerning the well-researched Mediterranean dietary pattern included in nutritional genomics studies. A literature review was performed in MEDLINE up to July 2015. The search aimed to identify current knowledge on nutritional genomics mechanisms that could explain the beneficial effects of the Mediterranean diet on preventing cardiovascular diseases. The following Medical Subject Heading Terms (MESH) were used: Mediterranean diet, humans, nutritional genomics, nutritigenomics, nutrigenetics, dietary pattern, epigenomics, interventions, studies. In the present review, we revised more than 70 English articles. Those describing nutritional genomics mechanisms, after adherence to the Mediterranean dietary pattern, in human intervention studies were finally included. Nutritional genomics mechanisms and studies on issues other than the Mediterranean dietary pattern were not the objective of the present review.

2. Nutritional Genomics Mechanisms

Our genetic predisposition is responsible for a percentage of CVD risk that varies among people. Genetic predisposition could explain a great part of the differential responses observed in individuals after the same dietary treatments, and could help health professionals personalize even more their recommendations. Nutritional genomics has emerged as a relatively new field of research assessing the mechanisms by which nutrients and dietary patterns interact with our genome at different stages. It embraces a systems biology approach to evaluate individual risk factors in the light of genetic diversity at the transcriptome, genetic, metabolome, and epigenome levels (Figure 1) [16].

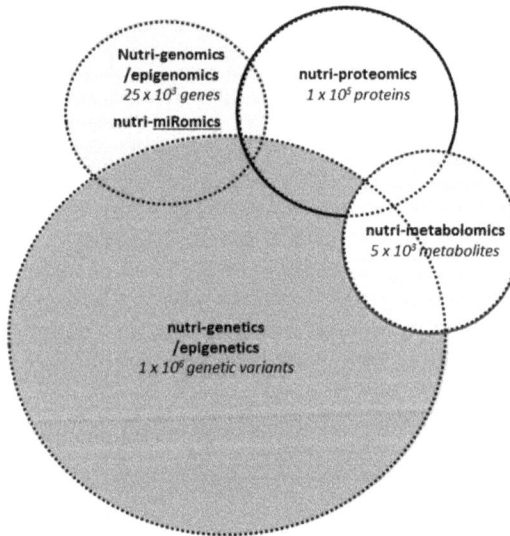

Figure 1. Proposed nutritional genomics mechanisms. The "Nutri-" prefix in the name of each of the 4 categories defines the influence of nutrition on genomics/epigenomics, proteomics, metabolomics and genetics/epigenomics.

The integration of data from all these areas of complexity needs advanced computational methodology to establish networks of interacting biological components and determine linked activities. The goal of nutritional genomics is to take into consideration the complexity of dietary patterns, culture, and metabolic processes that lead to health or disease, and to provide personalized and precise recommendations to prevent common, multifactorial diseases decades before their clinical manifestation.

To the best of our knowledge, conclusive evidence for the effects of interactions between genes and dietary patterns on cardiovascular health is lacking. Genome-wide interaction studies (GWIS) are a real possibility in order to identify specific gene-diet interactions even though providing the necessary sample size presents some difficulty [17]. We review here the current results of nutrigenetics, nutrigenomics, nutri-metabolomics, nutri-epigenomics, nutri-epigenetics, and nutri-miRomics related to Mediterranean diet interventions in humans. Table 1 summarizes the relevant studies. The majority of these studies include mainly Spanish populations and have been performed in the framework of PREDIMED study. We strongly encourage the design and performance of similar studies, in terms of design and follow-up duration, in different populations, to further confirm current results.

2.1. Nutrigenetics

Nutrigenetics aims to gain greater understanding of the mechanisms associated with inter-variability among individuals and to develop more personalized dietary recommendations. Genetic predisposition in humans is arising as a main factor to identify sub-groups that would benefit from dietary interventions. There is increasing evidence that individuals with different genotypes respond differently to diet. Genotyping methods detect the most common form of genetic variants, called single nucleotide polymorphisms (SNPs), in the human DNA sequence. The SNPs constitute the genetic fingerprint of each person, and genome-wide association studies (GWAS) assess the relationships between SNPs and concrete observable traits (phenotypes) [18].

The PREDIMED results support the notion that individual genetic predisposition toward CVD risk could be influenced by dietary components, mainly by a stricter adherence to the Mediterranean diet pattern. Corella *et al.* studied the genetic predisposition to present increased fasting glucose, total cholesterol, LDL cholesterol, triglyceride (TG) concentrations, and stroke incidence in homozygote individuals for the T allele of the rs7903146 polymorphism in the TCF7L2 (transcription factor 7-like 2) gene. They found that this predisposition could be attenuated by adherence to the Mediterranean diet [19].

Other genetic variants were also found to be protective. This is the case of the rs3812316 functional single nucleotide polymorphism (SNP) at the MLXIPL (Max-like protein X interacting protein-like) gene [20]. This SNP has been associated with lower systemic TG concentrations. Using data from the PREDIMED study, Ortega-Azorin replicated previous associations with TG concentrations and showed that they were modified by adherence to a Mediterranean diet. Thus, the potential CVD protection was enhanced in individuals who had higher adherence to the Mediterranean diet. Most importantly, the reduction in CVD risk that was associated with the Mediterranean diet, as shown in the whole PREDIMED study [10], was significantly enhanced in carriers of the minor, G allele, at this MLXIPL locus.

Recently, leukocyte telomere length, considered as a potential biomarker of biological age, has also been described as being involved in the gene-diet interaction in the PREDIMED study [21]. In this work, DNA from 521 participants of the PREDIMED Study was genotyped for the presence of the Ala allele in rs1801282 SNP of the PPARγ2 (peroxisome proliferator-activated receptor gamma) gene. It was observed that the presence of the Ala allele prevented telomere attrition associated with aging. Higher adherence to the Mediterranean dietary pattern showed benefits after a 5-year follow-up in subjects with the Ala allele because they had longer telomeres. The authors concluded that this gene-diet interaction (rs1801282-Mediterranean diet) could have an added value in the improvement of personalized dietary recommendations based on genetic predisposition to achieve healthy aging and lower CVD risk.

Table 1. Nutrigenetics, nutrigenomics, nutri-metabolomics, and nutri-miRomics studies related to Mediterranean diet interventions in humans.

Nutrigenetics	SNPs Tested	Outcome	Reference
	rs7903146 (homozygotes for the T risk allele) at the TCF7L2 gene.	Increased fasting glucose, total cholesterol, LDL-C, TG, stroke incidence	[19]
	rs3812316 (carriers of the G protective allele) at the MLXIPL gene.	Lower TG, reduction in CVD risk	[20]
	rs1801282 (carriers of the Ala-G protective allele) at the PPARγ2 gene.	Higher adherence to the Mediterranean diet strengthens the prevention of telomere shortening	[21]
	rs1801260 in the CLOCK gene (homozygous for the major T allele).	Triggering glucose metabolism in patients with metabolic syndrome	[22]
	rs1801260 in the CLOCK gene (carriers of the minor C allele)	Less weight loss for the C carriers with high emotional score (emotional eaters).	[23]
Nutri-Genomics	**Gene Expression**	**Gene groups Affected**	
	Protective modulation (*i.e.*, ADRB2, IL7R, IFNγ, MCP1, TNFα *etc.*).	Pro-atherosclerotic in vascular inflammation, foam cell formation, thrombosis, oxidative stress	[24–26]
	Protective modulation (*i.e.*, IFNγ, ARHGAP15, IL7R, POLK, ADRB2 *etc.*).	Artery wall production of inflammatory mediators	[26,27]
	Canonical pathways modulation.	Atherosclerosis, hypertension, renin-angiotensin, nitric oxide, angiopoietin signaling, hypoxia, eNOS signaling pathways	[28]
Nutri-Metabolomics	**Sample Type/Population Characteristics**	**Results**	
	Plasma from individuals with MetS.	altered metabolic profile	[29]
	Urine from non-diabetic adults.	Classification of individuals by evaluating changes in the urinary metabolome at different time points	[30]
	Spot urine samples of free-living population.	Predictive model of dietary walnut exposure	[31]
	Urinary metabolome in free-living population.	Improved predictive model of dietary exposure to cocoa by combining different metabolites as biomarkers	[32]
	Urinary metabolome in elderly men and women.	Greater hippurate after Med+CoQ and higher phenylacetylglycine levels after SFA diet in women	[33]
Nutri-miRomics	**MicroRNA/Target SNP**	**Effect**	
	miRNA-410/rs13702 in the 3'untranslated region (3'UTR) of the lipoprotein lipase (LPL) gene.	Disruption of the recognition element seed site, gain-of-function, and lower TG.	[34]
	miRNA-410/rs13702 C allele carriers.	Stroke incidence modulated by diet by decreasing TG and stroke risk after a high-unsaturated fat Mediterranean diet	[35]

ADRB2: adrenoreceptor beta 2, surface; ARHGAP15: Rho GTPase activating protein 15; CLOCK: circadian locomotor output cycles kaput; CVD: cardiovascular disease; IFNγ: interferon gamma; IL7R: interleukin 7 receptor; LDL-C: low density lipoprotein cholesterol; MCP1: chemokine (C-C motif) ligand 2; MetS: Metabolic Syndrome; MLXIPL: Max-like protein X interacting protein-like; POLK: polymerase (DNA directed) kappa; PPARγ2: peroxisome proliferator-activated receptor gamma; TCF7L2: transcription factor 7-like 2; TG: triglycerides; TNFα: tumor necrosis factor α.

Garcia-Rios *et al.* have proposed that dietary recommendations in individuals with metabolic syndrome may also require a more personalized approach [22]. They have studied genetic variation at the CLOCK (circadian locomotor output cycles kaput) gene and their data support the hypothesis that a habitual consumption of a healthy diet, such as the Mediterranean one, could contribute to triggering glucose metabolism through interactions with the rs1801260 SNP in the CLOCK gene. Lopez-Guimera *et al.* have analyzed the role of emotional eating behavior and the interaction of the same CLOCK 3111 T/C polymorphism on the effectiveness of a weight-loss program. In a 30-week follow-up with a Mediterranean population, they reported that the CLOCK 3111 T/C SNP interacted with emotional eating behavior to modulate total weight loss [23].

Glycaemia, lipid profile, stroke incidence, telomeres length, and emotional eating behavior are some of the characteristics that have been seen to be affected by genetic predisposition and adherence to the Mediterranean diet. Thus, taking into account individual genetic make-up can be useful in the management and control of these traits and their subsequent consequences in CVD development.

2.2. Nutrigenomics

Nutrition researchers have acknowledged that gene–diet interactions could play a major role in the development of and protection against chronic degenerative diseases [24]. Although the mechanisms behind statistically significant associations and interactions remain unclear, given the continuous novel knowledge being obtained about the genome [36], some of the ambiguities are being resolved. Nutrients may influence gene expression directly as ligands for nuclear receptors or indirectly by inducing epigenetic modifications without changing the underlying DNA sequence. Gene expression changes are measured in the level of messenger RNA (mRNA) by transcriptomic techniques [37] such as, but not limited to, microarrays and real-time reverse transcription PCR [38].

The high antioxidant content of the Mediterranean diet could be one of its protective mechanisms of action. Antioxidants have the capacity to modulate gene, protein expression [25] and subsequently, metabolite production [29]. Oxidation and inflammation are intertwined processes, and when sustained for a long period may be involved in the physiopathology of many diseases [39]. Indeed, chronic inflammation is another key patho-physiological factor in the development of obesity, type-2 diabetes, and CVD. Previous nutrigenomic intervention studies have shown that the Mediterranean diet pattern has a protective effect on the expression of pro-atherosclerotic genes involved in vascular inflammation, foam cell formation, and thrombosis [24–26]. In addition, adherence to a Mediterranean dietary pattern may protect against artery wall production of inflammatory mediators [26,27]. Moreover, recent nutrition research has indicated that our diet is able to influence, directly or indirectly, the immune system and well-being, and thus affects inflammatory disease development [40–42].

In an overall transcriptomic study within the PREDIMED study, the principal pathways in the physiopathology of cardiovascular events, such as atherosclerosis, renin-angiotensin, nitric oxide and angiopoietin signaling, were modulated by TMD + EVOO, whereas hypoxia and eNOS signaling pathways were modified by TMD enriched with EVOO or nuts [28]. After simultaneous testing adjustment, 9 pathways were modulated by TMD + EVOO and 4 by TMD+Nuts while none of the pathways changed in the control group. Thus, a higher overall modulation of gene expression was observed after adherence to a Mediterranean diet. In this regard, it can also be considered as a better adaptive response to detrimental factors, such as a mechanism for hormesis [43].

Gene expression changes have been reported in humans, both after the Mediterranean diet and olive oil consumption at postprandial or sustained time [24]. Changes in the regulation of gene expression are reflected in fingerprinting patterns that could prove very useful for the future development of biomarkers. However, caution should be exercised due to heterogeneity of the studies assessing gene expression changes in human tissues and body fluids. Further research on larger population sizes, with robust designs and standardized methodologies, is required before definite nutrigenomic-based recommendations can be formed.

2.3. Nutri-Metabolomics

Metabolomics aims to study the entire small molecule (metabolite) complement of a system. Metabolites are defined as possessing an atomic mass inferior to 1.5 kDa and can be exogenous, endogenous, or derived from microbiome metabolism. A huge variety of metabolites exists, including peptides, lipids, nucleotides, carbohydrates, amino acids, and carbohydrates [44,45].

The effects of an intervention based on the Mediterranean dietary pattern were assessed by Bondia-Pons *et al.* [29]. They used liquid chromatography coupled to the quadrupole-time of a flight-MS (LQ-QTOF/MS) metabolic profiling technique to screen plasma from individuals with MetS features who participated in the Metabolic Syndrome Reduction Study in Navarra (RESMENA), a randomized, controlled trial. It was reported that a two-month pattern based on the Mediterranean diet produced significant changes in plasma metabolic profile. However, and in spite of the fact there were associations between metabolic and clinical variables, these changes disappeared after six months, suggesting that compliance had declined during the self-control period.

Nutri-metabolomic effects were also assessed within the frame of the PREDIMED study. Metabolomics results enabled the classification of individuals according to their specific food consumption or dietary patterns. Vazquez-Fresno *et al.* studied the metabolomics pattern of non-diabetic participants in the PREDIMED study after one and three years of follow-up [30]. The Proton nuclear magnetic resonance (^{1}H NMR) urinary metabolome profile was analyzed in the participants who were classified as consuming either a low fat diet or a Mediterranean one. Results showed that the most prominent hallmarks in the groups that followed the Mediterranean diet were related to the metabolism of carbohydrates (3-hydroxybutyrate, citrate, and cis-aconitate), creatine, creatinine, amino acids (proline, *N*-acetylglutamine, glycine, branched-chain amino acids, and derived metabolites), lipids (oleic and suberic acids), and microbial co-metabolites (phenylacetylglutamine and p-cresol). In addition, the dietary walnut fingerprinting by an HPLC-q-ToF-MS untargeted metabolomics approach has been assessed [31]. Walnut consumption was characterized by 18 metabolites, such as markers of fatty acid metabolism, ellagitannin-derived microbial compounds, and intermediate metabolites of the tryptophan/serotonin pathway. Likewise, the urinary metabolome signature of cocoa intake in PREDIMED participants has been reported [32].

Metabolomic profile has been also characterized in the elderly. Gonzalez-Guardia *et al.* investigated the effect of the Mediterranean diet when supplemented with coenzyme Q10 in elderly men and women after 4 weeks of intervention [33]. Greater hippurate urine levels were described after the Mediterranean diet + CoQ and higher phenylacetylglycine levels after saturated fat diet consumption in women. These results suggest that the long-term consumption of a Mediterranean diet supplemented with Q10 could exert benefits on healthy aging and on the prevention of processes related to chronic oxidative stress.

Gut microbiota play a key role in CVD; having being identified as a possible novel CVD risk factor, they represent a realistic therapeutic target [46]. The microbiome-gut-brain axis links human physiology (and pathology) to millions of other microorganisms that share the same host. The microbiome is affected by dietary intake [47] and specific dietary factors (carbohydrate, protein, and Mediterranean foods) seem to regulate CVD risk factors through the modulation of microbial populations and activities [48].

Microbiota also appear to play a critical role in the clock–nutrition interplay. Our circadian clock is a highly specialized and stratified network that drives and orchestrates proper rhythms for organism homeostasis. It operates as a critical interface between nutrition and homeostasis. The circadian clock is a mechanism calling for more attention concerning the beneficial effects of dietary patterns on disease prevention and health maintenance; in addition, the disruption of the circadian rhythm may cause manifestations of metabolic syndrome [49].

Metabolomics results that could serve as future biomarkers of consumption and/or adherence are increasing. Moreover, nutri-metabolomics studies could offer another level of knowledge for nutritional personalization based on our gut microbiota although, once again, further studies are necessary before solid conclusions can be reached.

2.4. Nutri-Epigenomics and Nutri-Epigenetics

Epigenetics studies the heritable DNA modifications able to regulate chromosome architecture and modulate gene expression without changing the underlying sequence. Epigenetic phenomena are critical for the aging process that takes place from embryonic development to later adult life. Increasing evidence supports the complex interactions that exist among food components, dietary patterns, and epigenetic modifications such as histone modifications, DNA methylation, non-coding RNA expression, and chromatin remodeling factors. Such alterations are among the hallmarks of age-related chronic inflammatory diseases including metabolic syndrome and diabetes [50]. In analogy to GWAS studies, epigenome-wide association studies (EWAS) have arisen [51]. The first results demonstrate the central role of epigenomic information and of epigenetic changes in response to diet and environmental conditions to understand human disease. Nutrition in early life can induce long-term changes in DNA methylation thus affecting individual susceptibility to a range of diseases [52].

Nutritional epigenetics is a novel mechanism underlying gene-diet interactions. Epigenetic phenomena are critical for the aging process, from embryonic development to later adult life, and the complexity of integrating all these data is a huge multidisciplinary challenge.

2.5. Nutri-miRomics

Nutrimiromics has emerged as a subsidiary field of nutritional genomics assessing how nutrients affect microRNAs (miRs) and their function. MiRs are small non-coding RNA sequences of single sequences of 19-24 nucleotides located in intra- or inter-regions of protein coding genes [53]. MiRs have emerged as the major regulators of a great number of physiological processes including cell differentiation, apoptosis, and lipid metabolism, and they have been reported to regulate glucose homeostasis, β-cell function, and insulin signaling. The main function of miRs is silencing their target genes by acting as specific inhibitors of mRNA [54]. The complementarity between miRs and mRNA is not always perfect and, depending on the grade of complementarity, miRs could induce mRNA degradation, de-adenylation, and transductional repression [55].

Numerous SNPs in miRs-target sites have also been demonstrated to have allele-specific effects. For example, the minor allele of the SNP rs13702 in the 3′ untranslated region (3′ UTR) of the lipoprotein lipase (LPL) gene disrupts a miRs recognition element seed site for the human miRNA-410, resulting in a gain-of-function and lower plasma TG [34]. This work has revealed that the molecular basis for some of the observed cardiovascular effects could involve differential regulation by miRs [34]. Corella *et al.* reported a novel association between a microRNA target site variant and stroke incidence, modulated by a high-unsaturated-fat Mediterranean diet in terms of decreasing TG levels and possibly stroke risk in rs13702 C allele carriers, within the frame of the PREDIMED Study [35]. MicroRNAs have emerged as relevant epigenetic regulators in cardiovascular diseases. The study of miRNA target site polymorphisms as functional variants could contribute to a better understanding of the mechanisms of physio-pathology of CVD, among others.

3. Conclusions

The interactions among food and nutrients, calorie intake, meal frequency and timing, single-nutrient modifications, microbiota, and genetic predisposition in modulating the key mechanisms that maintain cellular tissue and organ function during aging are not yet well-established. However, individual genetic variation should definitely be taken into account before developing personalized recommendations. The Mediterranean dietary pattern, which is more than just a diet, is to date most studied at the level of evidence-based medicine. Nutritional genomics embraces and researches different aspects of nutrition-related molecular mechanisms at all levels of systems biology approach such as transcriptomics, genomics, genetics, and metabolomics. Although the benefits of the traditional Mediterranean diet in the prevention of cardiovascular disease have been assessed, the nutritional genomics mechanisms are yet to be fully elucidated. Data reported in the present review has not yet been fully replicated in different ethnic populations, ages, genders, and physiopathological conditions. The nutritional genomics field is quickly advancing but a great deal of effort is yet required from the scientific community, in different disciplines, to establish the subjacent mechanisms linked to the nutritional genomics of the healthy benefits of Mediterranean diet on cardiovascular diseases. The integration of OMICS, both at a single-OMICS level or preferably at a multi-OMICS one, will be crucial to better understand the inter-individual mechanisms behind the conferred protection of the traditional Mediterranean diet as well as to gain greater knowledge with respect to personalized nutrition. An integrative approach is necessary to extract conclusions from large-scale data. Further nutritional genomics research, at all levels, will be necessary to evaluate optimal "doses" of this dietary pattern, from an early stage *in utero* gestation until later adult life, to control diet-related disease, and to promote healthy living and aging.

Acknowledgments: MF was supported by a joint contract of the ISCIII and Health Department of the Catalan Government (Generalitat de Catalunya) (CP 06/00100). CIBEROBN is an initiative of Institute of Health Carlos III of Spain which is supported by FEDER funds (CB06/03).

Conflicts of Interest: The founding sponsors had no role in the design of the study, in the writing of the manuscript, and in the decision to publish the results. VK and MF declare no conflict of interest.

References

1. Scoditti, E.; Capurso, C.; Capurso, A.; Massaro, M. Vascular effects of the Mediterranean diet-part II: Role of omega-3 fatty acids and olive oil polyphenols. *Vascul. Pharmacol.* **2014**, *63*, 127–134. [CrossRef] [PubMed]
2. Simpson, S.J.; Le Couteur, D.G.; Raubenheimer, D. Putting the balance back in diet. *Cell* **2015**, *161*, 18–23. [CrossRef] [PubMed]
3. Estruch, R.; Martínez-González, M.A.; Corella, D.; Salas-Salvadó, J.; Ruiz-Gutiérrez, V.; Covas, M.I.; Fiol, M.; Gómez-Gracia, E.; López-Sabater, M.C.; Vinyoles, E.; *et al.* Effects of a Mediterranean-style diet on cardiovascular risk factors: A randomized trial. *Ann. Intern. Med.* **2006**, *145*, 1–11. [CrossRef] [PubMed]
4. Harnden, K.E.; Frayn, K.N.; Hodson, L. Dietary Approaches to Stop Hypertension (DASH) diet: Applicability and acceptability to a UK population. *J. Hum. Nutr. Diet.* **2010**, *23*, 3–10. [CrossRef] [PubMed]
5. Konstantinidou, V.; Ruiz, L.A.; Ordovás, J.M. Personalized nutrition and cardiovascular disease prevention: From Framingham to PREDIMED. *Adv. Nutr.* **2014**, *5*, 368S–371S. [CrossRef] [PubMed]
6. Keys, A.; Menotti, A.; Karvonen, M.J.; Aravanis, C.; Blackburn, H.; Buzina, R.; Djordjevic, B.S.; Dontas, A.S.; Fidanza, F.; Keys, M.H.; *et al.* The diet and 15-year death rate in the seven countries study. *Am. J. Epidemiol.* **1986**, *124*, 903–991. [PubMed]
7. Donini, L.M.; Serra-Majem, L.; Bulló, M.; Gil, A.; Salas-Salvadó, J. The Mediterranean diet: Culture, health and science. *Br. J. Nutr.* **2015**, *113*, S1–S3. [CrossRef] [PubMed]
8. Trichopoulou, A.; Costacou, T.; Bamia, C.; Trichopoulos, D. Adherence to a Mediterranean diet and survival in a Greek population. *N. Engl. J. Med.* **2003**, *348*, 2599–2608. [CrossRef] [PubMed]
9. De Lorgeril, M.; Salen, P.; Martin, J.L.; Monjaud, I.; Boucher, P.; Mamelle, N. Mediterranean dietary pattern in a randomized trial: Prolonged survival and possible reduced cancer rate. *Arch. Intern. Med.* **1998**, *158*, 1181–1187. [CrossRef] [PubMed]
10. Estruch, R.; Ros, E.; Salas-Salvadó, J.; Covas, M.I.; Corella, D.; Arós, F.; Gómez-Gracia, E.; Ruiz-Gutiérrez, V.; Fiol, M.; Lapetra, J.; *et al.* Primary prevention of cardiovascular disease with a Mediterranean diet. *N. Engl. J. Med.* **2013**, *368*, 1279–1290. [CrossRef] [PubMed]
11. Ros, E.; Martínez-González, M.A.; Estruch, R.; Salas-Salvadó, J.; Fitó, M.; Martínez, J.A.; Corella, D. Mediterranean diet and cardiovascular health: Teachings of the PREDIMED study. *Adv. Nutr.* **2014**, *5*, 330S–336S. [CrossRef] [PubMed]
12. Guasch-Ferré, M.; Hu, F.B.; Martínez-González, M.A.; Fitó, M.; Bulló, M.; Estruch, R.; Ros, E.; Corella, D.; Recondo, J.; Gómez-Gracia, E.; *et al.* Olive oil intake and risk of cardiovascular disease and mortality in the PREDIMED Study. *BMC Med.* **2014**, *12*, 78.

13. Martínez-González, M.Á.; Toledo, E.; Arós, F.; Fiol, M.; Corella, D.; Salas-Salvadó, J.; Ros, E.; Covas, M.I.; Fernández-Crehuet, J.; Lapetra, J.; *et al.* PREDIMED Investigators. Extravirgin olive oil consumption reduces risk of atrial fibrillation: The PREDIMED (Prevención con Dieta Mediterránea) trial. *Circulation* **2014**, *130*, 18–26.

14. Salas-Salvadó, J.; Bulló, M.; Babio, N.; Martínez-González, M.Á.; Ibarrola-Jurado, N.; Basora, J.; Estruch, R.; Covas, M.I.; Corella, D.; Arós, F.; *et al.* Reduction in the incidence of type 2 diabetes with the Mediterranean diet: Results of the PREDIMED-Reus nutrition intervention randomized trial. *Diabetes Care* **2011**, *34*, 14–19.

15. Corella, D.; Salas-Salvadó, J.; Martínez-González, M.A. Association of Mediterranean diet with peripheral artery disease: The PREDIMED randomized trial. *JAMA* **2014**, *311*, 415–417.

16. Corella, D.; Ordovás, J.M. How does the Mediterranean diet promote cardiovascular health? Current progress toward molecular mechanisms: Gene-diet interactions at the genomic, transcriptomic, and epigenomic levels provide novel insights into new mechanisms. *Bioessays* **2014**, *36*, 526–537. [CrossRef] [PubMed]

17. Khoury, M.J.; Wacholder, S. Invited Commentary: From Genome-Wide Association Studies to Gene-Environment-Wide Interaction Studies-Challenges and Opportunities. *Am. J. Epidemiol.* **2009**, *169*, 227–230. [CrossRef] [PubMed]

18. Pearson, T.A.; Manolio, T.A. How to Interpret a Genome wide Association Study. *JAMA* **2008**, *299*, 1335–1344. [CrossRef] [PubMed]

19. Corella, D.; Carrasco, P.; Sorlí, J.V.; Estruch, R.; Rico-Sanz, J.; Martínez-González, M.Á.; Salas-Salvadó, J.; Covas, M.I.; Coltell, O.; Arós, F.; *et al.* Mediterranean diet reduces the adverse effect of the TCF7L2-rs7903146 polymorphism on cardiovascular risk factors and stroke incidence: A randomized controlled trial in a high-cardiovascular-risk population. *Diabetes Care* **2013**, *36*, 3803–3811. [CrossRef] [PubMed]

20. Ortega-Azorín, C.; Sorlí, J.V.; Estruch, R.; Asensio, E.M.; Coltell, O.; González, J.I.; Martínez-González, M.Á.; Ros, E.; Salas-Salvadó, J.; Fitó, M.; *et al.* Amino acid change in the carbohydrate response element binding protein is associated with lower triglycerides and myocardial infarction incidence depending on level of adherence to the Mediterranean diet in the PREDIMED trial. *Circ. Cardiovasc. Genet.* **2014**, *7*, 49–58.

21. García-Calzón, S.; Martínez-González, M.A.; Razquin, C.; Corella, D.; Salas-Salvadó, J.; Martínez, J.A.; Zalba, G.; Marti, A. Pro12Ala polymorphism of the PPARγ2 gene interacts with a mediterranean diet to prevent telomere shortening in the PREDIMED-NAVARRA randomized trial. *Circ. Cardiovasc. Genet.* **2015**, *8*, 91–99. [CrossRef] [PubMed]

22. Garcia-Rios, A.; Gomez-Delgado, F.J.; Garaulet, M.; Alcala-Diaz, J.F.; Delgado-Lista, F.J.; Marin, C.; Rangel-Zuñiga, O.A.; Rodriguez-Cantalejo, F.; Gomez-Luna, P.; Ordovas, J.M.; *et al.* Beneficial effect of CLOCK gene polymorphism rs1801260 in combination with low-fat diet on insulin metabolism in the patients with metabolic syndrome. *Chronobiol. Int.* **2014**, *31*, 401–408. [CrossRef] [PubMed]

23. López-Guimerà, G.; Dashti, H.S.; Smith, C.E.; Sánchez-Carracedo, D.; Ordovas, J.M.; Garaulet, M. CLOCK 3111 T/C SNP interacts with emotional eating behavior for weight-loss in a Mediterranean population. *PLoS ONE* **2014**, *9*, e99152.

24. Konstantinidou, V.; Covas, M.I.; Sola, R.; Fito, M. Up-to date knowledge on the *in vivo* transcriptomic effect of the Mediterranean diet in humans. *Mol. Nutr. Food Res.* **2013**, *57*, 772–783. [CrossRef] [PubMed]

25. Llorente-Cortés, V.; Estruch, R.; Mena, M.P.; Ros, E.; González, M.A.; Fitó, M.; Lamuela-Raventós, R.M.; Badimon, L. Effect of Mediterranean diet on the expression of pro-atherogenic genes in a population at high cardiovascular risk. *Atherosclerosis* **2010**, *208*, 442–450. [CrossRef] [PubMed]

26. Konstantinidou, V.; Covas, M.I.; Muñoz-Aguayo, D.; Khymenets, O.; de la Torre, R.; Saez, G.; Tormos, M.C.; Toledo, E.; Marti, A.; Ruiz-Gutiérrez, V.; *et al.* *In vivo* nutrigenomic effects of virgin olive oil polyphenols within the frame of the Mediterranean diet: A randomized controlled trial. *FASEB J.* **2010**, *24*, 2546–2557. [CrossRef] [PubMed]

27. Serrano-Martinez, M.; Palacios, M.; Martinez-Losa, E.; Lezaun, R.; Maravi, C.; Prado, M.; Martínez, J.A.; Martinez-Gonzalez, M.A. A Mediterranean dietary style influences TNF-alpha and VCAM-1 coronary blood levels in unstable angina patients. *Eur. J. Nutr.* **2005**, *44*, 348–354. [CrossRef] [PubMed]

28. Castañer, O.; Corella, D.; Covas, M.I.; Sorlí, J.V.; Subirana, I.; Flores-Mateo, G.; Nonell, L.; Bulló, M.; de la Torre, R.; Portolés, O.; *et al.* *In vivo* transcriptomic profile after a Mediterranean diet in high-cardiovascular risk patients: A randomized controlled trial. *Am. J. Clin. Nutr.* **2013**, *98*, 845–853.

29. Bondia-Pons, I.; Martinez, J.A.; de la Iglesia, R.; Lopez-Legarrea, P.; Poutanen, K.; Hanhineva, K.; Zulet, M.L. Effects of short- and long-term Mediterranean-based dietary treatment on plasma LC-QTOF/MS metabolic profiling of subjects with metabolic syndrome features: The Metabolic Syndrome Reduction in Navarra (RESMENA) randomized controlled trial. *Mol. Nutr. Food Res.* **2015**, *59*, 711–728. [CrossRef] [PubMed]

30. Vázquez-Fresno, R.; Llorach, R.; Urpi-Sarda, M.; Lupianez-Barbero, A.; Estruch, R.; Corella, D.; Fitó, M.; Arós, F.; Ruiz-Canela, M.; Salas-Salvadó, J.; et al. Metabolomic pattern analysis after mediterranean diet intervention in a nondiabetic population: A 1- and 3-year follow-up in the PREDIMED study. *J. Proteome Res.* **2015**, *14*, 531–540.

31. Garcia-Aloy, M.; Llorach, R.; Urpi-Sarda, M.; Tulipani, S.; Estruch, R.; Martínez-González, M.A.; Corella, D.; Fitó, M.; Ros, E.; Salas-Salvadó, J.; et al. Novel multimetabolite prediction of walnut consumption by a urinary biomarker model in a free-living population: The PREDIMED study. *J. Proteome Res.* **2014**, *13*, 3476–3483. [CrossRef] [PubMed]

32. Garcia-Aloy, M.; Llorach, R.; Urpi-Sarda, M.; Jáuregui, O.; Corella, D.; Ruiz-Canela, M.; Salas-Salvadó, J.; Fitó, M.; Ros, E.; Estruch, R.; et al. A metabolomics-driven approach to predict cocoa product consumption by designing a multimetabolite biomarker model in free-living subjects from the PREDIMED study. *Mol. Nutr. Food Res.* **2015**, *59*, 212–220. [CrossRef] [PubMed]

33. González-Guardia, L.; Yubero-Serrano, E.M.; Delgado-Lista, J.; Perez-Martinez, P.; Garcia-Rios, A.; Marin, C.; Camargo, A.; Delgado-Casado, N.; Roche, H.M.; Perez-Jimenez, F.; et al. Effects of the Mediterranean diet supplemented with coenzyme q10 on metabolomic profiles in elderly men and women. *J. Gerontol. A Biol. Sci. Med. Sci.* **2015**, *70*, 78–84.

34. Richardson, K.; Nettleton, J.A.; Rotllan, N.; Tanaka, T.; Smith, C.E.; Lai, C.Q.; Parnell, L.D.; Lee, Y.C.; Lahti, J.; Lemaitre, R.N.; et al. Gain-of-function lipoprotein lipase variant rs13702 modulates lipid traits through disruption of a microRNA-410 seed site. *Am. J. Hum. Genet.* **2013**, *92*, 5–14. [CrossRef] [PubMed]

35. Corella, D.; Sorlí, J.V.; Estruch, R.; Coltell, O.; Ortega-Azorín, C.; Portolés, O.; Martínez-González, M.Á.; Bulló, M.; Fitó, M.; Arós, F.; et al. MicroRNA-410 regulated lipoprotein lipase variant rs13702 is associated with stroke incidence and modulated by diet in the randomized controlled PREDIMED trial. *Am. J. Clin. Nutr.* **2014**, *100*, 719–731. [CrossRef] [PubMed]

36. ENCODE Project Consortium. An integrated encyclopedia of DNA elements in the human genome. *Nature* **2012**, *489*, 57–74.

37. Müller, M.; Kersten, S. Nutrigenomics: Goals and strategies. *Nat. Rev. Genet.* **2003**, *4*, 315–322. [CrossRef] [PubMed]

38. Bünger, M.; Hooiveld, G.J.; Kersten, S.; Müller, M. Exploration of PPAR functions by microarray technology—A paradigm for nutrigenomics. *Biochim Biophys. Acta* **2007**, *1771*, 1046–1064. [CrossRef] [PubMed]

39. Lee, S.; Park, Y.; Zuidema, M.Y.; Hannink, M.; Zhang, C. Effects of interventions on oxidative stress and inflammation of cardiovascular diseases. *World J. Cardiol.* **2011**, *3*, 18–24. [CrossRef] [PubMed]

40. Sala-Vila, A.; Romero-Mamani, E.S.; Gilabert, R.; Núñez, I.; de la Torre, R.; Corella, D.; Ruiz-Gutiérrez, V.; López-Sabater, M.C.; Pintó, X.; Rekondo, J.; et al. Changes in ultrasound-assessed carotid intima-media thickness and plaque with a Mediterranean diet: A substudy of the PREDIMED trial. *Arterioscler. Thromb. Vasc. Biol.* **2014**, *34*, 439–445. [CrossRef] [PubMed]

41. Rytter, M.J.; Kolte, L.; Briend, A.; Friis, H.; Christensen, V.B. The immune system in children with malnutrition-a systematic review. *PLoS ONE* **2014**, *9*, e105017.

42. Veldhoen, M.; Ferreira, C. Influence of nutrient-derived metabolites on lymphocyte immunity. *Nat. Med.* **2015**, *21*, 709–718. [CrossRef] [PubMed]

43. Calabrese, V.; Scapagnini, G.; Davinelli, S.; Koverech, G.; Koverech, A.; De Pasquale, C.; Salinaro, A.T.; Scuto, M.; Calabrese, E.J.; Genazzani, A.R. Sex hormonal regulation and hormesis in aging and longevity: Role of vitagenes. *J. Cell Commun. Signal.* **2014**, *8*, 369–384. [CrossRef] [PubMed]

44. Rankin, N.J.; Preiss, D.; Welsh, P.; Burgess, K.E.; Nelson, S.M.; Lawlor, D.A.; Sattar, N. The emergence of proton nuclear magnetic resonance metabolomics in the cardiovascular arena as viewed from a clinical perspective. *Atherosclerosis* **2014**, *237*, 287–300. [CrossRef] [PubMed]

45. Ganna, A.; Salihovic, S.; Sundström, J.; Broeckling, C.D.; Hedman, A.K.; Magnusson, P.K.; Pedersen, N.L.; Larsson, A.; Siegbahn, A.; Zilmer, M.; et al. Large-scale metabolomic profiling identifies novel biomarkers for incident coronary heart disease. *PLoS Genet.* **2014**, *10*, e1004801. [CrossRef] [PubMed]

46. Tuohy, K.M.; Fava, F.; Viola, R. The way to a man's heart is through his gut microbiota'—dietary pro—and prebiotics for the management of cardiovascular risk. *Proc. Nutr. Soc.* **2014**, *73*, 172–185. [CrossRef] [PubMed]

47. Zuker, C.S. Food for the brain. *Cell* **2015**, *161*, 9–77. [CrossRef] [PubMed]

48. Lopez-Legarrea, P.; Fuller, N.R.; Zulet, M.A.; Martinez, J.A.; Caterson, I.D. The influence of Mediterranean, carbohydrate and high protein diets on gut microbiota composition in the treatment of obesity and associated inflammatory state. *Asia Pac. J. Clin. Nutr.* **2014**, *23*, 360–368. [PubMed]

49. Asher, G.; Sassone-Corsi, P. Time for food: The intimate interplay between nutrition, metabolism and the circadian clock. *Cell* **2015**, *161*, 84–92. [CrossRef] [PubMed]

50. Szarc vel Szic, K.; Declerck, K.; Vidaković, M.; Vanden Berghe, W. From inflammaging to healthy aging by dietary lifestyle choices: Is epigenetics the key to personalized nutrition? *Clin. Epigenet.* **2015**, *7*, 33. [CrossRef] [PubMed]

51. Roadmap Epigenomics Consortium; Kundaje, A.; Meuleman, W.; Ernst, J.; Bilenky, M.; Yen, A.; Heravi-Moussavi, A.; Kheradpour, P.; Zhang, Z.; Wang, J.; *et al.* Integrative analysis of 111 reference human epigenomes. *Nature* **2015**, *518*, 317–330. [CrossRef] [PubMed]

52. Lillycrop, K.A.; Hoile, S.P.; Grenfell, L.; Burdge, G.C. DNA methylation, ageing and the influence of early life nutrition. *Proc. Nutr. Soc.* **2014**, *73*, 413–421. [CrossRef] [PubMed]

53. Winter, J.; Jung, S.; Keller, S.; Gregory, R.I.; Diederichs, S. Many roads to maturity: MicroRNA biogenesis pathways and their regulation. *Nat. Cell Biol.* **2009**, *11*, 228–234. [CrossRef] [PubMed]

54. Filipowicz, W.; Bhattacharyya, S.N.; Sonenberg, N. Mechanisms of post-transcriptional regulation by microRNAs: Are the answers in sight? *Nat. Rev. Genet.* **2008**, *9*, 102–114. [CrossRef] [PubMed]

55. Gallach, S.; Calabuig-Fariñas, S.; Jantus-Lewintre, E.; Camps, C. MicroRNAs: Promising new antiangiogenic targets in cancer. *Biomed. Res. Int.* **2014**, *2014*, 878450. [CrossRef] [PubMed]

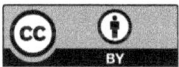

nutrients

MDPI

Review

Mediterranean Diet and Cardiovascular Disease: A Critical Evaluation of *A Priori* Dietary Indexes

Annunziata D'Alessandro [1,*] and Giovanni De Pergola [2]

[1] Endocrinologist, General Practitioner, General Medicine ASL BA/4 D.S.S. 8, viale Japigia 38/G, Bari 70126, Italy

[2] Department of Biomedical Sciences and Human Oncology, Section of Internal Medicine and Oncology, School of Medicine, Policlinico, Piazza Giulio Cesare 11, University of Bari "Aldo Moro", Bari 70124, Italy; E-Mail: gdepergola@libero.it

* Author to whom correspondence should be addressed; E-Mail: a.dalessandro2011@libero.it; Tel.: +39-080-2021905.

Received: 11 July 2015 / Accepted: 1 September 2015 / Published: 16 September 2015

Abstract: The aim of this paper is to analyze the *a priori* dietary indexes used in the studies that have evaluated the role of the Mediterranean Diet in influencing the risk of developing cardiovascular disease. All the studies show that this dietary pattern protects against cardiovascular disease, but studies show quite different effects on specific conditions such as coronary heart disease or cerebrovascular disease. *A priori* dietary indexes used to measure dietary exposure imply quantitative and/or qualitative divergences from the traditional Mediterranean Diet of the early 1960s, and, therefore, it is very difficult to compare the results of different studies. Based on real cultural heritage and traditions, we believe that the *a priori* indexes used to evaluate adherence to the Mediterranean Diet should consider classifying whole grains and refined grains, olive oil and monounsaturated fats, and wine and alcohol differently.

Keywords: Mediterranean diet; cardiovascular disease; coronary heart disease; cerebrovascular disease; *a priori* dietary indexes

1. Introduction

Diet is a very complex exposure variable in nutritional epidemiology. In the last years, the attention of scientists has moved from single foods or nutrients to dietary patterns, namely, the overall food consumption in the diet, that is, a holistic approach to study items that are highly interrelated and influence their impact on the risk of non-communicable chronic diseases [1]. There are two distinct approaches to examine overall dietary exposure: *a priori* and *a posteriori*. The first is based on the construction of an index on the basis of knowledge about the relationship between foods and diseases (sometimes synthesized in dietary guidelines) [2] or food consumption models (Mediterranean type diet, prudent diet, step I American Heart Association diet, and so on) [3]. The index is then used as a dietary exposure variable in epidemiological studies [2]. Conversely, the *a posteriori* approach is based on multivariate statistical techniques that identify sets of dietary exposures strongly correlated together and not previously known [3].

The *a priori* approach has been widely used in epidemiological studies to evaluate the relationship between the Mediterranean Diet and several outcomes such as cardiovascular incidence and mortality, risk factors for cardiovascular diseases, and incidence of major chronic non-communicable diseases.

We present a description of *a priori* dietary indexes used in the epidemiological studies that examined the relationship between the Mediterranean Diet and cardiovascular disease in this article. Then, we proceed to critically evaluate them.

2. Methods

PubMed was searched until May 2015 to find publications on the Mediterranean Diet and cardiovascular disease, using "Mediterranean Diet" matched with "coronary heart disease", "cerebrovascular disease", "stroke", "cardiovascular disease", "dietary score" and "dietary index" as key words.

3. Results

We found 26 studies that evaluated the relationship between the Mediterranean Diet and cardiovascular disease (Table 1). We also found five original *a priori* dietary indexes used to evaluate dietary exposure in such studies: *Mediterranean Diet Score* [4], *Dietary Score* [5], *Mediterranean Adequacy Index* [6], *a priori Mediterranean Dietary Pattern* [7], *PREvención con DIeta MEDiterránea* (PREDIMED) score [8]. Moreover, we found nine indexes derived from the original Mediterranean Diet Score (Table 2). We found only one index, the Mediterranean-Style Dietary Pattern Score, used to assess the conformity of an individual's diet to a traditional Mediterranean Diet [9].

Table 1. *A priori* dietary indexes and main results of the studies that evaluated the relationship between the Mediterranean Diet and CVD, CHD and cerebrovascular disease.

Authors (Year) (Reference)	A priori Index	Subjects, Number, Age	Study's Name, Type of Study and Follow-Up	Main Results
Bilenko et al., (2005) [10] °	MDS	Israeli Jewish population, 1159 adults, ≥35 year	NNS, transverse study	In men for each MDS decrease significant increased risk for MI, CABG, PTCA, CVD. In women similar trend, but not statistical significance.
Hoşcan et al., (2015) [11] °	MDS	Turkish population, 900 adults, 25–70 year	Cohort, (5.1 year)	Men with a lower adherence to the Mediterranean Diet had a significantly higher risk of CHD morbidity compared to men with a higher adherence. No association was found in women.
Trichopoulou et al., (2003) [12]	t-MED	Greek population, 22,043 adults, 20–86 year	EPIC, cohort, (3.7 year)	A 2-point increase in t-MED is associated with a CHD mortality reduction by 33%.
Dilis et al., (2012) [13]	t-MED	Greek population, 23,572 adults, 20–86 year	EPIC, cohort, (10 year)	A 2-point increase in t-MED was associated with a decrease in CHD mortality by 22% (*p* = 0.003) and a non-significant reduction in CHD incidence
Misirli et al., (2012) [14]	t-MED	Greek population, 23,601 adults, 20–86 year	EPIC, cohort, (10.6 year)	A 2-point increase in t-MED was associated with a significant decrease in cerebrovascular disease incidence and a non-significant decrease in cerebrovascular disease mortality
Tsivgoulis et al., (2015) * [15]	t-MED	U.S. population, 20,197 adults, 65 ± 9 year	REGARDS, cohort, (6.5 year)	A 1-point increase in t-MED was independently associated with a 5% reduction in the risk of incident ischemic stroke. No association with incident hemorrhagic stroke
Martínez-González et al., (2011) [16]	t-MED	Spanish population, 13,609 young, mean 38 year	SUN, cohort, (4.9 year)	A 2-point increase in t-MED was associated with a 20% decrease in total CVD risk and to a 26% reduction in CHD risk
Gardener et al., (2011) * [17]	t-MED	U.S. population, 2568 adult, mean 69 ± 10 year	NOMAS, cohort (9 year)	A 1-point increase in t-MED was associated with a 9% (*p* < 0.05) decrease in risk of vascular death. No association was found for vascular events (ischemic stroke and MI)
Agnoli et al., (2011) [18]	t-MED	Italian population, 40,681 adults, 35–74 year	EPICOR, cohort, (7.89 year)	t-MED was inversely associated with the risk of ischemic stroke and positively with the risk of hemorrhagic stroke without statistical significance
Turati et al., (2015) [19]	t-MED	Italian population, 760 patients with a first episode of non-fatal MI/682 controls, 16–79 year	Case-control	A 1-point increase in the t-MED was associated with a reduced risk of a first episode of MI by 9%
Knoops et al., (2004) [20]	The score according to Knoops	European population (11 European countries), 2339 elderly people, 70–90 year	HALE study, cohort, (10 year)	A score of at least four points reduced the CHD mortality by 39% and the CVD mortality by 29%
Agnoli et al., (2011) [18]	The Italian Mediterranean Index	Italian population, 40,681 adults, 35–74 year	EPICOR, cohort, (7.89 year)	The Italian Mediterranean Index was inversely associated with ischemic stroke (*p* for trend = 0.001) and hemorrhagic stroke (*p* for trend = 0.07)
Fung et al., (2009) [21]	a-MED	U.S. population, 74,886 females nurses, 38–63 year	NHS, cohort, (20 year)	Women in the highest a-MED quintile were at lower risk for both total CHD and total stroke compared with those in the lowest quintile (*p* for trend = 0.001 and = 0.03, respectively)

Table 1. Cont.

Authors (Year) (Reference)	A priori Index	Subjects, Number, Age	Study's Name, Type of Study and Follow-Up	Main Results
Mitrou et al., (2007) [22]	a-MED	U.S. population, 380,296 adults, median age 62 year	NIH-AARP Diet and Health Study, cohort (5 year)	The risk of mortality for CVD was lower in men and women with higher adherence to the Mediterranean Diet compared to those with a lower adherence ($p < 0.001$ and $p = 0.01$, respectively)
Buckland et al., (2009) [23]	r-MED	Spanish population, 41,078 adults, 29–69 year	EPIC, cohort, (10.4 year)	A 1-point increase in the r-MED was associated with a 6% lower risk of total CHD (p for trend < 0.001)
Hoevenaar-Blom et al., (2012) [24]	m-MED	Dutch population, 34,708 adults, 20–70 year	EPIC, cohort, (10–15 year)	A 2-point increase in the m-MED was inversely and significantly associated with fatal CVD, composite CVD, incident MI, incident stroke, and pulmonary embolism
Sjögren et al., (2010) [25]	The score according to Sjögren	Swedish men, 924 elderly, 71 ± 1 year	Cohort, (10.2 year)	A higher adherence to the Mediterranean Diet was associated with a lower risk of CVD mortality as compared to lower adherence (p for trend = 0.009)
Tognon et al., (2012) [26]	The score according to Tognon 2012	Sweden population, 77,151 adults, 30–70 year	VIP, cohort, (median 9 year)	The score according to Tognon 2012 was significantly associated only in women but not in men with mortality for CVD and mortality for MI. No association was found with stroke mortality in both genders.
Tognon et al., (2014) [27]	The score according to Tognon 2014	Danish population, 1849 adults	MONICA project, longitudinally	The score according to Tognon 2014 was inversely associated with CVD incidence and mortality. The strength of the associations depended on the way in which the score was built (see text)
Panagiotakos et al., (2015) [28]	DS	Greek population, 2583 adults, 18–89 year	ATTICA study, cohort, (10 year)	A 1-point increase in the DS decrease CVD risk by 4%
Panagiotakos et al., (2015) [29]	DS	Greek population, 848 patients with a first symptom of CHD/1078 controls	CARDIO 2000, case-control	An 11/55 unit increase in DS was associated with a reduced odds of having a first acute coronary syndrome by 27%
Kastorini et al., (2011) [30]	DS	Greek population, 250 patients with a first episode of acute coronary syndrome and 250 patients with a first ischemic stroke/500 controls	Case-control	A 1-point increase in the DS reduced the odds of having acute coronary syndrome by 9% and of having a stroke by 12%
Kastorini et al., (2012) [31]	DS	Greek population, 250 patients with a first ischemic stroke/250 controls	Case-control	A 1-point increase in DS reduced the odds of having a first ischemic stroke by 17% in non-hypercholesterolemic participant and by 10% in hypercholesterolemic participants
Fidanza et al., (2004) [32]	MAI	USA, Europe, Japan, 12,763 men, 40–59 year	Seven Countries Study, cohort, (25 year)	The MAI was inversely correlated with death rates from CHD ($p = 0.001$) in 16 cohorts of Seven Countries Study
Menotti et al., (2012) [33]	MAI	Italian population, 1139 men, 45–64 year	Seven Countries Study, two Italian cohorts, (20–40 year)	The hazard ratio for 2.7 units of MAI was associated with a CHD mortality reduction of 26% in 20y and 21% in 40y of follow-up

31

Table 1. *Cont.*

Authors (Year) (Reference)	A priori Index	Subjects, Number, Age	Study's Name, Type of Study and Follow-Up	Main Results
Martínez-González et al., (2002) [7]	a priori Mediterranean Dietary Pattern	Spanish population, 171 patients with a first MI/171 controls, <80 year	Case-control	A 1-point increase in the a priori Mediterranean Dietary Pattern was associated with a reduced risk of 8% for a first MI ($p < 0.01$)
Estruch et al., (2013) [34]	PREDIMED score	Spanish population, 7447 adults, 50–80 year	Randomized trial (4.8 year)	The rate of major CVD events was reduced by 30% ($p = 0.01$) in the group assigned to the Mediterranean Diet with extra-virgin olive oil and by 28% ($p = 0.33$) in the group assigned to the Mediterranean Diet with nuts compared with the control group. In subgroup analyses the supplemented Mediterranean Diet was significantly protective towards stroke but not towards MI and CVD deaths in comparison with the control diet

MDS, Mediterranean Diet Score; t-MED, Trichoupoulou Mediterranean Diet Index; a-MED, alternate Mediterranean Diet Index; r-MED, relative Mediterranean Diet Index; m-MED, modified Mediterranean Diet Index; DS, Dietary Score; MAI, Mediterranean Adequacy Index; PREDIMED, PREvencion con DIeta MEDiterranea; NNS, Negev Nutrition Study; EPIC, European Prospective Investigation into Cancer and Nutrition; REGARDS, Reasons for Geographic and Racial Differences in Stroke; SUN, Seguimiento Universidad de Navarra; NOMAS, Northern Manhattan Study; HALE, Healthy Ageing: a Longitudinal study in Europe; NHS, Nurses Health Study; NIH-AARP Diet and Health Study, National Institutes of Health-AARP Diet and Health Study; MONICA, MONItoring trends and determinants of CArdiovascular disease. MI, myocardial infarction; CABG, coronary artery bypass grafting; PTCA, percutaneus transluminal coronary angioplasty; CVD, cardiovascular disease; CHD, coronary heart disease; ° In this study, the food group of cereals was not clearly defined (bread and potatoes); * With the exception of potatoes, the used dietary and t-MED and t-MED scores had the same components in this study but were built differently.

Table 2. *A priori* dietary indexes and studies in which they have been evaluated or used to study the relationship between Mediterranean Diet and CVD, CHD, and cerebrovascular disease.

A priori Index	Authors (Year) (Reference)	Index Components	Score Range
MDS	Trichopoulou et al., (1995) [4] Bilenko et al., (2005) [10] ° Hoşcan et al., (2015) [11] °	8 components: M/S ratio; cereals (including bread and potatoes); vegetables; fruit; legumes; alcohol; meat and meat products; milk and dairy products	0–8
Other indexes adapted from the MDS: t-MED	Trichopoulou et al., (2003) [12] Dilis et al., (2012) [13] Misirli et al., (2012) [14] Tsivgoulis et al., (2015) [15] * Martínez-González (2011) [16] Gardener et al., (2011) [17] * Agnoli et al., (2011) [18] Turati et al., (2015) [19]	9 components: M/S ratio; cereals (including bread and potatoes); vegetables; fruit and nuts; legumes; fish; alcohol; meat and meat products; milk and dairy products	0–9
Other indexes adapted from the t-MED			

Table 2. *Cont.*

A priori Index	Authors (Year) (Reference)	Index Components	Score Range
the score according to Knoops	Knoops et al., (2004) [20]	the score according to Knoops 8 components: M/S ratio; legumes, nuts and seeds; cereals; fruits; vegetables and potatoes; fish; meat and meat products; dairy products	0–8
the Italian Mediterranean Index	Agnoli et al., (2011) [18]	the Italian Mediterranean Index 11 components: pasta, typical Mediterranean vegetables; fruit; legumes; olive oil; fish, soft drinks; butter; red meat; potatoes; alcohol	0–11
a-MED	Fung, et al., (2009) [21] Mitrou et al., (2007) [22]	a-MED 9 components: M/S ratio; legumes; fruits; vegetables (excluding potatoes); nuts; whole grains; fish; red and processed meats; alcohol	0–9
r-MED	Buckland et al., (2009) [23]	r-MED 9 components: Fruit, nuts, seeds (excluding fruit juices); vegetables (excluding potatoes); legumes; cereals; fish, sea foods; olive oil; meat and meat products, dairy products, alcohol	0–18
m-MED	Trichopoulou et al., (2005) [35] Hoevenaar-Blom et al., (2012) [24]	m-MED 9 components: M + P/S ratio; vegetables; legumes; fruit; cereals; fish; meat; dairy products; alcohol	0–9
Other indexes adapted from the m-MED			
the score according to Sjögren	Sjögren et al., (2010) [25]	the score according to Sjögren 8 components: P/S ratio; vegetables and legumes, fruit; cereals and potatoes; fish; meat and meat products; milk and milk products; alcohol	0–8
the scores according to Tognon	Tognon et al., (2012) [26]	the score according to Tognon (2012) 8 components: M − P/S ratio; vegetables and potatoes; fruit and juices; whole grain cereals; fish and fish products, meat and meat products; dairy products; alcohol	0–8
	Tognon et al., (2014) [27]	the score according to Tognon (2014) 8 components: M − P/S ratio; vegetables; fruit; cereal grains; fish and fish products, meat, meat products and eggs; dairy products; alcohol	0–8
DS	Pitsavos et al., (2005) [5] Panagiotakos et al., (2015) [28] Panagiotakos et al., (2006) [29] Kastorini et al., (2011) [30] Kastorini et al., (2012) [31]	DS 11 components: olive oil; whole grains; fruit; vegetables; potatoes; legumes; fish meat and meat products; poultry; full fat dairy; alcohol	0–55
MAI	Alberti-Fidanza et al., (1999) [6] Fidanza et al., (2004) [32] Menotti et al., (2012) [33]	MAI 18 components: bread; cereals; legumes; potatoes; vegetables; fresh fruit; nuts; fish; wine; vegetable oils; milk; cheese; meat; eggs; animal fat and margarines; sweet beverages; cakes, pies, cookies; sugar	0.6–11.6 #

Table 2. *Cont.*

A priori Index	Authors (Year) (Reference)	Index Components	Score Range
a priori Mediterranean Dietary Pattern		*a priori* Mediterranean Dietary Pattern	
	Martínez-González, *et al.*, (2002) [7]	8 components: olive oil; fiber; fruit; vegetables; fish; alcohol; meat and meat products; bread, pasta and rice	0–40
		PREDIMED score	0–14
PREDIMED score	Schröder *et al.*, (2011) [8] Estruch *et al.*, (2013) [34]	14-components: olive oil; vegetables; fruit (including natural fruit juices); red meat and meat products; animal fats; sugar sweetened beverages; red wine; legumes; fish and shell fish; sweets and pastries; nuts; sofrito; white meat; olive oil as main culinary fat	

MDS, Mediterranean Diet Score; t-MED, Trichoupoulou Mediterranean Diet Index; a-MED, alternate Mediterranean Diet Index; r-MED, relative Mediterranean Diet Index; m-MED, modified Mediterranean Diet Index; DS, Dietary Score; MAI, Mediterranean Adequacy Index; PREDIMED, PREvención con DIeta MEDiterranea; CVD, cardiovascular disease; CHD, coronary heart disease; M, monounsaturated fat; P, polyunsaturated fat; S, saturated fat; ° In this study, the food group of cereals was not clearly defined (bread and potatoes); * With the exception of potatoes, the used dietary and t-MED scores had the same components in this study but were built differently; # Score range among 16 cohorts of the Seven Countries Study (Fidanza *et al.*) [32].

4. Review

4.1. The Mediterranean Diet Score (MDS)

The MDS was the first index used to study adherence to the Mediterranean Diet in the population and it was developed by Trichopoulou *et al.* in 1995 [4]. It was based on eight main characteristics: monounsaturated fats (MUFAs) (from olive oil): saturated fats (SFAs) ratio; cereals (with inclusion of bread and potatoes); vegetables; fruit and nuts; legumes; alcohol; meat and meat products; and milk and dairy products. The score did not take into account sugars and syrups since, at that time, they had not been documented as dangerous for the health except for the total energy intake. The gender-specific median value was used as a cut-off point for each component. The hypothesis to be verified was that a diet with a high intake of cereals, vegetables, fruit, olive oil and legumes, a low intake of meat and dairy and a moderate intake of alcohol was healthy. The index was applied to elderly people, inhabitants of three rural Greek villages, who still followed the traditional Mediterranean Diet, with the aim of evaluating the relationship between adherence to diet and overall mortality [4].

The MDS was then used to examine the adherence to Mediterranean Diet and its relationship with coronary heart disease (CHD) in a random sample of 1159 Jewish people in Israel. In men, the odds ratio (ORs) for myocardial infarction, coronary bypass, angioplasty and any other cardiovascular disease (CVD) were 1.23 ($p = 0.04$), 1.56 ($p = 0.01$), 1.42 ($p = 0.003$), and 1.28 ($p < 0.01$), respectively, for each decrease in the MDS (score 0–8) in the logistic regression models adjusted for hypertension, hypercholesterolemia, diabetes mellitus, age, education, body mass index, and place of birth. A similar trend was observed in women, but no statistically significance was evident. In this study the mean consumption of olive oil was 0.82 g per day per person and the major contributors to MUFAs were canola oil, sunflower oil and dairy [10].

Very recently, the MDS was applied to a population study of 900 Turkish people in Alanya. After 5.1 years of follow-up, men with lower adherence to the Mediterranean Diet (score 0–4) had a higher risk of CHD morbidity (multivariate adjusted OR: 2.2; 95% CI (confidence interval): 1.03, 3.9; $p = 0.03$) compared to men with higher adherence (score 5–8). No association was found in women. In this study CHD was defined as myocardial infarction or coronary bypass or coronary angioplasty. Note that fish consumption was very low (2%) in this cohort and the consumption of olive oil was 0.9 g per day per person; the majors contributors to MUFAs were corn and sunflower oils [11].

In 2003 the MDS was updated by Trichopoulou *et al.* with the inclusion of another component, a moderate fish consumption and, just like in the previous study [4], each component received a value of 0 or 1 using the cut-off value of the gender-specific median. Subjects were assigned a value of 0 if the consumption of components considered beneficial (vegetables, legumes, fruit and nuts, cereals, fish, MUFAs:SFAs ratio) was below the median, whereas individuals were assigned a value of 1 if they had a consumption of beneficial food at or above the median. Otherwise, people with consumption of components considered harmful (meat, poultry, and dairy products) below the median were assigned a value of 1, whereas people with consumption at or above the median were assigned a value of 0. With regards to alcohol, a value of 1 was assigned to subjects consuming a moderate amount (*i.e.*, between 10 and 50 g per day for men and between 5 and 25 g per day for women) and a value of 0 otherwise. Therefore, this MDS with fish (t-MED) ranged from 0 (minimal adherence to Mediterranean Diet) to 9 (maximal adherence to Mediterranean Diet) [12]. In the Greek cohort of the *European Prospective Investigation into Cancer and Nutrition* (EPIC) study, 22,043 adults were followed for a median of 44 months, examining the relationship among diet and total mortality, CHD mortality and cancer mortality. A two-point increase in the t-MED was associated with a reduction in CHD mortality by 33% (multivariate adjusted hazard ratio (HR): 0.67; 95% CI: 0.47, 0.94) [12]. A contemporary study showed that dietary habits resembling the traditional Mediterranean Diet were widespread in Greece [36].

The Greek EPIC cohort has been followed in relation to CHD [13] and cerebrovascular disease [14]. During a median period of 10 years, a two-point increase in the t-MED was associated with a decrease in CHD mortality by 22% (multivariate adjusted HR: 0.78; 95% CI: 0.66, 0.92; p for trend = 0.003) and a non-significant reduction in CHD incidence (multivariate adjusted HR: 0.92; 95% CI: 0.84, 1.02; p for trend = 0.115) [13]. A two-point increase in t-MED was inversely associated with cerebrovascular disease incidence (multivariate adjusted HR: 0.85; 95% CI: 0.74, 0.96) during a median period of 10.6 years. In the subgroups analyzed by gender, the association was significant in women (multivariate adjusted HR: 0.81; 95% CI: 0.67, 0.98) but not in men. Overall, the protective effect of adherence to the Mediterranean Diet, evaluated by the t-MED, was evident in the incidence of ischemic (multivariate adjusted HR: 0.54; 95% CI: 0.29, 1.01; p for trend = 0.048) but not on the incidence of hemorrhagic cerebrovascular disease. The association between t-MED and cerebrovascular disease mortality was not significant [14].

Very recently, the t-MED was evaluated in 20,197 subjects enrolled in the *Reasons for Geographic and Racial Differences in Stroke* (REGARDS) study. In this population-based sample of US black and white adults, during a mean follow-up period of 6.5 years, a higher adherence to the Mediterranean Diet (score 5–9) was associated with a lower risk of incident ischemic stroke in comparison with a lower adherence (score 0–4) (multivariate adjusted HR: 0.79; 95% CI: 0.65, 0.96; p = 0.016). A one-point increase in t-MED was independently associated with a 5% reduction in the risk of incident ischemic stroke (95% CI: 0%, 11%). No association was found between incident hemorrhagic stroke and t-MED [15]. With the exception of potatoes, the used dietary and the t-MED scores had the same components in this study but they were built differently.

The t-MED, applied to the *Seguimiento Universidad de Navarra* (SUN) study, a Spanish cohort of 13,609 young graduates, followed for a median of 4.9 years, was inversely associated with CVD and CHD. CVD was a composite outcome of myocardial infarction mortality, stroke mortality, acute coronary syndromes, revascularization procedures, and stroke. A higher adherence to the Mediterranean Diet (score 7–9) was associated with a lower risk of developing CVD (multivariate adjusted HR: 0.41; 95% CI: 0.18, 0.95; p for trend = 0.07) and CHD (multivariate adjusted HR: 0.42; 95% CI: 0.16, 1.11; p for trend = 0.04). A two-point increase in the t-MED was associated with a 20% decrease in CVD risk (multivariate adjusted HR: 0.80; 95% CI: 0.62, 1.02) and a 26% reduction in CHD risk (multivariate adjusted HR: 0.74; 95% CI: 0.55, 0.99). It is noteworthy that using a t-MED built without cereals, namely a score with eight components, the inverse association between adherence to the Mediterranean Diet and CVD became significant (p for trend = 0.03) and the negative relationship between adherence to the Mediterranean Diet and CHD became more evident (p for trend = 0.01). Since both refined cereals and whole grains are considered a unique category in the t-MED, the authors hypothesized a negative impact from refined cereals on CVD risk [16]. Refined cereals have a negative impact on CVD risk because they raise the diet glycemic load, which has been associated with a decrease in HDL cholesterol, increase in fasting plasma triglycerides and fasting insulin, promotion of oxidative stress, low-grade systemic inflammation, and procoagulant activity [37].

In the *Northern Manhattan Study* (NOMAS), a multiethnic cohort of 2568 subjects followed for a mean period of 9 years, the association between adherence to Mediterranean Diet (estimated by the t-MED) and CVD events was not statistically significant for ischemic stroke and myocardial infarction but it was for vascular death (multivariate adjusted HR: 0.71; 95% CI: 0.49, 1.04; p for trend = 0.04 between the highest and the lowest quintile of the t-MED). A one-point increase in the t-MED was associated with a 9% decrease of the risk of vascular death (multivariate adjusted HR: 0.91; 95% CI: 0.85, 0.98; p for trend < 0.05). Consumption of alcohol, fish and legumes were the components driving the inverse association of t-MED with vascular death [17]. Also in this study, with the exception of potatoes, the used dietary and the t-MED scores had the same components but were built differently.

The t-MED applied to the Italian cohort of the *long-tErm follow-up of antithrombotic management Patterns In acute CORonary syndrome patients* (EPICOR) study involving 40,681 volunteers recruited from five cities uniformly distributed in the Italian territory and followed for a mean of 7.9 years was inversely associated with the risk of ischemic stroke, but the trend among the tertiles of intake was not significant. The association with the risk of hemorrhagic stroke was positive without a statistic significance [18].

In a hospital-based case-control study performed in a northern Italian City, 760 patients with a first episode of non-fatal myocardial infarction were matched with 682 controls by gender and age, admitted to the hospital for non-neoplastic conditions, unrelated to known risks for myocardial infarction or dietary modification. Adherence to the Mediterranean Diet was assessed by the t-MED. The risk of a first episode of myocardial infarction was reduced by 45% (multivariate adjusted OR: 0.55; 95% CI: 0.40, 0.75; p for trend < 0.01) in subjects with higher adherence to the Mediterranean Diet (score ≥ 6) as compared to subjects with lower adherence (score < 4). A one-point increase in the t-MED was associated with a reduced risk of a first episode of myocardial infarction by 9% (multivariate adjusted OR: 0.91; 95% CI: 0.85, 0.98). High consumption of vegetables and legumes were inversely associated with non-fatal myocardial infarction risk [19].

A modification of the t-MED was proposed by Trichopoulou *et al.* in 2005, with the aim of making the application of t-MED to non-Mediterranean populations, in which the intake of MUFAs from olive oil was minimal, possible. The modified t-MED (m-MED) was achieved by replacing the MUFAs: SFAs ratio with the MUFAs + Polyunsaturated fats (PUFAs): SFAs ratio [35].

The m-MED was applied to the Dutch cohort of the EPIC study, EPIC-NL, that included 34,708 participants followed for a mean of 11.8 years. A two-point increase in the m-MED was inversely and significantly associated with fatal CVD (multivariate adjusted HR: 0.78; 95% CI: 0.69, 0.88), composite CVD (fatal CVD, non-fatal myocardial infarction, non-fatal stroke) (multivariate adjusted HR: 0.85; CI 95%: 0.80, 0.91), incident myocardial infarction (multivariate adjusted HR: 0.86; 95% CI: 0.79, 0.93), incident stroke (multivariate adjusted HR: 0.88; 95% CI: 0.78, 1.00) and pulmonary embolism (multivariate adjusted HR: 0.74; 95% CI: 0.59, 0.92). No association was found between m-MED and incident angina pectoris, transient ischemic attack and peripheral arterial disease. Interestingly, the association of m-MED to fatal CVD, CVD incidence, composite CVD and myocardial infarction was mostly mitigated when alcohol was excluded from m-MED [24].

In the literature, we identified four variants of t-MED—the score according to Knoops *et al.* [20], the alternate Mediterranean Diet Index (a-MED) [38], the relative Mediterranean Diet Index (r-MED) [23], and the Italian Mediterranean Index [18]—and three variants of m-MED: the score according to Sjögren *et al.* [25] and the scores according to Tognon *et al.* [26,27].

In the *Healthy Ageing: a Longitudinal study in Europe* (HALE) study, performed in 2339 elderly people of 11 European countries, Knoops *et al.* used a modified t-MED based on eight components: MUFAs: SFAs ratio; legumes, nuts and seeds; cereals; fruit; vegetables and potatoes; fish; meat and meat products; and dairy products. The intake of each component was adjusted to daily intakes of 2500 kcal for men and 2000 kcal for women. For the first six components considered to be healthy, a value of 1 was assigned to people whose consumption was at least as high as the gender-specific median value, and a value of 0 to the others. Reverse values were assigned to the last two components considered unhealthy. Alcohol was evaluated as a separate lifestyle factor since many studies observed an independent effect of alcohol on survival. The score ranged from 0 (minimal adherence to the Mediterranean Diet) to 9 (maximal adherence to the Mediterranean Diet). A score of at least four points was associated with lower CHD mortality (multivariate adjusted HR: 0.61; 95% CI: 0.43, 0.88) and CVD mortality (multivariate adjusted HR: 0.71; 95% CI: 0.58, 0.88). The combination of four healthy lifestyles (high adherence to the Mediterranean Diet, moderate alcohol intake, moderate-high physical activity levels, nonsmoking) reduced the CHD mortality and the CVD mortality more than 50% in comparison with none or one healthy lifestyle [20].

The a-MED is a t-MED modified by excluding potatoes from the vegetable group, separating fruit and nuts into two groups, eliminating the dairy group, including whole-grain products only, including only red and processed meats for the meat group, and assigning alcohol intake between 5 and 15 g per day for 1 point. These changes were based on dietary patterns that were consistently associated with lower risk of chronic disease in clinical and epidemiological studies. The a-MED ranged from 0 to 9 [38].

In the *Nurses Health Study* (NHS) a cohort of 74,886 female nurses followed for 20 years, the risk of total (non-fatal and fatal cases) CHD was lower in the highest quintile of the a-MED compared with the lowest quintile (multivariate adjusted relative risk (RR): 0.71; 95% CI: 0.62, 0.82; *p* for trend < 0.0001). Total stroke (non-fatal and fatal cases) was lower in the highest quintile compared with the lowest quintile of a-MED (multivariate adjusted RR: 0.87; 95% CI: 0.73, 1.02; *p* for trend = 0.03). In the a-MED, alcohol intake could result from regular consumption of beer, spirits or wine while MUFAs resulted mainly from meat and only minimally from olive oil [21].

In the *National Institutes of Health-AARP Diet and Health Study cohort*, consisting of 380,296 people followed for 5 years, the risk of mortality for CVD was significantly lower in men and women with a higher adherence to the Mediterranean Diet (score 6–9) compared to those with a lower adherence (score 0–3), evaluated by the a-MED (men: multivariate adjusted HR: 0.78; 95% CI 0.69, 0.87; *p* for trend < 0.001; women: multivariate adjusted HR: 0.71; 95% CI: 0.68, 0.97; *p* for trend = 0.01) [22].

The r-MED was used to evaluate the exposure to the Mediterranean Diet in the Spanish cohort of EPIC. It derived from t-MED and consisted of nine components. Among these, six components were considered typical of Mediterranean diet: fruit (including nuts and seeds but excluding fruit juices); vegetables (excluding potatoes); legumes; cereals (whole and refined grains); fresh fish and sea foods; and olive oil. Two components were considered not typical of the Mediterranean Diet: meat and meat products; and dairy products (including low-fat and high-fat milk, yogurt, cheese, cream desserts, and dairy and nondairy creams). Each component, except alcohol, was measured as grams per 1000 kcal/day and was divided into tertiles of dietary intakes. A value of 0, 1 and 2 to the first, second and third tertiles of intake, respectively was assigned to typical components. Non-typical components were assigned with an inverted score. Alcohol was scored as a dichotomous variable and 2 points was assigned for an intake from 5 to 25 g per day for women and from 10 to 50 g per day for men. Intakes above or below these ranges were scored 0 points. Then, the theoretical r-MED ranged between 0 (no adherence) to 18 (maximal adherence). In the multivariate analysis performed on data for 40,757 subjects of the cohort, followed for a mean of 10.4 years, the risk of fatal and non-fatal (myocardial infarction or unstable angina requiring revascularization) incident CHD was lower in subjects with higher adherence to the Mediterranean Diet (score 11–18) compared to subjects with lower adherence (score 0–6) (multivariate adjusted HR: 0.60; 95% CI: 0.47, 0.77; *p* for trend < 0.001). A one-point increase in the r-MED was associated with a 6% lower risk of CHD (multivariate adjusted HR: 0.94; 95% CI: 0.91, 0.97; *p* for trend < 0.001). The use of t-MED instead of r-MED was associated with an almost identical decrease in CHD risk for a two-point increase in both scores [23].

The *Italian Mediterranean Index* was developed to adapt the t-MED to Italian eating behavior [18]. It consisted of 11 components: six typical Mediterranean food (pasta; typical Mediterranean vegetables; fruit; legumes; olive oil; and fish), four non-Mediterranean foods (soft drinks; butter; red meat; and potatoes), and alcohol. People whose consumption of typical Mediterranean foods was in the 3rd tertile of distribution received 1 point whereas all others received 0 points. People whose consumption of non-Mediterranean foods was in the first tertile of the distribution, received 1 point, and all others received 0 points. For alcohol, people whose consumption was up to 12 g per day received 1 point, whereas abstainers and people whose consumption was >12 g per day received 0 points. The theoretical score ranged from 0 to 11. This score applied to 40,681 subjects of EPICOR study, followed for a mean of 7.9 years, was inversely associated with ischemic stroke (multivariate adjusted HR: 0.37; 95% CI: 0.19–0.70; *p* for trend = 0.001) and hemorrhagic stroke (multivariate adjusted HR: 0.51; 95% CI: 0.22–1.20; *p* for trend = 0.07) [18].

The score according to Sjögren *et al.* was a variant of the m-MED and was applied to a population-based longitudinal study of 924 Swedish men. Due to a very low intake, nuts and seeds were excluded by the score and leguminous plants were pooled with vegetables. PUFAs replaced MUFAs because the consumption of the olive oil in this population was very low and SFAs and MUFAs had similar food origins and therefore strongly correlated. During a mean follow-up of 10 years, a higher adherence to the Mediterranean Diet (score 6–8) was associated with a lower risk of CVD mortality by 81%

(multivariate adjusted HR: 0.19; 95% CI: 0.04, 0.86; *p* for trend = 0.009) as compared to lower adherence (score 0–2) [25].

The score according to Tognon *et al.* was based on eight components: vegetables and potatoes; fruit and juices; whole grain cereals; fish and fish products; MUFAs + PUFAs:SFAs ratio; alcohol intake; meat and meat products; and dairy products. The cut-off points were the gender-specific medians and the value of 0 was assigned to people whose consumption was under the gender-specific median for the first six components and above for the last two components. The value of 1 was assigned to people whose consumption was above the gender-specific median for the first six components and under the gender-specific median for the last two components. The final score varied from 0 (low adherence) to 8 (high adherence) [26]. In a population based study performed in Västerbotten, a North Sweden County with 77,151 subjects followed for 17 years, the score was significantly associated, only in women and not in men, with CVD mortality (multivariate adjusted HR: 0.90; 95% CI: 0.82, 0.99; *p* for trend < 0.05), and with mortality for myocardial infarction (multivariate adjusted HR: 0.84; 95% CI: 0.71, 0.99; *p* for trend < 0.05). The mortality for stroke was not associated with the Mediterranean Diet in men and women. Only alcohol intake was independently and inversely associated with CVD mortality among the eight components of the score [26].

A score that was very similar to the previous one [26] was used to evaluate the relationship between Mediterranean Diet and CVD in a Danish cohort of the *MONItoring trends and determinants of Cardiovascular disease* (MONICA) project [27]. It was based on eight components: MUFAs + PUFAs: SFAs ratio; alcohol intake; vegetables; fruit; cereal grains; fish and fish products; meat, meat products and eggs; and dairy products. The cut-off points were the gender-specific medians and the value of 0 was assigned to people whose consumption was under the median for the first six components and above for the last two components. The value of 1 was assigned to people whose consumption was above the median for the first six components and under the median for the last two components. Two different procedures were used to produce two different scores. The first procedure excluded mixed dishes (score 1), and the second included ingredients extrapolated from mixed dishes or recipes (score 2). A third score was created in the same way as score 2 except considering wine instead of total alcohol intake (score 3). None of the scores were associated with stroke mortality and incidence (fatal and non-fatal cases) in the multivariate analysis. The score 1 was inversely associated with CVD mortality and incidence (fatal and non-fatal cases) and with myocardial infarction but without statistical significance. The score 2 was associated with CVD incidence (fatal and non-fatal cases) (multivariate adjusted HR: 0.94; 95% CI:0.89, 0.99; *p* for trend < 0.05), CVD mortality (multivariate adjusted HR: 0.90; 95% CI: 0.82, 0.99; *p* for trend < 0.05), myocardial infarction incidence (fatal and non-fatal cases) (multivariate adjusted HR: 0.89; 95% CI: 0.80, 1.00; *p* for trend < 0.05), and myocardial infarction mortality (multivariate adjusted HR: 0.80; 95% CI 0.67, 0.96; *p* for trend < 0.05). Score 3 was associated with the same outcomes slightly more than score 2 [27].

4.2. The Dietary Score (DS)

The DS, proposed in 2005 and inspired by the dietary guidelines of the Greek Mediterranean Diet pyramid for adults [39], was directly associated with antioxidant capacity and inversely correlated with oxidized LDL-cholesterol serum concentrations, in a random sample of healthy adults in the *ATTICA* study [5]. It consisted of 11 components: whole grains; fruit; vegetables; potatoes; legumes; olive oil; fish; meat and meat products; poultry; full fat dairy; and alcohol. With the exclusion of alcohol, the frequency of intakes was categorized as never, rare (1–4 servings per month), frequent (5–8 servings per month), very frequent (9–12 servings per month), weekly (13–18 servings per month) and daily (>18 servings per month). For these intake frequencies a value of 0, 1, 2, 3, 4, and 5 respectively was assigned for the first seven components. The values were reversed for frequency of intakes of red meat, poultry, and full fat dairy foods. The alcohol intake was scored 5 if <300 mL per day of wine, 0 for consumption >700 mL per day or none, and scored 4, 3, 2, 1, for intakes of 300–400, 400–500, 500–600, and 600–700 mL per day, respectively. It was stated that

100 mL of wine contained 12 g of alcohol. The theoretical range of the score varied from 0 to 55. The adherence to the Mediterranean Diet decreased the CVD risk in the *ATTICA* study that involved 2583 participants: during 10 years of follow-up, a one-point increase in the score decreased the risk by 4% (multivariate adjusted RR: 0.96; 95% CI: 0.93, 1.00) independently of socio-demographic variables, lifestyle, and clinical factors. The protective effect of Mediterranean Diet was also evident in participants at risk such as smokers, sedentary individuals, and obese people. No component of the dietary score was significantly associated with CVD risk, in line with the hypothesis that the Mediterranean pattern acts as a whole [28].

This score was also applied in some case-control studies.

In the *CARDIO2000*, a case-control study, 848 patients who had been hospitalized for a first symptom of coronary heart disease were matched with 1078 controls by age, gender and the region they came from. The subjects in the highest tertile of the score had a reduced odds of having acute coronary syndromes by 46% (multivariate adjusted OR: 0.54; 95% CI: 0.44, 0.66) compared with subjects in the lowest tertile. An 11/55-unit increase in DS was associated with a reduced odds of having acute coronary syndromes by 27% (multivariate adjusted OR: 0.73; 95% CI: 0.66–0.89) [29].

In a case-control study of 250 consecutive patients with a first episode of acute coronary syndrome and 250 consecutive patients with a first ischemic stroke, matched with 500 healthy subjects by gender and age, a one-point increase in the score reduced the odds of having acute coronary syndrome (multivariate adjusted OR: 0.91; 95% CI: 0.87, 0.96) and ischemic stroke (multivariate adjusted OR: 0.88; 95% CI: 0.82, 0.94) [30].

In a case-control study of 250 consecutive patients with a first ischemic stroke matched with 250 controls by gender, age and region, a one-point increase in DS reduced the odds of having a first ischemic stroke by 17% (multivariate adjusted OR: 0.83; 95% CI: 0.72, 0.96) in non-hypercolesterolemic participants and by 10% (multivariate adjusted OR: 0.90; 95% CI: 0.81, 0.99) in hypercolesterolemic participants [31].

4.3. The Mediterranean Adequacy Index (MAI)

The MAI is a dietary score built taking into account the Mediterranean Diet of Nicotera as a reference. In the early 1960s this diet was very similar to the Corfu and Crete diets [6], with low CHD mortality rate at 25-year of follow-up of the *Seven Countries Study* [40]. This score, consisting of 18 food or food groups, is computed by dividing the sum of the total energy percentages of the food groups typical of the reference Mediterranean Diet (bread; cereals; legumes; potatoes; vegetables; fresh fruit; nuts; fish; wine; and vegetable oil) by the sum of the total energy percentages of the food groups less typical of the reference Mediterranean Diet (milk; cheese; meat; eggs; animal fats and margarines; sweet beverages; cakes, pies, cookies; and sugar). The higher the MAI, the greater the amount of energy derived from typical Mediterranean foods [6]. The MAI could be expressed as g per day, or g per 1000 kcal, or g per 4.2 MJ [32].

The MAI, computed in random samples of men surveyed for their eating habits and belonging to 16 cohorts of the *Seven Countries Study*, was inversely associated with the 25-year death rates from CHD ($r = -0.72$; $p = 0.001$) [32]. The HR for 1 unit of natural log of MAI (approximately corresponding to 2.7 units of MAI) was associated with a CHD mortality decrease of 26% (multivariate adjusted RR: 0.74; 95% CI: 0.55, 0.99) in 20 years of follow-ups and of 21% (multivariate adjusted RR: 0.79; 95% CI: 0.64, 0.97) in 40 years of follow-ups in two Italian rural cohorts of the *Seven Countries Study*, Crevalcore and Montegiorgio. The statistical analysis was multivariate adjusted for the covariates [33].

4.4. A Priori Mediterranean Dietary Pattern

This score was applied to a case-control study of 171 patients with a first myocardial infarction matched with 171 controls by gender and age, hospitalized for diseases considered not to be related to the diet. It is based on six food groups or nutrients considered as protective, and two groups of foods of the Mediterranean Diet considered harmful. The first consisted of: olive oil; fibers; fruit;

vegetables; fish; and alcohol. For each of these items the distribution according to quintiles within the study was calculated and each subject received points from 1 to 5 corresponding to the quintile of intake from the lowest to the highest quintile. The latter consisted of: meat and meat products; foods with high glycemic load as white bread, pasta and rice. For these components each subject received 1 for the highest quintile and 5 for the lowest quintile. For each subject the score was obtained summing the eight quintiles values. The theoretical score ranged between 0 and 40. This score was applied to 342 subjects of the study. The subjects with score ⩾30 had a risk of a first myocardial infarction lower of 79% (multivariate adjusted OR: 0.21; 95% CI: 0.06, 0.73; p for trend = 0.01) compared with subjects scored <20. The risk was reduced by 8% for a one-point increase in the score (multivariate adjusted OR: 0.92; 95% CI: 0.86, 0.98; p for trend = 0.01) [7].

4.5. The (PREDIMED) Score

The PREDIMED is a Spanish multi center trial of 7447 people at high risk for CVD, randomly assigned to one of three groups: participants that received advise to reduce dietary fat (control diet); participants that received advice on Mediterranean Diet and provision of extra-virgin olive oil (approximately 1 liter per week); participants that received advice on Mediterranean Diet and provision of mixed nuts (30 g per day: 15 g of walnuts, 7.5 g of hazelnuts, and 7.5 g of almonds) [34]. The adherence to the Mediterranean Diet was evaluated at baseline and during the study by a 14-point Mediterranean Diet Adherence Screener (MEDAS). It consists of 12 questions on food intake frequency and two questions on dietary habits characteristic of the Spanish Mediterranean Diet [8]. A value of 1 point was assigned if these criteria were met:

- ⩾4 tablespoons of olive oil per day (including that used in frying, salado etc.) (1 tablespoon = 13.5 g)
- ⩾2 servings of vegetables per day (at least 1 portion raw or as salad) (1 serving = 200 g)
- ⩾3 fruit units (including natural fruit juices) per day
- <1 serving of red meat or meat products (1 serving =100–150 g) per day
- <1 serving of animal fat per day (1 serving = 12 g)
- <1 cup of sugar-sweetened beverage per day (1 cup = 100 mL)
- ⩾7 glasses of red wine per week
- ⩾3 servings of legumes per week (1 serving = 150 g)
- ⩾3 servings of fish or shellfish per week (1 serving: 100–150 g fish, or 4–5 units, 200 g shellfish)
- <3 commercial sweets or pastries per week (not homemade)
- ⩾3 servings of nuts (including peanuts) per week
- ⩾2 times per week of a dish with a traditional sauce of tomatoes, garlic, onion, or leeks sautéed in olive oil
- olive oil as main culinary fat
- preferential consumption of chicken, turkey, rabbit meat instead of veal, pork, hamburger or sausage

A value of 0 point was assigned if these criteria were not met. The final PREDIMED score ranged from 0 to 14.

The participants in the three groups at the beginning of the study had a similar score. During the study, the score of participants in the Mediterranean Diet group increased in comparison with the control group, and after three years the differences were significant for 12 out of 14 components of the score. An evaluation of biomarkers (urinary hydroxytyrosol in the group receiving extra-virgin oil, plasma alpha-linolenic acid levels in the group receiving nuts) confirmed the compliance to dietary advice. After a median follow-up of 4.8 years, the rate of major CVD events (myocardial infarction, stroke, death for CVD) was reduced by 30% (multivariate adjusted OR: 0.70; 95% CI: 0.54, 0.92; p = 0.01) in the group assigned to the Mediterranean Diet with extra-virgin olive oil and by 28% (multivariate adjusted OR: 0.72; 95% CI: 0.54, 0.96; p = 0.03) in the group assigned to the Mediterranean Diet with nuts, compared with the control group. In the subgroup analysis, the supplemented Mediterranean Diet had a clear protective effect on stroke (multivariate adjusted OR: 0.61; 95% CI: 0.44, 0.86; p = 0.005) but the protective effect on myocardial infarction and CVD death in comparison with the control diet did not reach statistical significance [34].

4.6. The Mediterranean-Style Dietary Pattern Score (MSDPS)

The MSDPS was elaborated by Rumawas *et al.* [9] using the Greek Mediterranean Diet pyramid for adults as a reference [39] and was based on 13 components corresponding to 13 food groups of the pyramid: whole grains; fruit; vegetables; milk and dairy products; wine; fish; poultry; olives, legumes, nuts; potatoes; eggs; sweets; meat; and olive oil. With the exception of olive oil, each group was scored from 0 to 10 depending on the compliance to the numbers of servings suggested in the pyramid. A penalty was assigned for a possible overconsumption by subtracting a point proportionally to the number of servings consumed that exceeded the recommended intake for the considered food group. If the score became negative it was defaulted to zero. Olive oil was scored 10 if its use was exclusive, 5 if its use was along with other vegetable oils, 0 for no use. For each subject the MSDPS was calculated by summing the values of 13 components, and dividing this sum by the theoretical maximum sum of 130 and multiplying by 100 by the aim to obtain a scale of standardized values ranging from 0 to 100. In view of the mixture of Mediterranean and non-Mediterranean foods that real patterns have, the previous score was corrected by a continuous factor ranging from 0 to 1 depending on the proportion of energy intake derived by foods not included in the pyramid. The MSDPS was applied to dietary data collected during the 7th examination of the Framingham Offspring Cohort. The quintiles of MSDPS were significantly and positively associated with the dietary intakes of fiber, *n*-3 PUFAs (linolenic acid, eicosapentaenoic acid, docosahexaenoic acid), antioxidant vitamins (β-carotene, folate, vitamin C, vitamin E, lycopene), calcium, magnesium, potassium, and inversely and significantly with added sugars, glycemic index, SFAs, trans-fat acids, *n*-6 PUFAs (linoleic acid and arachidonic acid): *n*-3 PUFAs ratio, MUFAs, and oleic acid. The inverse association of MSDPS with MUFAs and oleic acid depended on a large intake of meat (including poultry). The authors concluded that the MSDPS was a useful tool to evaluate the adherence to traditional Mediterranean Diet in a non-Mediterranean population [9].

We could not find any study investigating the relationship between Mediterranean Diet and CVD risk using this score.

5. Critical Appraisal

From the analysis of the above data it is evident that all the studies show a protective effect of Mediterranean Diet on CVD. Nevertheless the protective effect of the Mediterranean Diet against CHD and stroke is very different across the studies. Are there different types of Mediterranean Diets with different protective effects on these outcomes?

Two questions should be taken into consideration: Which Mediterranean Diet is the object of evaluation? How was exposure to the diet measured?

In most of the studies mentioned above, the score of dietary exposure was not established using traditional Mediterranean Diet of the early 1960s as a reference, and there are major deviations from the early dietary pattern that provides the best scientific evidence of a protective role against CVD [40,41]. The divergences observed are both qualitative and quantitative.

5.1. Qualitative Score Divergences from Traditional Mediterranean Diet

Fidanza *et al.* described the diet of Nicotera, a rural small town in the Calabria Region in Southern Italy. It was a cohort of the *Seven Countries Study,* but because of both a shortage of funds and similarity with the two cohorts of Greece, Creta and Corfu, it was not followed longitudinally [42]. The various components of the Nicotera diet, evaluated using the weighed method for seven days in three different seasons of 1960 and expressed as percentages of caloric intake provided, were the following: cereals (50%–59%), extra virgin olive oil (13%–17%), vegetables (2.2%–3.6%), potatoes (2.3%–3.6%), legumes (3%–6%), fruit (2.6%–3.6%, including nuts representing about 3% of the weight of all fruit), fish (1.6%–2.0%), and red wine (1%–6%). Meat (2.6%–5.0%), dairy products (2%–4%), eggs and animal fats were rarely eaten [31]. The bread was homemade from stone ground wheat [42] and was sourdough leavened [43].

Another source of dietary epidemiological data is that provided by the *Etude des consommations alimentaires des populations de onze regions de la communauté europeenne en vue de la determination des niveaux de contamination radioactive* (EURATOM), a study carried out in the early 1960s in 11 areas of seven European countries. Two areas were in Southern Italy, in Campania and Basilicata. The study was very accurate, using the weighed inventory method over seven consecutive days [44]. Here, the intake of pasta and bread was about 490 g per day providing 60% of total energy intake, the intake of fruit and vegetables was 426 g per day providing 9% of total energy intake, the intake of meat and fish was 62 g per day providing 5% of total energy intake, the intake of fats and oils was 51 g per day providing 18% of total energy intake, the intake of milk and dairy products was 87 g per day providing 4% of total energy intake, the intake of sugar was 15 g per day providing 2% of total energy intake, the intake of sweets was 1 g per day. The fiber intake was 24.4 g per day and 60% was derived from wheat while the remaining part came from tomatoes, onions, artichokes, pulses, eggplants and fruit. Added oils were almost exclusively vegetable oils, namely olive oil, whereas lard and butter were hardly ever used. Margarine was not used at all. The total of dietary lipids was 73 g per day, *i.e.*, 28% of total energy intake. Only the olive oil was used as vegetable oil and in quantity of 49 g per day. If it was considered only added lipids, the MUFAs:SFAs ratio was 3.9 while the PUFAs/SFAs ratio was 0.53. If it was considered total lipids the MUFAs:SFAs ratio was 2.29 while the PUFAs:SFAs ratio was 0.41 [45].

To sum up, the traditional Mediterranean Diet is well described by the Greek Mediterranean Diet pyramid for adults. It recommends a daily intake of 8 servings of whole grains, 3 servings of fruit, 6 servings of vegetables, 2 servings of dairy products, 3 glasses of wine for men and 1.5 glasses of wine for women; weekly intakes of 6 servings of fish, 4 servings of poultry, 4 servings of olives, pulses and nuts, 3 servings of potatoes, 3 serving of eggs, 3 servings of sweets; a monthly intake of 4 servings of red meat; and olive oil as the main added lipid [39].

Whole grains are, together with extra virgin olive oil and red wine, a peculiar characteristic of the Mediterranean Diet. The inclusion of whole grains into the score of dietary exposure to the Mediterranean Diet is consistent with the characteristics of traditional Mediterranean Diet but also with the scientific evidence of their protective role against CVD. In a pioneering study by Morris *et al.*, a high intake of fiber from cereals was a protective factor for CHD incidence during 20 years of follow-up in 337 healthy English men. It was not evident that CHD was associated with refined cereals intakes [46]. In a recent exhaustive review of pooled/meta-analyses and systematic reviews, the protective effect of whole grains against CVD was higher than that of fruit and vegetables with a risk reduction by a maximum of 29%, 23% and 23% respectively, for the highest levels of consumption [47].

Whole grains have a recognized protective effect against CVD risk factors, such as type 2 diabetes mellitus [48–53], total and LDL cholesterol [54,55], hypertension [56–58], and low grade systemic inflammation [59,60]. Besides, a higher intake of whole grains has been associated with a better body weight [61–64]. Cereal fiber partly accounts for the protective effects against CVD mortality [65]. If whole grains cereals seem to be protective, refined cereals have either a neutral or harmful effect on CVD and other diet-related chronic diseases [47]. However a review of 135 relevant articles evaluating the relationship between consumption of refined cereal grains and health outcomes, shows that a consumption of up to 50% of all grain foods as refined grain foods (without high levels of added fat, sugar, or sodium) is not associated with increased CVD and other diet-related chronic diseases risk [66]. According to some authors whole grains products should be distinguished from refined food in the score of dietary exposure [67].

Seemingly, the substitution of MUFAs for olive oil in the indexes of Mediterranean Diet creates some concern since many healthy effects depend on minor components [68–70] and because of doubts raised by some authors on the cardio-protective effect of MUFAs [71]. Indeed, dietary MUFAs can come from other vegetable oils (high-oleic safflower and sunflower oils, canola oil), mostly nuts, peanuts, avocados, and from animal products (meat, eggs, lard) [72]. In a systematic review and meta-analysis of cohort studies, the comparison of the top *versus* bottom third of the distribution of a combination of MUFAs (of both plant and animal derived from), olive oil, oleic acid, and MUFAs:SFAs ratio resulted in a significant risk reduction for CVD mortality, CVD events, stroke and all-cause mortality. However, in subgroup analyses, only higher intakes of olive oil were associated with a significant decrease of risk for CVD events, stroke and all-cause mortality. By contrast, MUFAs of mixed animal and vegetable sources *per se* were not associated with these outcomes [73].

In the same way, the substitution of alcohol for wine in Mediterranean Diet indexes deserves to be evaluated as there is some evidence that wine offers greater CVD protection in comparison to other alcoholic beverages, possibly because of phenolic compounds [74–76]. The score proposed by Tognon *et al.* including wine instead of total alcohol intake was better associated with CVD outcomes [27].

The *a priori* indexes used to evaluate the adherence to the Mediterranean Diet should consider whole grains and refined grains, olive oil and MUFAs, and wine and alcohol in a different way. Whole cereal grains, extra virgin olive oil, and wine characterize the Mediterranean Diet of the early 1960s beyond the plant-based foods diets (rich in fruit, vegetable, nuts, whole grains, fats from natural liquid vegetable oils, adequate intake of *n*-3 PUFAs) that are important to prevent CVD and other diet-related chronic diseases [77]. Among the scores examined in this review, only the DS and MSDPS are coherent with qualitative characteristics of Mediterranean Diet of the early 1960s.

5.2. Quantitative Score Divergences from Traditional Mediterranean Diet

In the MDS and some of its variants (Table 2) the gender-specific medians are used as cut-offs to distinguish between levels of intakes of each score component that will be scored 0 or 1. However, the value of the median does not necessarily reflect a level of intake of foods that is consistent with a positive or negative effect on health [67]. For example, it is well established that the intake at least of 3 servings of whole grains replacing refined grains is necessary to have CVD benefits [52,78]. If the intake of whole grains is low in the examined population, the value of 1 point assigned to people with a consumption level at or above the median should be inappropriate in any case, since it does not meet the protective value. In the same way, if there is a large intake of a non-Mediterranean food in the population, assigning a value of 1 point to people whose consumption is below the median should not be considered adequate since the intake could still be excessive. In agreement with the concept expressed by other authors, the median is just a value of position that divides a distribution in 50% below and 50% above the value of the median [67]. Besides, since the median values may be different among populations, the results of one study could not be comparable with those of another study performed in a different population [67]. It is noteworthy that the yes/no approach of this score implies an important loss of information. Indeed, the use of a large number of cut-off points (at least more than two) is recommended to improve the diagnostic capacity of a score [79] since the diagnostic accuracy of an index increases as the number of partitions of its components increases [80]. The DS, the r-MED, the Italian Mediterranean Index, the a priori Mediterranean Dietary Pattern, the MAI, and the MSDPS are consistent with this concept. The diagnostic accuracy of an index increases also when each component of the score is assigned with a specific "weight" that depends on the strength of the relationship that each component has with the binary outcome under study. Each component of a composite score contributes differently to the risk of a specific disease [80]. For example, there is some evidence that vegetables have a lower protective effect on CVD than whole grains or fruit [47]. So, "the development of weighted dietary indexes that adequately assess a dietary pattern and its relationship to the burden of a disease is considered essential" [81]. Some authors propose that the "weights" are the ORs obtained from univariate logistic regression [80], or from multiple logistic regression models with each component of the score entering as an independent variable and total score made by remaining components entered in the model, or by multiplying the "weights" obtained from the ORs with the inverse of the variance of the specific OR, which represents the effect size of the association [82].

6. Conclusions

In conclusion, our study shows that the Mediterranean Diet is a useful tool to reduce the risk of CVD as clearly shown by some systematic reviews and meta-analyses [83,84]. In a recent meta-analysis, Sofi *et al.* found that a two-point increase in adherence score for the Mediterranean Diet leads to a 10% reduced risk of CVD [84]. However, published studies show quite different effects from the Mediterranean Diet with regard to specific conditions such as CHD and cerebrovascular disease. We cannot exclude that several factors are responsible for these differences, such as a small number of cases in some studies, different control of confounders, or a different dietary assessment among the studies, and a lack of repeated measurement of a Mediterranean-style diet [85]. In our opinion, the use of *a priori* dietary indexes established to comply with the characteristics of the Mediterranean Diet of the early 1960s could be useful to better understand the effectiveness of this dietary pattern in managing CVD risk. A valid score for studying the relationship between the traditional Mediterranean Diet of the early 1960s and CVD should have the quantitative and qualitative characteristics of the true early dietary pattern as a reference. However, some of the health effects of the traditional Mediterranean Diet might be due to some characteristics which are not easily quantified: some cooking styles that preserve water-soluble nutrients, the consumption of fresh and not greenhouse vegetables which are poorer in phytochemicals, the consumption of fresh fruit at the end of meal which can counteract the pro-inflammatory and pro-oxidant effect of foods [86], the use of spices and herbs that may improve CVD risk factors [87], the use of stone ground sourdough bread whose richness in fiber and low glycemic index make it very healthy [88], and so on.

Acknowledgments: We acknowledge Giovanni Misciagna for his critical review.

Author Contributions: Annunziata D'Alessandro drafted the manuscript. Giovanni De Pergola helped to review the manuscript. Both authors read and approved the final version of the manuscript.

Conflicts of Interest: The authors declare no conflict of interest.

References

1. Hu, F.B. Dietary pattern analysis: A new direction in nutritional epidemiology. *Curr. Opin. Lipidol.* **2002**, *13*, 3–9. [CrossRef] [PubMed]
2. Kant, A.K. Dietary patterns and health outcomes. *J. Am. Diet. Assoc.* **2004**, *104*, 615–635. [CrossRef] [PubMed]
3. Panagiotakos, D.B.; Pitsavos, C.; Stefanadis, C. Alpha priori and alpha-posterior dietary pattern analyses have similar estimating and discriminating ability in predicting 5-Y incidence of cardiovascular disease: Methodological issues in nutrition assessment. *J. Food Sci.* **2009**, *74*, H218–H224. [CrossRef] [PubMed]
4. Trichopoulou, A.; Kouris-Blazos, A.; Wahlqvist, M.L.; Gnardellis, C.; Lagiou, P.; Polychronopoulos, E.; Vassilakou, T.; Lipworth, L.; Trichopoulos, D. Diet and overall survival in elderly people. *BMJ* **1995**, *311*, 1457–1460. [CrossRef] [PubMed]
5. Pitsavos, C.; Panagiotakos, D.B.; Tzima, N.; Chrysohoou, C.; Economou, M.; Zampelas, A.; Stefanadis, C. Adherence to the Mediterranean diet is associated with total antioxidant capacity in healthy adults: The ATTICA study. *Am. J. Clin. Nutr.* **2005**, *82*, 694–699. [PubMed]
6. Alberti-Fidanza, A.; Fidanza, F.; Chiuchiù, M.P.; Verducci, G.; Fruttini, D. Dietary studies on two rural Italian population groups of the Seven Countries Study. 3. Trend of food and nutrient intake from 1960 to 1991. *Eur. J. Clin. Nutr.* **1999**, *53*, 854–860. [CrossRef] [PubMed]
7. Martínez-González, M.A.; Fernández-Jarne, E.; Serrano-Martínez, M.; Marti, A.; Martinez, J.A.; Martín-Moreno, J.M. Mediterranean diet and reduction in the risk of a first acute myocardial infarction: An operational healthy dietary score. *Eur. J. Nutr.* **2002**, *41*, 153–160. [CrossRef] [PubMed]
8. Schröder, H.; Fitó, M.; Estruch, R.; Martínez-González, M.A.; Corella, D.; Salas-Salvadó, J.; Lamuela-Raventós, R.; Ros, E.; Salaverría, I.; Fiol, M.; *et al.* A short screener is valid for assessing Mediterranean diet adherence among older Spanish men and women. *J. Nutr.* **2011**, *141*, 1140–1145. [CrossRef] [PubMed]

9. Rumawas, M.E.; Dwyer, J.T.; McKeown, N.M.; Meigs, J.B.; Rogers, G.; Jacques, P.F. The development of the Mediterranean-style dietary pattern score and its application to the American diet in the Framingham Offspring Cohort. *J. Nutr.* **2009**, *139*, 1150–1156. [CrossRef] [PubMed]

10. Bilenko, N.; Fraser, D.; Vardi, H.; Shai, I.; Shahar, D.R. Mediterranean diet and cardiovascular diseases in an Israeli population. *Prev. Med.* **2005**, *40*, 299–305. [CrossRef] [PubMed]

11. Hoşcan, Y.; Yiğit, F.; Müderrisoğlu, H. Adherence to Mediterranean diet and its relation with cardiovascular diseases in Turkish population. *Int. J. Clin. Exp. Med.* **2015**, *8*, 2860–2866. [PubMed]

12. Trichopoulou, A.; Costacou, T.; Bamia, C.; Trichopoulos, D. Adherence to a Mediterranean diet and survival in a Greek population. *N. Engl. J. Med.* **2003**, *348*, 2599–2608. [CrossRef] [PubMed]

13. Dilis, V.; Katsoulis, M.; Lagiou, P.; Trichopoulos, D.; Naska, A.; Trichopoulou, A. Mediterranean diet and CHD: The Greek European Prospective Investigation into Cancer and Nutrition cohort. *Br. J. Nutr.* **2012**, *108*, 699–709. [CrossRef] [PubMed]

14. Misirli, G.; Benetou, V.; Lagiou, P.; Bamia, C.; Trichopoulos, D.; Trichopoulou, A. Relation of the traditional Mediterranean diet to cerebrovascular disease in a Mediterranean population. *Am. J. Epidemiol.* **2012**, *176*, 1185–1192. [CrossRef] [PubMed]

15. Tsivgoulis, G.; Psaltopoulou, T.; Wadley, V.G.; Alexandrov, A.V.; Howard, G.; Unverzagt, F.W.; Moy, C.; Howard, V.J.; Kissela, B.; Judd, S.E. Adherence to a Mediterranean diet and prediction of incident stroke. *Stroke* **2015**, *46*, 780–785. [CrossRef] [PubMed]

16. Martínez-González, M.A.; García-López, M.; Bes-Rastrollo, M.; Toledo, E.; Martínez-Lapiscina, E.H.; Delgado-Rodriguez, M.; Vazquez, Z.; Benito, S.; Beunza, J.J. Mediterranean diet and the incidence of cardiovascular disease: A Spanish cohort. *Nutr. Metab. Cardiovasc. Dis.* **2011**, *21*, 237–244. [PubMed]

17. Gardener, H.; Wright, C.B.; Gu, Y.; Demmer, R.T.; Boden-Albala, B.; Elkind, M.S.; Sacco, R.L.; Scarmeas, N. Mediterranean-style diet and risk of ischemic stroke, myocardial infarction, and vascular death: The Northern Manhattan Study. *Am. J. Clin. Nutr.* **2011**, *94*, 1458–1464. [CrossRef] [PubMed]

18. Agnoli, C.; Krogh, V.; Grioni, S.; Sieri, S.; Palli, D.; Masala, G.; Sacerdote, C.; Vineis, P.; Tumino, R.; Frasca, G.; *et al.* A priori-defined dietary patterns are associated with reduced risk of stroke in a large Italian cohort. *J. Nutr.* **2011**, *141*, 1552–1558. [CrossRef] [PubMed]

19. Turati, F.; Pelucchi, C.; Galeone, C.; Praud, D.; Tavani, A.; La Vecchia, C. Mediterranean diet and non-fatal acute myocardial infarction: A case-control study from Italy. *Public Health Nutr.* **2015**, *18*, 713–720. [CrossRef] [PubMed]

20. Knoops, K.T.; de Groot, L.C.; Kromhout, D.; Perrin, A.E.; Moreiras-Varela, O.; Menotti, A.; van Staveren, W.A. Mediterranean diet, lifestyle factors, and 10-year mortality in elderly European men and women: The HALE project. *JAMA* **2004**, *292*, 1433–1439. [CrossRef] [PubMed]

21. Fung, T.T.; Rexrode, K.M.; Mantzoros, C.S.; Manson, J.E.; Willett, W.C.; Hu, F.B. Mediterranean diet and incidence of and mortality from coronary heart disease and stroke in women. *Circulation* **2009**, *119*, 1093–1100. [CrossRef] [PubMed]

22. Mitrou, P.N.; Kipnis, V.; Thiébaut, A.C.; Reedy, J.; Subar, A.F.; Wirfält, E.; Flood, A.; Mouw, T.; Hollenbeck, A.R.; Leitzmann, M.F.; *et al.* Mediterranean dietary pattern and prediction of all-cause mortality in a US population: Results from the NIH-AARP Diet and Health Study. *Arch. Intern. Med.* **2007**, *167*, 2461–2468. [CrossRef] [PubMed]

23. Buckland, G.; González, C.A.; Agudo, A.; Vilardell, M.; Berenguer, A.; Amiano, P.; Ardanaz, E.; Arriola, L.; Barricarte, A.; Basterretxea, M.; *et al.* Adherence to the Mediterranean diet and risk of coronary heart disease in the Spanish EPIC Cohort Study. *Am. J. Epidemiol.* **2009**, *170*, 1518–1529. [CrossRef] [PubMed]

24. Hoevenaar-Blom, M.P.; Nooyens, A.C.; Kromhout, D.; Spijkerman, A.M.; Beulens, J.W.; van der Schouw, Y.T.; Bueno-de-Mesquita, B.; Verschuren, W.M. Mediterranean style diet and 12-year incidence of cardiovascular diseases: The EPIC-NL cohort study. *PLoS ONE* **2012**, *7*, e45458. [CrossRef] [PubMed]

25. Sjögren, P.; Becker, W.; Warensjö, E.; Olsson, E.; Byberg, L.; Gustafsson, I.B.; Karlström, B.; Cederholm, T. Mediterranean and carbohydrate-restricted diets and mortality among elderly men: A cohort study in Sweden. *Am. J. Clin. Nutr.* **2010**, *92*, 967–974. [CrossRef] [PubMed]

26. Tognon, G.; Nilsson, L.M.; Lissner, L.; Johansson, I.; Hallmans, G.; Lindahl, B.; Winkvist, A. The Mediterranean diet score and mortality are inversely associated in adults living in the subarctic region. *J. Nutr.* **2012**, *142*, 1547–1553. [CrossRef] [PubMed]

27. Tognon, G.; Lissner, L.; Sæbye, D.; Walker, K.Z.; Heitmann, B.L. The Mediterranean diet in relation to mortality and CVD: A Danish cohort study. *Br. J. Nutr.* **2014**, *111*, 151–159. [CrossRef]

28. Panagiotakos, D.B.; Georgousopoulou, E.N.; Pitsavos, C.; Chrysohoou, C.; Skoumas, I.; Pitaraki, E.; Georgiopoulos, G.A.; Ntertimani, M.; Christou, A.; Stefanadis, C. Exploring the path of Mediterranean diet on 10-year incidence of cardiovascular disease: The ATTICA study (2002–2012). *Nutr. Metab. Cardiovasc. Dis.* **2015**, *25*, 327–335. [CrossRef] [PubMed]

29. Panagiotakos, D.B.; Pitsavos, C.; Stefanadis, C. Dietary patterns: A Mediterranean diet score and its relation to clinical and biological markers of cardiovascular disease risk. *Nutr. Metab. Cardiovasc. Dis.* **2006**, *16*, 559–568. [CrossRef] [PubMed]

30. Kastorini, C.M.; Milionis, H.J.; Ioannidi, A.; Kalantzi, K.; Nikolaou, V.; Vemmos, K.N.; Goudevenos, J.A.; Panagiotakos, D.B. Adherence to the Mediterranean diet in relation to acute coronary syndrome or stroke nonfatal events: A comparative analysis of a case/case-control study. *Am. Heart J.* **2011**, *162*, 717–724. [CrossRef] [PubMed]

31. Kastorini, C.M.; Milionis, H.J.; Kantas, D.; Bika, E.; Nikolaou, V.; Vemmos, K.N.; Goudevenos, J.A.; Panagiotakos, D.B. Adherence to the mediterranean diet in relation to ischemic stroke nonfatal events in nonhypercholesterolemic and hypercholesterolemic participants: Results of a case/case–control study. *Angiology* **2012**, *63*, 509–515. [CrossRef] [PubMed]

32. Fidanza, F.; Alberti, A.; Lanti, M.; Menotti, A. Mediterranean Adequacy Index: Correlation with 25-year mortality from coronary heart disease in the Seven Countries Study. *Nutr. Metab. Cardiovasc. Dis.* **2004**, *14*, 254–258. [CrossRef]

33. Menotti, A.; Alberti-Fidanza, A.; Fidanza, F. The association of the Mediterranean Adequacy Index with fatal coronary events in an Italian middle-aged male population followed for 40 years. *Nutr. Metab. Cardiovasc. Dis.* **2012**, *22*, 369–375. [CrossRef] [PubMed]

34. Estruch, R.; Salas-Salvadó, J.; Corella, D.; Arós, F.; Gómez-Gracia, E.; Ruiz-Gutiérrez, V.; Fiol, M.; Lapetra, J.; Lamuela-Raventos, R.M.; Serra-Majem, L.; *et al.* Primary prevention of cardiovascular disease with a Mediterranean diet. *N. Engl. J. Med.* **2013**, *368*, 1279–1290. [CrossRef] [PubMed]

35. Trichopoulou, A.; Orfanos, P.; Norat, T.; Bueno-de-Mesquita, B.; Ocké, M.C.; Peeters, P.H.; van der Schouw, Y.T.; Boeing, H.; Hoffmann, K.; Boffetta, P.; *et al.* Modified Mediterranean diet and survival: EPIC-elderly prospective cohort study. *BMJ* **2005**, *330*, 991–995. [CrossRef] [PubMed]

36. Costacou, T.; Bamia, C.; Ferrari, P.; Riboli, E.; Trichopoulos, D.; Trichopoulou, A. Tracing the Mediterranean diet through principal components and cluster analyses in the Greek population. *Eur. J. Clin. Nutr.* **2003**, *57*, 1378–1385. [CrossRef] [PubMed]

37. Brand-Miller, J.; Dickinson, S.; Barclay, A.; Celermajer, D. The glycemic index and cardiovascular disease risk. *Curr. Atheroscler. Rep.* **2007**, *9*, 479–485. [CrossRef] [PubMed]

38. Fung, T.T.; McCullough, M.L.; Newby, P.K.; Manson, J.E.; Meigs, J.B.; Rifai, N.; Willett, W.C.; Hu, F.B. Diet-quality scores and plasma concentrations of markers of inflammation and endothelial dysfunction. *Am. J. Clin. Nutr.* **2005**, *82*, 163–173. [PubMed]

39. Supreme Scientific Health Council, Ministry of Health and Welfare. Dietary guidelines for adults in Greece. *Arch. Hell. Med.* **1999**, *16*, 516–524.

40. Menotti, A.; Kromhout, D.; Blackburn, H.; Fidanza, F.; Buzina, R.; Nissinen, A. Food intake patterns and 25-year mortality from coronary heart disease: Cross-cultural correlations in the Seven Countries Study. *Eur. J. Epidemiol.* **1999**, *15*, 507–515. [CrossRef] [PubMed]

41. Keys, A.; Menotti, A.; Karvonen, M.J.; Aravanis, C.; Blackburn, H.; Buzina, R.; Djordjevic, B.S.; Dontas, A.S.; Fidanza, F.; Keys, M.H.; *et al.* The diet and 15-year death rate in the seven countries study. *Am. J. Epidemiol.* **1986**, *124*, 903–915. [PubMed]

42. Fidanza, F.; Alberti, A.; Fruttini, D. The Nicotera diet: The reference Italian Mediterranean diet. *World Rev. Nutr. Diet.* **2005**, *95*, 115–121. [PubMed]

43. Istituto Nazionale Per la Dieta Mediterranea e la Nutrigenomica (I.N.Di.M.); Barbalace, P. Pietanze di un Tempo. Saperi e Sapori Della Cucina Nicoterese. Available online: http://www.indim.it/Documenti/Capitolo-I-II.pdf (accessed on 11 February 2013).

44. Cresta, M.; Ledermann, S.; Garnier, A.; Lombardo, E.; Lacourly, G. *Etude des Consommations Alimentaires des Populations de Onze Regions de la Communaute Europeenne en vue de la Determination des Niveaux de Contamination Radioactive. Rapport Établi au Centre d'Etude Nucléaire de Fontenay-Aux-Roses-France*; EURATOM: Bruxelles, Belgium, 1969; pp. 1–589.

45. Ferro-Luzzi, A.; Sette, S. The Mediterranean Diet: An attempt to define its present and past composition. *Eur. J. Clin. Nutr.* **1989**, *43* (Suppl. S2), 13–29. [PubMed]

46. Morris, J.N.; Marr, J.W.; Clayton, D.G. Diet and heart: A postscript. *BMJ* **1977**, *2*, 1307–1314. [CrossRef] [PubMed]

47. Fardet, A.; Boirie, Y. Associations between food and beverage groups and major diet-related chronic diseases: An exhaustive review of pooled/meta-analyses and systematic reviews. *Nutr. Rev.* **2014**, *72*, 741–762. [CrossRef] [PubMed]

48. Fung, T.T.; Hu, F.B.; Pereira, M.A.; Liu, S.; Stampfer, M.J.; Colditz, G.A.; Willett, W.C. Whole-grain intake and the risk of type 2 diabetes: A prospective study in men. *Am. J. Clin. Nutr.* **2002**, *76*, 535–540. [PubMed]

49. Murtaugh, M.A.; Jacobs, D.R., Jr.; Jacob, B.; Steffen, L.M.; Marquart, L. Epidemiological support for the protection of whole grains against diabetes. *Proc. Nutr. Soc.* **2003**, *62*, 143–149. [CrossRef] [PubMed]

50. Montonen, J.; Knekt, P.; Järvinen, R.; Aromaa, A.; Reunanen, A. Whole-grain and fiber intake and the incidence of type 2 diabetes. *Am. J. Clin. Nutr.* **2003**, *77*, 622–629. [PubMed]

51. De Munter, J.S.; Hu, F.B.; Spiegelman, D.; Franz, M.; van Dam, R.M. Whole grain, bran, and germ intake and risk of type 2 diabetes: A prospective cohort study and systematic review. *PLoS Med.* **2007**, *4*, e261. [CrossRef] [PubMed]

52. Ye, E.Q.; Chacko, S.A.; Chou, E.L.; Kugizaki, M.; Liu, S. Greater whole-grain intake is associated with lower risk of type 2 diabetes, cardiovascular disease, and weight gain. *J. Nutr.* **2012**, *142*, 1304–1313. [CrossRef] [PubMed]

53. Aune, D.; Norat, T.; Romundstad, P.; Vatten, L.J. Whole grain and refined grain consumption and the risk of type 2 diabetes: A systematic review and dose-response meta-analysis of cohort studies. *Eur. J. Epidemiol.* **2013**, *28*, 845–858. [CrossRef] [PubMed]

54. Newby, P.K.; Maras, J.; Bakun, P.; Muller, D.; Ferrucci, L.; Tucker, K.L. Intake of whole grains, refined grains, and cereal fiber measured with 7-d diet records and associations with risk factors for chronic disease. *Am. J. Clin. Nutr.* **2007**, *86*, 1745–1753. [PubMed]

55. Giacco, R.; Clemente, G.; Cipriano, D.; Luongo, D.; Viscovo, D.; Patti, L.; di Marino, L.; Giacco, A.; Naviglio, D.; Bianchi, M.A.; et al. Effects of the regular consumption of wholemeal wheat foods on cardiovascular risk factors in healthy people. *Nutr. Metab. Cardiovasc. Dis.* **2010**, *20*, 186–194. [CrossRef] [PubMed]

56. Wang, L.; Gaziano, J.M.; Liu, S.; Manson, J.E.; Buring, J.E.; Sesso, H.D. Whole- and refined-grain intakes and the risk of hypertension in women. *Am. J. Clin. Nutr.* **2007**, *86*, 472–479. [PubMed]

57. Flint, A.J.; Hu, F.B.; Glynn, R.J.; Jensen, M.K.; Franz, M.; Sampson, L.; Rimm, E.B. Whole grains and incident hypertension in men. *Am. J. Clin. Nutr.* **2009**, *90*, 493–498. [CrossRef] [PubMed]

58. Tighe, P.; Duthie, G.; Vaughan, N.; Brittenden, J.; Simpson, W.G.; Duthie, S.; Mutch, W.; Wahle, K.; Horgan, G.; Thies, F. Effect of increased consumption of whole-grain foods on blood pressure and other cardiovascular risk markers in healthy middle-aged persons: A randomized controlled trial. *Am. J. Clin. Nutr.* **2010**, *92*, 733–740. [CrossRef] [PubMed]

59. Esposito, K.; Giugliano, D. Whole-grain intake cools down inflammation. *Am. J. Clin. Nutr.* **2006**, *83*, 1440–1441. [PubMed]

60. Montonen, J.; Boeing, H.; Fritsche, A.; Schleicher, E.; Joost, H.G.; Schulze, M.B.; Steffen, A.; Pischon, T. Consumption of red meat and whole-grain bread in relation to biomarkers of obesity, inflammation, glucose metabolism and oxidative stress. *Eur. J. Nutr.* **2013**, *52*, 337–345. [CrossRef] [PubMed]

61. Liu, S.; Willett, W.C.; Manson, J.E.; Hu, F.B.; Rosner, B.; Colditz, G. Relation between changes in intakes of dietary fiber and grain products and changes in weight and development of obesity among middle-aged women. *Am. J. Clin. Nutr.* **2003**, *78*, 920–927. [PubMed]

62. Harland, J.I.; Garton, L.E. Whole-grain intake as a marker of healthy body weight and adiposity. *Public Health Nutr.* **2008**, *11*, 554–563. [CrossRef] [PubMed]

63. Good, C.K.; Holschuh, N.; Albertson, A.M.; Eldridge, A.L. Whole grain consumption and body mass index in adult women: An analysis of NHANES 1999–2000 and the USDA pyramid servings database. *J. Am. Coll. Nutr.* **2008**, *27*, 80–87. [CrossRef] [PubMed]

64. O'Neil, C.E.; Zanovec, M.; Cho, S.S.; Nicklas, T.A. Whole grain and fiber consumption are associated with lower body weight measures in US adults: National Health and Nutrition Examination Survey 1999–2004. *Nutr. Res.* **2010**, *30*, 815–822. [CrossRef] [PubMed]

65. Huang, T.; Xu, M.; Lee, A.; Cho, S.; Qi, L. Consumption of whole grains and cereal fiber and total and cause-specific mortality: Prospective analysis of 367,442 individuals. *BMC Med.* **2015**, *13*, 59. [CrossRef] [PubMed]

66. Williams, P.G. Evaluation of the evidence between consumption of refined grains and health outcomes. *Nutr. Rev.* **2012**, *70*, 80–99. [CrossRef] [PubMed]

67. Waijers, P.M.; Feskens, E.J.; Ocké, M.C. A critical review of predefined diet quality scores. *Br. J. Nutr.* **2007**, *97*, 219–231. [CrossRef] [PubMed]

68. Visioli, F.; Galli, C. The effect of minor constituents of olive oil on cardiovascular disease: New findings. *Nutr. Rev.* **1998**, *56*, 142–147. [CrossRef] [PubMed]

69. Huang, C.L.; Sumpio, B.E. Olive oil, the mediterranean diet, and cardiovascular health. *J. Am. Coll. Surg.* **2008**, *207*, 407–416. [CrossRef] [PubMed]

70. Covas, M.I.; Konstantinidou, V.; Fitó, M. Olive oil and cardiovascular health. *J. Cardiovasc. Pharmacol.* **2009**, *54*, 477–482. [CrossRef] [PubMed]

71. Degirolamo, C.; Rudel, L.L. Dietary monounsaturated fatty acids appear not to provide cardioprotection. *Curr. Atheroscler. Rep.* **2010**, *12*, 391–396. [CrossRef] [PubMed]

72. Banca Dati di Composizione Degli Alimenti Per Gli Studi Epidemiologici in Italia. Available online: http://www.ieo.it/bda (accessed on 9 April 2015).

73. Schwingshackl, L.; Hoffmann, G. Monounsaturated fatty acids, olive oil and health status: A systematic review and meta-analysis of cohort studies. *Lipids Health Dis.* **2014**, *13*, 154. [CrossRef] [PubMed]

74. Grønbaek, M. Alcohol, type of alcohol, and all-cause and coronary heart disease mortality. *Ann. N. Y. Acad. Sci.* **2002**, *957*, 16–20. [CrossRef] [PubMed]

75. Arranz, S.; Chiva-Blanch, G.; Valderas-Martínez, P.; Medina-Remón, A.; Lamuela-Raventós, R.M.; Estruch, R. Wine, beer, alcohol and polyphenols on cardiovascular disease and cancer. *Nutrients* **2012**, *4*, 759–781. [CrossRef] [PubMed]

76. Chiva-Blanch, G.; Arranz, S.; Lamuela-Raventos, R.M.; Estruch, R. Effects of wine, alcohol and polyphenols on cardiovascular disease risk factors: Evidences from human studies. *Alcohol Alcohol.* **2013**, *48*, 270–277. [CrossRef] [PubMed]

77. Hu, F.B. Plant-based foods and prevention of cardiovascular disease: An overview. *Am. J. Clin. Nutr.* **2003**, *78*, S544–S551.

78. Mozaffarian, D.; Appel, L.J.; van Horn, L. Components of a cardioprotective diet: New insights. *Circulation* **2011**, *123*, 2870–2891. [CrossRef] [PubMed]

79. Kourlaba, G.; Panagiotakos, D.B. Dietary quality indices and human health: A review. *Maturitas* **2009**, *62*, 1–8. [CrossRef] [PubMed]

80. Kourlaba, G.; Panagiotakos, D. The diagnostic accuracy of a composite index increases as the number of partitions of the components increases and when specific weights are assigned to each component. *J. Appl. Stat.* **2010**, *37*, 537–554. [CrossRef]

81. Arvaniti, F.; Panagiotakos, D.B. Healthy indexes in public health practice and research: A review. *Crit. Rev. Food. Sci. Nutr.* **2008**, *48*, 317–327. [CrossRef] [PubMed]

82. Panagiotakos, D. Health measurement scales: Methodological issues. *Open Cardiovasc. Med. J.* **2009**, *3*, 160–165. [CrossRef] [PubMed]

83. Sofi, F.; Abbate, R.; Gensini, G.F.; Casini, A. Accruing evidence on benefits of adherence to the Mediterranean diet on health: An updated systematic review and meta-analysis. *Am. J. Clin. Nutr.* **2010**, *92*, 1189–1196. [CrossRef] [PubMed]

84. Sofi, F.; Macchi, C.; Abbate, R.; Gensini, G.F.; Casini, A. Mediterranean diet and health status: An updated meta-analysis and a proposal for a literature-based adherence score. *Public Health Nutr.* **2014**, *17*, 2769–2782. [CrossRef] [PubMed]

85. Hoevenaar-Blom, M.P.; Spijkerman, A.M.; Boshuizen, H.C.; Boer, J.M.; Kromhout, D.; Verschuren, W.M. Effect of using repeated measurements of a Mediterranean style diet on the strength of the association with cardiovascular disease during 12 years: The Doetinchem Cohort Study. *Eur. J. Nutr.* **2014**, *53*, 1209–1215. [CrossRef] [PubMed]

86. Hoffman, R.; Gerber, M. Evaluating and adapting the Mediterranean diet for non-Mediterranean populations: A critical appraisal. *Nutr. Rev.* **2013**, *71*, 573–584. [CrossRef] [PubMed]

87. West, S.G.; Skulas-Ray, A.C. Spices and herbs may improve cardiovascular risk factors. *Nutr. Today* **2014**, *49*, S8–S9. [CrossRef]

88. D'Alessandro, A.; De Pergola, G. Mediterranean Diet Pyramid: A Proposal for Italian People. *Nutrients* **2014**, *6*, 4302–4316. [CrossRef] [PubMed]

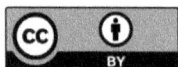

nutrients

MDPI

Review

Food Processing and the Mediterranean Diet

Richard Hoffman [1,*] and Mariette Gerber [2]

[1] School of Life and Medical Sciences, University of Hertfordshire, Hatfield AL10 9AB, UK
[2] Expert at French Food, Environment and Work Safety Agency (ANSES), Former INSERM Senior Scientist, Cancer Institute, 34298 Montpellier cedex 5, France; E-Mail: mariette.gerber@sfr.fr
* Author to whom correspondence should be addressed; E-Mail: r.hoffman@herts.ac.uk; Tel.: +44-1707-284526; Fax: +44-1707-285046.

Received: 18 August 2015 / Accepted: 9 September 2015 / Published: 17 September 2015

Abstract: The benefits of the Mediterranean diet (MD) for protecting against chronic disorders such as cardiovascular disease are usually attributed to high consumption of certain food groups such as vegetables, and low consumption of other food groups such as meat. The influence of food processing techniques such as food preparation and cooking on the nutrient composition and nutritional value of these foods is not generally taken into consideration. In this narrative review, we consider the mechanistic and epidemiological evidence that food processing influences phytochemicals in selected food groups in the MD (olives, olive oil, vegetables and nuts), and that this influences the protective effects of these foods against chronic diseases associated with inflammation. We also examine how the pro-inflammatory properties of meat consumption can be modified by Mediterranean cuisine. We conclude by discussing whether food processing should be given greater consideration, both when recommending a MD to the consumer and when evaluating its health properties.

Keywords: Mediterranean diet; food processing; food preparation; cooking; phytochemicals; inflammation; oxidative stress

1. Introduction

Food preparation and cooking influence the nutritional qualities of foods, and potentially their health benefits. These processes can have beneficial effects, for example by improving the digestibility and bioavailability of nutrients, and by enhancing attractiveness to the consumer because of improved texture and taste [1], and also deleterious effects due to loss of nutrients or the formation of toxic compounds [2]. The Mediterranean diet (MD) is well-known for its health benefits and this diet is increasingly being recommended in non-Mediterranean countries [3]. However, food preparation and cooking customs in non-Mediterranean countries may be quite different from those in Mediterranean countries. This is rarely considered when applying findings on the MD derived from one population to a different population with a different cuisine, and the extent to which differences in food preparation practices between populations impacts on the nutritional qualities of the MD is not well understood.

The traditional MD is characterized by plenty of fruits, vegetables and nuts, legumes, cereals (preferably whole grain), herbs and spices, fish and seafood, moderate amounts of meat and dairy produce (mainly from sheep and goats), olive oil (for dressing and cooking) and moderate amounts of wine with meals [4]. This rich diversity of foods results in the MD having a unique compendium of nutrients that contributes to its protective effects against chronic disease [5,6]. Because the MD is essentially a plant-based diet, phytochemicals are considered to be major contributors to the overall health benefits of this diet [7], and this group of nutrients is strongly influenced by food preparation and cooking [8,9]. A major property of phytochemicals that contributes to their health benefits is their ability to reduce oxidative stress and inflammation (reviewed in [10]), and a reduction in inflammation by phytochemicals has been linked to the benefits of phytochemicals for the MD [11].

In this review, we first consider the anti-inflammatory effects of the MD, and we then go on to discuss antioxidant and anti-inflammatory phytochemicals in some of the main food groups of the MD (olives and olive oil, vegetables and nuts). We then discuss how these phytochemicals are influenced by food preparation and cooking and the effects of these processes on health outcomes. Since the overall oxidative stress and inflammation in the body is due to factors that increase as well as decrease oxidative stress and inflammation, we also consider food preparation and cooking procedures that are pro-oxidant and pro-inflammatory, particularly in relation to meat. Because some traditional Mediterranean cooking practices may be less common in non-Mediterranean countries, we conclude by discussing whether advice on food preparation should be given when recommending the MD in non-Mediterranean countries.

2. Oxidation, Inflammation and the MD

Inflammation is now recognized as a major factor in the pathology of many chronic diseases including cardiovascular disease (CVD), cancer, type 2 diabetes, metabolic syndrome and Alzheimer's disease, and inflammation is also associated with obesity [10,12–15]. The inflammation that contributes to these diseases may occur systemically in the body, such as the low grade chronic inflammation that is also linked with aging (inflammaging) and obesity, or it may be more localized. Another source of inflammation with potentially harmful consequences is the acute inflammation that can occur during the postprandial state as a result of hyperlipemia and hyperglycemia [16].

A number of epidemiological studies have demonstrated that consuming a MD reduces inflammation [14]. Barbaresko and colleagues in a recent systematic review reported that among *a priori* healthy dietary patterns, the MD was the most consistent in showing a decrease in C reactive protein (CRP) and an increase in adiponectin [17]. In the large Italian Moli-sani study, a decrease in white blood cell and platelet counts (measured as markers of low grade inflammation) was shown to be associated with a greater adherence to a Mediterranean-like diet [18]. Adherence to a traditional MD was also shown to be associated with a reduction of CRP and IL-6 in survivors of a myocardial infarct, independently of the medication [19]. The potential role of the MD in reducing low grade chronic inflammation in the elderly (inflammaging) is currently being studied in the NU-AGE project [20].

As well as low grade inflammation, there is also good evidence that consuming a MD reduces postprandial inflammation [21–23], and the postprandial oxidative stress that can result from postprandial hyperglycemia and hyperlipemia [23]. One link between oxidative stress and inflammation is through the transcription factors NF-κB. This is because NF-κB is induced by oxidative stress, which in turn increases the expression of pro-inflammatory genes for cytokines and chemokines [24]. Hence, not surprisingly, antioxidant phytochemicals can reduce inflammatory responses. For example, in a short term intervention it was shown that polyphenols from virgin olive oil (VOO) decreased postprandial gene expression of the NF-κB-mediated pro-inflammatory cytokines *IL1B*, *IL6* and *CXCL1* in peripheral blood mononuclear cells [22]. In the Predimed (Prevención con Dieta Mediterránea) study, adherence to a MD was associated with increased total antioxidant capacity (TAC) [25], and high dietary anti-oxidant levels lowered CRP and IL-6 [26]. Total dietary antioxidants independently explained the relationship between adherence to a MD pattern with better health-related quality of life (especially mental rather than physical health) in the Moli-sani study [27].

Many of the nutrients, such as saturated fats, *trans* fats and refined carbohydrates, that are associated in *in vitro* models with inflammatory responses are present at far lower levels in the MD than are typically found in the western diet [28]. In order to quantify the overall inflammatory potential of dietary patterns, a Dietary Inflammatory Index (DII) has been developed [29]. The DII is computed from the inflammatory activity of 45 foods and nutrients. Some studies suggest that DII is positively associated with an increased risk of various diseases such as pancreatic cancer [30] and colon cancer [31]. Using data from the Predimed study, a DII was computed from a measure of adherence to the MD (a MD score) and, as expected, the MD score was found to be inversely associated with DII [32]. In this cross-sectional analysis of the Predimed study, a lower DII was associated with a lower prevalence of obesity [32] and in a prospective one with incidence of CVD [33]. Based on nutritional data from Luxembourg, higher adherence to a MD score was associated with a favorable cardio-metabolic, hepatic and renal risk profile, whereas the relationship with DII was weaker suggesting that other foods and nutrients than the ones used in the construction of the DII are necessary for greater prevention [34]. Hence, in summary, it can be concluded that there is good evidence that antioxidant phytochemicals in the MD have anti-inflammatory effects in the body, and there is increasing evidence that this is important for the health benefits of the MD.

3. Food Processing and Phytochemicals—General Considerations

When establishing associations between adherence to the MD and the inflammatory status of the diet (e.g., using DII), the nutritional data are based on food composition tables that usually do not take into consideration possible effects of food preparation and cooking. Loss of anti-oxidant phytochemicals can occur during cooking due to thermal degradation and from leaching of substances (especially of more polar compounds) into the cooking medium. As well as loss of antioxidants, the formation of pro-oxidants can occur, especially when cooking at high temperatures, notably as a consequence of the Maillard reaction. Food preparation can also have beneficial effects by increasing the bioavailability of antioxidant phytochemicals [35]. For some phytochemicals, this is because of enhanced release from the food matrix, although the extent to which this occurs may vary widely. Carotenoids can be released from their association with proteins inside chromoplasts, and folate from proteins [36,37]. However, some polyphenols such as phenolic acids are more tightly bound to dietary fiber and protein [38]. Bound polyphenols can constitute a significant proportion of total daily intake. In fruits (apples, peaches and nectarines), 80%–90% of polyphenols were in the bound form [39], and it was estimated that bound polyphenols constituted 78% of the total phenolics in the Spanish diet [40]. Hence, factors that release bound polyphenols may have a significant impact on the overall level of bioavailable polyphenols. Poor bioavailability is not, however, necessarily detrimental. Components of the food matrix can act as carriers enabling phytochemicals to reach the colon where they may be released by the actions of gut bacteria. For example, grain fiber carries polyphenols to the colon and releasing polyphenols here, rather than higher up the gastrointestinal tract, may have health benefits either in the colon itself or after being absorbed there into the body [41,42].

Because it is difficult to predict the consequences on health of food processing simply based on model systems, we consider a wide range of studies (biochemical studies, biomarkers and health outcomes) that address how food processing may influence both the bioavailability and health consequences of consuming antioxidant and anti-inflammatory phytochemicals present in the main foods groups of the MD.

4. Olive Oil and Olives

Antioxidant and anti-inflammatory compounds in extra virgin olive oil (EVOO) include tocopherols, carotenoids and polyphenols. Polyphenols are especially important because of their number, diversity and particular properties. At least 36 phenolic compounds have so far been identified in EVOO [43]. The most abundant polyphenols in EVOO include secoiridoids such as oleuropein derivatives (especially the dialdehydic form of decarboxymethyl elenolic acid linked to hydroxytyrosol), phenolic derivatives of secoiridoids such as tyrosol and hydroxytyrosol, lignans, flavonoids, and decarboxy methyl ligstroside aglycone—known as oleocanthal [44,45]. The antioxidant activities of EVOOs have been shown to correlate with their polyphenol content [46,47], one study finding a better correlation with diphenol content than with overall phenol content [47]. Ortho-diphenols such as hydroxytyrosol and oleuropein derivatives are more potent phenolic antioxidants [46,48]. Oleocanthal is an inhibitor of cyclooxygenase activity and is best known for its anti-inflammatory properties [44]. The major polyphenols hydroxytyrosol and tyrosol have high bioavailability (40%–95%) when present in olive oil [49], although there is less information for other EVOO polyphenols.

The health benefits of olive oil have been extensively reviewed [50–52]. When compared with olive oils with low polyphenol concentrations, most clinical studies demonstrated that olive oils containing high polyphenol concentrations resulted in greater reductions in inflammatory biomarkers, better protection of low-density lipoprotein-cholesterol (LDL-cholesterol) from oxidation, and greater decreases in isoprostanes [43]. EVOO has been shown to be superior to ordinary olive oil (which is lower in polyphenols) in preventing CVD [53]. Although there is suggestive evidence for a protective effect of olive oil against breast cancer [54], studies have not distinguished between ordinary olive oil and EVOO. The antioxidant properties of polyphenols are implicated in reducing CVD and some cancers (with levels of evidence categorized as possible to probable) by preventing LDL oxidation and neutralizing free radicals respectively [55]. The anti-inflammatory properties of polyphenols from EVOO may also contribute to these beneficial effects [56]. Oleocanthal has neuro-protective effects and attenuates markers of inflammation implicated in Alzheimer's disease, and has also been shown to have anti-proliferative effects against human breast and prostate cancer cell lines [44,57].

Table olives are extremely rich sources of antioxidant polyphenols, comprising 1%–3% of the fresh pulp weight [48]. For most types of olives, the major polyphenols are oleuropein and hydroxytyrosol. In one study, levels of hydroxytyrosol were estimated to be 250–760 mg/kg in Kalamata olives, 170–510 mg/kg in Spanish-style green olives, and 100–340 mg/kg in Greek-style naturally black olives [58]. Thus, one Kalamata olive (4 g flesh) provides approx. 1–3 mg of hydroxytyrosol. In comparison, data from the Phenol-Explorer database gives an average content in EVOO of 7.7 mg hydroxytyrosol/kg oil [59]. Not surprisingly, olive extracts exhibit high antioxidant activity in *in vitro* assays [60,61]. Despite the high levels of hydroxytyrosol in table olives compared to EVOO, the bioavailability in humans of hydroxytyrosol and other polyphenols from table olives is currently unknown and to the best of our knowledge there are no human studies on their health effects, possibly because of their frequent high salt content (although this can be reduced by rinsing).

4.1. Effects of Processing

Concentrations of total polyphenols in olive oils vary considerably—between 50 to 800 mg/kg depending on the quality and type of the oil [62]. The extraction technique is generally considered to have the greatest impact; the first extraction at low temperatures produces virgin olive oil and this has the highest level of polyphenols. However, other factors also influence polyphenol levels including the geographical location, growing conditions and cultivar of the olive trees, ripeness of the olive at harvest, possible infestation with the olive fly, extraction method for the oil, and storage of the oil [46]. For example, a 13-fold difference in diphenol content was found between EVOOs from different cultivars from various regions in Italy [47].

Antioxidant levels in table olives also vary widely. A 10-fold or more difference was found in levels of hydroxytyrosol between olive cultivars [48]. The production method for the olives is also very influential. Particularly dramatic is the almost complete loss of hydroxytyrosol, due to oxidation and polymerization, during the California-style oxidation method for converting green olives into black olives [48,63]. Pitting of olives is also influential: an additional washing step is required when olives are pitted, and this process was found to almost half the content of hydroxytyrosol that had been present in the un-pitted olives [64].

In relation to olive oil, a major influence for the consumer is how the oil is used for cooking. Common domestic cooking conditions include shallow frying (which is at approx. 140–160 °C), in soups and stews (which may include an initial frying period, followed by boiling at 100 °C or at a higher temperature if the dish is cooked in the oven), and as an addition towards the end of cooking, for example in the "lathera" dishes from Greece and Turkey. In Portugal, vegetable soups with added olive oil are very popular, and in a study that mimicked domestic conditions there was found to be less loss of tyrosol and hydroxytyrosol from the oil and phenolics from the vegetables if the oil was added towards the end of the cooking period rather than at the beginning [65]. However, not all studies have replicated conditions likely to be encountered during normal domestic cooking.

When olive oil is used for frying, the stability of olive oil polyphenols is strongly influenced by cooking temperature and time, the type of food present and the composition of the oil (including antioxidants and polyunsaturated fatty acid (PUFA) content) [52,66]. In a study that simulated frying by heating olive oil (although in the absence of food) to 180 °C, there was a significant decrease in hydroxytyrosol derivatives (60% reduction after 30 min and 90% reduction after 60 min) [67]. Similar results were reported for the mass-produced Bertolli EVOO [68]. A study from Spain found far higher loss of hydroxytyrosol derivatives from oils made from Arbequina olives than for Piqual olives [69], and it has been suggested that the higher rates of loss may reflect a higher PUFA (linoleic acid) content of oils derived from Arbequina olives [66].

In contrast to the secoiridoids, lignans and oleocanthal are relatively heat stable [69]. For example, 12 frying cycles of 10 min each at 180 °C only reduced oleocanthal levels by 20% [70], although the degree of loss may depend on the initial concentration of oleocanthal in the oil [71].

In a short term human study that compared the effects of heated oils on the postprandial inflammatory response in obese subjects, VOO repeatedly heated to 180 °C was found to suppress postprandial inflammation in obese subjects (determined as NF-κB activation in peripheral blood monocytes) [72]. Hydroxytyrosol was completely depleted by the heating process and so cannot be responsible for the observed effect. By contrast, some other polyphenols were preserved, including about 75% of tyrosol and 20% of oleuropein aglycones. Further work is required to establish the mechanism for the protective effect. Other than this study, most intervention studies in humans with olive oil have either used raw olive oil, such as EUROLIVE (the effect of olive oil consumption on oxidative damage in European countries) with oxidized LDL-cholesterol as an endpoint, or have not specified the use of the oil, e.g., Predimed with cardiovascular death as the primary endpoint. Moreover, none of the large number of prospective epidemiological studies examining the health benefits of consuming olive oil have distinguished between the consumption of raw and cooked olive oil. A recent systematic review concluded that there is no epidemiological evidence that consuming fried foods is associated with an increased risk of cardiovascular disease, although there was some evidence for weight gain [73]. Many of the studies used olive oil as the frying oil, but, as the authors point out, the precise outcome is likely to be influenced by the type of oil, frying technique (shallow frying or deep frying), frying duration and temperature, and use of new or reused oils.

Acrylamide has been found in black olives prepared by the California-style processing method [74]. Acrylamide is classified as a probable human carcinogen by the International Agency for Research on Cancer. Concentrations of acrylamide in California-style black olives varied between 410–512 µg/kg in this study and these concentrations are comparable to levels of acrylamide found in French fries, a better known dietary source of acrylamide. The acrylamide appears to be generated during the sterilization process of the olives [74]. By comparison, in this study, Spanish olives and Greek olives were found to have very low levels of acrylamide (<1.4 µg/kg). This is probably because these olives were not sterilized, and this is the normal case with black olives from some countries.

4.2. Implications

The European Food Safety Authority (EFSA) recently upheld a health claim that EVOO reduces LDL oxidation if "a minimum of 5 mg of hydroxytyrosol and its derivatives is consumed per day" [75]. However, because information on the polyphenol content of EVOOs is not at present commonly available to consumers, they are unlikely to know whether or not they have attained the goal recommended by EFSA. Labeling bottles of olive oil with their content of secoiridoids and making consumers aware of the possible losses of hydroxytyrosol due to high temperature cooking would facilitate implementing the EFSA guideline without requiring excessive intake of olive oil. There may already be some public understanding of possible losses of active compounds in olive oil: Portuguese consumers are apparently aware that adding olive oil towards the end of cooking is more beneficial [65]. As well as recommending EVOO for cooking, the use of raw EVOO could also be encouraged.

Due to the absence of human studies, there are currently no guidelines from EFSA recommending olives as a source of hydroxytyrosol and its derivatives. However the high levels of these compounds in certain types of olives, and because olives are mostly eaten raw, suggests that consumption of only a few olives could achieve the EFSA recommended levels and without consuming many calories (assuming there is good bioavailability). However, olives have markedly different levels of hydroxytyrosol and hence specific types of olives would need to be recommended. In particular, California-style black olives are not comparable to many other types of olives because of their low levels of hydroxytyrosol and quite high levels of acrylamide.

Because of the good evidence that polyphenols in EVOO contribute to its health benefits, it has been suggested that EVOO should be specifically recommended as part of a MD, rather than a more general recommendation of "olive oil" [76]. Although concentrations of hydroxytyrosol will vary depending on whether EVOO is consumed raw or after frying, how EVOO is used is not currently incorporated into estimates of consumption for calculating MD scores. Upper *versus* lower quantiles of olive oil intake in health studies mostly vary between 2–3 fold (see [52]). This variation is lower than the potential influence of food processing practices on hydroxytyrosol levels. Hence, variation in usage of olive oil is a potential confounding factor when evaluating the link between its consumption and health benefits. However, it should be noted that several other olive oil polyphenols are more stable than hydroxytyrosol.

5. Vegetables—General

Vegetables contain a wide range of antioxidant phytochemicals. The levels of these phytochemicals are influenced by environmental conditions such as exposure to sunshine, and by agronomic practices such as the choice of cultivar, use of fertilizers and whether the produce is grown organically or conventionally (see [77–79] for recent reviews). Epidemiological studies have compared the health benefits of raw and cooked vegetables, and this is particularly relevant to the MD since consumption of raw vegetables as a proportion of total vegetable consumption was reported to be higher in southern cohorts from the EPIC (European Prospective Investigation into Cancer and Nutrition) study compared to their northern counterparts [80]. In a recent review of case-control studies from Southern European countries, both raw and cooked vegetables protected against various cancers, especially upper digestive tract cancers, but there was greater protection with raw vegetable consumption [81]. In the case of breast cancer, only raw was beneficial [81]. However, since this analysis was based on case-control studies, it is possible that cases may have modified their intakes. In a large prospective study with a follow-up > 10 years, raw vegetables was the only category of fruit and vegetables that was significantly and strongly (50%) associated with a risk reduction for stroke [82].

Salads are a significant source of raw vegetables in the MD. In an analysis of the traditional Cretan Mediterranean diet, salads were found to be consumed several times per week [83]. This way of eating not only preserves heat labile nutrients, but dressing salads with olive oil, vinegar, herbs or spices can greatly increase the antioxidant capacity of the dish. For example, the herbs lemon balm and marjoram (1.5% w/w) increased the antioxidant capacity of a salad by 150% and 200% respectively [84]. Many herbs are consumed in high amounts in the MD compared to a typical western diet, and they are frequently consumed raw or with minimal cooking. Herbs are particularly high in antioxidant and anti-inflammatory compounds, especially polyphenols [84,85]. Herbs and spices contributed significantly to the overall dietary intake of flavonols and flavones of traditional Greek cuisine, and this was linked to their frequent consumption despite only being used in small quantities [86]. There is increasing recognition of the importance of herbs and spices for good health [87,88], and although herbs and spices are recommended foods in the MD, they are not currently assessed when measuring adherence to the MD.

Cooking processes can strongly influence antioxidant phytochemical levels in fruits vegetables and herbs [84,89]. Amongst the many ways of preparing vegetables, perhaps the most frequent and traditional way in Mediterranean cuisine is to present the vegetables in olive oil, either by cooking the vegetables in olive oil or by dressing the vegetables with raw oil. Olive oil enhances taste and acceptability and, it has been proposed, is an important reason for the high levels of consumption of vegetables in Mediterranean countries [90]. Another beneficial effect of EVOO is that when vegetables are cooked in this medium they may absorb significant levels of antioxidants from the oil [91]. In addition, the bioavailability and absorption of many phytochemicals in vegetables, especially carotenoids, is significantly enhanced and this may increase the health benefits. We now consider how food processing may influence the nutritional value of vegetables pertinent to the MD.

6. Tomato and Other Carotenoid-Containing Vegetables

The six main carotenoids usually reported to be present in human blood plasma are α-carotene, β-carotene, lycopene, β-cryptoxanthin, zeaxanthin and lutein. In the MD, these are obtained from a wide range of green leafy and other types of vegetables, fruits, cereals and olives [92]. Other potentially significant, but usually overlooked, carotenoids in the MD are the red pigment capsanthin and the yellow carotenoids crocin and crocetin. Capsanthin is the main carotenoid in red peppers and paprika, comprising 29.2–36.2 μg/g fresh weight in red pepper [93]. This compares with levels of lycopene—the main carotenoid in tomato—of 8.5–127.0 μg/g fresh weight [94]. The health significance of capsanthin is not known, and it does have a rather short half life in human plasma (20 h) compared to that of lycopene (222 h) [95]. Crocin and crocetin are the two main carotenoids in saffron and have anti tumor effects in *in vitro* and *in vivo* models [96]. Carotenoids are highly reactive towards oxygen and free radicals and have antioxidant and anti-inflammatory effects in the body [97]. Lycopene also suppresses carcinogenesis by inducing apoptosis and inhibiting proliferation and metastasis, and by inducing cyto-protective enzymes [98].

6.1. Food Processing

In many green leafy vegetables carotenoids are associated with proteins, whereas in carrots and tomatoes carotenoids exist in a semi-crystalline form. Chopping, blending and cooking help release carotenoids from the food matrix. Subsequently, carotenoids must be incorporated into lipid micelles in the gut lumen in order to be absorbed across the gut wall. The effects of cooking techniques on levels of carotenoids was evaluated in a meta-analysis by Murador and colleagues [99]. From the pooled data, stewing (a widely used technique in Mediterranean cuisine) increased overall carotenoid content by 36%. The apparent increase in carotenoid concentrations during stewing may be due to a combination of little thermal degradation and high water loss. Other techniques either had no effect or decreased levels—by 41% in the case of frying.

Whereas chopping and the use of sauces are widely used in different national cuisines for carotenoid-containing vegetables, especially tomatoes, it is the predominance of olive oil as the main dietary fat that characterizes the traditional MD. There is evidence from *in vitro* and animal studies of carotenoid micelle formation and uptake that olive oil enhances the bioavailability of carotenoids to a greater extent that some other fats [100]. In particular, long chain fatty acids are superior to medium chain fatty acids and oleic acid is superior to PUFAs (linoleic acid) [100]. There was greater bioavailability of carotenoids (lycopene and astaxanthin) in rats given oral doses of carotenoids in olive oil compared to corn oil [101] and higher levels of the photo-protective carotenoids lutein and zeaxanthin were found in the eyes of rats given these carotenoids in an emulsion with olive oil compared to an emulsion of sunflower oil or groundnut oil [102].

Despite these observations, their significance for humans is unclear since the amount of lipid in the meal may be a more significant factor for carotenoid bioavailability than the actual lipid composition [103]. It has been estimated that 3–5 g of dietary fat is required in order to significantly enhance the bioavailability of dietary carotenoids [104,105]. Certainly, excluding lipid altogether can significantly reduce carotenoid uptake. For example, cooking diced tomatoes in EVOO increased plasma concentrations of *cis*-lycopene (the more biologically active isomer [106]) and *trans*-lycopene by 40% and 82% respectively, whereas cooking the tomatoes without EVOO increased plasma concentrations of *cis*-lycopene by only 15% and there was no increase in *trans*-lycopene levels [107]. Similarly, refined olive oil enhanced the absorption of *cis* and *trans* isomers of lycopene (as determined by plasma levels and AUC) in tomato juice in healthy volunteers compared to when the oil was absent [108].

Olive oil has also been shown to enhance the bioavailability of more polar phenolic compounds. For example, the extraction of phenolic compounds such as chlorogenic acid and naringenin (the main polyphenol in tomatoes) from a tomato sauce were enhanced when the tomato sauce was prepared with VOO [109]. In a cross-over study, there was some evidence of higher bioavailability of naringenin when human subjects were given a tomato sauce prepared with VOO compared to when they were given a tomato sauce prepared in the absence of VOO [110]. However, in a prospective randomized, cross-over intervention study, mechanical and thermal treatments during tomato sauce processing enhanced the bioavailability of various phenolics including naringenin to a greater extent than added lipid (refined olive oil) [111] Hence, added lipid may be less important for phenolic bioavailability from tomatoes compared with lycopene bioavailability.

A number of studies have also examined if processing tomatoes affects disease outcomes, although it is not usually specified if the consumption of the tomatoes also included olive oil consumption. A Greek case-control study examined the relationship between tomato consumption and risk of prostate cancer. Olive oil is likely to have been the main dietary fat in this Mediterranean population. Intake of either raw or cooked tomatoes reduced prostate cancer risk, although there was a significant and greater risk reduction for cooked tomatoes (OR lowest *versus* highest tertile 1.91; CI 1.20–3.04 for cooked, *versus* OR 1.55; CI 1.00–2.52 for raw) [112]. Chen *et al.* recently conducted a meta-analysis of prospective studies of prostate cancer incidence and tomato consumption but there were too few studies on raw and cooked tomatoes (3 studies in each category) to draw firm conclusions regarding the effects of processing [113]. The lipid content of the meals was not known and so could be a confounding factor in the analysis of these data. The roles of various phytochemicals in tomato as preventive agents against prostate cancer and the importance of other dietary constituents for increasing the bioavailability of these phytochemicals also requires clarification [114]. However, in the meta-analysis conducted by Chen *et al.* there were enough studies with no heterogeneity to show that there was no association between lycopene and prostate cancer incidence [113].

Bioavailability of carotenoids is modified by factors besides food processing such as the adiposity of the subject, and exposure to tobacco or air pollution. This is an important aspect when assessing risk reduction of cancers through dietary questionnaires, and, since these factors are not always taken into consideration, this might explain some of the inconsistencies observed in epidemiological studies. Studies using biomarkers show stronger and more significant associations between plasma carotenoids and cancer risk than if only dietary intake of carotenoids is assessed. This has been shown clearly for the association with breast cancer [115,116]. It is also noteworthy that the enzymes that metabolize lycopene are polymorphic. This contributes to wide inter-individual variations in lycopene plasma levels and so will influence health outcomes potentially associated with this carotenoid [106].

In relation to CVD, a short term study found that enhancing carotenoid bioavailability favorably influenced biomarkers for CVD as end points. In a small (11 subjects) randomized cross-over trial, LDL cholesterol and total cholesterol decreased significantly after the consumption of tomato with olive oil, and this was associated with an increase of *trans*-lycopene and 5-*cis*-lycopene, respectively [108].

6.2. Implications

Food processing and the presence of fat increase carotenoid bioavailability and there is some limited evidence that increasing carotenoid bioavailability may improve health benefits, at least in relation to CVD. It is less clear if preparing the food with fat is superior to simply having fat in the meal. Also, more work is needed to clarify if olive oil has benefits over other types of oils in relation to carotenoid absorption. Nevertheless, EVOO does have the added advantage that when vegetables are fried in it they may absorb beneficial micronutrients from the oil.

7. Cruciferous Vegetables

Cruciferous vegetables (e.g., cabbages, broccoli, cauliflower), also known as brassicas, contain a wide range of health promoting compounds including polyphenols, carotenoids, tocopherols and vitamin C. However, it is the presence of glucosinolates (GSLs) in crucifers that distinguishes them from other vegetables, and it is these compounds that have received the most attention. Most GSLs are considered to be inactive, but when they come into contact with the enzyme myrosinase GSLs are converted into various bioactive products including isothiocyanates and nitriles.

Sulforaphane, the breakdown product of the GSL glucoraphanin, is found in a wide range of crucifers. Sulforaphane has anti-carcinogenic and cyto protective effects through its ability to activate the transcription factor nuclear factor erythroid 2-related factor 2 (Nrf-2) that in turn induces phase 2 metabolizing enzymes and antioxidant proteins [117,118]. In animal models, sulforaphane protects not only against carcinogenesis but also against organ damage and various neurodegenerative diseases [117,119]. A number of clinical studies have shown an effect of supplementation with various crucifers or glucosinolates on factors implicated in carcinogenesis such as cytoprotective enzymes (e.g., glutathione transferase) and markers of *Helicobacter pylori* colonization and gastric inflammation [118]. Some prospective studies on breast cancer showed a risk reduction associated with crucifer consumption [120,121], and also some evidence for a risk reduction of for gastric cancer, although the evidence is limited [122].

7.1. Food Processing

Because of their pungent taste, most crucifers are cooked prior to consumption. Two major cooking processes that reduce GSL breakdown products are leaching of the water-soluble GSLs into cooking water and heat inactivation of myrosinase. McNaughton and Marks estimated that on average 36% of GSLs are lost following processing of crucifers [123]. However, actual losses will vary widely depending on the precise cooking technique employed. Leaching of GSLs during boiling in water, the most common cooking technique for crucifers in western countries, is estimated to lead to losses of between 25%–75% of GSLs [124]. It is therefore noteworthy that in Mediterranean cuisine crucifer leaves are commonly consumed as part of composite dishes in which the cooking liquor is also consumed (soups and stews).

Myrosinase is progressively inactivated by heat, hence reducing its capacity to generate bioactive GSL breakdown products. Consuming crucifers raw will not only ensure that myrosinase remains active but also avoid losses from leaching. Rocket (arugula) is the most common crucifer leaf consumed in salads. In Mediterranean countries, both the cultivated form *Eruca sativa* and the wild form *Diplotaxis tenuifolia* are consumed. Extracts of *E. sativa* reduced benzo(a)pyrene-induced genotoxicity against human hepatoma (HepG2) cells [125] and had a range of cancer chemopreventive effects in cell culture and animal models [126]. An isothiocyanate-rich extract of *E. sativa* was found to inhibit melanoma growth and angiogenesis in mice [127]. A wide range of glucosinolates has been identified in *E. sativa* and *D. tenuifolia* [128]. Unlike other glucosinolates, glucoerucin, the main glucosinolate found in *Eruca* species, has direct antioxidant activity as well as acting as a precursor for the isothiosulphanate erucin [129].

7.2. Implications

Since food processing strongly influences the levels of GSL breakdown products in cruciferous vegetables this may impact on the health benefits of consuming these vegetables. This is suggested in a case-control study that found that consuming raw crucifers was associated with a risk reduction of bladder cancer (OR 0.64; 95% CI 0.42–0.97) whereas this was not observed for total crucifer consumption [130]. Apart from plant myrosinase, GSL breakdown products are also generated by the action of gut bacteria. However, this is less efficient than by plant myrosinase [131]. Moreover, relying on this as a means of generating GSL breakdown products is also less desirable because of the wide variations between individuals in their capacity to breakdown GSLs; this has been attributed to inter-individual variations in gut microflora composition [132].

Preparation techniques that retain cooking liquid (e.g., soups and stews) or that do not inactivate myrosinase (e.g., consuming raw) will maximize available GSL breakdown products. Providing myrosinase in the form of crucifer leaves is one way to compensate for losses of myrosinase activity. Providing myrosinase in the form of a few raw crucifer leaves (broccoli sprouts) was found to enhance conversion of a glucoraphanin-rich powder [133]. In Italy and Provence, salads that include a few rocket leaves are popular and may be able to act in a similar way by enhancing the conversion of glucosinolates from a dish of cooked crucifers in which the myrosinase has been inactivated. Blanching prior to freezing is another process that inactivates myrosinase, and adding raw crucifer (0.25% daikon root) was able to restore 100% of sulforaphane formation in frozen broccoli [134]. Hence, a few raw crucifer leaves may also be useful when consuming frozen crucifers.

Although retaining GSLs might be desirable from a health point of view, GSL breakdown products are responsible for the pungent taste of crucifers and hence many cultures prefer to consume these vegetables cooked, a process which will reduce pungency but also GSLs. Both taste and texture affect the cooking time chosen by consumers and the impact of these decisions on GSL content has been modeled for broccoli consumption. This study found that the most common boiling time compatible with optimal sensory acceptability (20 min) corresponded to a 20% to 80% reduction in GSL content (depending on the amount of water added) [135]. In contrast to this usual convention in western cuisine of consuming crucifers as a separate vegetable, crucifers in Mediterranean cuisine are frequently consumed as part of composite dishes such as stews or soups. Here the taste of GSL breakdown products is complemented by other flavors and higher levels of GSLs in the dish may be more acceptable. In the case of raw rocket leaves where levels of GSL breakdown products cannot be manipulated by cooking, a sweetened salad dressing may be added, although in a sensory analysis by a group of panelists the bitterness of rocket was perceived as a positive attribute in itself [136]. Another source of GSLs in the traditional MD is wild greens. The collection and consumption of wild greens remains an important part of the traditional Mediterranean diet [137], and wild greens belonging to the crucifer family, such as wild mustards, will add to the overall dietary intake of GSLs.

8. Alliums

The MD typically includes high consumption of onions and garlic. Two groups of phytochemicals in alliums that have received particular attention for their putative health benefits are organo-sulfur phytochemicals (thiosulfinates) and flavonoids. Thiosulfinates are volatile, unstable compounds generated by the enzyme alliinase from precursors (S-alk(en)yl-L-cysteine sulfoxides). In garlic, alliin is first converted by alliinase to allicin which then degrades to various compounds including ajoene, diallyl sulfides and vinyldithiins. These compounds are rapidly metabolized *in vivo* [138], and one metabolite of diallyl disulfide and diallyl trisulfide, hydrogen sulfide, is implicated in the vasoactive effects of garlic [139]. Allicin has *in vitro* anti-bacterial action against *H. pylori* which is incriminated in stomach cancer [140]. High levels of flavonoids are present in onions and garlic; onions contain particularly high levels of quercetin and kaempferol glucosides and garlic contains myricetin glucosides [141]. Both organo-sulfur compounds and quercetin have antioxidant and anti-inflammatory properties [142,143].

As is the case for many individual fruits and vegetables, epidemiological studies of all sites cancer risk and garlic intake are inconsistent because most cancer sites have specific modifying factors. The World Cancer Research Fund/American Institute for Cancer Research (WCRF/AICR) qualified the level of evidence for a causal relationship between allium vegetable consumption and prevention of stomach cancer and for colorectal cancer as probable [144]. For colorectal cancer, this was confirmed in the WCRF/AICR Systematic Literature Continuous Update Project (CUP) of 2011 [145]. These collective expertise reports have subsequently been confirmed by several studies. A recent review of Southern European case-control studies (mostly Italian cohorts) suggested that high intakes of onion and garlic decreased the risk for cancers of the oral cavity and pharynx, oesophagus, colorectum, larynx, endometrium, ovary and kidney (garlic only) [81]. In addition, in a case control study raw garlic consumption (two or more times per week) was inversely associated with lung cancer (OR 0.56; 95% CI 0.44–0.72) [146]. The authors speculated that this may have been because the volatile oil from raw garlic (which includes allicin and diallyl sulfides) is largely excreted in the lungs and hence may be able to exert a beneficial effect there. In another meta-analysis of mostly case-control studies, combined allium intake (garlic, onions and others) was significantly associated with reduced gastric cancer risk (OR 0.54; 95% CI 0.43–0.65) [147]. However, a recent meta-analysis found no overall protective effect of garlic consumption, even in the cohort studies which included garlic supplements [148]. There was considerable heterogeneity between studies and when only the case-control studies were analyzed (excluding the cohort studies and supplements) there was a 37% risk reduction (combined risk estimate = 0.63; 95% CI 0.48–0.82) in spite of significant heterogeneity in this sub-group analysis.

Garlic is also linked to reducing cardiovascular risk based on favorable effects *in vitro* and in animal studies in preventing vascular inflammation and reactive oxygen species (ROS) production, increasing nitric oxide, and inhibiting platelet aggregation. [149]. However, only modest effects on blood pressure were described, and a recent Cochrane review of epidemiological studies found insufficient evidence to determine if garlic provides a therapeutic advantage *versus* placebo in terms of reducing the risk of mortality and cardiovascular morbidity in patients diagnosed with hypertension [150].

8.1. Food Processing

Although there is also some rationale from experimental studies that raw garlic may have beneficial effects over and above cooked garlic for the prevention of cancer and CVD, there are too few epidemiological studies to undertake this analysis [149,151]. Nevertheless, food processing may differentially affect flavonoids and organo-sulfur compounds since they have distinct properties. Leaching of water soluble compounds is less of an issue for onions and garlic since they usually form the base of a dish that is consumed in its entirety. However, onions and garlic are frequently subject to high temperature cooking by frying. After moderate frying (5 min), concentrations of quercetin glucosides (quercetin 4-glucoside and quercetin 3,4 di-glucoside) in onions increased even when expressed on a dry weight basis which may possibly be explained by loss of other soluble solids and/or increased extractability due to plant cell wall degradation [152]. Longer heat treatments (>10 min) decreased levels of the quercetin glucosides.

The alliinase system is analogous to myrosinase in crucifers by being activated by damage to the plant tissue and also by being susceptible to inactivation by heat. Crushing garlic and allowing time for allicin to accumulate before heating improved the *in vitro* antiplatelet activity of garlic compared to heating garlic without crushing. [153], and, similarly, conditions that retained thiosulfinate generation in onions, such as heating whole intact onions, enhanced their anti-platelet activity [154]. However, the relevance of these *in vitro* findings to *in vivo* is unclear because of the rapid metabolism of allicin that occurs *in vivo*.

8.2. Implications

Whereas moderate cooking may enhance the bioavailability of quercetin glucosides in onions, cooking is deleterious to the generation of organo-sulfur compounds. There is no evidence that alliin is converted by gut bacteria to allicin, hence food processing is an important way of generating bioactive organo-sulfur compounds. Although epidemiological evidence is currently lacking, evidence from experimental studies suggests that typical Mediterranean dishes that include raw garlic or raw onions may have greater protective effects than for heated garlic or onions where alliinase has been inactivated. Crushing garlic (common in Spain) rather than chopping, and finely processing onion (such as the custom of using grated onions in tagines) may also be beneficial by causing greater plant cell disruption which increases alliinase activity.

9. Nuts

Nuts are an important component of the MD and have been shown to have significant health benefits, especially against CVD and all-cause mortality (see [155,156] for recent meta-analyses). The Predimed study found that when nuts (a combination of walnuts, almonds and hazelnuts) were given to enrich a MD, they reduced the risk of incident CVD and of diabetes [157]. Data on cancer are currently too limited to draw conclusions [158].

Nuts contain broadly similar constituents, and most nuts are rich sources of unsaturated fats (and low in saturated fatty acids (SFA)), protein, arginine (a precursor of nitric oxide (NO), important for vascular tone), fiber and a variety of minerals and vitamins including tocopherols, folate, Mg and Ca. However, there are important differences between nuts. For example, although the predominant FA in most nuts is MUFA (oleic acid), walnuts contain only low levels of MUFA and are high in PUFA (linoleic acid and α-linolenic acid). α-Tocopherol predominates in almonds and hazelnuts but γ-tocopherol is the main form in walnuts and pistachios [159]. Nuts are also excellent sources of antioxidant phenolics, with some nuts having particularly high levels of proanthocyanidins and hydrolysable tannins (gallotannins and ellagitannins) (see [160] for recent review). The stilbene *trans*-resveratrol occurs in peanuts and resveratrol-3-β-glucoside (piceid) has recently been identified in almonds [161].

9.1. Food Processing

Two common processing techniques that may influence the health benefits of nuts are removal of the skins (pellicles) and roasting. The pellicle is a major source of "total antioxidant capacity" (TAC) as measured by the FRAP (ferric reducing antioxidant potential) assay, particularly in walnuts where, by one estimate, 95% of TAC was present in the pellicle [162]. In another study, removal of the pellicle reduced TAC by approximately 36% in hazelnuts, 90% in walnuts and 55% in pistachios [163]. This reduction in TAC can be explained because the pellicle is the location for the majority of phenolic antioxidants. For example, pistachio skins contain 70.27 mg of flavonoids/g fresh weight (expressed as catechin equivalents) whereas the kernel contains only 0.46 mg of catechin equivalents/g fresh weight [164]. Some nuts such as walnuts are almost always eaten with their pellicle whereas others, such as peanuts, are usually eaten without it. Peanuts are the main type of nut consumed in some non-Mediterranean countries, and so nut-derived antioxidant polyphenols may be lower in these countries. However, nuts without their skins still contain various fat soluble antioxidants such as tocopherols since these are present in the kernel [160].

Almond skin is an effective inhibitor of copper-induced oxidation of human LDL cholesterol [165]. However, the benefits of consuming the whole nut may be greater since antioxidant polyphenols from almond skins were shown synergise with α-tocopherol to increase the resistance of LDL to oxidation [166]. This may be explained by flavonoids recycling the radical generated by α-tocopherol during inhibition of LDL oxidation [167]. Beneficial effects have been observed even for nuts without their pellicles. For example, a recent crossover clinical study on 15 moderately hypercholesterolemic subjects examined the differential effects of whole walnut, walnut oil, meat and skin on biomarkers for cardiovascular disease risk [168]. Walnut oil favorably affected endothelial function, and whole walnuts increased cholesterol efflux.

Nuts are sometimes consumed after roasting (which is typically between 140–180 °C). Roasting may cause changes to nut lipids and phytochemicals and generate new products through the Maillard reaction. Some studies [169] but not others [170] found small increases in *trans*-FAs after roasting, although levels were not considered to be of a concern to health. Increases in lipid oxidation products (as measured by Thiobarbituric Acid Reactive Substances—TBARs) following roasting correlated with the PUFA content, and tocopherol levels were reduced by prolonged roasting [170]. Although roasting can reduce antioxidant polyphenols in the nut skins, prolonged roasting can increase overall TAC. Possible reasons for this have been suggested by Bullo and colleagues and include breakdown of polymeric polyphenols to monomers, hydrolysis of glycosylated flavonoids, the decomposition of aglycones and the formation of Maillard reaction products (MRPs) with antioxidant activity [171]. The Maillard reaction can also lead to the production of harmful products. One such product, acrylamide, is produced by roasting, especially in almonds at high temperatures, which is probably due to their high asparagine and reducing sugar content [172]. Advanced glycation endproducts (AGEs), which are mostly pro-inflammatory, also form when almonds [173] and other nuts [174] are roasted.

Although complex changes can occur to antioxidants in nuts during roasting, the effects of roasting on oxidative stress have not been examined in clinical studies to the best of the authors' knowledge. A few clinical studies have examined the consequences of roasting on other health parameters. One study comparing the effects of unprocessed with processed peanuts (whole raw, roasted unsalted, roasted salted or honey roasted peanuts, or ground peanut butter) found that none of the forms of peanuts induced a change in body weight or lipid parameters (total, LDL-cholesterol and triglycerides) [175]. In a few hypercholesterolemic subjects, total cholesterol, LDL-cholesterol and triglyceride concentrations were reduced in the same way by unprocessed and by processed forms of peanuts. Similarly, both raw and roasted almonds lowered LDL-cholesterol and total cholesterol [176].

9.2. Implications

It is likely that the health benefits of nuts result from many components in nuts such as their healthy fat profile, high level of antioxidants, and high levels of arginine (which acts as a source of NO). *In vitro* studies suggest that whole nuts (with their skins) that are either unroasted or only moderately roasted will be optimal for health although clinical studies suggest that some lipid parameters are influenced similarly by roasted or unroasted nuts. Although assessments of nut intake in the MD do not distinguish between the type of nut, this could be a confounder, for example because of the significantly different fatty acid profile for walnuts. Retaining the skin also improves storage since the skin acts as a protective shield against oxidation of unsaturated fatty acids [177].

10. Meat

Low meat consumption is recommended as part of a MD. Red meat consumption was shown to increase inflammatory biomarkers in healthy women [178] and thus meat may work in opposition to the anti-inflammatory effects of many plant foods. Not only does a low meat diet reduce the DII [179], but aspects of Mediterranean cuisine may also contribute to reducing the inflammatory effects of meat as discussed below.

Red meat consumption is consistently associated in prospective studies with an increased risk of obesity [180–183] and diabetes [184–190]. For CVD, two recent meta-analyses showed an increased risk with red and processed meat, with a level of evidence of "probable" [191,192]. Cancers have also been associated with meat consumption particularly colorectal cancer. Red meat and processed meat have been analyzed separately, and the WCRF/AICR CUP qualified the level of evidence for a causal association between red meat and processed meat and colorectal cancer as convincing [145]. Since this study, six prospective studies [193–198], three meta-analyses [199–201] and one analysis of pooled studies [202] have shown some inconsistencies in relation to processed meat which might be related to different processing methods of meat between countries. However, the level of evidence for the association remains probable to convincing and underlines the importance of processing methods. Two prospective studies analyzed the relationship between prostate cancer and processed meat, and both showed a significantly increased risk suggesting a positive association [203,204].

One group of compounds implicated in the adverse effects of cooked meat is MRPs. Most MRPs in meat result from cooking at high temperatures, and although some MRPs contribute to the desirable flavor of cooked meat, others, including heterocyclic amines (HCAs) and advanced glycation endproducts (AGEs), are potentially harmful. HCAs are suspected carcinogens, whereas many AGEs have pro-inflammatory activities and are incriminated in a wide range of chronic diseases [205].

Although below median consumption of meat is positively scored for in the MD, there is no consideration of how cooking techniques, such as the degree of cooking or foodstuffs cooked with the meat, may modify the formation of pro-inflammatory or pro-carcinogenic MRPs. Here we briefly discuss the evidence for adverse health effects of MRPs in meat especially in relation to inflammation, and we then discuss if food processing techniques relevant to the MD may reduce their formation.

10.1. Heterocyclic Amines

Cooking meat at high temperatures generates a wide range of HCAs, and more than 25 have so far been identified [206]. PhIP (2-amino-1-methyl-6-phenylimidazo(4,5-b)pyridine) is the most abundant HCA detected in the human diet, followed by MeIQx (2-amino-3,8-dimethylimidazo(4,5-f)quinoxaline) and DiMeIQx (2 amino 3,4,8-trimethylimidazo(4,5-t)quinoxaline). In 1993 the International Agency for Research on Cancer concluded that the evidence from animal studies was sufficient to claim that PhIP and MeIQx are carcinogenic. Studies examining if HCAs contribute to the association between cooked meat and colorectal cancer risk are inconsistent (reviewed in [207]). The results of a case-control study strongly suggested an association with increased risk of breast cancer with high intake of well-done red meat and MeIQx among postmenopausal women only (P-trend = 0.002 and 0.003, respectively) [208]. The evidence for a causal relationship between processed meat and breast cancer is limited and mainly observed in case-control studies where a genetic polymorphism in N-acetyltransferase 2 has been investigated in relation to the presence of HCA in foods (e.g., [209]). However, recent evidence does not suggest that polymorphisms in genes that metabolize HCAs (N-acetyltransferase 2 and CYP 1A12) modify colon or breast cancer risk [210,211]. In the National Institutes of Health (NIH)—AARP Diet and Health prospective study, there is suggestive evidence implicating HCAs found in red meat cooked at high temperatures in gastric cardia and non-cardia adenocarcinomas although the association never reached statistical significance [212].

10.2. Advanced Glycation Endproducts

AGEs result from dicarbonyl groups from carbohydrate degradation products reacting with an amino terminal group. Although AGEs are mainly products of the Maillard reaction, they can also be formed from the auto-oxidation of glucose or from the peroxidation of lipids into dicarbonyl groups due to oxidative stress [213,214]. As well as coming from the diet, AGEs are also produced endogenously in the body. Cooked meat is the major dietary source of AGEs in most countries, with fish, aged cheese and roasted nuts being other sources [215].

Many *in vitro* studies have shown that AGEs increase oxidative stress and inflammation and this may at least in part be mediated by binding of AGEs to a receptor (RAGE) [205]. A number of human studies have demonstrated a link between dietary intake of AGEs and inflammation, although results are not conclusive. From a recent systematic review of human intervention studies in both healthy individuals and patients with an underlying disease (mostly commonly type 2 diabetes), the authors concluded that the main effect was a decrease in inflammatory status on a low AGE diet, whereas results for an increase in inflammatory status on a high AGE diet were less consistent [216]. The response to AGEs may be related to the inflammatory status of the individual and the level of circulating AGEs [216]. AGEs have been implicated as causal factors for a wide range of diseases, in particular for type 2 diabetes [217,218] and also for memory decline and Alzheimer's disease [219,220]. In a recent study, a high level of circulating methylglyoxal (MG)—an AGE precursor—was shown to correlate with impaired cognition in humans and impaired learning and memory function and enhanced amyloid-β accumulation in mice [221]. In addition, high dietary consumption of AGEs has been shown to be associated with pancreatic cancer [222]. Despite this accumulating evidence, the role of AGEs in disease pathology remains controversial and there are conflicting results both in preclinical and clinical studies, not least because of the lack of a fully validated assay for measuring the AGE content of foods [14,214].

There is some limited evidence linking AGEs with the MD. In a population of Italian students, loss of adherence to a MD correlated with an increased intake of AGEs [223]. A recent study that retrospectively estimated AGE intake from various ecological and cohort studies showed that high adherence to a MD resulted in a lower meat and dairy intake, both of which contained high levels of AGEs [215]. This study then compared the extrapolated AGE intake to Alzheimer's disease incidence in two cohorts (Washington Heights-Inwood Community Aging Project cohorts from 1992 and 1999). They proposed a correlation between AGE intake and Alzheimer's disease incidence although further studies are required to validate this study.

10.3. Food Processing

Several aspects of Mediterranean cuisine may contribute to reducing the inflammatory and carcinogenic effects of meat that are mediated by MRPs. The Maillard reaction is a non-enzymatic reaction that is influenced by a large range of factors. The reaction accelerates significantly at high temperatures, with a doubling in the rate with a 10 °C increase in temperature [224] and levels of AGEs in foods cooked at high temperatures are typically up to 100-fold above those found in uncooked foods [174]. This is an important consideration for meat since it is cooked at a wide range of temperatures ranging from 100 °C for poaching/stewing, 140–190 °C for frying, to over 200 °C for roasting and barbecuing. For example, levels of carboxymethyl lysine (CML) (an AGE precursor) determined by UPLC/MS were up to twice as high in roasted chicken compared to boiled chicken [225]. The degree of "doneness" also influences AGE formation, and CML levels were twice as high in a well-done roasted beef joint compared to one roasted rare [225].

The Maillard reaction is low at acidic pH [214] and marinating beef with lemon juice or vinegar has been shown to reduce subsequent AGE formation during roasting [214]. Marinating is commonly used in traditional Mediterranean cooking to tenderize tough meat. Besides effects on pH, constituents in commonly used marinades have been found to reduce the formation of MRPs including some types of HCAs. In most cases, the reduction in HCA formation was attributed to the antioxidant activities of the marinades. For example, marinating chicken breasts with red wine reduced PhIP by up to 88% [226], marinating beef patties with garlic was especially effective at reducing the formation of MeIQx and 4,8-DiMeIQx [227], both MeIQx and PhIP were reduced by a rosemary extract [228]. VOO reduced the formation of various HCAs in fried burgers to a greater extent than non-VOO [229]. Various components in VOO may contribute to its ability to inhibit MRPs. Oleanolic acid—a main terpene in olive oil and especially in olives [230]—has anti-glycative effects in diabetic mice [231]. There is a good deal of interest in the development of oleanolic acid for the treatment of diabetes although multiple mechanisms may be involved in its action [232]. Olive phenolics, added as olive mill waste water, trap dicarbonyl compounds and are being studied as anti-glycative agents, but it is not known if VOO has similar properties to the olive mill waste water [233].

In Mediterranean cooking, meat is often cooked with other ingredients such as vegetables, fruits, herbs and spices. A wide range of these foodstuffs have been shown to inhibit MRP formation, including both HCAs [206] and AGEs [234]. For example, HCA formation in model systems comprising mixtures of sugars and amino acids or meat extracts was inhibited by carotenoids from tomatoes [235] and a cherry extract inhibited PhIP formation in beef patties by up to 93% [236]. However, not all studies have been positive, and no significant differences in HCA levels were found between meat samples cooked in the typical Portuguese way with garlic, wine, olive oil, onion, and tomato and in control meat samples (cooked without other ingredients) [237]. Many foodstuffs typically used in Mediterranean meat dishes including cinnamon, garlic and rosemary have been shown to inhibit the formation of AGEs in *in vitro* and animal models [234].

10.4. Implications

Not only is the MD low in foods with potentially high HCA and AGE contents—such as cooked meat, it is also high in foods with a low content of these MRPs—such as fish, grains, low-fat milk products, fruits, and vegetables. Lamb—the meat traditionally consumed most frequently in the MD—has low levels of AGEs compared to other meats [174]. The wide range of studies demonstrating that cooking meat with plant foods such as vegetables, fruit, herbs and spices lowers HCA/AGE formation, suggests that this could be a healthful attribute of Mediterranean cuisine in comparison to some other cuisines where meat is more typically cooked on its own. The overall composition of a dish, rather than any single factor such as cooking temperature, can be important for determining the formation of MRPs. Not only can many foodstuffs inhibit MRP formation but there may also be a negative impact of combining meat with sources of sugars. For example, fried battered/breaded cod (not a traditional technique in Mediterranean cuisine) had significantly higher CML levels than when the fish was grilled/roasted, and casseroled chicken had higher levels of CML than portions roasted on their own. This may be because reducing sugars in the prepared dish are reacting with lysine residues in the protein [225]. The consequences of heating food are complex and not all MRPs are equally harmful; indeed some are beneficial and some MRPs have antioxidant and anti-inflammatory properties [238]. MRPs from foods rich in protein and fat appear to be more damaging than MRPs from roasted coffee and the crust of bread. This may be related to the higher content of the AGE precursors CML and MG in foods rich in protein and fat [213].

Since the Maillard reaction generates products with favorable attributes such as color and aroma, the aim—for optimum consumer acceptability—should not be to eliminate the Maillard reaction altogether but rather to use cooking techniques that direct the reaction towards favorable products rather than towards harmful ones [214]. Further research is clearly required to elucidate the roles of HCAs and AGEs in health and their relation to food processing. The WCRF/AICR CUP in 2010 stated that "it is probable that HCAs found on the surface of well-done meat can cause colon cancer in people with genetic predisposition" but no recommendation was made to the general public [239]. In relation to AGEs, recommendations for reducing AGE formation are strongest for diabetic patients and those with kidney disease [214].

11. Discussion

The importance of considering the MD as more than just its food components is widely recognized. According to UNESCO's broad definition, the MD includes "a set of skills, knowledge, rituals, symbols and traditions concerning crops, harvesting, fishing, animal husbandry, conservation, processing, cooking, and particularly the sharing and consumption of food" [240]. Other commentators have also emphasized the importance to the MD of practices such as food preparation methods and physical activity [241], eating patterns and the absence of, or type of, snacking between meals [242,243]. Recent updates of the MD pyramid also emphasize "the production, selection, processing and consumption of foods" and other aspects of the Mediterranean lifestyle [244] and this is summarized in Table 1. In this review, we provide further evidence of the importance of these wider considerations. In particular, we have identified several examples of food processing pertinent to the MD that can have a significant impact on the nutritional qualities of foods such as olives, olive oil and vegetables that are consumed as part of a MD.

Table 1. Selected examples of how food processing techniques influence the levels of phytochemicals in foods in the Mediterranean diet and levels of biomarkers.

Food	Food Processing Technique	Resulting Change			
		Phytochemicals & Other Compounds	Ref.	Biomarkers	Ref.
Olives	California-style Processing	↓ Hydroxytyrosol, ↑ acrylamide	[48,63]		
	Pitting	↓ Hydroxytyrosol	[64]		
Olive oil	Refining	↓ Polyphenols	[51]	↓ Protection of LDL-cholesterol from oxidation in humans	[51]
Extra virgin olive oil	Deep frying (heating to 180 °C)	↓ Hydroxytyrosol	[67]		
		Small ↓ in oleocanthal	[70]		
		Small ↓ in lignans	[69]		
		↓ Hydroxytyrosol, oleuropein aglycone, luteolin	[72]		
Tomatoes	Cooked in olive oil	↑ Lycopene bioavailability	[107,108]		
		↑ Naringenin bioavailability	[110]		
	Mechanical processing	↑ Naringenin bioavailability	[111]		
Crucifers	Boiling	↓ Glucosinolates	[124]		
	Chopping	↑ Isothiocyanates	[123]		
Onions	Frying 5 min	↑ Quercetin glucosides	[152]		
	Frying > 10 min	↓ Quercetin glucosides	[152]		
Garlic	Crushing	↑ Allicin	[153]	↑ *In vitro* antiplatelet activity	[153]
Nuts	Removal of pellicle	↓ Anti-oxidant polyphenols	[162–164]	↓ Total plasma antioxidant capacity in overweight and obese adults	[168]
	Roasting	↑ or ↓ Total antioxidant activity	[171]	No change in LDL-cholesterol lowering effect	[176]

Contrasting with this perspective, it is often considered that effectively promoting a MD in non-Mediterranean countries requires taking into consideration the cultural cuisine of the country in question, and allowing for the ways food items are typically prepared and cooked in the adopting country [3,245]. This potentially creates a mismatch between tailoring the MD to non-Mediterranean cuisines whilst at the same time respecting the specific cultural aspects of traditional Mediterranean cuisine. Fortunately, advice on food processing pertinent to the MD is, in most cases, still compatible with the cultural cuisine of consumers in non-Mediterranean countries, since it merely involves changing cooking practices (such as stewing rather than boiling vegetables) or selecting healthier variants of foods (e.g., of olives and olive oil). Further implications of food processing on the nutritional qualities of foods are discussed more fully in the sections of this review for each food group.

At present, there is only limited information regarding the extent to which changing food preparation and cooking practices influences levels of consumption of antioxidant and anti-inflammatory phytochemicals. However, significant steps in this direction have been taken with the development of a Retention Factor (RF) for polyphenols [246]. The RF is a measure of how levels of polyphenols in foods change with food processing, and RF values have been incorporated into recent estimates of polyphenol intake in cohorts from the EPIC study [247].

Further work is also required to establish if food processing influences health outcomes, and whether or not this information should be incorporated into measures of adherence to the MD. Adherence to the MD is usually determined by establishing a MD score for a population based on median consumption of various food groups and then grouping subjects into quantiles based on their score above or below the median value [248]. Upper *versus* lower quantile values typically vary 2–3 fold for olive oil (in populations where olive oil is commonly consumed) [52] and 2–3 fold for vegetable consumption [249]. This narrative review, and the more quantitative data from RF values from the Phenol Explorer database [9], indicate that different cooking methods can also give rise to several-fold differences in polyphenol content between vegetables, depending on the type of polyphenol and type of vegetable. Hence, food processing practices may have a significant impact on the nutritional quality of some foods in the MD, comparable in some circumstances to differences in intake between low and high consumers. The use of the RF database will help capture the influence of food processing on the nutritional values of some food groups within the MD. However, this database only applies to polyphenols and, as discussed in this review, there are many other influences on the nutritional value of food groups, and there are currently no databases that quantify these. In addition, there are practical difficulties in capturing a level of precision in epidemiological studies beyond "raw" and "cooked" for vegetables and "boiled" and "fried" for animal products, and this information is of limited value if it is not translated by food composition tables. In the same way, the use of herbs and spice might be evaluated by "yes" or "no" or, at the most, by frequency, but never quantitatively.

12. Conclusions

In this review, we have highlighted aspects of food processing pertinent to the MD that can influence the nutritional quality of foods, and we also provide evidence that this may impact on health outcomes, especially in relation to oxidative stress and inflammation. Currently, it is difficult to quantify this impact. Nevertheless, recognizing that food processing influences the nutritional quality of foods may be important for public health campaigns promoting the MD and for epidemiological studies comparing the health benefits of the MD between populations with different cooking practices.

Acknowledgments: The present review received no specific grant from any funding agency in the public, commercial or not-for-profit sectors.

Author Contributions: R.H. conceived the review; M.G. wrote the sections on epidemiology and R.H. wrote the other sections.

Conflicts of Interest: The authors declare no conflict of interest.

References

1. Van Boekel, M.; Fogliano, V.; Pellegrini, N.; Stanton, C.; Scholz, G.; Lalljie, S.; Somoza, V.; Knorr, D.; Jasti, P.R.; Eisenbrand, G. A review on the beneficial aspects of food processing. *Mol. Nutr. Food Res.* **2010**, *54*, 1215–1247. [CrossRef] [PubMed]
2. Seal, C.J.; de Mul, A.; Eisenbrand, G.; Haverkort, A.J.; Franke, K.; Lalljie, S.P.; Mykkanen, H.; Reimerdes, E.; Scholz, G.; Somoza, V.; *et al.* Risk-benefit considerations of mitigation measures on acrylamide content of foods—A case study on potatoes, cereals and coffee. *Br. J. Nutr.* **2008**, *99* (Suppl. S2), S1–S46. [PubMed]
3. Hoffman, R.; Gerber, M. Evaluating and adapting the Mediterranean diet for non-Mediterranean populations: A critical appraisal. *Nutr. Rev.* **2013**, *71*, 573–584. [CrossRef] [PubMed]
4. Gerber, M.; Hoffman, R. The Mediterranean diet: Health, science and society. *Br. J. Nutr.* **2015**, *113* (Suppl. S2), S4–S10. [CrossRef]
5. Castro-Quezada, I.; Roman-Vinas, B.; Serra-Majem, L. The Mediterranean diet and nutritional adequacy: A review. *Nutrients* **2014**, *6*, 231–248. [CrossRef] [PubMed]
6. Maillot, M.; Issa, C.; Vieux, F.; Lairon, D.; Darmon, N. The shortest way to reach nutritional goals is to adopt Mediterranean food choices: Evidence from computer-generated personalized diets. *Am. J. Clin. Nutr.* **2011**, *94*, 1127–1137. [CrossRef] [PubMed]
7. Tresserra-Rimbau, A.; Rimm, E.B.; Medina-Remon, A.; Martinez-Gonzalez, M.A.; Lopez-Sabater, M.C.; Covas, M.I.; Corella, D.; Salas-Salvado, J.; Gomez-Gracia, E.; Lapetra, J.; *et al.* Polyphenol intake and mortality risk: A re-analysis of the predimed trial. *BMC Med.* **2014**, *12*, 77–88. [CrossRef] [PubMed]
8. Ruiz-Rodriguez, A.; Marín, F.R.; Ocaña, A.; Soler-Rivas, C. Effect of domestic processing on bioactive compounds. *Phytochem. Rev.* **2008**, *7*, 345–384. [CrossRef]
9. Rothwell, J.A.; Medina-Remon, A.; Perez-Jimenez, J.; Neveu, V.; Knaze, V.; Slimani, N.; Scalbert, A. Effects of food processing on polyphenol contents: A systematic analysis using phenol-explorer data. *Mol. Nutr. Food Res.* **2015**, *59*, 160–170. [CrossRef] [PubMed]
10. Ostan, R.; Lanzarini, C.; Pini, E.; Scurti, M.; Vianello, D.; Bertarelli, C.; Fabbri, C.; Izzi, M.; Palmas, G.; Biondi, F.; *et al.* Inflammaging and cancer: A challenge for the Mediterranean diet. *Nutrients* **2015**, *7*, 2589–2621. [CrossRef] [PubMed]

11. Kontogiorgis, C.A.; Bompou, E.M.; Ntella, M.; Berghe, W.V. Natural products from Mediterranean diet: From anti-inflammatory agents to dietary epigenetic modulators. *Anti-Inflamm. Anti-Allergy Agents Med. Chem.* **2010**, *9*, 101–124. [CrossRef]

12. Schulze, M.B.; Hoffmann, K.; Manson, J.E.; Willett, W.C.; Meigs, J.B.; Weikert, C.; Heidemann, C.; Colditz, G.A.; Hu, F.B. Dietary pattern, inflammation, and incidence of type 2 diabetes in women. *Am. J. Clin. Nutr.* **2005**, *82*, 675–684. [PubMed]

13. Ahluwalia, N.; Andreeva, V.A.; Kesse-Guyot, E.; Hercberg, S. Dietary patterns, inflammation and the metabolic syndrome. *Diabetes Metab.* **2013**, *39*, 99–110. [CrossRef] [PubMed]

14. Calder, P.C.; Ahluwalia, N.; Brouns, F.; Buetler, T.; Clement, K.; Cunningham, K.; Esposito, K.; Jonsson, L.S.; Kolb, H.; Lansink, M.; *et al.* Dietary factors and low-grade inflammation in relation to overweight and obesity. *Br. J. Nutr.* **2011**, *106* (Suppl. S3), S5–S78. [CrossRef] [PubMed]

15. Holmes, C.; Butchart, J. Systemic inflammation and Alzheimer's disease. *Biochem. Soc. Trans.* **2011**, *39*, 898–901. [CrossRef] [PubMed]

16. Herieka, M.; Erridge, C. High-fat meal induced postprandial inflammation. *Mol. Nutr. Food Res.* **2014**, *58*, 136–146. [CrossRef] [PubMed]

17. Barbaresko, J.; Koch, M.; Schulze, M.B.; Nothlings, U. Dietary pattern analysis and biomarkers of low-grade inflammation: A systematic literature review. *Nutr. Rev.* **2013**, *71*, 511–527. [CrossRef] [PubMed]

18. Bonaccio, M.; Cerletti, C.; Iacoviello, L.; de Gaetano, G. Mediterranean diet and low-grade subclinical inflammation: The moli-sani study. *Endocr. Metab. Immune Disord. Drug Targets* **2015**, *15*, 18–24. [PubMed]

19. Panagiotakos, D.B.; Dimakopoulou, K.; Katsouyanni, K.; Bellander, T.; Grau, M.; Koenig, W.; Lanki, T.; Pistelli, R.; Schneider, A.; Peters, A.; *et al.* Mediterranean diet and inflammatory response in myocardial infarction survivors. *Int. J. Epidemiol.* **2009**, *38*, 856–866. [CrossRef] [PubMed]

20. Santoro, A.; Pini, E.; Scurti, M.; Palmas, G.; Berendsen, A.; Brzozowska, A.; Pietruszka, B.; Szczecinska, A.; Cano, N.; Meunier, N.; *et al.* Combating inflammaging through a Mediterranean whole diet approach: The NU-AGE project's conceptual framework and design. *Mech. Ageing Dev.* **2014**, *136–137*, 3–13. [CrossRef]

21. Camargo, A.; Delgado-Lista, J.; Garcia-Rios, A.; Cruz-Teno, C.; Yubero-Serrano, E.M.; Perez-Martinez, P.; Gutierrez-Mariscal, F.M.; Lora-Aguilar, P.; Rodriguez-Cantalejo, F.; Fuentes-Jimenez, F.; *et al.* Expression of proinflammatory, proatherogenic genes is reduced by the Mediterranean diet in elderly people. *Br. J. Nutr.* **2012**, *108*, 500–508. [CrossRef] [PubMed]

22. Camargo, A.; Rangel-Zuniga, O.A.; Haro, C.; Meza-Miranda, E.R.; Pena-Orihuela, P.; Meneses, M.E.; Marin, C.; Yubero-Serrano, E.M.; Perez-Martinez, P.; Delgado-Lista, J.; *et al.* Olive oil phenolic compounds decrease the postprandial inflammatory response by reducing postprandial plasma lipopolysaccharide levels. *Food Chem.* **2014**, *162*, 161–171. [CrossRef] [PubMed]

23. Yubero-Serrano, E.M.; Delgado-Casado, N.; Delgado-Lista, J.; Perez-Martinez, P.; Tasset-Cuevas, I.; Santos-Gonzalez, M.; Caballero, J.; Garcia-Rios, A.; Marin, C.; Gutierrez-Mariscal, F.M.; *et al.* Postprandial antioxidant effect of the Mediterranean diet supplemented with coenzyme q10 in elderly men and women. *Age (Dordr)* **2011**, *33*, 579–590. [CrossRef] [PubMed]

24. Reuter, S.; Gupta, S.C.; Chaturvedi, M.M.; Aggarwal, B.B. Oxidative stress, inflammation, and cancer: How are they linked? *Free Radic. Biol. Med.* **2010**, *49*, 1603–1616. [CrossRef] [PubMed]

25. Razquin, C.; Martinez, J.A.; Martinez-Gonzalez, M.A.; Mitjavila, M.T.; Estruch, R.; Marti, A. A 3 years follow-up of a Mediterranean diet rich in virgin olive oil is associated with high plasma antioxidant capacity and reduced body weight gain. *Eur. J. Clin. Nutr.* **2009**, *63*, 1387–1393. [CrossRef] [PubMed]

26. Estruch, R. Anti-inflammatory effects of the Mediterranean diet: The experience of the predimed study. *Proc. Nutr. Soc.* **2010**, *69*, 333–340. [CrossRef] [PubMed]

27. Bonaccio, M.; di Castelnuovo, A.; Bonanni, A.; Costanzo, S.; de Lucia, F.; Pounis, G.; Zito, F.; Donati, M.B.; de Gaetano, G.; Iacoviello, L.; *et al.* Adherence to a Mediterranean diet is associated with a better health-related quality of life: A possible role of high dietary antioxidant content. *BMJ Open* **2013**. [CrossRef] [PubMed]

28. Giugliano, D.; Ceriello, A.; Esposito, K. The effects of diet on inflammation: Emphasis on the metabolic syndrome. *J. Am. Coll Cardiol.* **2006**, *48*, 677–685. [CrossRef] [PubMed]

29. Shivappa, N.; Steck, S.E.; Hurley, T.G.; Hussey, J.R.; Hebert, J.R. Designing and developing a literature-derived, population-based dietary inflammatory index. *Public Health Nutr.* **2014**, *17*, 1689–1696. [CrossRef] [PubMed]

30. Shivappa, N.; Bosetti, C.; Zucchetto, A.; Serraino, D.; la Vecchia, C.; Hebert, J.R. Dietary inflammatory index and risk of pancreatic cancer in an italian case-control study. *Br. J. Nutr.* **2014**, *113*, 292–298. [CrossRef] [PubMed]

31. Tabung, F.K.; Steck, S.E.; Ma, Y.; Liese, A.D.; Zhang, J.; Caan, B.; Hou, L.; Johnson, K.C.; Mossavar-Rahmani, Y.; Shivappa, N.; *et al.* The association between dietary inflammatory index and risk of colorectal cancer among postmenopausal women: Results from the women's health initiative. *Cancer Causes Control* **2015**, *26*, 399–408. [CrossRef] [PubMed]

32. Ruiz-Canela, M.; Zazpe, I.; Shivappa, N.; Hebert, J.R.; Sanchez-Tainta, A.; Corella, D.; Salas-Salvado, J.; Fito, M.; Lamuela-Raventos, R.M.; Rekondo, J.; *et al.* Dietary inflammatory index and anthropometric measures of obesity in a population sample at high cardiovascular risk from the predimed (prevencion con dieta mediterranea) trial. *Br. J. Nutr.* **2015**, *113*, 984–995. [CrossRef] [PubMed]

33. Garcia-Arellano, A.; Ramallal, R.; Ruiz-Canela, M.; Salas-Salvado, J.; Corella, D.; Shivappa, N.; Schroder, H.; Hebert, J.R.; Ros, E.; Gomez-Garcia, E.; *et al.* Dietary inflammatory index and incidence of cardiovascular disease in the predimed study. *Nutrients* **2015**, *7*, 4124–4138 [CrossRef] [PubMed]

34. Alkerwi, A.; Vernier, C.; Crichton, G.E.; Sauvageot, N.; Shivappa, N.; Hebert, J.R. Cross-comparison of diet quality indices for predicting chronic disease risk: Findings from the observation of cardiovascular risk factors in luxembourg (oriscav-lux) study. *Br. J. Nutr.* **2014**, *113*, 259–269. [CrossRef] [PubMed]

35. Sensoy, I. A review on the relationship between food structure, processing, and bioavailability. *Crit. Rev. Food Sci. Nutr.* **2014**, *54*, 902–909. [CrossRef] [PubMed]

36. Parada, J.; Aguilera, J.M. Food microstructure affects the bioavailability of several nutrients. *J. Food Sci.* **2007**, *72*, R21–R32. [CrossRef] [PubMed]

37. Mcnulty, H.; Pentieva, K. Folate bioavailability. *Proc. Nutr. Soc.* **2004**, *63*, 529–536. [CrossRef] [PubMed]

38. Saura-Calixto, F. Concept and health-related properties of nonextractable polyphenols: The missing dietary polyphenols. *J. Agric. Food Chem.* **2012**, *60*, 11195–11200. [CrossRef] [PubMed]

39. Arranz, S.; Saura-Calixto, F.; Shaha, S.; Kroon, P.A. High contents of nonextractable polyphenols in fruits suggest that polyphenol contents of plant foods have been underestimated. *J. Agric. Food Chem.* **2009**, *57*, 7298–7303. [CrossRef] [PubMed]

40. Arranz, S.; Silvan, J.M.; Saura-Calixto, F. Nonextractable polyphenols, usually ignored, are the major part of dietary polyphenols: A study on the spanish diet. *Mol. Nutr. Food Res.* **2010**, *54*, 1646–1658. [CrossRef] [PubMed]

41. Vitaglione, P.; Mennella, I.; Ferracane, R.; Rivellese, A.A.; Giacco, R.; Ercolini, D.; Gibbons, S.M.; la Storia, A.; Gilbert, J.A.; Jonnalagadda, S.; *et al.* Whole-grain wheat consumption reduces inflammation in a randomized controlled trial on overweight and obese subjects with unhealthy dietary and lifestyle behaviors: Role of polyphenols bound to cereal dietary fiber. *Am. J. Clin. Nutr.* **2015**, *101*, 251–261. [CrossRef] [PubMed]

42. Vitaglione, P.; Napolitano, A.; Fogliano, V. Cereal dietary fibre: A natural functional ingredient to deliver phenolic compounds into the gut. *Trends Food Sci. Technol.* **2008**, *19*, 451–463. [CrossRef]

43. Cicerale, S.; Lucas, L.; Keast, R. Biological activities of phenolic compounds present in virgin olive oil. *Int. J. Mol. Sci.* **2010**, *11*, 458–479. [CrossRef] [PubMed]

44. Parkinson, L.; Keast, R. Oleocanthal, a phenolic derived from virgin olive oil: A review of the beneficial effects on inflammatory disease. *Int. J. Mol. Sci.* **2014**, *15*, 12323–12334. [CrossRef] [PubMed]

45. Bulotta, S.; Celano, M.; Lepore, S.M.; Montalcini, T.; Pujia, A.; Russo, D. Beneficial effects of the olive oil phenolic components oleuropein and hydroxytyrosol: Focus on protection against cardiovascular and metabolic diseases. *J. Transl. Med.* **2014**, *12*, 219. [CrossRef] [PubMed]

46. Baiano, A.; Gambacorta, G.; Terracone, C.; Previtali, M.A.; Lamacchia, C.; la Notte, E. Changes in phenolic content and antioxidant activity of Italian extra-virgin olive oils during storage. *J. Food Sci.* **2009**, *74*, C177–C183. [CrossRef] [PubMed]

47. Del Monaco, G.; Officioso, A.; D'angelo, S.; la Cara, F.; Ionata, E.; Marcolongo, L.; Squillaci, G.; Maurelli, L.; Morana, A. Characterization of extra virgin olive oils produced with typical Italian varieties by their phenolic profile. *Food Chem.* **2015**, *184*, 220–228. [CrossRef] [PubMed]

48. Charoenprasert, S.; Mitchell, A. Factors influencing phenolic compounds in table olives (*Olea europaea*). *J. Agric. Food Chem.* **2012**, *60*, 7081–7095. [CrossRef] [PubMed]

49. Vissers, M.N.; Zock, P.L.; Roodenburg, A.J.; Leenen, R.; Katan, M.B. Olive oil phenols are absorbed in humans. *J. Nutr.* **2002**, *132*, 409–417. [PubMed]

50. Buckland, G.; Gonzalez, C.A. The role of olive oil in disease prevention: A focus on the recent epidemiological evidence from cohort studies and dietary intervention trials. *Br. J. Nutr.* **2015**, *113* (Suppl. S2), S94–S101. [CrossRef] [PubMed]

51. Covas, M.I.; de la Torre, R.; Fito, M. Virgin olive oil: A key food for cardiovascular risk protection. *Br. J. Nutr.* **2015**, *113* (Suppl. S2), S19–S28. [CrossRef] [PubMed]

52. Hoffman, R.; Gerber, M. Can rapeseed oil replace olive oil as part of a Mediterranean-style diet? *Br. J. Nutr.* **2014**, *112*, 1882–1895. [CrossRef] [PubMed]

53. Buckland, G.; Travier, N.; Barricarte, A.; Ardanaz, E.; Moreno-Iribas, C.; Sanchez, M.J.; Molina-Montes, E.; Chirlaque, M.D.; Huerta, J.M.; Navarro, C.; *et al.* Olive oil intake and CHD in the European prospective investigation into cancer and nutrition spanish cohort. *Br. J. Nutr.* **2012**, *108*, 2075–2082. [CrossRef] [PubMed]

54. Buckland, G.; Travier, N.; Agudo, A.; Fonseca-Nunes, A.; Navarro, C.; Lagiou, P.; Demetriou, C.; Amiano, P.; Dorronsoro, M.; Chirlaque, M.D.; *et al.* Olive oil intake and breast cancer risk in the Mediterranean countries of the European prospective investigation into cancer and nutrition study. *Int. J. Cancer* **2012**, *131*, 2465–2469. [CrossRef] [PubMed]

55. Tripoli, E.; Giammanco, M.; Tabacchi, G.; di Majo, D.; Giammanco, S.; la Guardia, M. The phenolic compounds of olive oil: Structure, biological activity and beneficial effects on human health. *Nutr. Res. Rev.* **2005**, *18*, 98–112. [CrossRef] [PubMed]

56. Cicerale, S.; Lucas, L.J.; Keast, R.S. Antimicrobial, antioxidant and anti-inflammatory phenolic activities in extra virgin olive oil. *Curr. Opin. Biotechnol.* **2012**, *23*, 129–135. [CrossRef] [PubMed]

57. Cicerale, S.; Lucas, L.J.; Keast, R.S.J. Oleocanthal: A naturally occurring anti-inflammatory agent in virgin olive oil. In *Virgin Olive Oil, Olive Oil—Constituents, Quality, Health Properties and Bioconversions*; Boskou, D., Ed.; Intech: Rijeka, Croatia, 2012; pp. 357–374.

58. Blekas, G.; Vassilakis, C.; Harizanis, C.; Tsimidou, M.; Boskou, D.G. Biophenols in table olives. *J. Agric. Food Chem.* **2002**, *50*, 3688–3692. [CrossRef] [PubMed]

59. Neveu, V.; Perez-Jimenez, J.; Vos, F.; Crespy, V.; du Chaffaut, L.; Mennen, L.; Knox, C.; Eisner, R.; Cruz, J.; Wishart, D.; *et al.* Phenol-explorer: An online comprehensive database on polyphenol contents in foods. *Database (Oxf.)* **2010**, *2010*. [CrossRef] [PubMed]

60. Boskou, G.; Salta, F.N.; Chrysostomou, S.; Mylona, A.; Chiou, A.; Andrikopoulos, N.K. Antioxidant capacity and phenolic profile of table olives from the Greek market. *Food Chem.* **2006**, *94*, 558–564. [CrossRef]

61. Pereira, J.A.; Pereira, A.P.; Ferreira, I.C.; Valentao, P.; Andrade, P.B.; Seabra, R.; Estevinho, L.; Bento, A. Table olives from portugal: Phenolic compounds, antioxidant potential, and antimicrobial activity. *J. Agric. Food Chem.* **2006**, *54*, 8425–8431. [CrossRef] [PubMed]

62. Boskou, D. Olive oil. In *Vegetable Oils in Food Technology: Composition, Properties and Uses*, 2nd ed.; Gunstone, F.D., Ed.; Wiley-Blackwell: Oxford, UK, 2011; pp. 243–271.

63. Marsilio, V.; Campestre, C.; Lanza, B. Phenolic compounds change during California-style ripe olive processing. *Food Chem.* **2001**, *74*, 55–60. [CrossRef]

64. Romero, C.; Brenes, M.; Yousfi, K.; Garcia, P.; Garcia, A.; Garrido, A. Effect of cultivar and processing method on the contents of polyphenols in table olives. *J. Agric. Food Chem.* **2004**, *52*, 479–484. [CrossRef] [PubMed]

65. Silva, L.; Garcia, B.; Paiva-Martins, F. Oxidative stability of olive oil and its polyphenolic compounds after boiling vegetable process. *Food Sci. Technol.* **2010**, *43*, 1336–1344. [CrossRef]

66. Santos, C.S.P.; Cruz, R.; Cunha, S.C.; Casal, S. Effect of cooking on olive oil quality attributes. *Food Res. Int.* **2013**, *54*, 2016–2024. [CrossRef]

67. Daskalaki, D.; Kefi, G.; Kotsiou, K.; Tasioula-Margari, M. Evaluation of phenolic compounds degradation in virgin olive oil during storage and heating. *J. Food Nutr. Res.* **2009**, *48*, 31–41.

68. Carrasco-Pancorbo, A.; Cerretani, L.; Bendini, A.; Segura-Carretero, A.; Lercker, G.; Fernandez-Gutierrez, A. Evaluation of the influence of thermal oxidation on the phenolic composition and on the antioxidant activity of extra-virgin olive oils. *J. Agric. Food Chem.* **2007**, *55*, 4771–4780. [CrossRef] [PubMed]

69. Brenes, M.; Garcia, A.; Dobarganes, M.C.; Velasco, J.; Romero, C. Influence of thermal treatments simulating cooking processes on the polyphenol content in virgin olive oil. *J. Agric. Food Chem.* **2002**, *50*, 5962–5967. [CrossRef] [PubMed]

70. Gomez-Alonso, S.; Fregapane, G.; Salvador, M.D.; Gordon, M.H. Changes in phenolic composition and antioxidant activity of virgin olive oil during frying. *J. Agric. Food Chem.* **2003**, *51*, 667–672. [CrossRef] [PubMed]

71. Cicerale, S.; Lucas, L.J.; Keast, R.S.J. Oleocanthal: A naturally occurring anti-inflammatory agent in virgin olive oil. In *Olive Oil—Constituents, Quality, Health Properties and Bioconversions*; Dimitrios, B., Ed.; Intech: Rijeka, Croatia, 2012; pp. 357–374.

72. Perez-Herrera, A.; Delgado-Lista, J.; Torres-Sanchez, L.A.; Rangel-Zuniga, O.A.; Camargo, A.; Moreno-Navarrete, J.M.; Garcia-Olid, B.; Quintana-Navarro, G.M.; Alcala-Diaz, J.F.; Munoz-Lopez, C.; *et al*. The postprandial inflammatory response after ingestion of heated oils in obese persons is reduced by the presence of phenol compounds. *Mol. Nutr. food Res.* **2012**, *56*, 510–514. [CrossRef] [PubMed]

73. Sayon-Orea, C.; Carlos, S.; Martinez-Gonzalez, M.A. Does cooking with vegetable oils increase the risk of chronic diseases?: A systematic review. *Br. J. Nutr.* **2015**, *113* (Suppl. S2), S36–S48. [CrossRef] [PubMed]

74. Charoenprasert, S.; Mitchell, A. Influence of California-style black ripe olive processing on the formation of acrylamide. *J. Agric. Food Chem.* **2014**, *62*, 8716–8721. [CrossRef] [PubMed]

75. EFSA. Scientific opinion on the substantiation of health claims related to polyphenols in olive and protection of ldl particles from oxidative damage (ID 1333, 1638, 1639, 1696, 2865), maintenance of normal blood hdl cholesterol concentrations (ID 1639), maintenance of normal blood pressure (ID 3781), "anti-inflammatory properties" (ID 1882), "contributes to the upper respiratory tract health" (ID 3468), "can help to maintain a normal function of gastrointestinal tract" (3779), and "contributes to body defences against external agents" (ID 3467) pursuant to article 13(1) of regulation (ec) no 1924/2006. *EFSA J.* **2011**, *9*, 2033–2057.

76. Estruch, R.; Salas-Salvado, J. Towards an even healthier Mediterranean diet. *Nutr. Metab. Cardiovasc. Dis.* **2013**, *23*, 1163–1166. [CrossRef] [PubMed]

77. Tiwari, U.; Cummins, E. Factors influencing levels of phytochemicals in selected fruit and vegetables during pre- and post-harvest food processing operations. *Food Res. Int.* **2013**, *50*, 497–506. [CrossRef]

78. Baranski, M.; Srednicka-Tober, D.; Volakakis, N.; Seal, C.; Sanderson, R.; Stewart, G.B.; Benbrook, C.; Biavati, B.; Markellou, E.; Giotis, C.; *et al*. Higher antioxidant and lower cadmium concentrations and lower incidence of pesticide residues in organically grown crops: A systematic literature review and meta-analyses. *Br. J. Nutr.* **2014**, *112*, 794–811. [CrossRef] [PubMed]

79. Lairon, D. Nutritional quality and safety of organic food. A review. *Agron. Sustain. Dev.* **2010**, *30*, 33–41. [CrossRef]

80. Agudo, A.; Slimani, N.; Ocke, M.C.; Naska, A.; Miller, A.B.; Kroke, A.; Bamia, C.; Karalis, D.; Vineis, P.; Palli, D.; *et al*. Consumption of vegetables, fruit and other plant foods in the European prospective investigation into cancer and nutrition (EPIC) cohorts from 10 European countries. *Public Health Nutr.* **2002**, *5*, 1179–1196. [CrossRef] [PubMed]

81. Turati, F.; Rossi, M.; Pelucchi, C.; Levi, F.; la Vecchia, C. Fruit and vegetables and cancer risk: A review of southern European studies. *Br. J. Nutr.* **2015**, *113* (Suppl. S2), S102–S110. [CrossRef]

82. Oude Griep, L.M.; Verschuren, W.M.; Kromhout, D.; Ocke, M.C.; Geleijnse, J.M. Raw and processed fruit and vegetable consumption and 10-year stroke incidence in a population-based cohort study in the Netherlands. *Eur. J. Clin. Nutr.* **2011**, *65*, 791–799. [CrossRef]

83. Kafatos, A.; Verhagen, H.; Moschandreas, J.; Apostolaki, I.; van Westerop, J.J. Mediterranean diet of crete: Foods and nutrient content. *J. Am. Diet. Assoc.* **2000**, *100*, 1487–1493. [CrossRef]

84. Ninfali, P.; Mea, G.; Giorgini, S.; Rocchi, M.; Bacchiocca, M. Antioxidant capacity of vegetables, spices and dressings relevant to nutrition. *Br. J. Nutr.* **2005**, *93*, 257–266. [CrossRef]

85. Rubio, L.; Motilva, M.J.; Romero, M.P. Recent advances in biologically active compounds in herbs and spices: A review of the most effective antioxidant and anti-inflammatory active principles. *Crit. Rev. Food Sci. Nutr.* **2013**, *53*, 943–953. [CrossRef]

86. Dilis, V.; Vasilopoulou, E.; Trichopoulou, A. The flavone, flavonol and flavan-3-ol content of the Greek traditional diet. *Food Chem.* **2007**, *105*, 812–821. [CrossRef]

87. Kaefer, C.M.; Milner, J.A. The role of herbs and spices in cancer prevention. *J. Nutr. Biochem.* **2008**, *19*, 347–361. [CrossRef]

88. Opara, E.I.; Chohan, M. Culinary herbs and spices: Their bioactive properties, the contribution of polyphenols and the challenges in deducing their true health benefits. *Int. J. Mol. Sci.* **2014**, *15*, 19183–19202. [CrossRef] [PubMed]

89. Palermo, M.; Pellegrini, N.; Fogliano, V. The effect of cooking on the phytochemical content of vegetables. *J. Sci. Food Agric.* **2014**, *94*, 1057–1070. [CrossRef] [PubMed]

90. Vasilopoulou, E.; Georga, K.; Bjoerkov Joergensen, M.; Naska, A.; Trichopoulou, A. The antioxidant properties of Greek foods and the flavonoid content of the Mediterranean menu. *Curr. Med. Chem. Immunol. Endocr. Metab. Agents* **2005**, *5*, 33–45. [CrossRef]

91. Del Pilar ramírez-Anaya, J.; Samaniego-Sánchez, C.; Castañeda-Saucedo, M.C.; Villalón-Mir, M.; lópez-García de la Serrana, H. Phenols and the antioxidant capacity of Mediterranean vegetables prepared with extra virgin olive oil using different domestic cooking techniques. *Food Chem.* **2015**, *188*, 430–438. [CrossRef] [PubMed]

92. Fernández-García, E.; Carvajal-Lérida, I.; Jarén-Galán, M.; Garrido-Fernández, J.; Pérez-Gálvez, A.; Hornero-Méndez, D. Carotenoids bioavailability from foods: From plant pigments to efficient biological activities. *Food Res. Int.* **2012**, *46*, 438–450. [CrossRef]

93. De Azevedo-Meleiro, C.H.; rodriguez-Amaya, D.B. Qualitative and quantitative differences in the carotenoid composition of yellow and red peppers determined by HPLC-DAD-MS. *J. Sep. Sci.* **2009**, *32*, 3652–3658. [CrossRef] [PubMed]

94. Maiani, G.; Caston, M.J.; Catasta, G., Toti, E.; Cambrodon, I.G.; Bysted, A.; Granado-Lorencio, F.; Olmedilla-Alonso, B.; Knuthsen, P.; Valoti, M.; *et al.* Carotenoids: Actual knowledge on food sources, intakes, stability and bioavailability and their protective role in humans. *Mol. Nutr. Food Res.* **2009**, *53* (Suppl. S2), S194–S218. [CrossRef] [PubMed]

95. Oshima, S.; Sakamoto, H.; Ishiguro, Y.; Terao, J. Accumulation and clearance of capsanthin in blood plasma after the ingestion of paprika juice in men. *J. Nutr.* **1997**, *127*, 1475–1479. [PubMed]

96. Bolhassani, A.; Khavari, A.; Bathaie, S.Z. Saffron and natural carotenoids: Biochemical activities and anti-tumor effects. *Biochim. Biophys. Acta* **2014**, *1845*, 20–30. [CrossRef] [PubMed]

97. Ciccone, M.M.; Cortese, F.; Gesualdo, M.; Carbonara, S.; Zito, A.; Ricci, G.; de Pascalis, F.; Scicchitano, P.; Riccioni, G. Dietary intake of carotenoids and their antioxidant and anti-inflammatory effects in cardiovascular care. *Mediat. Inflamm.* **2013**. [CrossRef] [PubMed]

98. Sporn, M.B.; Liby, K.T. Is lycopene an effective agent for preventing prostate cancer? *Cancer Prev. Res. (Phila.)* **2013**, *6*, 384–386. [CrossRef] [PubMed]

99. Murador, D.C.; da Cunha, D.T.; de Rosso, V.V. Effects of cooking techniques on vegetable pigments: A meta-analytic approach to carotenoid and anthocyanin levels. *Food Res. Int.* **2014**, *65*, 177–183. [CrossRef]

100. Lakshminarayana, R.; Baskara, V. Influence of olive oil on the bioavailability of carotenoids. *Eur. J. Lipid Sci. Technol.* **2013**, *115*, 1085–1093. [CrossRef]

101. Clark, R.M.; Yao, L.; She, L.; Furr, H.C. A comparison of lycopene and astaxanthin absorption from corn oil and olive oil emulsions. *Lipids* **2000**, *35*, 803–806. [CrossRef] [PubMed]

102. Lakshminarayana, R.; Raju, M.; Krishnakantha, T.P.; Baskaran, V. Lutein and zeaxanthin in leafy greens and their bioavailability: Olive oil influences the absorption of dietary lutein and its accumulation in adult rats. *J. Agric. Food Chem.* **2007**, *55*, 6395–6400. [CrossRef] [PubMed]

103. Goltz, S.R.; Campbell, W.W.; Chitchumroonchokchai, C.; Failla, M.L.; Ferruzzi, M.G. Meal triacylglycerol profile modulates postprandial absorption of carotenoids in humans. *Mol. Nutr. Food Res.* **2012**, *56*, 866–877. [CrossRef] [PubMed]

104. Jayarajan, P.; Reddy, V.; Mohanram, M. Effect of dietary fat on absorption of β carotene from green leafy vegetables in children. *Indian J. Med Res.* **1980**, *71*, 53–56. [PubMed]

105. Van het Hof, K.H.; West, C.E.; Weststrate, J.A.; Hautvast, J.G. Dietary factors that affect the bioavailability of carotenoids. *J. Nutr.* **2000**, *130*, 503–506. [PubMed]

106. Moran, N.E.; Erdman, J.W., Jr.; Clinton, S.K. Complex interactions between dietary and genetic factors impact lycopene metabolism and distribution. *Arch. Biochem. Biophys.* **2013**, *539*, 171–180. [CrossRef] [PubMed]

107. Fielding, J.M.; Rowley, K.G.; Cooper, P.; O'Dea, K. Increases in plasma lycopene concentration after consumption of tomatoes cooked with olive oil. *Asia Pac. J. Clin. Nutr.* **2005**, *14*, 131–136. [PubMed]

108. Arranz, S.; Martinez-Huelamo, M.; Vallverdu-Queralt, A.; Valderas-Martinez, P.; Illan, M.; Sacanella, E.; Escribano, E.; Estruch, R.; Lamuela-Raventos, R.M. Influence of olive oil on carotenoid absorption from tomato juice and effects on postprandial lipemia. *Food Chem.* **2015**, *168*, 203–210. [CrossRef] [PubMed]

109. Vallverdu-Queralt, A.; Regueiro, J.; Rinaldi de Alvarenga, J.F.; Torrado, X.; Lamuela-Raventos, R.M. Home cooking and phenolics: Effect of thermal treatment and addition of extra virgin olive oil on the phenolic profile of tomato sauces. *J. Agric. Food Chem.* **2014**. [CrossRef] [PubMed]

110. Tulipani, S.; Martínez-Huélamo, M.; Rotchés-Ribalta, M.; Estruch, R.; Escribano-Ferrer, E.; Andres-Lacueva, C.; Illan, M.; Lamuela-Raventós, R.M. Oil matrix effects on plasma exposure and urinary excretion of phenolic compounds from tomato sauces: Evidence from a human pilot study. *Food Chem.* **2011**, *130*, 581–590. [CrossRef]

111. Martinez-Huelamo, M.; Tulipani, S.; Estruch, R.; Escribano, E.; Illan, M.; Corella, D.; Lamuela-Raventos, R.M. The tomato sauce making process affects the bioaccessibility and bioavailability of tomato phenolics: A pharmacokinetic study. *Food Chem.* **2015**, *173*, 864–872. [CrossRef] [PubMed]

112. Bosetti, C.; Tzonou, A.; Lagiou, P.; Negri, E.; Trichopoulos, D.; Hsieh, C.C. Fraction of prostate cancer incidence attributed to diet in Athens, Greece. *Eur. J. Cancer Prev.* **2000**, *9*, 119–123. [CrossRef] [PubMed]

113. Chen, J.; Song, Y.; Zhang, L. Lycopene/tomato consumption and the risk of prostate cancer: A systematic review and meta-analysis of prospective studies. *J. Nutr. Sci. Vitaminol. (Tokyo)* **2013**, *59*, 213–223. [CrossRef] [PubMed]

114. Tan, H.L.; Thomas-Ahner, J.M.; Grainger, E.M.; Wan, L.; Francis, D.M.; Schwartz, S.J.; Erdman, J.W., Jr.; Clinton, S.K. Tomato-based food products for prostate cancer prevention: What have we learned? *Cancer Metastasis Rev.* **2010**, *29*, 553–568. [CrossRef] [PubMed]

115. Eliassen, A.H.; Hendrickson, S.J.; Brinton, L.A.; Buring, J.E.; Campos, H.; Dai, Q.; Dorgan, J.F.; Franke, A.A.; Gao, Y.T.; Goodman, M.T.; *et al.* Circulating carotenoids and risk of breast cancer: Pooled analysis of eight prospective studies. *J. Natl. Cancer Inst.* **2012**, *104*, 1905–1916. [CrossRef] [PubMed]

116. Aune, D.; Chan, D.S.; Vieira, A.R.; Navarro Rosenblatt, D.A.; Vieira, R.; Greenwood, D.C.; Norat, T. Dietary compared with blood concentrations of carotenoids and breast cancer risk: A systematic review and meta-analysis of prospective studies. *Am. J. Clin. Nutr.* **2012**, *96*, 356–373. [CrossRef] [PubMed]

117. Guerrero-Beltran, C.E.; Calderon-Oliver, M.; Pedraza-Chaverri, J.; Chirino, Y.I. Protective effect of sulforaphane against oxidative stress: Recent advances. *Exp. Toxicol. Pathol.* **2012**, *64*, 503–508. [CrossRef] [PubMed]

118. Dinkova-Kostova, A.T.; Kostov, R.V. Glucosinolates and isothiocyanates in health and disease. *Trends Mol. Med.* **2012**, *18*, 337–347. [CrossRef] [PubMed]

119. Tarozzi, A.; Angeloni, C.; Malaguti, M.; Morroni, F.; Hrelia, S.; Hrelia, P. Sulforaphane as a potential protective phytochemical against neurodegenerative diseases. *Oxid. Med. Cell. Longev.* **2013**. [CrossRef] [PubMed]

120. Boggs, D.A.; Palmer, J.R.; Wise, L.A.; Spiegelman, D.; Stampfer, M.J.; Adams-Campbell, L.L.; Rosenberg, L. Fruit and vegetable intake in relation to risk of breast cancer in the black women's health study. *Am. J. Epidemiol.* **2010**, *172*, 1268–1279. [CrossRef] [PubMed]

121. Suzuki, R.; Iwasaki, M.; Hara, A.; Inoue, M.; Sasazuki, S.; Sawada, N.; Yamaji, T.; Shimazu, T.; Tsugane, S.; Japan Public Health Center-Based Prospective Study Group. Fruit and vegetable intake and breast cancer risk defined by estrogen and progesterone receptor status: The Japan public health center-based prospective study. *Cancer Causes Control* **2013**, *24*, 2117–2128. [CrossRef] [PubMed]

122. Herr, I.; Buchler, M.W. Dietary constituents of broccoli and other cruciferous vegetables: Implications for prevention and therapy of cancer. *Cancer Treat. Rev.* **2010**, *36*, 377–383. [CrossRef] [PubMed]

123. Mcnaughton, S.A.; Marks, G.C. Development of a food composition database for the estimation of dietary intakes of glucosinolates, the biologically active constituents of cruciferous vegetables. *Br. J. Nutr.* **2003**, *90*, 687–697. [CrossRef]

124. Nugrahedi, P.Y.; Verkerk, R.; Widianarko, B.; Dekker, M. A mechanistic perspective on process-induced changes in glucosinolate content in brassica vegetables: A review. *Crit. Rev. Food Sci. Nutr.* **2015**, *55*, 823–838. [CrossRef] [PubMed]

125. Lamy, E.; Schroder, J.; Paulus, S.; Brenk, P.; Stahl, T.; Mersch-Sundermann, V. Antigenotoxic properties of *Eruca sativa* (rocket plant), erucin and erysolin in human hepatoma (HepG2) cells towards benzo(a)pyrene and their mode of action. *Food Chem. Toxicol.* **2008**, *46*, 2415–2421. [CrossRef]

126. Melchini, A.; Traka, M.H. Biological profile of erucin: A new promising anticancer agent from cruciferous vegetables. *Toxins* **2010**, *2*, 593–612. [CrossRef] [PubMed]

127. Khoobchandani, M.; Ganesh, N.; Gabbanini, S.; Valgimigli, L.; Srivastava, M.M. Phytochemical potential of *Eruca sativa* for inhibition of melanoma tumor growth. *Fitoterapia* **2011**, *82*, 647–653. [CrossRef] [PubMed]

128. Cavaiuolo, M.; Ferrante, A. Nitrates and glucosinolates as strong determinants of the nutritional quality in rocket leafy salads. *Nutrients* **2014**, *6*, 1519–1538. [CrossRef] [PubMed]

129. Barillari, J.; Canistro, D.; Paolini, M.; Ferroni, F.; Pedulli, G.F.; Iori, R.; Valgimigli, L. Direct antioxidant activity of purified glucoerucin, the dietary secondary metabolite contained in rocket (*Eruca sativa* mill.) seeds and sprouts. *J. Agric. Food Chem.* **2005**, *53*, 2475–2482. [CrossRef] [PubMed]

130. Tang, L.; Zirpoli, G.R.; Guru, K.; Moysich, K.B.; Zhang, Y.; Ambrosone, C.B.; Mccann, S.E. Consumption of raw cruciferous vegetables is inversely associated with bladder cancer risk. *Cancer Epidemiol. Biomark. Prev.* **2008**, *17*, 938–944. [CrossRef] [PubMed]

131. Traka, M.; Mithen, R. Glucosinolates, isothiocyanates and human health. *Phytochem. Rev.* **2009**, *8*, 269–282. [CrossRef]

132. Li, F.; Hullar, M.A.; Beresford, S.A.; Lampe, J.W. Variation of glucoraphanin metabolism *in vivo* and *ex vivo* by human gut bacteria. *Br. J. Nutr.* **2011**, *106*, 408–416. [CrossRef] [PubMed]

133. Cramer, J.M.; Teran-Garcia, M.; Jeffery, E.H. Enhancing sulforaphane absorption and excretion in healthy men through the combined consumption of fresh broccoli sprouts and a glucoraphanin-rich powder. *Br. J. Nutr.* **2012**, *107*, 1333–1338. [CrossRef] [PubMed]

134. Dosz, E.B.; Jeffery, E.H. Modifying the processing and handling of frozen broccoli for increased sulforaphane formation. *J. Food Sci.* **2013**, *78*, H1459–H1463. [CrossRef] [PubMed]

135. Bongoni, R.; Steenbekkers, L.P.A.; Verkerk, R.; van Boekel, M.A.J.S.; Dekker, M. Studying consumer behaviour related to the quality of food: A case on vegetable preparation affecting sensory and health attributes. *Trends Food Sci. Technol.* **2013**, *33*, 139–145. [CrossRef]

136. Pasini, F.; Verardo, V.; Cerretani, L.; Caboni, M.F.; D'antuono, L.F. Rocket salad (*Diplotaxis* and *Eruca* spp.) sensory analysis and relation with glucosinolate and phenolic content. *J. Sci. Food Agric.* **2011**, *91*, 2858–2864. [CrossRef] [PubMed]

137. Salvatore, S.; Pellegrini, N.; Brenna, O.V.; del Rio, D.; Frasca, G.; Brighenti, F.; Tumino, R. Antioxidant characterization of some Sicilian edible wild greens. *J. Agric. Food Chem.* **2005**, *53*, 9465–9471. [CrossRef] [PubMed]

138. Yun, H.M.; Ban, J.O.; Park, K.R.; Lee, C.K.; Jeong, H.S.; Han, S.B.; Hong, J.T. Potential therapeutic effects of functionally active compounds isolated from garlic. *Pharmacol. Ther.* **2014**, *142*, 183–195. [CrossRef] [PubMed]

139. Benavides, G.A.; Squadrito, G.L.; Mills, R.W.; Patel, H.D.; Isbell, T.S.; Patel, R.P.; Darley-Usmar, V.M.; Doeller, J.E.; Kraus, D.W. Hydrogen sulfide mediates the vasoactivity of garlic. *Proc. Natl. Acad. Sci. USA* **2007**, *104*, 17977–17982. [CrossRef] [PubMed]

140. Canizares, P.; Gracia, I.; Gomez, L.A.; Garcia, A.; de Argila, C.M.; Boixeda, D.; de Rafael, L. Thermal degradation of allicin in garlic extracts and its implication on the inhibition of the *in vitro* growth of *Helicobacter pylori*. *Biotechnol. Prog.* **2004**, *20*, 32–37. [CrossRef] [PubMed]

141. Lanzotti, V. The analysis of onion and garlic. *J. Chromatogr. A* **2006**, *1112*, 3–22. [CrossRef] [PubMed]

142. Jan, A.T.; Kamli, M.R.; Murtaza, I.; Singh, J.B.; Ali, A.; Haq, Q. Dietary flavonoid quercetin and associated health benefits: An overview. *Food Rev. Int.* **2010**, *26*, 302–317. [CrossRef]

143. Santhosha, S.G.; Jamuna, P.; Prabhavathi, S.N. Bioactive components of garlic and their physiological role in health maintenance: A review. *Food Biosci.* **2013**, *3*, 59–74. [CrossRef]

144. World Cancer Research Fund/American Institute for Cancer Research. *Food, Nutrition, Physical Activity, and the Prevention of Cancer: A Global Perspective*; AICR: Washington, DC, USA, 2007.

145. World Cancer Research Fund/American Institute for Cancer Research. *Continuous Update Project Report. Food, Nutrition, Physical Activity, and the Prevention of Colorectal Cancer*; AICR: Washington, DC, USA, 2011.

146. Jin, Z.Y.; Wu, M.; Han, R.Q.; Zhang, X.F.; Wang, X.S.; Liu, A.M.; Zhou, J.Y.; Lu, Q.Y.; Zhang, Z.F.; Zhao, J.K. Raw garlic consumption as a protective factor for lung cancer, a population-based case-control study in a Chinese population. *Cancer Prev. Res. (Phila.)* **2013**, *6*, 711–718. [CrossRef] [PubMed]

147. Zhou, Y.; Zhuang, W.; Hu, W.; Liu, G.J.; Wu, T.X.; Wu, X.T. Consumption of large amounts of allium vegetables reduces risk for gastric cancer in a meta-analysis. *Gastroenterology* **2011**, *141*, 80–89. [CrossRef] [PubMed]

148. Chiavarini, M.; Minelli, L.; Fabiani, R. Garlic consumption and colorectal cancer risk in man: A systematic review and meta-analysis. *Public Health Nutr.* **2015**, 1–10. [CrossRef] [PubMed]

149. Vazquez-Prieto, M.A.; Miatello, R.M. Organosulfur compounds and cardiovascular disease. *Mol. Aspects Med.* **2010**, *31*, 540–545. [CrossRef] [PubMed]

150. Stabler, S.N.; Tejani, A.M.; Huynh, F.; Fowkes, C. Garlic for the prevention of cardiovascular morbidity and mortality in hypertensive patients. *Cochrane Database Syst. Rev.* **2012**, *8*. [CrossRef]
151. Fleischauer, A.T.; Arab, L. Garlic and cancer: A critical review of the epidemiologic literature. *J. Nutr.* **2001**, *131*, 1032S–1040S. [PubMed]
152. Harris, S.; Brunton, N.; Tiwari, U.; Cummins, E. Human exposure modelling of quercetin in onions (*Allium cepa* L.) following thermal processing. *Food Chem.* **2015**, *187*, 135–139. [CrossRef] [PubMed]
153. Cavagnaro, P.F.; Camargo, A.; Galmarini, C.R.; Simon, P.W. Effect of cooking on garlic (*Allium sativum* L.) antiplatelet activity and thiosulfinates content. *J. Agric. Food Chem.* **2007**, *55*, 1280–1288. [CrossRef] [PubMed]
154. Cavagnaro, P.F.; Galmarini, C.R. Effect of processing and cooking conditions on onion (*Allium cepa* L.) induced antiplatelet activity and thiosulfinate content. *J. Agric. Food Chem.* **2012**, *60*, 8731–8737. [CrossRef] [PubMed]
155. Luo, C.; Zhang, Y.; Ding, Y.; Shan, Z.; Chen, S.; Yu, M.; Hu, F.B.; Liu, L. Nut consumption and risk of type 2 diabetes, cardiovascular disease, and all-cause mortality: A systematic review and meta-analysis. *Am. J. Clin. Nutr.* **2014**, *100*, 256–269. [CrossRef] [PubMed]
156. Afshin, A.; Micha, R.; Khatibzadeh, S.; Mozaffarian, D. Consumption of nuts and legumes and risk of incident ischemic heart disease, stroke, and diabetes: A systematic review and meta-analysis. *Am. J. Clin. Nutr.* **2014**, *100*, 278–288. [CrossRef] [PubMed]
157. Ros, E. Nuts and CVD. *Br. J. Nutr.* **2015**, *113* (Suppl. S2), S111–S120. [CrossRef] [PubMed]
158. Wu, L.; Wang, Z.; Zhu, J.; Murad, A.L.; Prokop, L.J.; Murad, M.H. Nut consumption and risk of cancer and type 2 diabetes: A systematic review and meta-analysis. *Nutr. Rev.* **2015**, *73*, 409–425. [CrossRef] [PubMed]
159. Lopez-Uriarte, P.; Bullo, M.; Casas-Agustench, P.; Babio, N.; Salas-Salvado, J. Nuts and oxidation: A systematic review. *Nutr. Rev.* **2009**, *67*, 497–508. [CrossRef] [PubMed]
160. Alasalvar, C.; Bolling, B.W. Review of nut phytochemicals, fat-soluble bioactives, antioxidant components and health effects. *Br. J. Nutr.* **2015**, *113* (Suppl. S2), S68–S78. [CrossRef] [PubMed]
161. Xie, L.; Bolling, B.W. Characterisation of stilbenes in California almonds (*Prunus dulcis*) by UHPLC-MS. *Food Chem.* **2014**, *148*, 300–306. [CrossRef] [PubMed]
162. Blomhoff, R.; Carlsen, M.H.; Andersen, L.F.; Jacobs, D.R., Jr. Health benefits of nuts: Potential role of antioxidants. *Br. J. Nutr.* **2006**, *96* (Suppl. S2), S52–S60. [CrossRef] [PubMed]
163. Arcan, I.; Yemenicioglu, A. Antioxidant activity and phenolic content of fresh and dry nuts with or without seed coat. *J. Food Compos. Anal.* **2009**, *22*, 184–188. [CrossRef]
164. Tomaino, A.; Martorana, M.; Arcoraci, T.; Monteleone, D.; Giovinazzo, C.; Saija, A. Antioxidant activity and phenolic profile of pistachio (*Pistacia vera* L., variety bronte) seeds and skins. *Biochimie* **2010**, *92*, 1115–1122. [CrossRef]
165. Wijeratne, S.S.; Abou-Zaid, M.M.; Shahidi, F. Antioxidant polyphenols in almond and its coproducts. *J. Agric. Food Chem.* **2006**, *54*, 312–318. [CrossRef]
166. Milbury, P.; Chen, C.-Y.; Kwak, H.-K.; Blumberg, J. Almond skins polyphenolics act synergistically with α-tocopherol to increase the resistance of low-density lipoproteins to oxidation. *Free Radic. Res.* **2002**, *36*, 78–80.
167. Chen, C.Y.; Milbury, P.E.; Lapsley, K.; Blumberg, J.B. Flavonoids from almond skins are bioavailable and act synergistically with vitamins C and E to enhance hamster and human LDL resistance to oxidation. *J. Nutr.* **2005**, *135*, 1366–1373. [PubMed]
168. Berryman, C.E.; Grieger, J.A.; West, S.G.; Chen, C.Y.; Blumberg, J.B.; Rothblat, G.H.; Sankaranarayanan, S.; Kris-Etherton, P.M. Acute consumption of walnuts and walnut components differentially affect postprandial lipemia, endothelial function, oxidative stress, and cholesterol efflux in humans with mild hypercholesterolemia. *J. Nutr.* **2013**, *143*, 788–794. [CrossRef] [PubMed]
169. Amaral, J.S.; Casal, S.; Seabra, R.M.; Oliveira, B.P. Effects of roasting on hazelnut lipids. *J. Agric. Food Chem.* **2006**, *54*, 1315–1321. [CrossRef] [PubMed]
170. Schlormann, W.; Birringer, M.; Bohm, V.; Lober, K.; Jahreis, G.; Lorkowski, S.; Muller, A.K.; Schone, F.; Glei, M. Influence of roasting conditions on health-related compounds in different nuts. *Food Chem.* **2015**, *180*, 77–85. [CrossRef] [PubMed]
171. Bullo, M.; Lamuela-Raventos, R.; Salas-Salvado, J. Mediterranean diet and oxidation: Nuts and olive oil as important sources of fat and antioxidants. *Curr. Top. Med. Chem.* **2011**, *11*, 1797–1810. [CrossRef] [PubMed]

172. Amrein, T.M.; Lukac, H.; Andres, L.; Perren, R.; Escher, F.; Amado, R. Acrylamide in roasted almonds and hazelnuts. *J. Agric. Food Chem.* **2005**, *53*, 7819–7825. [CrossRef] [PubMed]

173. Zhang, G.; Huang, G.; Xiao, L.; Mitchell, A.E. Determination of advanced glycation endproducts by LC-MS/MS in raw and roasted almonds (*Prunus dulcis*). *J. Agric. Food Chem.* **2011**, *59*, 12037–12046. [CrossRef] [PubMed]

174. Uribarri, J.; Woodruff, S.; Goodman, S.; Cai, W.; Chen, X.; Pyzik, R.; Yong, A.; Striker, G.E.; Vlassara, H. Advanced glycation end products in foods and a practical guide to their reduction in the diet. *J. Am. Diet. Assoc.* **2010**, *110*, 911–916. [CrossRef] [PubMed]

175. Mckiernan, F.; Lokko, P.; Kuevi, A.; Sales, R.L.; Costa, N.M.; Bressan, J.; Alfenas, R.C.; Mattes, R.D. Effects of peanut processing on body weight and fasting plasma lipids. *Br. J. Nutr.* **2010**, *104*, 418–426. [CrossRef] [PubMed]

176. Spiller, G.A.; Miller, A.; Olivera, K.; Reynolds, J.; Miller, B.; Morse, S.J.; Dewell, A.; Farquhar, J.W. Effects of plant-based diets high in raw or roasted almonds, or roasted almond butter on serum lipoproteins in humans. *J. Am. Coll. Nutr.* **2003**, *22*, 195–200. [CrossRef] [PubMed]

177. Lin, X.; Wu, J.; Zhu, R.; Chen, P.; Huang, G.; Li, Y.; Ye, N.; Huang, B.; Lai, Y.; Zhang, H.; *et al.* California almond shelf life: Lipid deterioration during storage. *J. Food Sci.* **2012**, *77*, C583–C593. [CrossRef] [PubMed]

178. Ley, S.H.; Sun, Q.; Willett, W.C.; Eliassen, A.H.; Wu, K.; Pan, A.; Grodstein, F.; Hu, F.B. Associations between red meat intake and biomarkers of inflammation and glucose metabolism in women. *Am. J. Clin. Nutr.* **2014**, *99*, 352–360. [CrossRef] [PubMed]

179. Turner-Mcgrievy, G.M.; Wirth, M.D.; Shivappa, N.; Wingard, E.E.; Fayad, R.; Wilcox, S.; Frongillo, E.A.; Hebert, J.R. Randomization to plant-based dietary approaches leads to larger short-term improvements in dietary inflammatory index scores and macronutrient intake compared with diets that contain meat. *Nutr. Res.* **2015**, *35*, 97–106. [CrossRef] [PubMed]

180. Bujnowski, D.; Xun, P.; Daviglus, M.L.; van Horn, L.; He, K.; Stamler, J. Longitudinal association between animal and vegetable protein intake and obesity among men in the United States: The Chicago Western Electric Study. *J. Am. Diet. Assoc.* **2011**, *111*, 1150–1155. [CrossRef] [PubMed]

181. Romaguera, D.; Angquist, L.; Du, H.; Jakobsen, M.U.; Forouhi, N.G.; Halkjaer, J.; Feskens, E.J.; Daphne, L.A.; Masala, G.; Steffen, A.; *et al.* Food composition of the diet in relation to changes in waist circumference adjusted for body mass index. *PLoS ONE* **2011**, *6*, e23384. [CrossRef] [PubMed]

182. Tucker, L.A.; Tucker, J.M.; Bailey, B.; Lecheminant, J.D. Meat intake increases risk of weight gain in women: A prospective cohort investigation. *Am. J. Health Promot.* **2014**, *29*, e43–e52. [CrossRef] [PubMed]

183. Vergnaud, A.C.; Norat, T.; Romaguera, D.; Mouw, T.; May, A.M.; Travier, N.; Luan, J.; Wareham, N.; Slimani, N.; Rinaldi, S.; *et al.* Meat consumption and prospective weight change in participants of the EPIC-PANACEA study. *Am. J. Clin. Nutr.* **2010**, *92*, 398–407. [CrossRef] [PubMed]

184. Fretts, A.M.; Howard, B.V.; Mcknight, B.; Duncan, G.E.; Beresford, S.A.; Mete, M.; Eilat-Adar, S.; Zhang, Y.; Siscovick, D.S. Associations of processed meat and unprocessed red meat intake with incident diabetes: The strong heart family study. *Am. J. Clin. Nutr.* **2012**, *95*, 752–758. [CrossRef] [PubMed]

185. Lajous, M.; Tondeur, L.; Fagherazzi, G.; de Lauzon-Guillain, B.; Boutron-Ruaualt, M.C.; Clavel-Chapelon, F. Processed and unprocessed red meat consumption and incident type 2 diabetes among French women. *Diabetes Care* **2012**, *35*, 128–130. [CrossRef] [PubMed]

186. Mannisto, S.; Kontto, J.; Kataja-Tuomola, M.; Albanes, D.; Virtamo, J. High processed meat consumption is a risk factor of type 2 diabetes in the Alpha-Tocopherol, Beta-Carotene Cancer Prevention study. *Br. J. Nutr.* **2010**, *103*, 1817–1822. [CrossRef] [PubMed]

187. Pan, A.; Sun, Q.; Bernstein, A.M.; Manson, J.E.; Willett, W.C.; Hu, F.B. Changes in red meat consumption and subsequent risk of type 2 diabetes mellitus: Three cohorts of US men and women. *JAMA Intern. Med.* **2013**, *173*, 1328–1335. [CrossRef] [PubMed]

188. Pan, A.; Sun, Q.; Bernstein, A.M.; Schulze, M.B.; Manson, J.E.; Willett, W.C.; Hu, F.B. Red meat consumption and risk of type 2 diabetes: 3 cohorts of US adults and an updated meta-analysis. *Am. J. Clin. Nutr.* **2011**, *94*, 1088–1096. [CrossRef] [PubMed]

189. Steinbrecher, A.; Erber, E.; Grandinetti, A.; Kolonel, L.N.; Maskarinec, G. Meat consumption and risk of type 2 diabetes: The multiethnic cohort. *Public Health Nutr.* **2011**, *14*, 568–574. [CrossRef] [PubMed]

190. Van Woudenbergh, G.J.; Kuijsten, A.; Tigcheler, B.; Sijbrands, E.J.; van Rooij, F.J.; Hofman, A.; Witteman, J.C.; Feskens, E.J. Meat consumption and its association with C-reactive protein and incident type 2 diabetes: The rotterdam study. *Diabetes Care* **2012**, *35*, 1499–1505. [CrossRef] [PubMed]

191. Chen, G.C.; Lv, D.B.; Pang, Z.; Liu, Q.F. Red and processed meat consumption and risk of stroke: A meta-analysis of prospective cohort studies. *Eur. J. Clin. Nutr.* **2013**, *67*, 91–95. [CrossRef] [PubMed]

192. Micha, R.; Wallace, S.K.; Mozaffarian, D. Red and processed meat consumption and risk of incident coronary heart disease, stroke, and diabetes mellitus: A systematic review and meta-analysis. *Circulation* **2010**, *121*, 2271–2283. [CrossRef] [PubMed]

193. Cross, A.J.; Ferrucci, L.M.; Risch, A.; Graubard, B.I.; Ward, M.H.; Park, Y.; Hollenbeck, A.R.; Schatzkin, A.; Sinha, R. A large prospective study of meat consumption and colorectal cancer risk: An investigation of potential mechanisms underlying this association. *Cancer Res.* **2010**, *70*, 2406–2414. [CrossRef] [PubMed]

194. Egeberg, R.; Olsen, A.; Christensen, J.; Halkjaer, J.; Jakobsen, M.U.; Overvad, K.; Tjonneland, A. Associations between red meat and risks for colon and rectal cancer depend on the type of red meat consumed. *J. Nutr.* **2013**, *143*, 464–472. [CrossRef] [PubMed]

195. Ollberding, N.J.; Wilkens, L.R.; Henderson, B.E.; Kolonel, L.N.; le Marchand, L. Meat consumption, heterocyclic amines and colorectal cancer risk: The multiethnic cohort study. *Int. J. Cancer* **2012**, *131*, e1125–e1133. [CrossRef] [PubMed]

196. Parr, C.L.; Hjartaker, A.; Lund, E.; Veierod, M.B. Meat intake, cooking methods and risk of proximal colon, distal colon and rectal cancer: The norwegian women and cancer (NOWAC) cohort study. *Int. J. Cancer* **2013**, *133*, 1153–1163. [CrossRef] [PubMed]

197. Ruder, E.H.; Thiebaut, A.C.; Thompson, F.E.; Potischman, N.; Subar, A.F.; Park, Y.; Graubard, B.I.; Hollenbeck, A.R.; Cross, A.J. Adolescent and mid-life diet: Risk of colorectal cancer in the NIR-AARP diet and health study. *Am. J. Clin. Nutr.* **2011**, *94*, 1607–1619. [CrossRef] [PubMed]

198. Takachi, R.; Tsubono, Y.; Baba, K.; Inoue, M.; Sasazuki, S.; Iwasaki, M.; Tsugane, S.; Japan Public Health Center-Based Prospective Study Group. Red meat intake may increase the risk of colon cancer in Japanese, a population with relatively low red meat consumption. *Asia Pac. J. Clin. Nutr.* **2011**, *20*, 603–612. [PubMed]

199. Alexander, D.D.; Miller, A.J.; Cushing, C.A.; Lowe, K.A. Processed meat and colorectal cancer: A quantitative review of prospective epidemiologic studies. *Eur. J. Cancer Prev.* **2010**, *19*, 328–341. [CrossRef] [PubMed]

200. Bastide, N.M.; Pierre, F.H.; Corpet, D.E. Heme iron from meat and risk of colorectal cancer: A meta-analysis and a review of the mechanisms involved. *Cancer Prev. Res. (Phila.)* **2011**, *4*, 177–184. [CrossRef] [PubMed]

201. Chan, D.S.; Lau, R.; Aune, D.; Vieira, R.; Greenwood, D.C.; Kampman, E.; Norat, T. Red and processed meat and colorectal cancer incidence: Meta-analysis of prospective studies. *PLoS ONE* **2011**, *6*, e20456. [CrossRef] [PubMed]

202. Spencer, E.A.; Key, T.J.; Appleby, P.N.; Dahm, C.C.; Keogh, R.H.; Fentiman, I.S.; Akbaraly, T.; Brunner, E.J.; Burley, V.; Cade, J.E.; *et al.* Meat, poultry and fish and risk of colorectal cancer: Pooled analysis of data from the UK dietary cohort consortium. *Cancer Causes Control* **2010**, *21*, 1417–1425. [CrossRef] [PubMed]

203. Major, J.M.; Cross, A.J.; Watters, J.L.; Hollenbeck, A.R.; Graubard, B.I.; Sinha, R. Patterns of meat intake and risk of prostate cancer among African-Americans in a large prospective study. *Cancer Causes Control* **2011**, *22*, 1691–1698. [CrossRef] [PubMed]

204. Sinha, R.; Park, Y.; Graubard, B.I.; Leitzmann, M.F.; Hollenbeck, A.; Schatzkin, A.; Cross, A.J. Meat and meat-related compounds and risk of prostate cancer in a large prospective cohort study in the United States. *Am. J. Epidemiol.* **2009**, *170*, 1165–1177. [CrossRef] [PubMed]

205. Stirban, A.; Gawlowski, T.; Roden, M. Vascular effects of advanced glycation endproducts: Clinical effects and molecular mechanisms. *Mol. Metab.* **2014**, *3*, 94–108. [CrossRef] [PubMed]

206. Alaejos, M.S.; Afonso, A.M. Factors that affect the content of heterocyclic aromatic amines in foods. *Compr. Rev. Food Sci. Food Saf.* **2011**, *10*, 52–108. [CrossRef]

207. Kim, E.; Coelho, D.; Blachier, F. Review of the association between meat consumption and risk of colorectal cancer. *Nutr. Res.* **2013**, *33*, 983–994. [CrossRef] [PubMed]

208. Fu, Z.; Deming, S.L.; Fair, A.M.; Shrubsole, M.J.; Wujcik, D.M.; Shu, X.O.; Kelley, M.; Zheng, W. Well-done meat intake and meat-derived mutagen exposures in relation to breast cancer risk: The Nashville breast health study. *Breast Cancer Res. Treat.* **2011**, *129*, 919–928. [CrossRef] [PubMed]

209. Rabstein, S.; Bruning, T.; Harth, V.; Fischer, H.P.; Haas, S.; Weiss, T.; Spickenheuer, A.; Pierl, C.; Justenhoven, C.; Illig, T.; *et al*. N-acetyltransferase 2, exposure to aromatic and heterocyclic amines, and receptor-defined breast cancer. *Eur. J. Cancer Prev.* **2010**, *19*, 100–109. [CrossRef] [PubMed]

210. Ananthakrishnan, A.N.; Du, M.; Berndt, S.I.; Brenner, H.; Caan, B.J.; Casey, G.; Chang-Claude, J.; Duggan, D.; Fuchs, C.S.; Gallinger, S.; *et al*. Red meat intake, NAT2, and risk of colorectal cancer: A pooled analysis of 11 studies. *Cancer Epidemiol. Biomark. Prev.* **2015**, *24*, 198–205. [CrossRef] [PubMed]

211. Lee, H.J.; Wu, K.; Cox, D.G.; Hunter, D.; Hankinson, S.E.; Willett, W.C.; Sinha, R.; Cho, E. Polymorphisms in xenobiotic metabolizing genes, intakes of heterocyclic amines and red meat, and postmenopausal breast cancer. *Nutr. Cancer* **2013**, *65*, 1122–1131. [CrossRef] [PubMed]

212. Cross, A.J.; Freedman, N.D.; Ren, J.; Ward, M.H.; Hollenbeck, A.R.; Schatzkin, A., Sinha, R.; Abnet, C.C. Meat consumption and risk of esophageal and gastric cancer in a large prospective study. *Am. J. Gastroenterol.* **2011**, *106*, 432–442. [CrossRef] [PubMed]

213. Luevano-Contreras, C.; Chapman-Novakofski, K. Dietary advanced glycation end products and aging. *Nutrients* **2010**, *2*, 1247–1265. [CrossRef] [PubMed]

214. Poulsen, M.W.; Hedegaard, R.V.; Andersen, J.M.; de Courten, B.; Bugel, S.; Nielsen, J.; Skibsted, L.H.; Dragsted, L.O. Advanced glycation endproducts in food and their effects on health. *Food Chem. Toxicol.* **2013**, *60*, 10–37. [CrossRef] [PubMed]

215. Perrone, L.; Grant, W.B. Observational and ecological studies of dietary advanced glycation end products in national diets and Alzheimer's disease incidence and prevalence. *J. Alzheimers Dis.* **2015**, *45*, 965–979. [PubMed]

216. Van Puyvelde, K.; Mets, T.; Njemini, R.; Beyer, I.; Bautmans, I. Effect of advanced glycation end product intake on inflammation and aging: A systematic review. *Nutr. Rev.* **2014**, *72*, 638–650. [CrossRef] [PubMed]

217. Vlassara, H.; Striker, G.E. Age restriction in diabetes mellitus: A paradigm shift. *Nat. Rev. Endocrinol.* **2011**, *7*, 526–539. [CrossRef] [PubMed]

218. Uribarri, J.; Cai, W.; Ramdas, M.; Goodman, S.; Pyzik, R.; Chen, X.; Zhu, L.; Striker, G.E.; Vlassara, H. Restriction of advanced glycation end products improves insulin resistance in human type 2 diabetes: Potential role of AGER1 and SIRT1. *Diabetes Care* **2011**, *34*, 1610–1616. [CrossRef] [PubMed]

219. Srikanth, V.; Maczurek, A.; Phan, T.; Steele, M.; Westcott, B.; Juskiw, D.; Munch, G. Advanced glycation endproducts and their receptor RAGE in Alzheimer's disease. *Neurobiol. Aging* **2011**, *32*, 763–777. [CrossRef] [PubMed]

220. West, R.K.; Moshier, E.; Lubitz, I.; Schmeidler, J.; Godbold, J.; Cai, W.; Uribarri, J.; Vlassara, H.; Silverman, J.M.; Beeri, M.S. Dietary advanced glycation end products are associated with decline in memory in young elderly. *Mech. Ageing Dev.* **2014**, *140*, 10–12. [CrossRef] [PubMed]

221. Cai, W.; Uribarri, J.; Zhu, L.; Chen, X.; Swamy, S.; Zhao, Z.; Grosjean, F.; Simonaro, C.; Kuchel, G.A.; Schnaider-Beeri, M.; *et al*. Oral glycotoxins are a modifiable cause of dementia and the metabolic syndrome in mice and humans. *Proc. Natl. Acad. Sci. USA* **2014**, *111*, 4940–4945. [CrossRef] [PubMed]

222. Jiao, L.; Stolzenberg-Solomon, R.; Zimmerman, T.P.; Duan, Z.; Chen, L.; Kahle, L.; Risch, A.; Subar, A.F.; Cross, A.J.; Hollenbeck, A.; *et al*. Dietary consumption of advanced glycation end products and pancreatic cancer in the prospective NIH-AARP diet and health study. *Am. J. Clin. Nutr.* **2015**, *101*, 126–134. [CrossRef] [PubMed]

223. Pasquali, R. Quality of diet, screened by the Mediterranean diet quality index and the evaluation of the content of advanced glycation endproducts, in a population of high school students from Emilia Romagna. *Mediterr. J. Nutr. Metab.* **2010**, *3*, 153–157.

224. Ledl, F.; Schleicher, E. New aspects of the maillard reaction in foods and in the human body. *Angew. Chem. Int. Ed.* **1990**, *29*, 565–594. [CrossRef]

225. Hull, G.L.J.; Woodside, J.V.; Ames, J.M.; Cuskelly, G.J. N^ϵ-((carboxymethyl)lysine content of foods commonly consumed in a western style diet. *Food Chem.* **2012**, *131*, 170–174. [CrossRef]

226. Busquets, R.; Puignou, L.; Galceran, M.T.; Skog, K. Effect of red wine marinades on the formation of heterocyclic amines in fried chicken breast. *J. Agric. Food Chem.* **2006**, *54*, 8376–8384. [CrossRef] [PubMed]

227. Gibis, M. Effect of oil marinades with garlic, onion, and lemon juice on the formation of heterocyclic aromatic amines in fried beef patties. *J. Agric. Food Chem.* **2007**, *55*, 10240–10247. [CrossRef] [PubMed]

228. Gibis, M.; Weiss, J. Antioxidant capacity and inhibitory effect of grape seed and rosemary extract in marinades on the formation of heterocyclic amines in fried beef patties. *Food Chem.* **2012**, *134*, 766–774. [CrossRef] [PubMed]

229. Persson, E.; Graziani, G.; Ferracane, R.; Fogliano, V.; Skog, K. Influence of antioxidants in virgin olive oil on the formation of heterocyclic amines in fried beefburgers. *Food Chem. Toxicol.* **2003**, *41*, 1587–1597. [CrossRef]

230. Romero, C.; García, A.; Medina, E.; Ruíz-Méndez, M.V.; de Castro, A.; Brenes, M. Triterpenic acids in table olives. *Food Chem.* **2010**, *118*, 670–674. [CrossRef]

231. Wang, Z.H.; Hsu, C.C.; Huang, C.N.; Yin, M.C. Anti-glycative effects of oleanolic acid and ursolic acid in kidney of diabetic mice. *Eur. J. Pharmacol.* **2010**, *628*, 255–260. [CrossRef] [PubMed]

232. Castellano, J.M.; Guinda, A.; Delgado, T.; Rada, M.; Cayuela, J.A. Biochemical basis of the antidiabetic activity of oleanolic acid and related pentacyclic triterpenes. *Diabetes* **2013**, *62*, 1791–1799. [CrossRef] [PubMed]

233. Navarro, M.; Fiore, A.; Fogliano, V.; Morales, F.J. Carbonyl trapping and antiglycative activities of olive oil mill wastewater. *Food Funct.* **2015**, *6*, 574–583. [CrossRef] [PubMed]

234. Wu, C.H.; Huang, S.M.; Lin, J.A.; Yen, G.C. Inhibition of advanced glycation endproduct formation by foodstuffs. *Food Funct.* **2011**, *2*, 224–234. [CrossRef] [PubMed]

235. Vitaglione, P.; Monti, S.M.; Ambrosino, P.; Skog, K.; Fogliano, V. Carotenoids from tomatoes inhibit heterocyclic amine formation. *Eur. Food Res. Technol.* **2002**, *215*, 108–113. [CrossRef]

236. Britt, C.; Gomaa, E.A.; Gray, J.I.; Booren, A.M. Influence of cherry tissue on lipid oxidation and heterocyclic aromatic amine formation in ground beef patties. *J. Agric. Food Chem.* **1998**, *46*, 4891–4897. [CrossRef]

237. Melo, A.; Viegas, O.; Eca, R.; Petisca, C.; Pinho, O.; Ferreira, I.M.P.L.V.O. Extraction, detection, and quantification of heterocyclic aromatic amines in portuguese meat dishes by HPLC/Diode array. *J. Liquid Chromatogr. Relat. Technol.* **2008**, *31*, 772–787. [CrossRef]

238. Chen, X.M.; Kitts, D.D. Antioxidant and anti-inflammatory activities of maillard reaction products isolated from sugar-amino acid model systems. *J. Agric. Food Chem.* **2011**, *59*, 11294–11303. [CrossRef] [PubMed]

239. Norat, T.; Aune, D.; Chan, D.; Lau, R.; Veira, R. *The Associations between Food, Nutrition and Physical Activity and the Risk of Colorectal Cancer*; Wcrf/Aicr Systematic Literature Review Continuous Update Project Report; AICR: Washington, DC, USA, 2010.

240. United Nations Educational, Scientific and Cultural Organization. Representative List of the Intangible Cultural Heritage of Humanity. Available online: http://www.unesco.org/culture/ich/ rl/00884 (accessed on 13 July 2015).

241. Ortega, R. Importance of functional foods in the Mediterranean diet. *Public Health Nutr.* **2006**, *9*, 1136–1140. [CrossRef] [PubMed]

242. Bellisle, F. Infrequently asked questions about the Mediterranean diet. *Public Health Nutr.* **2009**, *12*, 1644–1647. [CrossRef] [PubMed]

243. Tessier, S.; Gerber, M. Comparison between Sardinia and Malta: The Mediterranean diet revisited. *Appetite* **2005**, *45*, 121–126. [CrossRef] [PubMed]

244. Bach-Faig, A.; Berry, E.M.; Lairon, D.; Reguant, J.; Trichopoulou, A.; Dernini, S.; Medina, F.X.; Battino, M.; Belahsen, R.; Miranda, G.; et al. Mediterranean diet pyramid today. Science and cultural updates. *Public Health Nutr.* **2011**, *14*, 2274–2284. [CrossRef] [PubMed]

245. Richter, C.K.; Skulas-Ray, A.C.; Kris-Etherton, P.M. Recent findings of studies on the Mediterranean diet: What are the implications for current dietary recommendations? *Endocrinol. Metab. Clin. N. Am.* **2014**, *43*, 963–980. [CrossRef] [PubMed]

246. Rothwell, J.A.; Perez-Jimenez, J.; Neveu, V.; Medina-Remon, A.; M'hiri, N.; Garcia-Lobato, P.; Manach, C.; Knox, C.; Eisner, R.; Wishart, D.S.; et al. Phenol-explorer 3.0: A major update of the phenol-explorer database to incorporate data on the effects of food processing on polyphenol content. *Database (Oxf.)* **2013**, *2013*. [CrossRef] [PubMed]

247. Zamora-Ros, R.; Knaze, V.; Rothwell, J.A.; Hemon, B.; Moskal, A.; Overvad, K.; Tjonneland, A.; Kyro, C.; Fagherazzi, G.; Boutron-Ruault, M.C.; et al. Dietary polyphenol intake in Europe: The European prospective investigation into cancer and nutrition (EPIC) study. *Eur. J. Nutr.* **2015**. [CrossRef] [PubMed]

248. Trichopoulou, A.; Costacou, T.; Bamia, C.; Trichopoulos, D. Adherence to a Mediterranean diet and survival in a Greek population. *N. Engl. J. Med.* **2003**, *348*, 2599–2608. [CrossRef] [PubMed]

249. Panagiotakos, D.B.; Pitsavos, C.; Stefanadis, C. Dietary patterns: A Mediterranean diet score and its relation to clinical and biological markers of cardiovascular disease risk. *Nutr. Metab. Cardiovasc. Dis.* **2006**, *16*, 559–568. [CrossRef] [PubMed]

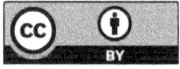

nutrients

MDPI

Article

Interpreting the Australian Dietary Guideline to "Limit" into Practical and Personalised Advice

Flavia Fayet-Moore * and Suzanne Pearson

Nutrition Research Australia, Level 13 167 Macquarie St, Sydney 2000, Australia; suzanne@nraus.com
* Author to whom correspondence should be addressed; flavia@nraus.com;
   Tel.: +61-2-8667-3072; Fax: +61-2-8667-3200.

Received: 2 February 2015; Accepted: 6 March 2015; Published: 20 March 2015

Abstract: Food-based dietary guidelines shift the focus from single nutrients to whole diet. Guideline 3 of the Australian Dietary Guidelines (ADG) recommends "limiting" discretionary foods and beverages (DF)—Those high in saturated fat, added sugars, salt, and/or alcohol. In Australia, DF contribute 35% of total energy intake. Using the ADG supporting documents, the aim of this study was to develop a food-based educational toolkit to help translate guideline 3 and interpret portion size. The methodology used to produce the toolkit is presented here. "Additional energy allowance" is specific to gender, age, height and physical activity level, and can be met from core foods, unsaturated fats/oils/spreads and/or DF. To develop the toolkit, additional energy allowance was converted to serves equaling 600 kJ. Common DF were selected and serves were determined based on nutrient profile. Portion sizes were used to calculate number of DF serves. A consumer brochure consisting of DF, portion sizes and equivalent number of DF serves was developed. A healthcare professional guide outlines the methodology used. The toolkit was designed to assist dietitians and consumers to translate guideline 3 of the ADF and develop a personalized approach to include DF as part of the diet.

Keywords: dietary guidelines; discretionary foods; ready reckoner; dietary advice

1. Introduction

Dietary guidelines provide health professionals, policy makers and the public with evidence-based recommendations that promote health and wellbeing and reduce chronic disease risk. They are developed to guide food choices to optimize nutrient intake and improve eating patterns. In recent years, there has been a shift away from nutrient-based recommendations to considering whole foods in the context of total diet and food intake patterns. Globally, food-based dietary guidelines (FBDG) have been promoted as an important part of national food and nutrition policies [1–3]. Dietary patterns proposed by FBDG help individuals meet their nutrient intakes by recommending intake of nutrient-dense foods and limiting intake of nutrient-poor foods. In order to be effective in optimizing health, there is a need for FBDG to be translated and personalized to facilitate compliance and ultimately behaviour change. Personalization of dietary advice can serve to empower individuals to make dietary changes relevant to them [4]. It is important that the behavior change be maintained. To implement FBDGs, the joint FAO/WHO consultation report recommends providing a qualitative version for the public and supporting quantitative materials aimed at dietitians and policy-makers [5].

FBDG typically include recommendations around nutrient-dense foods and beverages, *i.e.*, those that are high in fat, sugar, salt and alcohol. The general consensus is to "limit", "avoid", "reduce" or consume these foods and beverages "sometimes" or "occasionally". For example, guideline 3 of the Australian dietary guidelines (ADG; Table 1) advises Australians to limit intake of foods containing saturated fat, added salt, added sugars and alcohol [6]. Similarly, Americans are told to consume fewer foods with sodium, saturated fats, trans fats, cholesterol, added sugars, and refined grains [7]; the Eat Well Plate of the UK suggests consuming just a small amount of high fat/sugar foods [8]; Canadians are guided to limit foods and beverages high in calories, fat, sugar or salt (sodium) [9]; and several European countries, including Switzerland, Austria and Luxemburg, recommend limiting intake of saturated fat, sugar and salt but do not quantify this recommendation [3]. While the advice is sound, its meaning can be lost in the absence of quantitative guidance. How exactly does one interpret terms like "limit", "small amounts" and "sometimes" to translate them into meaningful, personalized advice?

Table 1. Guideline 3 of the 2013 Australian dietary guidelines [6].

Limit intake of foods containing saturated fat, added salt, added sugars and alcohol.

a.   Limit intake of foods high in saturated fat such as many biscuits, cakes, pastries, pies, processed meats, commercial burgers, pizza, fried foods, potato chips, crisps and other savoury snacks.
   ● Replace high-fat foods, which contain predominantly saturated fats such as butter, cream, cooking margarine, coconut and palm oil with foods, which contain predominantly polyunsaturated and monounsaturated fats such as oils, spreads, nut butters/pastes and avocado.
   ● Low-fat diets are not suitable for children under the age of 2 years.

b.   Limit intake of foods and drinks containing added salt.
   ● Read labels to choose lower sodium options among similar foods.
   ● Do not add salt to foods in cooking or at the table.

c.   Limit intake of foods and drinks containing added sugars such as confectionary, sugar-sweetened soft drinks and cordials, fruit drinks, vitamin waters, energy and sports drinks.
d.   If you choose to drink alcohol, limit intake. For women who are pregnant, planning a pregnancy or breastfeeding, not drinking alcohol is the safest option.

In the U.S., these nutrient-dense foods and beverages are considered foods and food components to reduce [7]; in Australia they are termed "discretionary foods" (DF) as they do not fit into the Five Food Groups, or core food groups of the ADG and are not needed to meet nutrient requirements. DF are not an essential part of dietary patterns. Nevertheless, as acknowledged by the ADG, "they [DF] can contribute to the overall enjoyment of eating, often in the context of social activities and family or cultural celebrations." Being part of the Australian diet, the ADG advise DF can be included occasionally if energy needs allow but that they should always be considered "extras" in the context of energy requirements and when selecting a healthy eating pattern [10]. Consumers are encouraged to check the nutrition information panel found on packaged foods and beverages to determine what amount of food contains 600 kJ and examples of DF are offered. However, there is no specific guidance on how many choices can be included in the diet of an individual based on their age, gender, height and physical activity level nor clear cut-offs or guidelines for what constitutes a DF.

There is a gap between dietary recommendations and actual consumer behaviour and compliance with the guidelines is generally poor. According to the most recent data from the 2011 to 2012 National Nutrition and Physical Activity Survey, Australians are consuming less vegetables, fruits, grains and dairy than recommended, while DF contribute 35% and 39% of the total daily energy intake for adults ($\geq$19 year) and children and adolescents (<18 year), respectively [11]. Comparatively, DF contributed 36% of daily energy intake of adults and 41% of energy intake of children and adolescents [12] in the nationally representative 1995 National Nutrition Survey (NNS) and 35% [13] in the 2007 Australian National Children's Nutrition and Physical Activity Survey for children. Similarly, the majority of the US population did not meet recommendations for all of the nutrient-rich food groups, except total grains and meat and beans. Concomitantly, overconsumption of energy from solid fats, added sugars, and alcoholic beverages was ubiquitous. Over 80% of adults 71-years and over, and 90% of all other sex-age groups had intakes exceeding the discretionary calorie allowances [14].

A dietary guideline implementation strategy is as equally important as the development of the evidence-base that inform the guidelines. The need for effective communications to assist in translating

Nutrients **2015**, *7*, 2026–2043

the recommendations into practical, actionable advice is widely acknowledged and has been included as part of the release of guidelines globally [2,5,15,16].

There is a need to develop food-based resources to assist in translating dietary recommendations into practice. With approximately 60% of Australian adults overweight and more than 25% obese [11], this is especially important when it comes to nutrient-dense DF. Therefore, the aim of this research was to develop a food-based educational toolkit to help dietitians and consumers translate guideline 3 of the ADG. Specifically, to calculate the maximum number of DF serves that can be included as part of the diet based on gender, age, height and physical activity level, and to provide guidance on the number of serves of common DF and their portion size.

2. Experimental Section

2.1. Resources Used

The ADG [6] and the following supporting documents were used to develop the toolkit:

(i) *A Modelling System to Inform the Revision of the Australian Guide to Healthy Eating (Modelling System)* [17]—A technical document that translates the nutrient reference values into dietary models. It describes the amounts of various foods needed to meet the estimated nutrient requirements of groups of Australian individuals of different age, gender and physical activity level.

(ii) *Eat for Health Educator Guide* [10]—Developed for dietitians, nutritionists, primary and secondary school teachers and other health educators with the aim of discussing food choices that minimise the risk of developing diet-related conditions and to contribute to overall health in the long term.

(iii) *The Eat for Health website* [18]—The online platform for the ADG.

2.2. Determining how DF Fit into the Diet: The "Additional Serves" Toolkit

To determine where DF fit into the diet, the *"Foundation Diets"* and *"Total Diets"* dietary models of the Modelling System were used. These diets demonstrate that while nutritional needs are met through the whole diet and not by single foods, the combination of foods is critical. The *Foundation Diets* are the dietary patterns that meet the nutrient and energy requirements for the smallest, youngest and least active individuals in each age and gender group accounting for chronic disease, food supply and social and cultural constraints. In addition to including foods from the Five Food groups (grain foods; vegetables and legumes/beans; fruit; lean meats and poultry, fish, eggs, tofu and nuts; milk, yoghurt, cheese and alternatives), or core foods of the ADG, an allowance for unsaturated fats, oils and spreads was used in the development of the *Foundation Diets*. The *Total Diets* provide a range of flexible options to add to the *Foundation Diets* to meet the higher energy requirements of people of varying body size and higher physical activity levels (PAL). Thus, the *Total Diets* includes the *Foundation Diets* and an "additional energy allowance". DF were considered in modelling *Total Diets* so that any "additional energy allowance" can be consumed from foods of the Five Food groups, unsaturated fats, oils and spreads and/or DF (Table 2).

Table 2. Rationale for determining how "discretionary foods" (DF) fit into the diet.

Total Diet = Foundation Diet + Additional Energy Allowance	
❖Meets energy & nutrient needs	✦ Age ✦ Height ✦ PAL
Five food groups	Five food groups
Unsaturated fats/oils/spread	Unsaturated fats/oils/spreads AND/OR ✓ Discretionary foods

2.3. Ready Reckoner

In order to develop the toolkit, the additional energy allowance had to be translated into additional serves. A ready reckoner (RR) was developed based on age, gender, height (for adults only) and physical activity level specific to additional serves so that dietitians and nutritionists could quickly determine maximum daily DF intake.

One additional serve was defined as the kilojoule content of a DF serve from the ADG (*i.e.*, 600 kJ; 143 kcal). Additional serves were calculated by dividing the additional energy allowance provided in the Educator Guide (Appendix) by 600 kJ (143 kcal) and rounding to the nearest whole number. For example, 1200 kJ (287 kcal) equals 2 serves.

Additional serves are based on gender, age, height (for adults only) and physical activity levels. The age and height categories for the RR were obtained from the Educator Guide. Adults were grouped into the following age bands: 19–30 years, 31–50 years, 51–70 years and >70 years. Height bands ranged from 160 cm to 190 cm for males and 150 cm to 180 cm for females. For children, an energy (kJ) value was provided for each single age between 2- and 18-years, independent of height. As there was a discrepancy in the terminology used to describe physical activity levels between the ADG, the Educator Guide and the Modelling System, a consistent definition based on those described on the Eat for Health website was established. Physical activity categories from the additional energy allowance tables were converted to those described online (Table 3).

Table 3. Physical activity categories for the ready reckoner (RR).

Educators Guide Additional Energy Tables	Modelling System Physical Activity Levels (PAL)	RR Physical Activity Categories	RR Physical Activity Definitions
Inactive	Very sedentary (PAL 1.4)	Sedentary	Sedentary work and no strenuous leisure activities (e.g., an office worker who drives to and from work and spends most of their leisure time sitting or standing).
Light	Light to moderate (PAL 1.5–1.7)	Light	Mostly sedentary work with little or no strenuous leisure activity (e.g., an office worker who only occasionally exercises (once or twice a week), lab assistants or drivers).
Moderate		Moderate	Moderately active work, predominantly standing or walking (e.g., waiters, shop assistants or teachers).
High	Heavy occupational or high activity (PAL 2.0)	Vigorous	Heavy activity (e.g., tradesperson or high performance athlete).

2.4. Consumer Brochure

A consumer-friendly brochure was developed to be used with the RR. The brochure outlines the number of additional serves in common DF and their equivalent portion size. To develop the consumer brochure it was necessary to define DF, group examples of popular DFs into simple, consumer-friendly categories and determine their typical serving sizes.

The ADG provides examples of DF, but no clear cut-offs for foods containing saturated fat, added salt and/or added sugars are described; except for alcohol, which is easily identified.

The Modelling System describes DF as "higher-fat", "higher-sugar" and "low energy density" but does not quantify these descriptors. For the purposes of the toolkit, DF inclusion criteria were defined based on the nutrient composition in the Modelling System:

Low fibre ($\leq$10 g/100 g)
High fibre (>10 g/100 g)
Low fat ($\leq$15 g/100 g)
High fat (>15 g/100 g)
High sugar (>30 g sugar; >35 g sugar if contains fruit per 100 g)
High sodium (>1000 mg/100 g)

All foods and beverages explicitly mentioned in any of the ADG documents as discretionary were automatically included as DF (*i.e.*, fruit drinks, honey, bacon, meat pies, cakes, chocolate, ice cream, muesli bar, and all alcoholic beverages). Only foods that were not part of the Five Food groups, or core foods, were assessed. Considering the cut-offs in the Modelling System, other popular foods and beverages were analyzed for nutrient composition using NUTTAB2010 [19], the most recent reference database from Food Standards Australia New Zealand at the time of this analysis, that contains data on the nutrient content of Australian foods. Their inclusion in the DF list was determined using the Modelling System cut-offs and by popularity of consumption. For example, banana cake was chosen over black forest cake and a croissant was chosen over apple strudel. Total fat, saturated fat, total sugars and sodium per 100 g were recorded for each DF under each category. Foods and beverages high in sugars were assessed by a dietitian to determine if they were typical sources of added sugars; those high in fat were assessed for their saturated fat content.

The DF list was then organized into consumer-friendly categories that reflect the current food supply. Food group terminology from NUTTAB2010 and online supermarket categories were used. A total of 10 DF groups and 72 foods and beverages were included. Examples of foods and beverages within each group are presented in Table 4.

Table 4. DF groups and examples of foods and beverages within each group.

Discretionary Food (DF) Group	Foods and Beverages	
Deli meats	Streaky bacon, fat not trimmed Ham, fat not trimmed (Prosciutto) Sliced luncheon meats (e.g., Mortadella)	Salami Sausages (including continental and frankfurter)
Take-away and frozen foods	Meat pie Sausage roll Dim sim (dumplings), spring roll, Pizza	Hamburger Hot chips Creamy style quiche (e.g., quiche Lorraine)
Confectionary	Chocolate bar/blocks Chocolate coated bars or wafers Chocolate coated fruit/nuts	Lollies/sugar confectionary Rocky road Jelly snakes
Dessert foods	Chocolate pudding Chocolate mousse Pavlova	Ice cream (regular fat) Ice blocks (fruit-juice based) Ice block, chocolate coated, cream-based
Sweet biscuits and bars	Plain biscuits Chocolate coated biscuits	Cream-filled biscuits Muesli or breakfast bars Puffed rice bars
Bakery products	Lamingtons Sponge cake (cream and jam-filled) Chocolate cake with icing Banana cake Cheesecake Fruit cake/pie	Sweet muffins Doughnuts Slices (e.g., caramel/chocolate/coconut) Fudge Cupcakes
Savoury foods and snacks	Potato crisps Corn chips Cheese rings	Savoury flavoured crackers Buttered popcorn Cracker/pea mixes and noodle snacks
Sauces, syrups, spreads and dips	Tomato sauce or other (e.g., sweet chilli, BBQ) Cream salad dressings Chocolate hazelnut spreads Honey/maple syrups/golden syrup	Jams Butter Cream (e.g., whipped, thickened *etc.*) Creamy dips (e.g., French onion)
Alcoholic beverages	Full strength beer (5%) Mid strength beer (3.5%) and light beer (2.1%) Red wine White wine/sparkling white wine	Spirits Cocktails Alcopop Cider
Non-alcoholic beverages	Sports drink Vitamin water Soft drink/diet soft drink	Fruit drink/iced tea Cordial/diet cordial Energy drink

As serve size remains consistent and portion size changes, the tool was developed to reflect real portion sizes as consumed. For each DF, a typical serve size was determined using the portion sizes of those foods as depicted by Food Works Professional [20] and in their corresponding consumer smartphone application Easy Diet Diary [21]—Two dietary recall tools commonly used by dietitians and nutritionists in Australia, as well as consumers.

Portion size for each DF in each category was recorded in grams, and the energy (kJ) content for all DF were calculated. In addition, a small, medium and large portion size for two specific DF (hot chips and muffin) were calculated to depict the effect that portion has on number of DF serves.

The kilojoule content of each DF portion was divided by 600 kJ and mathematically rounded to the nearest 0.5 to convert it to a serve. For example, chocolate pudding has 1272 kJ/100 g; one portion equals one "regular serve" or 90 g. There are 1145 kJ per regular serve; divided by 600 kJ equals 1.91, or 2 DF serves.

2.5. Healthcare Professional Guide

The healthcare professional guide details the ADG guideline 3 and explains additional serves. Included in the toolkit is a step-by-step guide detailing how to use the educational materials. It describes the RR and client brochure, suggests steps on how to use the toolkit and provides an example case study.

3. Results

The Additional Serves toolkit consists of three resources:

1. *The Additional Serves Ready Reckoner*
2. A consumer brochure describing "*How discretionary foods fit into a healthy diet*"

3.   A *Health Professional Guide to Additional Serves Resources*

The *Additional Serves Ready Reckoner (RR)* is used to estimate the additional serves allowance (Figure 1). Applying gender, age, height and physical activity level, the RR readily provides a maximum daily number of additional serves that can be selected from the Five Foods groups, or core foods, unsaturated fats/oils/spreads and/or DF.

A separate RR was developed for adults and for children and adolescents. When using the RR, if a client falls between two height bands, then the serves can be estimated as a value between the two corresponding values. Additional serves are recommended to meet additional energy requirements only for people who are taller or more physically active. Additional serves, and therefore a DF allowance, are not recommended for those who are overweight or who fall in the shortest, least active category. Children and adolescents who are overweight or obese are encouraged to adhere to the Foundation Diets and avoid additional serves in order to maintain body weight while the child grows in height, thus "normalizing" BMI for age.

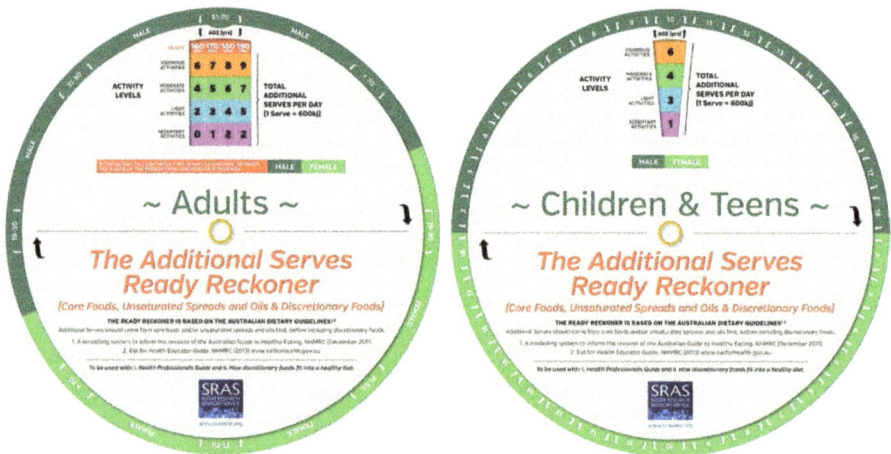

Figure 1. The additional serves ready reckoner.

The physical activity measure of the RR is reflective of occupation, or usual daily physical activity, rather than planned physical activity. Thus, an individual could step up to the next physical activity category if they exercise 30 to 60 min, 4 to 5 times a week.

To accompany the RR, a consumer brochure describing *"How discretionary foods fit into a healthy diet"* was developed to assist consumers in understanding how many DF serves are contained in common portions of DF (Figure 2). The consumer brochure was designed as an interactive educational tool and can be personalized to help encourage consumers to assess their DF intake relative to their maximum allowance. The brochure depicts 72 foods and beverages in 10 categories and states the equivalent number of DF for a typical portion size. It includes a descriptor of each DF and its equivalent portion size in grams or mL and using common household measures (e.g., 1 can/375 mL; 2–3 small/10 g; 1 regular bucket/100 g). Two sections called *"Portion distortion: How portion size impacts on DF serves"* illustrate the food/beverage, energy content (kJ) and total number of DF serves for that portion size. For example, hot chips are illustrated as small (1 small bucket—70 g; 720 kJ), medium (1 regular bucket/100 g; 1028 kJ) and large (1 large bucket—240 g; 2467 kJ); corresponding to 1, $1\frac{1}{2}$ and 4 DF serves. The consumer brochure includes *"Healthy Lifestyle Tips"*, which outline four key recommendations from the Eat for Health website [18] on how to *"Get more active"*, *"Get portion size right"* *"Eat mindfully"* and *"Be prepared when away from home"*.

The *Health Professional Guide to Additional Serves Resources* was developed to assist dietitians in using the RR and the accompanying consumer brochure to translate the guideline "to limit" into practical and ersonalized advice (Figure 3). It includes information on guideline 3 of the ADG, explains how to use the additional serves resources and provides an example as a case study.

3.1. How to Use the Additional Serves Resources

Applying gender, age, height and physical activity level to the RR results in a number ranging from 0 to 11. The number is not a recommendation, rather it provides the maximum number of additional serves that can be included in the diet per day providing a starting point for personalized dietary recommendations based on an individual food habits, needs and goals. Additional serves should preferably be consumed as core foods and/or unsaturated fats/oils/spreads over DF [10].

The following is the step-by-step process suggested to dietitians when using the RR:

1. Assess how many and how much (*i.e.*, portion size) DF serves the client is currently consuming.
2. Use the RR to calculate number of additional serves based on age, height and physical activity level. Depending on the client, the number of DF serves can be averaged for those individuals who fall between two height bands. DF serves are not recommended for those who are overweight or obese.
3. Make recommendations of how the additional serves can be met using a combination of core foods, unsaturated fats/oils/spreads and/or DF serves. It is important to highlight how portion size impacts greatly on kilojoules and DF serves.

3.2. Case Study

A 35-year-old woman, 170 cm tall and very active (*i.e.*, high activity) requires an extra 4100 kJ, or 7 additional serves, per day to meet her dietary needs. These additional serves can be consumed through intake of core foods, unsaturated fats/oils/spreads and/or DF. For example, 4 × grains (3.5 serves), 2 × fruit (1 serve), 1 × starchy vegetable (0.5 serve), 1 × legume (0.5 serve), 1 × salad vegetable (0.5 serve) and 1 × DF (1 serve) or any other preferred combination at the discretion of the healthcare professional and/or consumer based on dietary patterns and preferences.

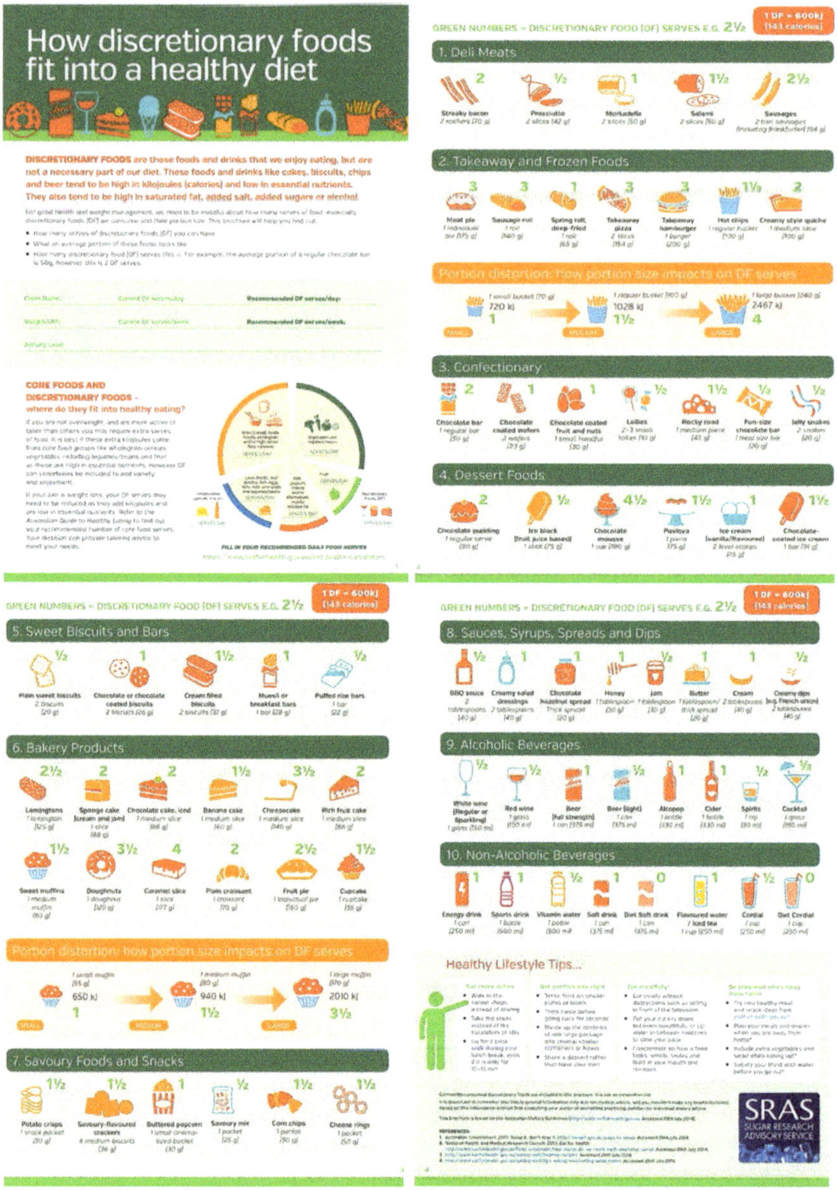

Figure 2. Consumer brochure.

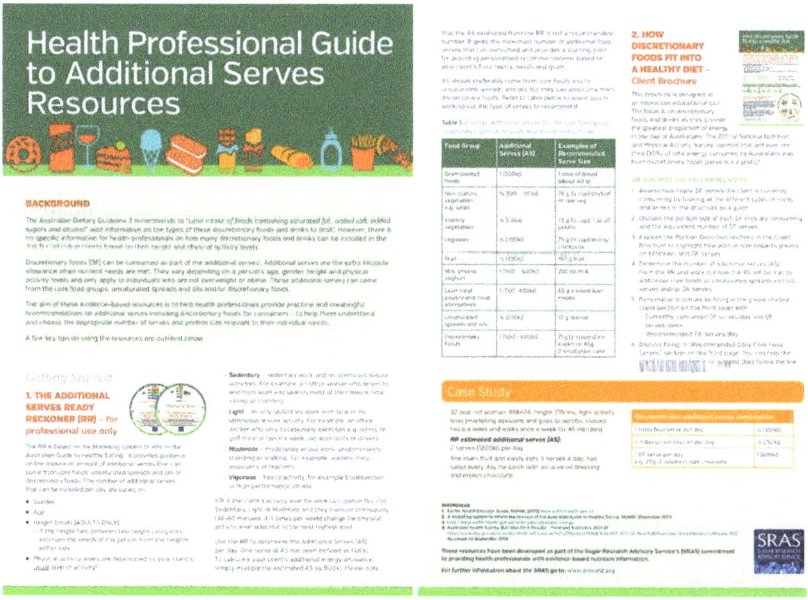

Figure 3. Health professional guide to additional serves resources

4. Discussion

A food-based educational toolkit that helps translates guideline 3 of the ADG into practical, actionable advice was developed. The toolkit includes a RR, a consumer brochure and a healthcare professional guide, and is used to estimate the additional serves allowance of an individual accounting for their gender, age, height and physical activity level. To our knowledge, this is the first tool of its kind; designed to assist dietitians start the dialogue and offer personalized, food-based advice on incorporating DF into the diet. It is intended that providing realistic targets to help consumers understand how to include DF into their diet will support behaviour change. With approximately 60% of Australians overweight and DF contributing 35% and 39% of the total daily energy intake of adults and children and adolescents, respectively, consumers need practical advice on how to translate "limit", "avoid", "reduce", or consume these foods and beverages "sometimes" or "occasionally".

DF have a place within the diets of Australians; however, when DF displace nutrient-rich core foods they can affect the nutrient profile of the diet and influence weight. Energy from nutrient-poor foods such as cookies, candy and sugar-sweetened beverages was shown to be more closely related to body mass index (kg/m^2) than fruit and vegetable consumption or physical activity suggesting these types of foods and beverages are important targets for obesity prevention campaigns [22]. In a cluster analysis using diet history data from two clinical weight loss trials, correcting exposure to DF was shown to be key to successful weight loss in individuals with a dietary pattern characterised by non-core foods and drinks, higher- and medium-fat dairy foods, fatty meats and alcohol. Subjects who reportedly consumed larger amounts of these foods and beverages at baseline were able to alter their dietary pattern more successfully to achieve an energy deficit [23]. Therefore, adequately quantifying DF and ensuring advice is given specifically regarding these foods within the diet prescription may increase awareness of appropriate food choices and portion size, and assist with compliance [23].

The toolkit not only determines how many additional serves can be included as part of a well-balanced diet but also provides guidance on where those additional serves should come from (*i.e.*, from one of the five core food groups, from unsaturated fats/oils/spreads or from DF). Offering individuals more choice can empower them to make decisions about their diet that work for them and foster compliance. While the ADG provide general recommendations for a population, the RR tailors advice to the individual that may facilitate dietary change.

FBDG worldwide include implementation strategies that attempt to translate recommendations into consumer-friendly advice. The ADG are complemented by a website that provides resources to support educators and consumers with implementing the recommendations, advice and tips on eating well, and calculators that estimate energy and nutrient needs and the number of serves to meet recommendations [18]. In the United States, federal agencies, regional and state offices, food assistance programs, food and health organization and local community educators communicate messages and implement guidance based on the 2010 dietary guidelines for Americans. Resources to help communicate the dietary guidelines, including consumer messages, tools, and educational materials, are also available at various websites, including ChooseMyPlate.gov and healthfinder.gov. Consumers are offered daily food plans, a BMI calculator and tips on healthy eating and on how to reduce certain foods and beverages (e.g., "Compare sodium in foods like soup, bread, and frozen meals and choose the foods with lower numbers." "Drink water instead of sugary drinks") [24]. The Chilean implementation strategy included the development of written educational materials and training for health professionals on using and communicating the dietary guidelines to the public [2]. The National Institute of Nutrition in India produced booklets, leaflets, posters and folders with emphasis on pictorial representation of the messages to coincide with the release of their food-based dietary guidelines [16]. And the Ministry of Health in Malaysia organized a series of advocacy and training workshops for nutritionists and other health care professionals, as well as the food industry, in an effort to widely disseminate their guidelines. Activities included provision of educational materials, seminars and workshops, as well as road shows and exhibitions at the community level [25].

Despite the well-recognised importance of translating dietary guidelines into practical advice for consumers, there is little research conducted in this area. Instead research considers population compliance to dietary recommendations rather than developing strategies to assist behaviour change [16,26–30]. "The need for translating the evidence into real behaviour change has never been greater, as has the need for appropriate communications to the public [31]."

The toolkit not only provides consumers with a personalized target intake for DF but it may assist with consumer education on how portion size and physical activity influence additional energy allowance. Advocating portion-control can be an effective strategy for weight loss. Obese adults were more likely to achieve and maintain meaningful weight loss when limiting portion sizes [32]. And obese children found a portion-controlled diet easier to follow compared with a reduced-carbohydrate diet [33].

Physical activity has also been shown as a successful intervention for weight loss and weight maintenance [4,34]. As age, gender and height are independent variables in the toolkit, it is physical activity level that has the greatest impact on the additional serves allowance. Although the physical activity category is based on occupation, the fact that a higher physical activity category results in a higher additional serves allowance may be one way of encouraging consumers to exercise more in order to include DF into their diets.

While every attempt was made to ensure accuracy in developing the RR, modelling of dietary intake has inherent limitations. All values were rounded, including height estimation, the additional energy allowance values given by the ADG, the kilojoule content of DF and the values for serves. Despite being derived from estimates, the RR provides consumers with a numerical understanding of the total additional serves that will fit into their diet per day based on variables relevant to them. Importantly, throughout development of the RR, it was tested on a group of 6 dietitians and advice was sought from both the Dietitians Association of Australia and the Australian Government Department of Health.

As with any implementation strategy, there is a need for the tool to be evaluated for effectiveness among dietitians and to be assessed for its impact on the actual eating behaviour in the general population. Efficacy cannot be determined in the absence of monitoring and critical evaluation.

Further research is needed to evaluate the effectiveness of the resource. Ideally, this would include some measure of dietary change by the individual.

5. Conclusions

In conclusion, this toolkit was designed to assist dietitians and consumers to translate guideline 3 of the ADG and develop a personalized approach to include DF as part of the diet.

Acknowledgments: A research grant from the Australian Sugar Alliance was provided for this work. Appetite Communications assisted with the development of the resource into a consumer-friendly toolkit.

Author Contributions: Flavia Fayet-Moore conducted the research, developed the information for the toolkit design and content, liaised with Appetite Communications, drafted and revised the manuscript. Suzanne Pearson conducted background research, assisted in drafting the manuscript, revised and reviewed the manuscript.

Appendix A

Table A1. Additional serves by age, gender and physical activity levels—Boys.

Age (Years)	Very Sedentary (PAL 1.4)		Sedentary		Moderate		Vigorous (PAL 2.0)	
	Per Day	Per Week	Per Day	Per Week	Per Day	Per Week	Per Day	Per Week
2	0	0	1	7	2	14	3	21
3	1	7	1	8	2	16	3	23
4	0	0	1	8	2	16	4	25
5	1	4	2	12	3	21	4	30
6	1	7	2	16	4	26	5	35
7	2	11	3	21	4	30	6	41
8	2	14	4	25	5	35	7	47
9	0	0	2	12	3	23	5	34
10	1	6	3	18	4	29	6	42
11	2	11	3	23	5	36	7	49
12	0	0	2	13	4	27	6	40
13	1	6	3	21	5	35	7	49
14	0	0	2	15	4	30	7	46
15	1	7	3	22	6	39	8	55
16	2	12	4	29	7	46	9	63
17	2	16	5	34	7	51	10	69
18	3	19	5	37	8	55	11	74

Table A2. Additional serves by age, gender and physical activity levels—Girls.

Age (Years)	Very Sedentary (PAL 1.4)		Sedentary		Moderate		Vigorous (PAL 2.0)	
	Per Day	Per Week	Per Day	Per Week	Per Day	Per Week	Per Day	Per Week
2	0	0	1	7	2	14	3	21
3	1	7	1	9	2	15	3	22
4	0	0	1	8	2	15	3	23
5	1	4	2	11	3	20	4	28
6	1	7	2	15	4	25	5	33
7	2	11	3	20	4	29	6	39
8	2	14	4	25	5	34	6	44
9	0	0	2	11	3	21	5	32
10	1	4	2	14	4	25	5	36
11	1	7	3	19	4	30	6	42
12	0	0	2	13	4	25	6	37
13	1	5	3	18	4	30	6	43
14	0	0	2	13	4	26	6	40
15	0	1	2	15	4	29	6	42
16	1	4	2	16	4	30	6	44
17	1	4	3	18	5	32	7	46
18	1	5	3	19	5	33	7	47

Table A3. Additional serves by age, gender and physical activity levels—Adult males.

Age (years)	Height (cm)	Very Sedentary (PAL 1.4)		Sedentary		Moderate		Vigorous (PAL 2.0)	
		Per Day	Per Week	Per Day	Per Week	Per Day	Per Week	Per Day	Per Week
19–30	160	0	0	2	15	4	30	7	46
	170	1	8	3	23	6	40	8	56
	180	2	15	5	33	7	50	10	68
	190	4	25	6	42	9	61	11	79
31–50	160	0	0	2	15	4	29	6	44
	170	1	6	3	21	5	37	8	53
	180	2	12	4	28	6	44	9	62
	190	3	18	5	35	8	53	10	70
51–70	160	0	0	2	13	4	26	6	39
	170	1	5	3	19	5	34	7	48
	180	2	11	4	26	6	41	8	57
	190	2	16	5	34	7	49	9	65
>70	160	0	0	2	12	4	25	5	36
	170	1	6	3	19	5	32	7	46
	180	2	12	4	26	6	40	8	54
	190	3	19	5	34	7	48	9	63

Table A4. Additional serves by age, gender and physical activity levels—Adult females.

Age (Years)	Height (cm)	Very Sedentary (PAL 1.4)		Sedentary		Moderate		Vigorous (PAL 2.0)	
		Per Day	Per Week	Per Day	Per Week	Per Day	Per Week	Per Day	Per Week
19–30	150	0	0	2	13	4	25	5	36
	160	1	7	3	20	5	33	7	47
	170	2	15	4	29	6	43	8	57
	180	3	22	5	37	8	53	10	68
31–50	150	0	0	2	13	4	25	5	36
	160	1	4	2	16	4	29	6	42
	170	1	8	3	21	5	35	7	48
	180	2	12	4	26	6	40	8	54
51–70	150	0	0	2	12	3	23	5	34
	160	1	5	2	16	4	28	6	41
	170	1	8	3	21	5	34	6	44
	180	2	13	4	26	6	40	8	53
>70	150	0	0	2	11	3	21	5	33
	160	1	5	2	15	4	27	6	39
	170	1	8	3	21	5	33	6	44
	180	2	14	4	26	6	39	7	51

Conflicts of Interest: The authors declare a perceived conflict of interest resulting from the financial support of the research from the Australian Sugar Alliance. The Australian Sugar Alliance had no influence in this research.

References

1. Brown, K.A.; Timotijevic, L.; Barnett, J.; Shepherd, R.; Lahteenmaki, L.; Raats, M.M. A review of consumer awareness, understanding and use of food-based dietary guidelines. *Br. J. Nutr.* **2011**, *106*, 15–26. [CrossRef] [PubMed]

2. Keller, I.; Lang, T. Food-based dietary guidelines and implementation: Lessons from four countries—Chile, Germany, New Zealand and South Africa. *Public Health Nutr.* **2008**, *11*, 867–874. [CrossRef] [PubMed]

3. WHO. *Food Based Dietary Guidelines in the WHO European Region*; WHO Regional Office: Copenhagen, Denmark, 2003.

4. Ramage, S.; Farmer, A.; Eccles, K.A.; McCargar, L. Healthy strategies for successful weight loss and weight maintenance: A systematic review. *Appl. Physiol. Nutr. Metab.* **2014**, *39*, 1–20. [CrossRef] [PubMed]

5. WHO. *Preparation and Use of Food-Based Dietary Guidelines*; Report of a Joint FAO/WHO Consultation; World Health Organization: Geneva, Switzerland, 1998; Volume 880, pp. 1–108.

6. NHMRC. *Australian Dietary Guidelines*; National Health and Medical Research Council: Canberra, Australia, 2013.

7. USDA; HSS. *Dietary Guidelines for Americans*; U.S. Department of Agriculture and U.S. Department of Health and Human Services: Washington, DC, USA, 2010.

8. NHS. The Eatwell Plate. Available onlie: http://www.nhs.uk/livewell/goodfood/pages/eatwell-plate.aspx (accessed on 13 October 2014).

9. Canada's Food Guide. Available online: http://www.hc-sc.gc.ca/fn-an/food-guide-aliment/index-eng.php (accessed on 13 October 2014).

10. NHMRC. *Eat for Health Educator Guide: Information for Nutrition Educators*; Department of Health and Ageing, National Health and Medical Research Council: Canberra, Australia, 2013.

11. ABS. *Australian Health Survey: First Results, 2011–2012*; Australian Bureau of Statistics: Canberra, Australia, 2014.

12. Rangan, A.M.; Schindeler, S.; Hector, D.J.; Gill, T.P.; Webb, K.L. Consumption of "extra" foods by australian adults: Types, quantities and contribution to energy and nutrient intakes. *Eur. J. Clin. Nutr.* **2009**, *63*, 865–871. [CrossRef] [PubMed]

13. Rangan, A.M.; Kwan, J.; Flood, V.M.; Louie, J.C.; Gill, T.P. Changes in "extra" food intake among australian children between 1995 and 2007. *Obes. Res. Clin. Pract.* **2011**, *5*, e1–e78. [CrossRef] [PubMed]

14. Krebs-Smith, S.M.; Guenther, P.M.; Subar, A.F.; Kirkpatrick, S.I.; Dodd, K.W. Americans do not meet federal dietary recommendations. *J. Nutr.* **2010**, *140*, 1832–1838. [CrossRef] [PubMed]

15. Dwyer, J.T. Nutrition guidelines and education of the public. *J. Nutr.* **2001**, *131*, 3074S–3077S. [PubMed]

16. Krishnaswamy, K. Developing and implementing dietary guidelines in india. *Asia Pac. J. Clin. Nutr.* **2008**, *17* (Suppl. S1), 66–69.

17. NHMRC. *A Modelling System to Inform the Revision of the Australian Guide to Healthy Eating*; National Health and Medical Research Council: Canberra, Australia, 2011.

18. NHMRC. Eat for Health. Available online: http://eatforhealth.gov.au (accessed on 13 October 2014).

19. FANZ. NUTTAB 2010—Food Standards Australia New Zeland. Available onlie: http://www.foodstandards. gov.au/science/monitoringnutrients/nutrientables/pages/default.asp (accessed on 12 November 2014).

20. Xyris. Foodworks Professional Edition. Available online: www.xyris.com.au/Foodworks (accessed on 12 November 2014).

21. Xyris. Easy Diet Diary Application. Available online: http://support.easydietdiary.com/hc/en-us (accessed on 12 November 2014).

22. Cohen, D.A.; Sturm, R.; Lara, M.; Gilbert, M.; Gee, S. Discretionary calorie intake a priority for obesity prevention: Results of rapid participatory approaches in low-income US communities. *J. Public Health* **2010**, *32*, 379–386. [CrossRef]

23. Grafenauer, S.J.; Tapsell, L.C.; Beck, E.J.; Batterham, M.J. Baseline dietary patterns are a significant consideration in correcting dietary exposure for weight loss. *Eur. J. Clin. Nutr.* **2013**, *67*, 330–336. [CrossRef] [PubMed]

24. USDA. Choosemyplate. Available online: http://www.choosemyplate.gov (accessed 13 October 2014).

25. Tee, E.S. Development and promotion of Malaysian dietary guidelines. *Asia Pac. J. Clin. Nutr.* **2011**, *20*, 455–461. [PubMed]

26. Brennan, D.S.; Singh, K.A. Compliance with dietary guidelines in grocery purchasing among older adults by chewing ability and socio-economic status. *Gerodontology* **2012**, *29*, 265–271. [CrossRef] [PubMed]

27. Kachan, D.; Lewis, J.E.; Davila, E.P.; Arheart, K.L.; LeBlanc, W.G.; Fleming, L.E.; Caban-Martinez, A.J.; Lee, D.J. Nutrient intake and adherence to dietary recommendations among US workers. *J. Occup. Environ. Med.* **2012**, *54*, 101–105. [CrossRef] [PubMed]

28. Knudsen, V.K.; Fagt, S.; Trolle, E.; Matthiessen, J.; Groth, M.V.; Biltoft-Jensen, A.; Sorensen, M.R.; Pedersen, A.N. Evaluation of dietary intake in Danish adults by means of an index based on food-based dietary guidelines. *Food Nutr. Res.* **2012**, *56*. [CrossRef]

29. Maillot, M.; Drewnowski, A. A conflict between nutritionally adequate diets and meeting the 2010 dietary guidelines for sodium. *Am. J. Prev. Med.* **2012**, *42*, 174–179. [CrossRef] [PubMed]

30. Russell, J.; Flood, V.; Rochtchina, E.; Gopinath, B.; Allman-Farinelli, M.; Bauman, A.; Mitchell, P. Adherence to dietary guidelines and 15-year risk of all-cause mortality. *Br. J. Nutr.* **2013**, *109*, 547–555. [CrossRef] [PubMed]

31. Rowe, S.; Alexander, N.; Almeida, N.; Black, R.; Burns, R.; Bush, L.; Crawford, P.; Keim, N.; Kris-Etherton, P.; Weaver, C. Food science challenge: Translating the dietary guidelines for Americans to bring about real behavior change. *J. Food Sci.* **2011**, *76*, 29–37. [CrossRef]

32. Abildso, C.G.; Schmid, O.; Byrd, M.; Zizzi, S.; Quartiroli, A.; Fitzpatrick, S.J. Predictors of weight loss maintenance following an insurance-sponsored weight management program. *J. Obes.* **2014**, *2014*. [CrossRef]

33. Kirk, S.; Brehm, B.; Saelens, B.E.; Woo, J.G.; Kissel, E.; D'Alessio, D.; Bolling, C.; Daniels, S.R. Role of carbohydrate modification in weight management among obese children: A randomized clinical trial. *J. Pediatr.* **2012**, *161*, 320–327. [CrossRef] [PubMed]
34. Nicklas, J.M.; Huskey, K.W.; Davis, R.B.; Wee, C.C. Successful weight loss among obese US adults. *Am. J. Prev. Med.* **2012**, *42*, 481–485. [CrossRef]

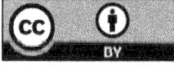

nutrients

MDPI

Article

Development of a Food Group-Based Diet Score and Its Association with Bone Mineral Density in the Elderly: The Rotterdam Study

Ester A. L. de Jonge [1,2], Jessica C. Kiefte-de Jong [1,3,*], Lisette C. P. G. M. de Groot [4], Trudy Voortman [1], Josje D. Schoufour [1], M. Carola Zillikens [2], Albert Hofman [1], André G. Uitterlinden [1,2], Oscar H. Franco [1] and Fernando Rivadeneira [2]

[1] Department of Epidemiology, Erasmus MC, University Medical Centre, P.O. box 2040, 3000 CA Rotterdam, The Netherlands; E-Mails: e.a.l.dejonge@erasmusmc.nl (E.A.L.J.); trudy.voortman@erasmusmc.nl (T.V.); j.schoufour@erasmusmc.nl (J.D.S.); a.hofman@erasmusmc.nl (A.H.); a.g.uitterlinden@erasmusmc.nl (A.G.U.); o.franco@erasmusmc.nl (O.H.F.)

[2] Department of Internal Medicine, Erasmus MC, University Medical Centre, P.O. box 2040, 3000 CA Rotterdam, The Netherlands; E-Mails: m.c.zillikens@erasmusmc.nl (M.C.Z.); f.rivadeneira@erasmusmc.nl (F.R.)

[3] Department of Global Public Health, Leiden University College The Hague, P.O. box 13228, 2501 EE The Hague, The Netherlands

[4] Department of Human Nutrition, Wageningen University, P.O. box 8129, 6700 EV Wageningen, The Netherlands; E-Mail: Lisette.deGroot@wur.nl

* Author to whom correspondence should be addressed; E-Mail: j.c.kiefte-dejong@erasmusmc.nl; Tel.: +31-10-7043536; Fax: +31-10-7044657.

Received: 9 June 2015 / Accepted: 11 August 2015 / Published: 18 August 2015

Abstract: No diet score exists that summarizes the features of a diet that is optimal for bone mineral density (BMD) in the elderly. Our aims were (a) to develop a BMD-Diet Score reflecting a diet that may be beneficial for BMD based on the existing literature, and (b) to examine the association of the BMD-Diet Score and the Healthy Diet Indicator, a score based on guidelines of the World Health Organization, with BMD in Dutch elderly participating in a prospective cohort study, the Rotterdam Study (n = 5144). Baseline dietary intake, assessed using a food frequency questionnaire, was categorized into food groups. Food groups that were consistently associated with BMD in the literature were included in the BMD-Diet Score. BMD was measured repeatedly and was assessed using dual energy X-ray absorptiometry. The BMD-Diet Score considered intake of vegetables, fruits, fish, whole grains, legumes/beans and dairy products as "high-BMD" components and meat and confectionary as "low-BMD" components. After adjustment, the BMD-Diet Score was positively associated with BMD (β (95% confidence interval) = 0.009 (0.005, 0.012) g/cm^2 per standard deviation). This effect size was approximately three times as large as has been observed for the Healthy Diet Indicator. The food groups included in our BMD-Diet Score could be considered in the development of future dietary guidelines for healthy ageing.

Keywords: dietary patterns; bone mineral density; BMD-Diet score; healthy diet indicator

1. Introduction

Osteoporosis, characterized by low bone mineral density (BMD), is a major determinant of fracture risk and can lead to a decreased quality of life and loss of independency in the elderly [1]. An important and modifiable risk factor for osteoporosis is an inadequate diet [2]. Although studies on single nutrients, such as calcium and Vitamin D, have provided important insights on the relationship between diet and bone health [3], investigating full dietary patterns has additional benefits because additive or antagonistic nutrient-interactions might occur [4]. Two main approaches of dietary pattern identification can be distinguished. The first is an *a posteriori* approach, in which statistical data reduction techniques, such as factor or cluster analysis, are used to identify dietary patterns in a specific population [4]. This approach can be particularly useful to identify the local and existing dietary patterns as they are shaped by a variety of lifestyle factors, including individual preferences and beliefs, cultural traditions, and food availability and affordability [5]. Second, an *a priori* approach can be used, in which diet scores or diet indices are developed based on current knowledge from literature and guidelines.

Examples of diet scores are the Alternate Healthy Eating Index (AHEI) and the Recommended Food Score (RFS), which reflect diet quality based on the Dietary Guidelines for Americans and the food guide pyramid developed by researchers at the US Department of Agriculture. However, these scores were recently shown not to be associated with BMD in pre-menopausal women [6]. Accordingly, it may be argued that existing dietary scores based on existing dietary recommendations may not fully capture or consider foods that influence bone health.

Adherence to the dietary guidelines of the World Health Organization (WHO) [1] has been translated into the Healthy Diet Indicator (HDI) by Jankovic *et al.*, (2014) [7]. This score reflects the overall quality of a subject's diet based on single nutrients (e.g., sodium) and some food groups (e.g., fruits and vegetables). The guidelines, and therefore the score, were developed based on existing evidence on dietary intake and chronic diseases, which included limited data from osteoporosis-related studies [1]. Moreover, as dietary guidelines are in transition to become food-group-based rather than nutrient-based, it would be valuable to develop a BMD-Diet Score based on the intake of food groups. By deriving these food groups from full dietary pattern analyses, this BMD-Diet Score might account for potential nutrient interactions. Eventually, it might serve the development of future food-group-based guidelines that sufficiently account for bone health.

In the present study, the first aim was to develop a BMD-Diet Score reflecting an overall diet that may be beneficial for BMD based on a narrative review of previously published *a priori* and *a posteriori* dietary pattern analyses on BMD. A second aim was to examine the association of the BMD-Diet Score and the Healthy Diet Indicator, a diet score based on current dietary guidelines of the WHO, with measured BMD and to compare these associations.

2. Experimental Section

2.1. Study Population

This study was embedded in the Rotterdam Study I (RS-I-1), a prospective cohort study among subject from the Ommoord district in Rotterdam, the Netherlands. Participants were elderly males and females of 55 years and older at baseline (1989–1993). Details on the design and main objectives of the Rotterdam Study have been published elsewhere [8]. The Rotterdam Study has been approved by the institutional review board (Medical Ethics Committee, MEC 89.230) of the Erasmus Medical Center and by the review board of The Netherlands Ministry of Health, Welfare and Sports [8]. Written informed consent was obtained from all subjects.

2.2. Dietary Assessment

All participants were interviewed at baseline for food intake assessment using an extensive semi-quantitative food frequency questionnaire (FFQ) at the study center, administered by a trained dietician. The questionnaire was validated and adapted for use in the elderly [9,10]. It consists of 170 food items and questions about dietary habits. The ability of the FFQ to rank subjects adequately according to their dietary intakes was demonstrated by results from a validation study comparing the FFQ to 15-day food records collected over a year to cover all seasons. Pearson's correlation coefficients of this comparison ranged from 0.4 to 0.8 after adjustment for sex, age, total energy intake, and within-person variability in daily intakes [9]. The dietary intake of nutrients was calculated using the Dutch Food Composition Database (NEVO) from 1993 and 2006.

2.3. Development of the BMD-Diet Score

We searched PubMed for publications (through March 2015) on studies examining the relationship between dietary patterns and BMD using the following search terms: "Dietary patterns" OR "diet score" AND "bone" OR "BMD" OR "osteoporosis". Studies included dietary patterns, derived by either cluster or factor analysis, or dietary indices as exposure and bone mineral density or loss thereof, or osteoporosis as outcome in adult populations. Selected studies on single food groups, single dietary nutrients or nutrient biomarkers as exposure and outcomes other than bone mineral density or osteoporosis were excluded. Furthermore, we excluded specific diseased populations, such as celiac disease patients and studies in children (because their dietary patterns may differ of those from adults and they are still undergoing bone accrual). We only considered original research (observational and experimental) and no case reports.

We extracted food groups from dietary patterns and labelled them as "high-BMD" or "low-BMD" food groups if significant associations ($p < 0.05$) were reported with high or low BMD, respectively. Characterization as well as labelling of dietary patterns derived by principal component analysis was based on their factor loadings, which represent the correlation between the food groups and the dietary patterns. However, different studies might use different factor loading- thresholds. Because not all studies reported smaller factor loadings, we only included food groups with a factor loading of >0.3 for positively correlated food groups and <−0.3 for negatively correlated food groups. Next, we created bar charts presenting the count of dietary patterns in which any of these food groups occurred. Only those with the highest frequency of occurrence (>25th percentile of cumulative count) were included for the BMD-Diet Score. The direction of the association (favorable or unfavorable) was considered consistent when more than two thirds (67%) of the studies showed an effect in the same direction. Only food groups with consistent associations with BMD were included in the BMD-Diet Score.

For each participant, the newly developed BMD-Diet Score was calculated as follows: first, dietary intake of all relevant food groups was categorized into quartiles. Next, each subject was assigned ascending values (1,2,3,4) for food groups that are assumed to increase BMD and descending values (4,3,2,1) for those assumed to decrease BMD, based on their quartiles of intakes. Only if the distribution of intake of a food group did not allow computation of quartiles (e.g., for groups with a high number of non-consumers such as legumes and beans), values were dichotomized. Intake of alcoholic beverages was not included in the BMD-Diet Score but considered a potential confounder in our analysis, because the relationship with BMD might be non-linear [11,12].

2.4. Computation of HDI, Based on Dietary Guidelines of the WHO

The computation of the HDI for each participant was based on WHO dietary guidelines of 2003. Briefly, the HDI consists of 12 dietary components, of which 5 are recommended to be consumed in moderation: saturated fatty acids (SFA), mono-and disaccharides, cholesterol, trans fat and sodium, three components which are recommened to consume within a specific range: polyunsaturated fatty acids (PUFAs), protein, total fat, *n*-6 PUFAs and *n*-3 PUFAs, and two components for which an adequate intake is recommended: dietary fiber and fruits and vegetables. Cut-offs and more detailed information regarding the scoring system are presented in Table 1. The HDI is coded as a continuous variable, proportionally ranging from 10 to 0 between the optimal intake and the lower or upper limit respectively per component. Therefore, the theoretical range of HDI is 0 to 120.

Table 1. Cut-offs used for computation of the Healthy Diet Indicator (HDI) (Jankovic, 2014 [7], adapted).

Components of the Healthy Diet Indicator	Lower Limit 0 Points	Optimal Intake * 10 Points	Upper Limit ** 0 Points
Moderation (unfavorable) components			
Saturated fatty acids	N.A.	<10	>15
Monosaccharides and disaccharides	N.A.	<10	>30
Cholesterol	N.A.	<300	>400
Trans fatty acids	N.A.	<1	>1.5
Sodium (grams, not sodium chloride)	N.A.	<2	>3.0
Moderation range components			
Polyunsaturated fatty acids (PUFAs)	0	6 to 10	>10
Protein	0	10 to 15	>20
Total fat	0	15 to 30	> 43
Moderation range components			
n-6 PUFA	0	5 to 8	>8.5
n-3 PUFA	0	1 to 2	N.A. **
Adequacy (favorable) components			
Dietary fiber (g)	0	>25	N.A.
Fruits and vegetables (g)	0	>400	N.A.

*: Representing the World Health Orgnization (WHO) recommendation; ** For *n*-3 PUFA's no upper level could be calculated as the 85th percentile of intake falls within the range of optimal intake in our population; Abbreviations: N.A. = not applicable, PUFA = polyunsaturated fatty acid; The Healthy Diet Indicator (HDI) is coded as a continuous variable, proportionally ranging from 10 to 0 between the optimal intake and the lower or upper limit respectively.

2.5. Assessment of BMD

BMD of the femoral neck was measured by dual energy X-ray absorptiometry (DXA) using a Lunar DPX- densitometer (Lunar Radiation Corp., Madison, WI, USA) at baseline (1989–1993) and at 3 subsequent visits (1993–1995, 1997–1999 and 2002–2004). DXA scans were analyzed with DPX-IQ software (v.4.7d) and BMD values are expressed in g/cm^2. A flowchart showing the numbers of subjects with available BMD data for each visit is shown in Figure S1.

2.6. Assessment of Covariates

We included covariates related to body composition, lifestyle, socioeconomic status (SES), prevalent metabolic diseases, use of medication and other indicators of overall health, of which the majority was assessed at baseline (1989–1993). Body height and weight were measured at the research center at baseline and three follow up visits (1993–1995, 1997–1999 and 2002–2004). Regarding lifestyle factors, smoking at baseline was calculated as "current" or "past or never". Physical activity was assessed at the 3rd visit (1997–1999), using the Zutphen Study Physical Activity Questionnaire including questions on walking, cycling, gardening, diverse sports, hobbies, and housekeeping [13–15]. Total time spend on physical activity was calculated by the sum of minutes per week for each type of activity. Dietary intake of alcoholic beverages and calcium were derived from the FFQ. Baseline use of any dietary supplement was assessed during the home interview, without specific questions on dose or duration and coded as "never" or "ever". Highest education and net household income were used as proxy for SES. Education was coded as "low" (primary education, primary + higher not completed, lower vocational and lower secondary education) or "high" (intermediate vocational, general secondary, higher vocational education and university). Household income was coded "above" or "below" the average of 2400 net Dutch Guilders (≈1600 Euro) per month. Regarding prevalent diseases at baseline, type 2 diabetes mellitus was determined as baseline serum glucose concentrations >11 mmol/L or use of glucose lowering drugs and cardiovascular disease included prevalent coronary heart disease, heart failure, stroke and arterial fibrillation at baseline. Methods of data collection and definitions of cardiac outcomes in the Rotterdam Study have been described in detail elsewhere [16]. Regarding medication, the use of serum lipid reducing agents, antihypertensive drugs, or drugs taken for calcium homeostasis and disorders of the musculoskeletal system was registered during the home interview by trained research assistants [17]. Use of hormone replacement therapy (HRT) in females was coded as "never" or "ever". Lower limb disability and Vitamin D status were included as remaining measures of overall health. Lower limb disability index, a combined index reflecting a subject's ability to stand up, walk, climb and bend [18] was based on the Stanford Health Assessment Questionnaire. Serum 25-hydroxyvitamin D (25(OH)D) was measured in a subgroup of participants (n = 3171) at the 3rd visit of the cohort to the visiting center using radioimmunoassays (IDS Ltd, Boldon, UK). The sensitivity of the test was 3 nmol/L which ranged from 4 to 400 nmol/L. Intra-assay accuracy was <8% and the inter-assay accuracy was <12%.

2.7. Statistical Analysis

Characteristics of the study population were provided for subjects with a BMD Diet-Score below or above the median separately. Median values (+ interquartile ranges) for continuous variables and percentages of the total population for categorical variables were provided. The association between the BMD-Diet Score and HDI with BMD was studied using linear mixed modelling with the diet scores, expressed in standard deviations (SDs) or in quartiles, as exposure and longitudinal measurements of BMD (expressed in g/cm^2 and sex-specific z-scores) as the outcome. Analyses in quartiles, using the lowest quartile as the reference category, were performed to explore potential non- linear relationships. We coded the time- variable in the mixed model 0, 2, 6.5 and 11, to correct for differences in the length of time- intervals between subjects. Basic models (model 1) were adjusted for age and sex only. Potential confounding was tested by adding covariates to the models separately. Only covariates that changed the effect estimates by >10% were kept in the final adjusted models [19]. Based on this criterion, analyses were adjusted for age, sex and total kilocalorie intake, plus body weight and height (model 2), education, household income, current smoking behavior, physical activity, prevalent type 2 diabetes at baseline, and use of lipid lowering drugs, alcohol consumption and dietary supplement use (model 3). To assess whether BMD Diet-score had additional value upon the HDI, we further adjusted the final model for the HDI diet score (model 4). The aim of this paper is to study associations between diet scores reflecting full dietary patterns, not single nutrients, in relation to BMD. However, as the nutrient calcium is one of the most important constituents of the bone, we investigated the effects of additional adjustment for calcium intake in a separate model (model 5). To be able to study whether the trajectories of BMD were different in subjects with low or high diet scores, we tested for interaction with time by adding the product term of BMD-Diet Score or HDI with time to model 3.

We used a multiple imputation procedure to estimate missing values for covariates (details in Tables S1 and S2). To facilitate proper comparison of the effect estimates of associations between the BMD-Diet Score (ranging from 0 to 30) with BMD with that of the HDI (ranging from 0 to 120) with BMD, the regression coefficients were shown per SD increase for both diet scores.

As the majority of studies that served as a basis for our BMD-Diet Score were performed in women only, we tested for interaction with sex, by adding the product term of the our main exposures (the two diet scores) and sex to our basic models. Additionally, we performed a sensitivity analysis excluding participants with type 2 diabetes at baseline. All analyses were performed using SPSS 22 (IBM, Chicago, IL, USA) and R 3.1.2 (The R Foundation for Statistical Computing, Vienna, Austria) statistical software.

3. Results

3.1. Food Groups Included in Our BMD-Diet Score

In summary, we identified 15 papers to be used for the development of our BMD-Diet Score. The majority of these studies investigated *a posteriori* defined dietary patterns using principal component analysis [20–31] or cluster analysis [32]. Details on these studies regarding their design, sample size and food group extracted are shown in Table S3 and S4. Studies on *a priori* defined diet scores and BMD showed positive effects for the Mediterranean Diet Score [33], the Dietary

Diversity Score [23,34] and the Diet and Lifestyle Score, based on guidelines of the American Heart Association [35] (Table S5).

After careful evaluation of the available evidence, eight food groups were included in the BMD Diet-score: vegetables, fruits, dairy products, whole grain products, fish and legumes & beans as "High-BMD" components and meat (including red, processed and organ meat) and confectionary (including candies, cakes and cookies) as "Low-BMD" components (Figure 1). An overview of food items included in each food group is shown in Table S6.

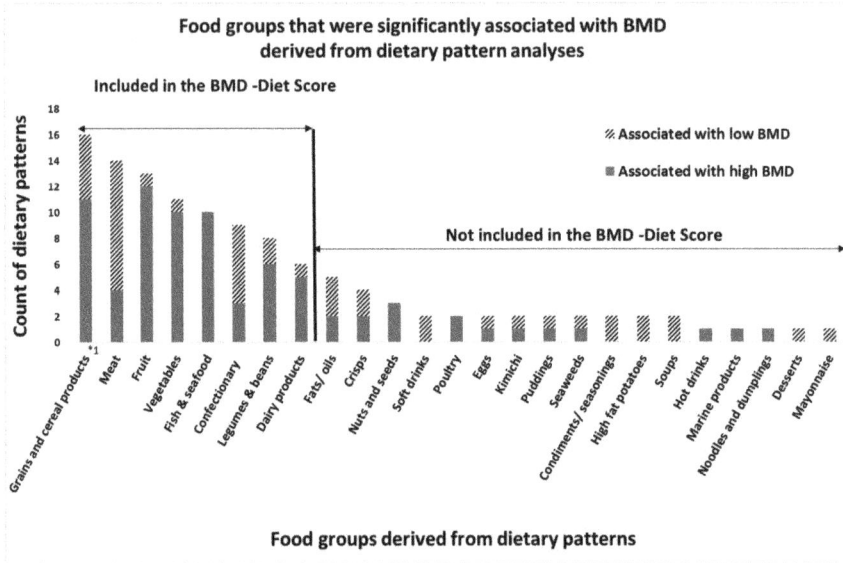

Figure 1. Results of the narrative review: Food groups that were associated with high or low bone mineral density (BMD) in dietary pattern analyses; The X-axis displays the food groups, derived from dietary patterns that were significantly associated with high or low BMD in the reviewed literature. The Y-axis displays the number of dietary patterns in which corresponding food group occurred (count of dietary patterns). As some studies report more than one dietary pattern to be associated with BMD, the number of patterns that was counted is slightly different from the number of studies that was counted. *1: Although not all studies distinguished between refined and whole grains, those that did found particularly beneficial associations with bone for whole grains only.

3.2. Characteristic of the Study Population

Characteristics of the study population are shown in Table 2. Subjects with a BMD-Diet Score above the median were more likely to be female (62% *vs.* 56%) and to have a higher income (54% *vs.* 49%) than those with a BMD-Diet Score below the median. Furthermore, they were less likely to be smokers (27% *vs.* 19%) and had higher calcium intakes (median of 1248 mg/day *vs.* 960 mg/day).

Table 2. Characteristics of the study population in participants with a BMD-Diet Score below or above the median.

	BMD-Diet Score below or Equal to the Median [2]	BMD-Diet Score above the Median	Total
n	2903	2241	5144
Age (year) [1]	68 (61, 73)	65 (60, 71)	67 (61, 73)
Total energy intake (kcal/day) [1]	1926 (1613, 2265)	1921 (1617, 2254)	1923 (1615, 2261)
Dietary calcium intake (mg/day) [1]	960 (769, 1170)	1248 (1032, 1497)	1079 (863, 1324)
Physical activity (h/day)	5.6 (4.0, 7.5)	6.0 (4.4, 8.0)	5.8 (4.2, 7.7)
Of which vigorous (h/day) [1]	0.4 (0.1, 0.9)	0.6 (0.2, 1.1)	0.5 (0.2, 1.0)
Height (cm) [1]	167 (161, 174)	167 (160, 174)	162 (157, 166)
Weight (kg) [1]	73 (65, 80)	74 (66, 81)	73 (66, 81)
Healthy Diet Indicator [1]	74 (66, 82)	79 (70, 86)	76 (68, 84)
Plasma Vitamin D (nmol/L) [1,3]	44 (29, 64)	45 (31, 65)	45 (30, 64)
Sex (% females)	56	62	57
Prevalent osteoporosis (%)	12	10	11
Prevalent type 2 diabetes (%)	9	10	10
Prevalent cardiovascular disease (%)	13	12	13
High education (%)	35	39	37
Monthly income > 1600 Euro (%)	49	54	51
Current smokers (%)	27	19	23
Current or past HRT use (%) [4]	8	11	9
Lipid lowering drug use (%)	2	3	3
Antihypertensive drug use (%)	13	13	13
Lower limb disabled (%)	19	16	17

[1]: median (interquartile range); [2]: the median of the BMD-Diet Score in our population is 19; [3]: assessed at the 3rd visit; [4]: expressed as percentages of the female population; Abbreviations: BMD = Bone mineral density; HRT = hormone replacement therapy.

The BMD-Diet Score and the HDI were weakly but significantly correlated (Pearson's $\rho = 0.18$). The HDI, but not the BMD-Diet Score, was significantly correlated with lower total energy intake (Pearson's $\rho = -0.23$). Median intake of each food group included in the BMD-Diet Score is shown in Table S7.

3.3. Longitudinal Associations between BMD-Diet Score, HDI and BMD

Associations between the BMD-Diet Score or the HDI and BMD, are shown in Table 3. Adjusted for age, sex and total energy intake (model 1), a high BMD-Diet Score was significantly associated with higher BMD (β (95% confidence interval (CI)) = 0.012 (0.008, 0.015) g/cm^2 per SD increase in the diet score). This association was slightly attenuated (β (95% CI) = 0.010 (0.007, 0.013) after adjustment for body height and weight (model 2) and after including additional confounders (β (95% CI) = 0.009 (0.005, 0.012), model 3). Additional adjustment for adherence to the HDI did not change the results (model 4). After further adjustment for dietary calcium intake effect sizes were diluted, but remained significant (β (95% CI) = 0.004 (0.001, 0.009) g/cm^2 per SD increase in the diet score). No significant interaction with time was observed (p for interaction = 0.25), indicating that the trajectories of BMD were comparable between subjects with high or low BMD-Diet Scores.

The HDI was significantly associated with higher BMD in the basic model. However, after adjustment for age, sex, height and weight (model 2) the standardized effect size decreased (β (95% CI) = 0.005 (0.002, 0.008) and was of a lesser magnitude than that of the BMD-Diet Score. After adjustment for confounders the association was diluted and became non-significant (β (95% CI) = 0.003 (−0.000, 0.007) in model 3). Further adjustment for adherence to the BMD-Diet Score did not change this effect (model 4), while a positive association was observed after additional adjustment for calcium intake (model 5). No significant interaction with time was observed (p for interaction = 0.18).

Categorical analyses, using the lowest quartile as the reference group, did not indicate the presence of a non- linear relationship between the BMD- Diet Score or the HDI with BMD (Table 3).

3.4. Additional Analysis

No interaction between the BMD-Diet Score or the HDI with sex was observed in relation to BMD (p all interactions > 0.12). Additionally, stratification by gender did not show different associations for males and females. Additional analyses with BMD in sex- specific z-scores as the outcome did not change the results. In addition, sensitivity analyses in which participants were excluded if they had type 2 diabetes at baseline did not change the results.

Table 3. Associations between the BMD-Diet Score or Healthy Diet Indicator and femoral neck BMD, using linear mixed modelling.

		Model 1		Model 2		Model 3		Model 4		Model 5	
		Basic		Model 1+		Model 2+		Model 3+		Model 3+	
				Height and Weight		Confounders		Other Score		Calcium Intake	
		β [1]	95% CI	β	95% CI	β	95% CI	β	95% CI	β	95% CI
Food group-based BMD-Diet Score	Per SD	0.012	(0.008, 0.015)	0.010	(0.007, 0.013)	0.009	(0.005, 0.012)	0.008	(0.004, 0.011)	0.004	(0.001, 0.008)
	Q2 vs. Q1	0.007	(−0.004, 0.018)	0.007	(−0.003, 0.016)	0.005	(−0.004, 0.015)	0.005	(−0.004, 0.015)	0.001	(−0.009, 0.012)
	Q3 vs. Q1	0.024	(0.014, 0.034)	0.020	(0.011, 0.030)	0.019	(0.009, 0.028)	0.018	(0.008, 0.028)	0.019	(0.002, 0.022)
	Q4 vs. Q1	0.029	(0.020, 0.040)	0.024	(0.016, 0.033)	0.022	(0.013, 0.031)	0.021	(0.012, 0.030)	0.010	(0.000, 0.020)
	P for trend	<0.001		<0.001		<0.001		<0.001		0.016	
WHO guidelines-based HDI	Per SD	0.004	(0.001, 0.008)	0.005	(0.002, 0.009)	0.003	(−0.000, 0.007)	0.003	(−0.000, 0.007)	0.005	(0.003, 0.010)
	Q2 vs. Q1	−0.006	(−0.017, 0.005)	−0.006	(−0.016, 0.005)	−0.008	(−0.018, 0.003)	−0.007	(−0.020, 0.002)	−0.007	(−0.018, 0.003)
	Q3 vs. Q1	0.006	(−0.026, 0.016)	0.007	(−0.012, 0.016)	0.004	(−0.004, 0.013)	0.002	(−0.007, 0.010)	0.005	(−0.004, 0.013)
	Q4 vs. Q1	0.011	(−0.000, 0.021)	0.012	(0.002, 0.022)	0.007	(−0.004, 0.017)	0.002	(−0.009, 0.012)	0.008	(−0.002, 0.018)
	P for trend	0.014		0.003		0.067		0.377		0.038	

[1] Regression coefficients (+95% confidence intervals) are shown for the fixed effects of the linear mixed model per SD increase or per quartile, using the first quartile as the reference, in the corresponding diet score. As the median BMD in this population is 0.86 g/cm², a regression coefficient of 0.012 g/cm² approximates a 1.4% higher BMD; Model 1: Adjusted for age, sex and total energy intake; Model 2: Model 1, additionally adjusted for body weight and height; Model 3: Model 2, additionally adjusted for education, household income, smoking behavior, physical activity, use of lipid lowering drugs + use of any dietary supplement + alcohol intake. *Additional adjustment for plasma vitamin D, use of antihypertensive drugs, drugs for calcium homeostasis or for disorders of the musculo-skeletal system, HRT, lower limb disability or CVD prevalence did not change these results;* Model 4: Model 3, additionally adjusted for the other diet Score (HDI for the BMD-Diet Score analysis and vice versa); Model 5: Model 3, additionally adjusted for calcium intake; Significant findings (*p* < 0.05) in **bold**. Abbreviations: BMD = bone mineral density, HDI = Healthy Diet Indicator, HRT = hormone replacement therapy, CVD = cardiovascular disease, SD = standard deviation; CI = Confidence interval; Q = quartile.

4. Discussion

4.1. Summary of Main Findings

This is the first study in which a food group-based BMD-Diet Score based on existing evidence from previous studies on full dietary patterns and BMD in several populations has been developed. We found that this newly developed BMD-Diet Score was significantly associated with high BMD, independent of adherence to the dietary recommendations of the WHO as assessed by the HDI. Our findings suggest that there is room for improvement of current dietary guidelines seeking optimal bone health.

4.2. Comparison to Existing Scores That were Shown to Favorably Affect Markers of Bone Turnover

Our BMD-Diet Score was developed based on studies investigating the effects of dietary patterns on BMD. However, the associations between existing diet scores have also been studied in relation to other bone-related outcomes, such as markers of bone turnover. For example, the "Dietary Approaches to Stop Hypertension" (DASH)-Diet score was shown to favorably affect osteocalcin, a serum marker of bone formation, which, if sustained, may improve bone mineral status [36] and reduce bone loss.

The DASH-Diet score and our BMD-Diet Score share common components, namely fruits, vegetables, fish, and whole grains as favorable (high-BMD) food groups and (red) meat as unfavorable (low-BMD) food groups. However, the DASH-Diet score does include dairy products as favorable components, similar to our BMD-Diet Score, but uses a more specific definition by including only low fat dairy products [36]. Additionally, the study by Karamati *et al.*, (2012) [28] showed a dietary pattern including low fat dairy to be associated with high BMD, and a pattern including high fat dairy to be associated with low BMD. Based on these findings, it could be argued that the BMD-Diet Score might be refined further by using low fat instead of all dairy products as a favorable component. The DASH-Diet score includes total fat as unfavorable nutrient-component (Table S8). Our BMD-Diet Score was based solely on food groups and therefore has no specific fatty acid-component. However, it includes foods as pork, cake, and chocolate bars, products high in saturated fatty acids, in the unfavorable "low BMD" components (Table S6), and fish, rich in polyunsaturated fatty acids, as favorable component. Therefore, our BMD-Diet Score could be considered a score in which the existing DASH-diet score was covered, but was fully translated into food groups.

4.3. Potential Nutrients Involved

The aim of this paper is to study the associations between complete dietary patterns, reflected by different diet scores in relation to BMD. However, calcium is a vital element of bone and a well-established dietary factor that influences BMD [3,37,38]. Our analysis showed the associations between the BMD-Diet Score and BMD were diluted, but remained significant after additional adjustment for dietary calcium. This indicates that calcium intake is important, but does not fully explain the favorable association between the BMD-Diet Score and BMD. This finding is in line with an earlier review by Ahmadieh *et al.*, (2001) who highlighted the positive contributions of a variety of nutrients to BMD, such as Vitamin B2, B6, Vitamin C and Vitamin K, in addition to calcium [2]. These nutrients can underlie our associations, since vitamin B2 and B6 might be reflected by the whole grain component of our BMD-diet Score and Vitamin C and K1 by the fruits and vegetable components.

4.4. Strengths and Limitations

Our study has several strengths. Firstly, the development of our BMD-Diet Score was based on a variety of study populations, including both Caucasian and Asian subjects. Despite the differences in dietary habits between these populations, we were able to identify common food groups that were consumed and were shown to be associated with BMD across populations. Secondly, by using full dietary pattern analyses as a basis for the BMD-Diet Score, we were able to take into account strong correlations and potential interactions between foods and nutrients. Thirdly, we had the opportunity to include repeated measurements of BMD, body weight, and height. Repeated BMD measurements provided more insights into long-term associations between dietary intake and BMD and the opportunity to study associations with BMD trajectories. Repeated measurements of body weight and height enabled a precise adjustment for changes in anthropometric measures, which are known to be important determinants of BMD. Lastly, our sample included both males and females, increasing the external validity of our results since most studies on dietary patterns and BMD focused on women only.

We do, however, also recognize some limitations. Our study population consisted of Dutch participants from one specific neighborhood, in which the vast majority of inhabitants were of Caucasian background, an aspect that is important to consider when extrapolating our findings to other populations. The absolute intakes of some components of the BMD-Diet Score (such as fish and legumes) were very low in our population, which might have affected the strength of our associations. However, for the main food groups, including fruits, vegetables, fish and whole grain products, we believe this concern is limited since items in these food groups are widely consumed in our population. It could be argued that using results from Rotterdam Study for the development of the BMD-Diet Score while subsequently testing the association between this score with BMD in the same cohort might have led to bias. However, the composition of the BMD-Diet Score would be similar with or without inclusion of our own previous results [24] (Tables S3 and S4) in its development. Therefore, we believe that inclusion of our previous results did not lead to bias in this study.

4.5. Future Steps and Implications

This is the first study that developed a BMD Diet Score that has been associated with BMD in a Dutch population of elderly subjects. Although the score is based on data from different populations, it is essential to study its performance in other populations, including Asian and other non-Caucasian populations. For example populations with (a) low dairy intake or (b) higher levels of Vitamin D or (c) high intake of foods that were hardly consumed in our population such as fish or legumes would be particularly interesting for replication. If future studies replicate positive associations with BMD, this BMD-Diet Score could help to shape food group-based dietary guidelines aiming to contribute to healthy ageing while considering a healthy BMD as important aspect of ageing. However, since dietary guidelines aim to promote overall healthy ageing by preventing all chronic diseases such as cardiometabolic diseases and cancer, our BMD-Diet Score should be studied in relation to these health outcomes as well. Calcium might favor BMD while adversely affecting cardiovascular disease risk [39], whereas an approach which evaluates the full diet, such as the BMD-Diet Score, might indicate benefit for various aspects of healthy ageing simultaneously.

For the development of our BMD-Diet Score we only used studies with BMD, and not fracture risk, as the primary outcome. However, as adherence to the Mediterranean Diet Score, for example, has been shown to be favorably associated with fracture risk in a cohort of adults from eight European countries [40], consumption of the food groups in our proposed BMD-Diet Score might favorably affect fracture risk as well.

5. Conclusions

We developed a new BMD-Diet Score composed of components representing high intake of vegetables, fruits, fish, whole grains, legumes and beans, and dairy products, and low intake of and meat and confectionary. This BMD-Diet Score is positively associated with BMD in our cohort of middle-aged and elderly subjects independent of adherence to the HDI based on dietary guidelines from the WHO. The food groups included in our BMD-Diet Score could be considered in the development of future dietary guidelines for healthy ageing.

Acknowledgments: Acknowledgments

Oscar H. Franco, Jessica C. Kiefte-de Jong, Ester A.L. de Jonge, Trudy Voortman and Josje D. Schoufour work at ErasmusAGE, a center for ageing research across the life course funded by Nestlé Nutrition (Nestec Ltd., Vevey, Switzerland) and Metagenics Inc., (Aliso Viejo, CA, USA). Nestlé Nutrition or Metagenics Inc. had no role in design and conduct of the study; collection, management, analysis, and interpretation of the data; and preparation, review or approval of the manuscript. Fernando Rivadeneira received a grant from the Netherlands Organization for Scientific Research (NWO, VIDI 016.136.367). Ester A.L. de Jongeis supported by a grant from the NWO for the graduate program of 2010 (project number: 022.002.023).

The Rotterdam Study is supported by the Erasmus MC University Medical Centre and Erasmus University Rotterdam; The Netherlands Organization for Scientific Research (NWO), The Netherlands Organization for Health Research and Development (ZonMw); the Research Institute for Diseases in the Elderly; the Netherlands Genomics Initiative (NGI); the Netherlands Consortium of Healthy ageing (NCHA); the Ministry of Education, Culture and Science; the Ministry of Health, Welfare and Sports; the European Commission (DG XII); and the Municipality of Rotterdam.

The contribution of inhabitants, general practitioners and pharmacists of the Ommoord district to the Rotterdam Study is gratefully acknowledged.

Author Contributions: Albert Hofman, André G. Uiterlinden and Oscar H. Franco designed the Rotterdam Study. Trudy Voortman, Lisette C.P.G.M. de Groot, Josje D. Schoufour, Ester A.L. de Jonge and Jessica C. Kiefte-de Jong developed the dietscore. Ester A.L. de Jonge and Jessica C. Kiefte-de Jong participated in the data acquisition related to dietary intake. Fernando Rivadeneira and M. Carola Zillikens were responsible for the data acquisition of bone parameters. Ester A.L. de Jonge, and Jessica C. Kiefte-de Jong formulated the research questions, Ester A.L. de Jonge and Jessica C. Kiefte-de Jong analyzed the data and wrote the article.

Conflicts of Interest: The authors declare no conflict of interest.

References

1. World Health Organisation. World Health Organisation Scientific Group on the Assessment of Osteoporosis at Primary Health Care Level. *Summary Meeting Report*, Brussels, Belgium, 5–7 May 2004. Avaliable online: http://www.who.int/chp/topics/Osteoporosis.pdf (accessed on 8 August 2015).
2. Ahmadieh, H.; Arabi, A. Vitamins and bone health: Beyond calcium and Vitamin D. *Nutr. Rev.* **2011**, *69*, 584–598. [CrossRef] [PubMed]
3. Zhu, K.; Prince, R.L. Calcium and bone. *Clin. Biochem.* **2012**, *45*, 936–942. [CrossRef] [PubMed]
4. Hu, F.B. Dietary pattern analysis: A new direction in nutritional epidemiology. *Curr. Opin. Lipidol.* **2002**, *13*, 3–9. [CrossRef] [PubMed]
5. Ocke, M.C. Evaluation of methodologies for assessing the overall diet: Dietary quality scores and dietary pattern analysis. *Proc. Nutr. Soc.* **2013**, *72*, 191–199. [CrossRef] [PubMed]
6. Zagarins, S.E.; Ronnenberg, A.G.; Gehlbach, S.H.; Lin, R.; Bertone-Johnson, E.R. Are existing measures of overall diet quality associated with peak bone mass in young premenopausal women? *J. Hum. Nutr. Diet.* **2012**, *25*, 172–179. [CrossRef] [PubMed]
7. Jankovic, N.; Geelen, A.; Streppel, M.T.; de Groot, L.C.; Orfanos, P.; van den Hooven, E.H.; Pikhart, H.; Boffetta, P.; Trichopoulou, A.; Bobak, M.; *et al.* Adherence to a healthy diet according to the world health organization guidelines and all-cause mortality in elderly adults from Europe and the United States. *Am. J. Epidemiol.* **2014**, *180*, 978–988. [CrossRef] [PubMed]
8. Hofman, A.; Murad, S.D.; van Duijn, C.M.; Franco, O.H.; Goedegebure, A.; Ikram, M.A.; Klaver, C.C.W.; Nijsten, T.E.C.; Peeters, R.P.; Stricker, B.H.C.; *et al.* The Rotterdam Study: 2014 objectives and design update. *Eur. J. Epidemiol.* **2013**, *28*, 889–926. [CrossRef] [PubMed]
9. Klipstein-Grobusch, K.; den Breeijen, J.H.; Goldbohm, R.A.; Geleijnse, J.M.; Hofman, A.; Grobbee, D.E.; Witteman, J.C.M. Dietary assessment in the elderly: Validation of a semiquantitative food frequency questionnaire. *Eur. J. Clin. Nutr.* **1998**, *52*, 588–596. [CrossRef] [PubMed]
10. Goldbohm, R.A.; van den Brandt, P.A.; Brants, H.A.; van't Veer, P.; Al, M.; Sturmans, F.; Hermus, R.J. Validation of a dietary questionnaire used in a large-scale prospective cohort study on diet and cancer. *Eur. J. Clin. Nutr.* **1994**, *48*, 253–265. [PubMed]

11. Sommer, I.; Erkkila, A.T.; Jarvinen, R.; Mursu, J.; Sirola, J.; Jurvelin, J.S.; Kroger, H.; Tuppurainen, M. Alcohol consumption and bone mineral density in elderly women. *Public Health Nutr.* **2013**, *16*, 704–712. [CrossRef] [PubMed]

12. Rapuri, P.B.; Gallagher, J.C.; Balhorn, K.E.; Ryschon, K.L. Alcohol intake and bone metabolism in elderly women. *Am. J. Clin. Nutr.* **2000**, *72*, 1206–1213. [PubMed]

13. Caspersen, C.J.; Bloemberg, B.P.; Saris, W.H.; Merritt, R.K.; Kromhout, D. The prevalence of selected physical activities and their relation with coronary heart disease risk factors in elderly men: The Zutphen Study, 1985. *Am. J. Epidemiol.* **1991**, *133*, 1078–1092. [PubMed]

14. Stel, V.S.; Smit, J.H.; Pluijm, S.M.; Visser, M.; Deeg, D.J.; Lips, P. Comparison of the LASA physical activity questionnaire with a 7-day diary and pedometer. *J. Clin. Epidemiol.* **2004**, *57*, 252–258. [CrossRef] [PubMed]

15. Voorrips, L.E.; Ravelli, A.C.; Dongelmans, P.C.; Deurenberg, P.; Van Staveren, W.A. A physical activity questionnaire for the elderly. *Med. Sci. Sports Exerc.* **1991**, *23*, 974–979. [CrossRef] [PubMed]

16. Leening, M.J.G.; Kavousi, M.; Heeringa, J.; van Rooij, F.J.A.; Verkroost-van Heemst, J.; Deckers, J.W.; Mattace-Raso, F.U.S.; Ziere, G.; Hofman, A.; Stricker, B.H.C.; *et al.* Methods of data collection and definitions of cardiac outcomes in the Rotterdam Study. *Eur. J. Epidemiol.* **2012**, *27*, 173–185. [CrossRef] [PubMed]

17. Sjahid, S.I.; van der Linden, P.D.; Stricker, B.H. Agreement between the pharmacy medication history and patient interview for cardiovascular drugs: The Rotterdam Elderly Study. *Br. J. Clin. Pharmacol.* **1998**, *45*, 591–595. [CrossRef] [PubMed]

18. Burger, H.; de Laet, C.E.D.H.; van Daele, P.L.A.; Weel, A.E.A.M.; Witteman, J.C.M.; Hofman, A.; Pols, H.A.P. Risk factors for increased bone loss in an elderly population—The Rotterdam Study. *Am. J. Epidemiol.* **1998**, *147*, 871–879. [CrossRef] [PubMed]

19. Mickey, R.M.; Greenland, S. The impact of confounder selection criteria on effect estimation. *Am. J. Epidemiol.* **1989**, *129*, 125–137. [PubMed]

20. Shin, S.; Joung, H. A dairy and fruit dietary pattern is associated with a reduced likelihood of osteoporosis in Korean postmenopausal women. *Br. J. Nutr.* **2013**, *110*, 1926–1933. [CrossRef] [PubMed]

21. Shin, S.; Sung, J.; Joung, H. A fruit, milk and whole grain dietary pattern is positively associated with bone mineral density in Korean healthy adults. *Eur. J. Clin. Nutr.* **2014**, *69*, 442–448. [CrossRef] [PubMed]

22. Mu, M.; Wang, S.F.; Sheng, J.; Zhao, Y.; Wang, G.X.; Liu, K.Y.; Hu, C.L.; Tao, F.B.; Wang, H.L. Dietary patterns are associated with body mass index and bone mineral density in Chinese freshmen. *J. Am. Coll. Nutr.* **2014**, *33*, 120–128. [CrossRef] [PubMed]

23. Whittle, C.R.; Woodside, J.V.; Cardwell, C.R.; McCourt, H.J.; Young, I.S.; Murray, L.J.; Boreham, C.A.; Gallagher, A.M.; Neville, C.E.; McKinley, M.C. Dietary patterns and bone mineral status in young adults: The Northern Ireland young hearts project. *Br. J. Nutr.* **2012**, *108*, 1494–1504. [CrossRef] [PubMed]

24. De Jonge, E.A.L.; Rivadeneira, F.; Erler, N.S.; Hofman, A.; Uitterlinden, A.G.; Franco, O.H.; Kiefte-de Jong, J.C. Dietary patterns in an elderly population and their relation with bone mineral density: The Rotterdam Study. 2015, submitted for publication.

25. Fairweather-Tait, S.J.; Skinner, J.; Guile, G.R.; Cassidy, A.; Spector, T.D.; MacGregor, A.J. Diet and bone mineral density study in postmenopausal women from the twinsuk registry shows a negative association with a traditional English dietary pattern and a positive association with wine. *Am. J. Clin. Nutr.* **2011**, *94*, 1371–1375. [CrossRef] [PubMed]

26. Hardcastle, A.C.; Aucott, L.; Fraser, W.D.; Reid, D.M.; Macdonald, H.M. Dietary patterns, bone resorption and bone mineral density in early post-menopausal Scottish women. *Eur. J. Clin. Nutr.* **2011**, *65*, 378–385. [CrossRef] [PubMed]

27. McNaughton, S.A.; Wattanapenpaiboon, N.; Wark, J.D.; Nowson, C.A. An energy-dense, nutrient-poor dietary pattern is inversely associated with bone health in women. *J. Nutr.* **2011**, *141*, 1516–1523. [CrossRef] [PubMed]

28. Karamati, M.; Jessri, M.; Shariati-Bafghi, S.E.; Rashidkhani, B. Dietary patterns in relation to bone mineral density among menopausal Iranian women. *Calcif. Tissue Intl.* **2012**, *91*, 40–49. [CrossRef] [PubMed]

29. Langsetmo, L.; Poliquin, S.; Hanley, D.A.; Prior, J.C.; Barr, S.; Anastassiades, T.; Towheed, T.; Goltzman, D.; Kreiger, N. Dietary patterns in Canadian men and women ages 25 and older: Relationship to demographics, body mass index, and bone mineral density. *BMC Musculoskelet. Disord.* **2010**, *11*, 20. [CrossRef] [PubMed]

30. Kontogianni, M.D.; Melistas, L.; Yannakoulia, M.; Malagaris, I.; Panagiotakos, D.B.; Yiannakouris, N. Association between dietary patterns and indices of bone mass in a sample of Mediterranean women. *Nutrition* **2009**, *25*, 165–171. [CrossRef] [PubMed]

31. Okubo, H.; Sasaki, S.; Horiguchi, H.; Oguma, E.; Miyamoto, K.; Hosoi, Y.; Kim, M.K.; Kayama, F. Dietary patterns associated with bone mineral density in premenopausal Japanese farmwomen. *Am. J. Clin. Nutr.* **2006**, *83*, 1185–1192. [PubMed]

32. Tucker, K.L.; Chen, H.; Hannan, M.T.; Cupples, L.A.; Wilson, P.W.; Felson, D.; Kiel, D.P. Bone mineral density and dietary patterns in older adults: The Framingham Osteoporosis Study. *Am. J. Clin. Nutr.* **2002**, *76*, 245–252. [PubMed]

33. Rivas, A.; Romero, A.; Mariscal-Arcas, M.; Monteagudo, C.; Feriche, B.; Lorenzo, M.L.; Olea, F. Mediterranean diet and bone mineral density in two age groups of women. *Intl. J. Food Sci. Nutr.* **2013**, *64*, 155–161. [CrossRef] [PubMed]

34. Go, G.; Tserendejid, Z.; Lim, Y.; Jung, S.; Min, Y.; Park, H. The association of dietary quality and food group intake patterns with bone health status among Korean postmenopausal women: A study using the 2010 Korean national health and nutrition examination survey data. *Nutr. Res. Pract.* **2014**, *8*, 662–669. [CrossRef] [PubMed]

35. Bhupathiraju, S.N.; Lichtenstein, A.H.; Dawson-Hughes, B.; Hannan, M.T.; Tucker, K.L. Adherence to the 2006 American heart association diet and lifestyle recommendations for cardiovascular disease risk reduction is associated with bone health in older Puerto Ricans. *Am. J. Clin. Nutr.* **2013**, *98*, 1309–1316. [CrossRef] [PubMed]

36. Lin, P.H.; Ginty, F.; Appel, L.J.; Aickin, M.; Bohannon, A.; Garnero, P.; Barclay, D.; Svetkey, L.P. The Dash diet and sodium reduction improve markers of bone turnover and calcium metabolism in adults. *J. Nutr.* **2003**, *133*, 3130–3136. [PubMed]

37. Cashman, K.D. Calcium intake, calcium bioavailability and bone health. *Br. J. Nutr.* **2002**, *87*, S169–S177. [CrossRef] [PubMed]

38. Wilczynski, C.; Camacho, P. Calcium use in the management of osteoporosis: Continuing questions and controversies. *Curr. Osteoporos. Rep.* **2014**, *12*, 396–402. [CrossRef] [PubMed]

39. Booth, A.; Camacho, P. A closer look at calcium absorption and the benefits and risks of dietary *versus* supplemental calcium. *Postgrad. Med.* **2013**, *125*, 73–81. [CrossRef] [PubMed]

40. Benetou, V.; Orfanos, P.; Pettersson-Kymmer, U.; Bergstrom, U.; Svensson, O.; Johansson, I.; Berrino, F.; Tumino, R.; Borch, K.B.; Lund, E.; *et al.* Mediterranean diet and incidence of hip fractures in a European cohort. *Osteoporos. Intl.* **2013**, *24*, 1587–1598. [CrossRef] [PubMed]

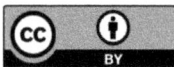

nutrients

MDPI

Article

The Association of a Mediterranean-Style Diet Pattern with Polycystic Ovary Syndrome Status in a Community Cohort Study

Lisa J. Moran [1,2,*], Jessica A. Grieger [1], Gita D. Mishra [3] and Helena J. Teede [2,4]

[1]   The Robinson Research Institute, University of Adelaide, 55 King William Road, North Adelaide,
     South Australia 5006, Australia; jessica.grieger@adelaide.edu.au
[2]   Monash Centre for Health Research Implementation, School of Public Health and Preventative Medicine,
     Monash University, Melbourne 3004, Australia; helena.teede@monash.edu
[3]   School of Public Health, University of Queensland, Herston, Queensland 4006, Australia:
     g.mishra@sph.uq.edu.au
[4]   Diabetes and Endocrine Unit, Monash Health, Clayton 3168, Australia
[*]   Correspondence: lisa.moran@adelaide.edu.au; Tel.: +61-8-313-1352; Fax: +61-8-3161-7652

Received: 31 August 2015 ; Accepted: 12 October 2015 ; Published: 16 October 2015

Abstract: Polycystic ovary syndrome (PCOS) is a common condition in reproductive-aged women. While lifestyle management is first-line treatment in PCOS, the dietary intake of women with PCOS is unclear and there is no research assessing dietary patterns of women with and without PCOS. The aim of this study was to examine dietary patterns in a large cohort of women with and without PCOS. Data were from 7569 participants in the 1973–1978 cohort of the Australian Longitudinal Study on Women's Health population assessed at 2009 (Survey 5) (n = 414 PCOS, n = 7155 non-PCOS). Dietary patterns were evaluated using factor analysis and multiple logistic regressions assessed their associations with PCOS status. Three dietary patterns were identified that explained 27% of the variance in food intake between women with and without PCOS: Non-core foods; Meats and take-away and Mediterranean-style. The Mediterranean-style dietary pattern was independently associated with PCOS status. On adjusted analysis for each 1 SD increase in the Mediterranean-style dietary pattern, there was a 26% greater likelihood that women had PCOS. This may indicate an improvement in the quality of dietary intake following a diagnosis of PCOS. Future research should examine the contribution of dietary patterns to the incidence and severity of PCOS and the potential for modification of dietary patterns in the lifestyle management of PCOS.

Keywords: polycystic ovary syndrome; diet; dietary patterns; Australia

---

1. Introduction

Polycystic ovary syndrome (PCOS) is a common endocrine condition affecting 12%–18% of reproductive-aged women [1]. It is associated with reproductive (hyperandrogenism, anovulation, menstrual irregularly, infertility and pregnancy complications) [2], metabolic (increased risk factors for and prevalence of impaired glucose tolerance, type 2 diabetes and cardiovascular disease) [3–5] and psychological (worsened quality of life and increased risk factors for depression and anxiety) [6] features. There is a proposed bidirectional relationship between obesity and PCOS [7]. Women with PCOS have an elevated prevalence of obesity [8] and increased longitudinal weight gain [7]. Obesity also worsens the presentation and prevalence of PCOS [9]. Mechanisms include increasing the pathophysiological factor insulin resistance, which increases hyperandrogenism through augmenting ovarian androgen production and decreasing hepatic production of the androgen binding-protein sex hormone binding globulin [10,11]. Due to the key aetiological role of obesity and insulin resistance in PCOS, weight management, defined as prevention of excess weight gain or achieving and maintaining a modest weight loss, is a key treatment strategy in PCOS. Evidence based guidelines recommend achieving this through a combination of diet, exercise or behavioural management [12].

The optimal dietary strategy as part of lifestyle management in PCOS remains controversial. We reported in a recent systematic review that the controlled clinical literature found no difference in the majority of anthropometric, reproductive, metabolic or psychological outcomes for a range of dietary approaches including higher protein, higher carbohydrate, lower glycaemic index or monounsaturated fat-enriched diets [13]. Despite this, a range of dietary approaches may be prescribed by health professionals [14]. While evidence-based National Health and Medical Council approved Australian guidelines outline the principles of dietary management for PCOS [12], the effect of these guidelines on actual dietary prescription by health professionals and subsequent dietary intake by women with PCOS is not known. In the absence of specific recommendations by health professionals, women with PCOS may also often seek non-evidence based sources of information on dietary management [15]. The effect of this on actual dietary intake is not known. We and others have reported subtle differences in dietary intake for women with PCOS compared to those without PCOS including a better dietary intake as indicated by elevated diet quality indices, fibre and micronutrient intake, lower glycaemic index and lower total fat or saturated fat intake or a poorer dietary intake indicated by poorer diet quality, increased fat, saturated fat and high glycaemic index food intake and decreased fibre intake compared to women without PCOS [16–21]. There however remains uncertainty as to the quality of dietary intake in women with PCOS.

Assessment of dietary patterns offers an additional way of comprehensively assessing dietary intake. Rather than assessing single nutrients in isolation, dietary pattern analysis identifies underlying dietary characteristics of the study population in which the consumption of foods that are eaten together can be derived. In particular, exploratory approaches or posteriori dietary pattern analyses such as principal components analysis, which are not hypothesis driven, groups correlated food groups into uncorrelated factors termed dietary patterns [22,23]. In pregnant populations, unhealthy dietary patterns in the pre-conception period were associated with increased risk for preterm birth [24] or gestational diabetes [25] and healthy, Mediterranean or prudent diet patterns were inversely associated with risk of developing hypertensive disorders during pregnancy [26] or gestational diabetes [27,28]. In non-pregnant populations, unhealthy/Western-type dietary patterns have been associated with increased risk of general and central obesity [29] and type 2 diabetes [30]; while a Mediterranean dietary pattern was associated with decreased prevalence of hypertension and metabolic syndrome [31] and a healthy dietary pattern containing vegetables, fruits and whole grains was associated with reduced risk for diabetes [30].

These findings are of potential relevance to PCOS given the increased prevalence of cardiometabolic conditions and pregnancy complications and the potential for clinical benefits with approaches such as the Mediterranean diet [32]. However, there has been limited research examining dietary patterns in women with and without PCOS. This could provide an understanding on both the association of dietary intake with the pathophysiology of PCOS as well as of the dietary changes that occur following a diagnosis of PCOS. The aim of this study was therefore to examine dietary patterns in a large cohort of women, with and without PCOS, participating in the Australian Longitudinal Study on Women's Health.

2. Experimental Section

2.1. Study Population

This study is based on data from the Australian Longitudinal Study on Women's Health (ALSWH), a longitudinal population-based study of three age cohorts of Australia women. Women were randomly selected from the national health insurance scheme (Medicare) database, which includes almost all people who are permanent residents of Australia, with national recruitment and intentional over-sampling from rural and remote areas [33]. Further details of the methods and characteristics of the sample have been reported elsewhere [34–36]. The Human Research Ethics Committees of the University of Newcastle and the University of Queensland approved the study methods and informed written consent was obtained from each participant.

The current study uses data from the cohort of younger women (born 1973–1978) ($n = 14{,}779$ at Survey 1) who first completed a mailed survey in 1996 [37]. For this analysis, data are from Survey 5 (2009, $n = 8200$, 58% retention of baseline participants and 84% retention of those who completed the second survey). The greatest drop out was from Survey 1 to Survey 2. However, the impact of attrition on associations between variables has been found to be minimal [36].

As with our prior publications on health outcomes in PCOS, we analysed data from $n = 7569$ women who completed Survey 5 and responded to the question on PCOS diagnosis ("In the last 3 years have you been diagnosed with or treated for Polycystic Ovary Syndrome") of which $n = 414$ were classified as PCOS and $n = 7155$ as non-PCOS [7]. The analyses in this study are based on cross-sectional analysis of dietary patterns in women with and without PCOS. No specific inclusion or exclusion criteria were applied to this cohort and all women were included irrespective of pregnancy, medication, country of birth and language spoken.

2.2. Anthropometric, Demographic and Physical Activity Variables

Self-reported height, weight and BMI were reported with overweight and obesity defined by the World Health Organization criteria (BMI $\geqslant 25$ kg/m^2 for overweight and obesity, BMI $\geqslant 30$ kg/m^2 for obesity) [38]. Demographic variables including parity, education, occupation and income were collected at Survey 5 and area of residence was measured at Survey 1. Physical activity was calculated as the sum of the products of total weekly minutes in categories of walking, moderate-intensity or vigorous-intensity physical activity and the metabolic equivalent value (MET) was assigned to each category: (walking minutes $\times$ 3.0 METs) + (moderate-intensity physical activity minutes $\times$ 4.0 METs) + (vigorous intensity physical activity minutes $\times$ 7.5 METs). Outliers were truncated at 28 h/day for total physical activity.

2.3. Food Group Consumption

At Survey 5, self-reported dietary intake data were collected from the Dietary Questionnaire for Epidemiological Studies (DQES) Version 2, a FFQ developed by The Cancer Council of Victoria previously validated in young Australian women [39] as previously reported [19]. One hundred different foods (grams per day) were obtained from the FFQ and were assigned into 33 food groups (grams per day) based on a previous Australian study [24,40] for use in the dietary pattern analysis.

2.4. Dietary Pattern Analysis

Dietary patterns were derived using factor analysis with factor loadings extracted using the principal component method and varimax/orthogonal rotation. The number of dietary patterns identified was based on eigenvalues >1.5, on identification of a break point in the scree plot, and on interpretability [41]. Using these criteria, a 3-factor solution was chosen and rerun with the resulting factor scores saved and converted to Z-scores for analysis. Items with factor loadings $\geqslant 0.25$ were considered as the items of relevance for the identified factor. These items represent the foods most highly related to the identified factor [42]. Foods that cross-loaded on several factors were retained.

2.5. Statistical Analyses

All statistical procedures were performed using SPSS version 22. Frequencies and descriptive statistics were expressed as n (%) and as means (SD), respectively. All reported P values were 2-tailed, and a p-value < 0.05 was considered to be statistically significant. Before hypothesis testing, data were examined for normality, in which all independent variables were normally distributed.

Data were analysed by independent *t*-test to compare continuous variables and chi-square test to compare categorical variables between women with and without PCOS. Binary logistic regression analyses were used to test the association between PCOS (yes/no) and the independent variables for each dietary pattern (Z-score), with values presented as OR (95% CI). All logistic regression analyses were undertaken adjusting for potential confounders identified a priori, including maternal age, BMI, currently breastfeeding, number of children and waist circumference, or statistically, from association with PCOS on univariate analysis ($p < 0.05$). Multicollinearity was tested with binary regression analysis using the variance inflation factor (<5); no multicollinearity was observed between any of the independent variables. All model assumptions were validated with residual plots. Analyses were conducted using survey commands for analysing data weighted by area of residence to adjust for the deliberate over sampling in rural and remote areas.

3. Results

3.1. Participant Characteristics

Participant characteristics are reported in Table 1. The women with PCOS were around two months younger, were more likely to not have children and had a lower prevalence of currently breastfeeding compared to women without PCOS. As reported previously, women with PCOS also reported a higher BMI, weight and waist circumference than women without PCOS [7]. As previously reported [19], women with PCOS had an elevated energy and fibre intake and lower glycaemic index and percent energy intake from saturated fat compared to women without PCOS (data not reported). As previously reported [19], women with and without PCOS had similar physical activity levels (814 ± 874 *vs.* 820 ± 895 MET/min, $p = 0.75$).

Table 1. Characteristics for women with and without polycystic ovary syndrome.

	All *n* = 8200	PCOS *n* = 414	Non-PCOS *n* = 7155	*p*
Age (years) *	33.7 (1.5)	33.5 ± 0.1	33.7 ± 0.02	0.015
BMI (kg/m^2) *	25.8 (5.9)	29.0 ± 0.4	25.4 ± 0.1	<0.001
Weight (kg) *	71.3 (16.7)	79.6 ± 1.2	70.3 ± 0.2	<0.001
Waist circumference (cm) *	86.0 (14.3)	91.9 ± 1.0	85.7 ± 0.2	<0.001
Smoking status †				0.729
Never smoker	4972 (60.4)	256 (59.1)	4341 (60.3)	
Ex-smoker	2112 (25.6)	121 (27.9)	1829 (25.6)	
Smoke <10 cigarettes/day	574 (6.9)	26 (6.0)	517 (7.1)	
Smoke 10–19 cigarettes/day	372 (4.5)	20 (4.6)	319 (4.4)	
Smoke ≥20 cigarettes/day	205 (2.5)	10 (2.3)	183 (2.5)	
Personal income †				0.765
No income	724 (9.5)	41 (9.8)	634 (9.1)	
Low (>$0–$36,399)	2923 (38.5)	156 (37.5)	2562 (36.3)	
Medium ($36,400–$77,999)	2737 (36.1)	137 (32.7)	2398 (34.0)	
High (>$78,000)	1207 (15.9)	71 (17.0)	1047 (14.9)	
Highest qualification †				0.762
No formal qual/year 10/12 Equiv	1492 (18.4)	76 (18.1)	1301 (17.3)	
Trade/diploma	2040 (21.2)	100 (23.8)	1793 (23.9)	
Degree or higher	4565 (56.4)	245 (58.2)	3986 (53.1)	

Table 1. Cont.

	All $n = 8200$	PCOS $n = 414$	Non-PCOS $n = 7155$	p
Marital status †				0.630
Married	5115 (62.2)	260 (59.9)	4455 (62.0)	
De facto	1233 (15.0)	64 (14.7)	1067 (14.9)	
Separated/divorced	422 (5.1)	21 (4.8)	373 (5.2)	
Widowed	14 (0.2)	0 (0)	14 (0.2)	
Never married	1445 (17.6)	89 (20.5)	1274 (17.7)	
Number of children †				0.002
0	3134 (38.1)	205 (47.2)	2748 (36.1)	
1	1630 (19.8)	86 (19.8)	1409 (18.5)	
2–3	3228 (39.2)	132 (30.4)	2818 (37.0)	
⩾4	243 (3.0)	11 (2.5)	213 (2.8)	
Currently breastfeeding †				0.003
No	4817 (58.4)	223 (51.3)	4193 (55.0)	
Yes	277 (3.4)	7 (1.6)	240 (3.2)	
No child	3149 (38.2)	205 (47.1)	2761 (36.2)	

* Values represent mean (SD); † Values represent *n* (%); Data were analysed by independent *t*-test to compare continuous variables and chi-square test to compare categorical variables between women with and without PCOS; BMI: Body mass index.

3.2. Dietary Patterns

The dietary pattern analysis revealed three distinct patterns explaining a total 27% variance (Table 2). The first pattern was labelled *Non-core foods* as there were high factor loadings for cakes, biscuits, sweet pastries; confectionary; refined grains and also take-away foods and crisps. The second pattern was labelled *High meat and take-away* as fish (fried, processed, canned and cooked), processed meat, red meat, but also take-away food highly correlated in this pattern. The final pattern was labelled *Mediterranean-style* as Mediterranean type foods highly correlated to this pattern including a variety of vegetables, fruit and nuts, small correlations with fish, while crisps were inversely correlated. Participant characteristics across the quartiles of dietary pattern score are presented in Supplemental Table 1.

Table 2. Factor loadings for each of the identified pre-conception dietary patterns for women with and without PCOS.

Food Group	Non-Core Foods	High Meat and Take-Away	Mediterranean-Style
Cakes, biscuits, sweet pastries	0.661	0.010	0.020
Confectionary	0.629	0.089	0.020
Refined grains	0.483	0.239	0.146
Vegemite	0.483	0.106	0.068
Takeaway	0.467	0.402	−0.138
Crisps	0.466	0.199	−0.262
Juice	0.408	0.007	0.071
Tomato sauce	0.380	0.018	0.029
Processed meat	0.359	0.567	−0.190
Red meat	0.330	0.595	−0.088
Added sugar	0.325	−0.023	−0.120
Wholegrains	0.319	−0.113	0.408
Saturated spreads	0.291	−0.117	0.111
Poultry	0.280	0.520	−0.098

Table 2. Cont.

Food Group	Non-Core Foods	High Meat and Take-Away	Mediterranean-Style
Potato	0.279	0.009	−0.199
Nuts and nut spread	0.260	0.137	0.493
Fried fish	0.212	0.649	−0.064
Fresh fruit	0.150	−0.020	0.539
Tomatoes	0.081	−0.137	0.355
Legumes	0.066	0.018	0.207
Other vegetables	−0.008	0.114	0.618
Leafy green vegetables	−0.038	0.082	0.503
Eggs	−0.039	0.202	0.271
Processed fish	−0.040	0.510	0.376
Other fish	−0.042	0.620	0.260
Garlic	−0.055	0.033	0.435
Soya	−0.082	−0.040	0.393
Alcohol	−0.185	0.287	0.060
Percentage variance explained	13%	8%	6%

Dietary patterns obtained using factor analysis with factor loadings extracted using the principal component method and varimax/orthogonal rotation. Food groups with factor loadings <0.25 for all factors are not included in the table (cruciferous vegetables; yellow or red vegetables; low fat dairy; full fat dairy; and canned fruit).

3.3. Dietary Patterns and PCOS

Table 3 reports the results from logistic regression. In the crude analysis, for each 1 SD increase in the *High meat, fish, poultry and take-away* pattern, there was a 9% greater likelihood for women to have PCOS, however this association did not remain in the adjusted analysis. In the crude analysis, for each 1 SD increase in the *Mediterranean-style* dietary pattern, there was a 15% greater likelihood for women to have PCOS. This association was strengthened after adjusting for maternal age, maternal BMI, current breastfeeding, number of children, such that for each 1 SD increase in the *Mediterranean-style* dietary pattern, there was a 26% greater likelihood that the women reported had PCOS. There were no associations between the *Unhealthy, non-core foods* pattern and PCOS.

Table 3. Odds ratios for likelihood of PCOS according to the dietary patterns identified.

	OR *	95% CI	p	Adjusted OR * †	95% CI	p
PCOS						
Unhealthy, non-core foods	1.06	0.97, 1.16	0.22	1.03	0.94, 1.13	0.55
High meat, fish, poultry and take-away	1.09	1.00, 1.17	0.03	1.04	0.95, 1.13	0.43
Mediterranean-style	1.15	1.05, 1.26	0.02	1.26	1.15, 1.39	<0.001
Maternal age	-			0.92	0.85, 0.98	0.014
Maternal BMI	-			1.09	1.07, 1.10	<0.001
Current breastfeeding	-			1.00	0.96, 1.05	0.97
Number of children	-			0.88	0.75, 1.04	0.13

Associations between PCOS and dietary patterns (Z-scores) in crude and adjusted analyses carried out using binary logistic regression analyses; Referent category is not having PCOS; * Indicates change in risk per 1 SD increase in factor score; † Adjusted for maternal age, maternal BMI, current breastfeeding, number of children.

4. Discussion

We report here for the first time that women with PCOS have different dietary patterns compared to women without PCOS, in a large population-based cohort of women. Women with PCOS were more likely to consume a dietary pattern consistent with the Mediterranean diet; however there were no differences in the other commonly consumed dietary patterns of unhealthy non-core foods or a pattern higher in meat.

The Mediterranean-style dietary pattern contains a number of foods similar to a Mediterranean diet which consists of fish, monounsaturated fats from olive oil, fruits, vegetables, wholegrains, legumes and nuts and moderate alcohol consumption [43]. It is also consistent with previously defined "Mediterranean" patterns in prior research comprising vegetables, fish, fruits, poultry, low-fat dairy products, and olive oil [44,45]. Surprisingly however, we found an inverse factor loading for poultry which is typically consumed in higher intakes in the Australian population compared to fish [46], which loaded on this pattern in moderate amounts for both processed (*i.e.*, tinned fish) and other fish (*i.e.*, cooked fish), while fried fish was inversely associated. It is to be noted that intake of olive oil is not collected in the food frequency questionnaire used in this study. Another surprising finding was that both low fat and high fat dairy foods did not correlate to any pattern. This might reflect the overall low consumption of dairy in men and women in the adult Australian population; yet this is consistent with a previous study in pregnant women where low fat dairy did not load on any of the three dietary patterns, and high fat dairy only moderately correlated with the vegetarian-type dietary pattern [24]. Nevertheless, non-core foods inversely loaded on this pattern such as take-away foods and crisps, as well as added sugar, which supports an overall healthier dietary pattern consisting of a number of Mediterranean foods. As we are the first to report that a Mediterranean-style dietary pattern was independently associated with increased likelihood of having PCOS, this discrepant finding may indicate the possible high level of women with PCOS seeking dietary knowledge with a subsequent adoption of healthy dietary patterns.

To date, there are few other studies reporting on the relationship between dietary patterns and other conditions co-existing with PCOS. In literature assessing infertile women, a large proportion of whom will likely have PCOS, a Mediterranean diet is associated with a higher chance of natural or assisted reproduction conception [44,47]. The adoption of a Mediterranean-style diet in PCOS may therefore have positive implications for the appropriate lifestyle management of chronic diseases associated with PCOS. Further studies are needed to expand on our findings on the association of dietary changes in those with a diagnosis of PCOS, the optimal means of conveying dietary education at diagnosis and the long-term maintenance of positive dietary changes.

We observed here that the two other identified dietary patterns, namely those consisting predominantly of non-core foods or a higher meat intake from either take-away/processed or non-processed sources explained a moderate proportion of variability in food intake in all participants (13% and 8% respectively). However, neither pattern was associated with PCOS status in the adjusted analysis. In association with higher weight and BMI in PCOS, this is a positive finding that is also consistent with the diagnosis of PCOS contributing to an improvement of dietary habits in keeping with population-based dietary guidelines of minimising discretionary or non-core food intake, reducing processed meats and consuming a moderate intake of protein [48].

While a Mediterranean diet is not a specifically recommended dietary intake for PCOS, emerging research suggests beneficial effects of certain components of this diet, such as elevated omega-3 fatty acids which are generally found in high amounts of oily fish. Although the specific types of fish consumed in our Mediterranean style dietary pattern cannot be extracted, both processed fish and cooked fish varieties contain some omega-3 fatty acids, likely contributing to a reasonable intake of omega-3 fatty acids in this population. The literature in PCOS focuses predominantly on omega-3 fatty acid supplementation studies which report improvements in outcomes including reductions in bioavailable androgens, triglycerides, blood pressure, glucose and surrogate markers of insulin resistance [49–52]. One recent study found that a Mediterranean diet pre-pregnancy was associated with a 42% reduced likelihood of developing hypertensive related disorders during pregnancy [26]; while higher consumption of sweets and seafood [25] or high intake of red meat, processed meat, refined grain products and sweets [27] during pregnancy was associated with a 23% and 63% increased risk of gestational diabetes. A Mediterranean dietary pattern has also been reported to be associated with improved health outcomes including decreased inflammation [53] and prevalence of the metabolic syndrome [54], abnormal glucose tolerance [55] or depression [45]. As adverse health outcomes are commonly associated with PCOS [3,4,6], this dietary pattern may therefore result in health benefits. However, we have previously reported in this cohort that this improved diet quality occurred in conjunction with a modest increase in energy intake (+215 kJ/day) which could contribute to additional longitudinal weight gain [19]. The potential benefits of an improved dietary pattern may not outweigh the effects of increased energy intake and consequent weight gain with regards to effects on reproductive, and potentially metabolic and psychological, parameters.

Strengths to our study include the large population of women with and without PCOS from a community-based population in contrast to the majority of the existing research assessing diet and PCOS. This minimises selection bias. This is also more likely to capture a lower proportion of women with PCOS with a more severe clinical phenotype and a higher BMI who typically present to clinical services and are captured in research studies [56]. While the use of self-report PCOS is a limitation, the nature of this research means that it is not feasible to clinically verify PCOS or control status. It is also not possible to determine the PCOS phenotype or which diagnostic criteria were used in diagnosis. However, given that the Rotterdam criteria were first published in 2004 [57], it is also most likely that the majority of women self-reporting diagnosed PCOS in Survey 4, conducted in 2006, would have been diagnosed based on NIH criteria. There are also some other limitations to our study. We report here 58% participant retention compared to baseline levels 13 years prior which may indicate bias and limit generalisability. However, no differences between completors and non-completors has previously been reported indicating a likely minimal effect of attrition on outcomes [36]. Although the FFQ is a validated measure of assessing nutritional intake, we are not able to assess the contribution of dietary patterns to the development or severity of PCOS due to the study design and report here only associations between dietary patterns and PCOS status. Further, the total variance explained by each factor was intermediate compared with previous factor analyses conducted in different age groups [29,58,59]; however, the Kaiser-Meyer-Olkin measure of sampling adequacy was 0.78, exceeding the recommended value of 0.6; and Bartlett's test of Sphericity achieved statistical significance indicating the correlations in the data set are appropriate for factor analysis. Moreover, the food groups loading on the factors were varied and many were greater than the 0.25 cut-off value suggesting that our population had a varied diet that was, nevertheless, still specific to the identified factors. As the present study is the first of its kind in this population, further studies are required to refute or support our findings and future work is warranted assessing the contribution of dietary pattern intake to the severity or incidence of PCOS.

5. Conclusions

In conclusion, we report for the first time the independent association of PCOS status with self-reported dietary patterns, specifically a Mediterranean diet pattern. This may indicate an improvement in the quality of dietary intake following a diagnosis of PCOS. We also report no increase in dietary patterns high in non-core, meat or take-away foods despite a higher body weight. Combined with our prior research showing healthier intake but higher caloric consumption, it appears that women with PCOS may have a greater appetite and are more overweight, despite a healthier diet. Future research should examine the contribution of dietary patterns to the incidence and severity of PCOS and the potential for modification of dietary patterns in the lifestyle management of PCOS.

Acknowledgments: The research on which this paper is based was conducted as part of the Australian Longitudinal Study on Women's Health, which was conceived and developed by groups of inter-disciplinary researchers at The University of Newcastle and The University of Queensland. We are grateful to the Australian Government Department of Health for funding and to the women who provided the survey data. The authors thank Professor Graham Giles of the Cancer Epidemiology Centre of The Cancer Council Victoria for permission to use the Dietary Questionnaire for Epidemiological Studies (version 2), Melbourne: The Cancer Council Victoria, 1996. We also thank all the participants for their valuable contribution to this project. L.J.M. is supported by a South Australian Cardiovascular Research Development Program Fellowship (ID AC11S374); a program collaboratively funded by the National Heart Foundation, the South Australian Department of Health and the South Australian Health and Medical Research Institute. J.A.G. is funded by a Robinson Research Institute Post-Doctoral Fellowship, G.D.M. is funded by the ARC Future fellowship (FT120100812) and H.J.T. is funded by an NHMRC fellowship (ID 545888).

Author Contributions: L.J.M., G.D.M.: Substantial contributions to conception and design, or acquisition of data; L.J.M., J.A.G.: Analysis and interpretation of data; L.J.M., J.A.G., G.D.M., H.J.T.: Drafting the article or revising it critically for important intellectual content; L.J.M., J.A.G., G.D.M., H.J.T.: Final approval of the version to be published.

Conflicts of Interest: The authors declare no conflict of interest.

References

1. March, W.A.; Moore, V.M.; Willson, K.J.; Phillips, D.I.; Norman, R.J.; Davies, M.J. The prevalence of polycystic ovary syndrome in a community sample assessed under contrasting diagnostic criteria. *Hum. Reprod.* **2010**, *25*, 544–551. [CrossRef] [PubMed]

2. Azziz, R.; Carmina, E.; Dewailly, D.; Diamanti-Kandarakis, E.; Escobar-Morreale, H.F.; Futterweit, W.; Janssen, O.E.; Legro, R.S.; Norman, R.J.; Taylor, A.E.; *et al.* The Androgen Excess and PCOS Society criteria for the polycystic ovary syndrome: The complete task force report. *Fertil. Steril.* **2009**, *91*, 456–488. [CrossRef] [PubMed]

3. Moran, L.J.; Misso, M.L.; Wild, R.A.; Norman, R.J. Impaired glucose tolerance, type 2 diabetes and metabolic syndrome in polycystic ovary syndrome: A systematic review and meta-analysis. *Hum. Reprod. Update* **2010**, *16*, 347–363. [CrossRef]

4. Toulis, K.A.; Goulis, D.G.; Mintziori, G.; Kintiraki, E.; Eukarpidis, E.; Mouratoglou, S.A.; Pavlaki, A.; Stergianos, S.; Poulasouchidou, M.; Tzellos, T.G.; *et al.* Meta-analysis of cardiovascular disease risk markers in women with polycystic ovary syndrome. *Hum. Reprod. Update* **2011**, *17*, 741–760. [CrossRef] [PubMed]

5. De Groot, P.C.; Dekkers, O.M.; Romijn, J.A.; Dieben, S.W.; Helmerhorst, F.M. PCOS, coronary heart disease, stroke and the influence of obesity: A systematic review and meta-analysis. *Hum. Reprod. Update* **2011**, *17*, 495–500. [CrossRef] [PubMed]

6. Barry, J.A.; Kuczmierczyk, A.R.; Hardiman, P.J. Anxiety and depression in polycystic ovary syndrome: A systematic review and meta-analysis. *Hum. Reprod.* **2011**, *26*, 2442–2451. [CrossRef] [PubMed]

7. Teede, H.J.; Joham, A.E.; Paul, E.; Moran, L.J.; Loxton, D.; Jolley, D.; Lombard, C. Longitudinal weight gain in women identified with Polycystic Ovary Syndrome: Results of an observational study in young women. *Obesity* **2013**, *21*, 1526–1532. [CrossRef] [PubMed]

8. Lim, S.S.; Davies, M.J.; Norman, R.J.; Moran, L.J. Overweight, obesity and central obesity in women with polycystic ovary syndrome: A systematic review and meta-analysis. *Hum. Reprod. Update* **2012**, *18*, 618–637. [CrossRef] [PubMed]

9. Lim, S.S.; Norman, R.J.; Davies, M.J.; Moran, L.J. The effect of obesity on polycystic ovary syndrome: A systematic review and meta-analysis. *Obes. Rev.* **2013**, *14*, 95–109. [CrossRef] [PubMed]

10. Pugeat, M.; Crave, J.C.; Elmidani, M.; Nicolas, M.H.; Garoscio-Cholet, M.; Lejeune, H.; Dechaud, H.; Tourniaire, J. Pathophysiology of sex hormone binding globulin (SHBG): Relation to insulin. *J. Steroid Biochem. Mol. Biol.* **1991**, *40*, 841–849. [CrossRef]

11. Poretsky, L.; Kalin, M.F. The gonadotropic function of insulin. *Endocr. Rev.* **1987**, *8*, 132–141. [CrossRef] [PubMed]

12. Teede, H.J.; Misso, M.L.; Deeks, A.A.; Moran, L.J.; Stuckey, B.G.A.; Wong, J.L.A.; Norman, R.J.; Costello, M.F. Assessment and management of polycystic ovary syndrome: Summary of an evidence-based guideline. *Med. J. Aust.* **2011**, *195*, S65–S112. [CrossRef] [PubMed]

13. Moran, L.J.; Ko, H.; Misso, M.; Marsh, K.; Noakes, M.; Talbot, M.; Frearson, M.; Thondan, M.; Stepto, N.; Teede, H.J. Dietary composition in the treatment of polycystic ovary syndrome: A systematic review to inform evidence-based guidelines. *J. Acad. Nutr. Diet.* **2013**, *113*, 520–545. [CrossRef] [PubMed]

14. Sharma, A.; Walker, D.M.; Atiomo, W. National survey on management of weight reduction in PCOS women in the United Kingdom. *Eur. J. Obstet. Gynecol. Reprod. Biol.* **2010**, *152*, 181–185. [CrossRef] [PubMed]

15. Humphreys, L.; Costarelli, V. Implementation of dietary and general lifestyle advice among women with polycystic ovarian syndrome. *J. R. Soc. Health* **2008**, *128*, 190–195. [CrossRef]

16. Douglas, C.C.; Norris, L.E.; Oster, R.A.; Darnell, B.E.; Azziz, R.; Gower, B.A. Difference in dietary intake between women with polycystic ovary syndrome and healthy controls. *Fertil. Steril.* **2006**, *86*, 411–417. [CrossRef] [PubMed]

17. Turner-McGrievy, G.; Davidson, C.R.; Billings, D.L. Dietary intake, eating behaviors, and quality of life in women with polycystic ovary syndrome who are trying to conceive. *Hum. Fertil. (Camb.)* **2015**, *18*, 16–21. [CrossRef] [PubMed]

18. Altieri, P.; Cavazza, C.; Pasqui, F.; Morselli, A.M.; Gambineri, A.; Pasquali, R. Dietary habits and their relationship with hormones and metabolism in overweight and obese women with polycystic ovary syndrome. *Clin. Endocrinol.* **2013**, *78*, 52–59. [CrossRef] [PubMed]

19. Moran, L.J.; Ranasinha, S.; Zoungas, S.; McNaughton, S.A.; Brown, W.J.; Teede, H.J. The contribution of diet, physical activity and sedentary behaviour to body mass index in women with and without polycystic ovary syndrome. *Hum. Reprod.* **2013**, *28*, 2276–2283. [CrossRef] [PubMed]

20. Wild, R.A.; Applebaum-Bowden, D.; Demers, L.M.; Bartholomew, M.; Landis, J.R.; Hazzard, W.R.; Santen, R.J. Lipoprotein lipids in women with androgen excess: Independent associations with increased insulin and androgen. *Clin. Chem.* **1990**, *36*, 283–289. [PubMed]

21. Sedighi, S.; Amir Ali Akbari, S.; Afrakhteh, M.; Esteki, T.; Alavi Majd, H.; Mahmoodi, Z. Comparison of lifestyle in women with polycystic ovary syndrome and healthy women. *Glob. J. Health Sci.* **2015**, *7*, 228–234. [CrossRef] [PubMed]

22. Newby, P.K.; Tucker, K.L. Empirically derived eating patterns using factor or cluster analysis: A review. *Nutr. Rev.* **2004**, *62*, 177–203. [CrossRef] [PubMed]

23. Hu, F.B. Dietary pattern analysis: A new direction in nutritional epidemiology. *Curr. Opin. Lipidol.* **2002**, *13*, 3–9. [CrossRef] [PubMed]

24. Grieger, J.A.; Grzeskowiak, L.E.; Clifton, V.L. Preconception dietary patterns in human pregnancies are associated with preterm delivery. *J. Nutr.* **2014**, *144*, 1075–1080. [CrossRef] [PubMed]

25. He, J.R.; Yuan, M.Y.; Chen, N.N.; Lu, J.H.; Hu, C.Y.; Mai, W.B.; Zhang, R.F.; Pan, Y.H.; Qiu, L.; Wu, Y.F.; *et al.* Maternal dietary patterns and gestational diabetes mellitus: A large prospective cohort study in China. *Br. J. Nutr.* **2015**, *113*, 1292–1300. [CrossRef] [PubMed]

26. Schoenaker, D.A.; Soedamah-Muthu, S.S.; Callaway, L.K.; Mishra, G.D. Prepregnancy dietary patterns and risk of developing hypertensive disorders of pregnancy: Results from the Australian Longitudinal Study on Women's Health. *Am. J. Clin. Nutr.* **2015**, *102*, 94–101. [CrossRef] [PubMed]

27. Zhang, C.; Schulze, M.B.; Solomon, C.G.; Hu, F.B. A prospective study of dietary patterns, meat intake and the risk of gestational diabetes mellitus. *Diabetologia* **2006**, *49*, 2604–2613. [CrossRef] [PubMed]

28. Schoenaker, D.A.; Soedamah-Muthu, S.S.; Callaway, L.K.; Mishra, G.D. Pre-pregnancy dietary patterns and risk of gestational diabetes mellitus: Results from an Australian population-based prospective cohort study. *Diabetologia* **2015**. in press. [CrossRef] [PubMed]

29. Yu, C.; Shi, Z.; Lv, J.; Du, H.; Qi, L.; Guo, Y.; Bian, Z.; Chang, L.; Tang, X.; Jiang, Q.; *et al.* Major dietary patterns in relation to general and central obesity among chinese adults. *Nutrients* **2015**, *7*, 5834–5849. [CrossRef] [PubMed]

30. Maghsoudi, Z.; Ghiasvand, R.; Salehi-Abargouei, A. Empirically derived dietary patterns and incident type 2 diabetes mellitus: A systematic review and meta-analysis on prospective observational studies. *Public Health Nutr.* **2015**, 1–12. [CrossRef] [PubMed]

31. Gadgil, M.D.; Anderson, C.A.; Kandula, N.R.; Kanaya, A.M. Dietary patterns are associated with metabolic risk factors in South asians living in the United States. *J. Nutr.* **2015**, *145*, 1211–1217. [CrossRef] [PubMed]

32. Orio, F.; Muscogiuri, G.; Palomba, S. Could the Mediterranean diet be effective in women with polycystic ovary syndrome? A proof of concept. *Eur. J. Clin. Nutr.* **2015**, *69*, 974. [CrossRef] [PubMed]

33. Dobson, A.J.; Hockey, R.; Brown, W.J.; Byles, J.E.; Loxton, D.J.; McLaughlin, D.; Tooth, L.R.; Mishra, G.D. Cohort Profile Update: Australian Longitudinal Study on Women's Health. *Int. J. Epidemiol.* **2015**. [CrossRef] [PubMed]

34. Brown, W.J.; Bryson, L.; Byles, J.E.; Dobson, A.J.; Lee, C.; Mishra, G.; Schofield, M. Women's Health Australia: Recruitment for a national longitudinal cohort study. *Women Health* **1998**, *28*, 23–40. [CrossRef]

35. Lee, C. *Women's Health Australia: Progress on the Australian Longitudinal Study on Women's Health 1995–2000*; Australian Academic Press Pty Ltd.: Brisbane, Australia, 2001.

36. Powers, J.; Loxton, D. The impact of attrition in an 11-year prospective longitudinal study of younger women. *Ann. Epidemiol.* **2010**, *20*, 318–321. [CrossRef] [PubMed]

37. Lee, C.; Dobson, A.J.; Brown, W.J.; Bryson, L.; Byles, J.; Warner-Smith, P.; Young, A.F. Cohort Profile: The Australian Longitudinal Study on Women's Health. *Int. J. Epidemiol.* **2005**, *34*, 987–991. [CrossRef] [PubMed]

38. WHO. *Obesity: Preventing and Managing the Global Epidemic. Report of a WHO Consultation*; WHO Technical Report Series 894 ed.; World Health Organisation: Geneva, Switzerland, 2000.

39. Hodge, A.; Patterson, A.J.; Brown, W.J.; Ireland, P.; Giles, G. The Anti Cancer Council of Victoria FFQ: Relative validity of nutrient intakes compared with weighed food records in young to middle-aged women in a study of iron supplementation. *Aust. N. Z. J. Public Health* **2000**, *24*, 576–583. [CrossRef] [PubMed]

40. Ambrosini, G.L.; Oddy, W.H.; Robinson, M.; O'Sullivan, T.A.; Hands, B.P.; de Klerk, N.H.; Silburn, S.R.; Zubrick, S.R.; Kendall, G.E.; Stanley, F.J.; *et al.* Adolescent dietary patterns are associated with lifestyle and family psycho-social factors. *Public Health Nutr.* **2009**, *12*, 1807–1815. [CrossRef] [PubMed]

41. Schulze, M.B.; Hoffmann, K.; Kroke, A.; Boeing, H. An approach to construct simplified measures of dietary patterns from exploratory factor analysis. *Br. J. Nutr.* **2003**, *89*, 409–419. [CrossRef] [PubMed]

42. Kline, P.K. *An Easy Guide to Factor Analysis*; Routledge: London, UK, 1994.

43. Widmer, R.J.; Flammer, A.J.; Lerman, L.O.; Lerman, A. The Mediterranean diet, its components, and cardiovascular disease. *Am. J. Med.* **2015**, *128*, 229–238. [CrossRef] [PubMed]

44. Toledo, E.; Lopez-del Burgo, C.; Ruiz-Zambrana, A.; Donazar, M.; Navarro-Blasco, I.; Martinez-Gonzalez, M.A.; de Irala, J. Dietary patterns and difficulty conceiving: A nested case-control study. *Fertil. Steril.* **2011**, *96*, 1149–1153. [CrossRef] [PubMed]

45. Rienks, J.; Dobson, A.J.; Mishra, G.D. Mediterranean dietary pattern and prevalence and incidence of depressive symptoms in mid-aged women: Results from a large community-based prospective study. *Eur. J. Clin. Nutr.* **2013**, *67*, 75–82. [CrossRef] [PubMed]

46. ABS. *4364.0.55.007—Australian Health Survey: Nutrition First Results—Foods and Nutrients, 2011–2012*; Statistics, A.B.O., Ed.; Australian Bureau of Statistics: Canberra, Australia, 2014.

47. Vujkovic, M.; de Vries, J.H.; Lindemans, J.; Macklon, N.S.; van der Spek, P.J.; Steegers, E.A.; Steegers-Theunissen, R.P. The preconception Mediterranean dietary pattern in couples undergoing *in vitro* fertilization/intracytoplasmic sperm injection treatment increases the chance of pregnancy. *Fertil. Steril.* **2010**, *94*, 2096–2101. [CrossRef] [PubMed]

48. NHMRC. *Australian Dietary Guidelines*; National Health and Medical Research Council: Canberra, Australia, 2013.

49. Mohammadi, E.; Rafraf, M.; Farzadi, L.; Asghari-Jafarabadi, M.; Sabour, S. Effects of omega-3 fatty acids supplementation on serum adiponectin levels and some metabolic risk factors in women with polycystic ovary syndrome. *Asia Pac. J. Clin. Nutr.* **2012**, *21*, 511–518. [PubMed]

50. Rafraf, M.; Mohammadi, E.; Asghari-Jafarabadi, M.; Farzadi, L. Omega-3 fatty acids improve glucose metabolism without effects on obesity values and serum visfatin levels in women with polycystic ovary syndrome. *J. Am. Coll. Nutr.* **2012**, *31*, 361–368. [CrossRef] [PubMed]

51. Cussons, A.J.; Watts, G.F.; Mori, T.A.; Stuckey, B.G. Omega-3 fatty acid supplementation decreases liver fat content in polycystic ovary syndrome: A randomized controlled trial employing proton magnetic resonance spectroscopy. *J. Clin. Endocrinol. Metab.* **2009**, *94*, 3842–3848. [CrossRef] [PubMed]

52. Phelan, N.; O'Connor, A.; Kyaw Tun, T.; Correia, N.; Boran, G.; Roche, H.M.; Gibney, J. Hormonal and metabolic effects of polyunsaturated fatty acids in young women with polycystic ovary syndrome: Results from a cross-sectional analysis and a randomized, placebo-controlled, crossover trial. *Am. J. Clin. Nutr.* **2011**, *93*, 652–662. [CrossRef] [PubMed]

53. Schwingshackl, L.; Hoffmann, G. Mediterranean dietary pattern, inflammation and endothelial function: A systematic review and meta-analysis of intervention trials. *Nutr. Metab. Cardiovasc. Dis* **2014**, *24*, 929–939. [CrossRef] [PubMed]

54. Steffen, L.M.; van Horn, L.; Daviglus, M.L.; Zhou, X.; Reis, J.P.; Loria, C.M.; Jacobs, D.R.; Duffey, K.J. A modified Mediterranean diet score is associated with a lower risk of incident metabolic syndrome over 25 years among young adults: The CARDIA (Coronary Artery Risk Development in Young Adults) study. *Br. J. Nutr.* **2014**, *112*, 1654–1661. [CrossRef] [PubMed]

55. Koloverou, E.; Esposito, K.; Giugliano, D.; Panagiotakos, D. The effect of Mediterranean diet on the development of type 2 diabetes mellitus: A meta-analysis of 10 prospective studies and 136,846 participants. *Metabolism* **2014**, *63*, 903–911. [CrossRef] [PubMed]

56. Ezeh, U.; Yildiz, B.O.; Azziz, R. Referral Bias in defining the phenotype and prevalence of obesity in polycystic ovary syndrome. *J. Clin. Endocrinol. Metab.* **2013**, *98*, 1088–1096. [CrossRef] [PubMed]

57. Rotterdam ESHRE ASRM-Sponsored PCOS Consensus Workshop Group. Revised 2003 consensus on diagnostic criteria and long-term health risks related to polycystic ovary syndrome (PCOS). *Hum. Reprod.* **2004**, *19*, 41–47.

58. Grieger, J.A.; Scott, J.; Cobiac, L. Dietary patterns and breast-feeding in Australian children. *Public Health Nutr.* **2011**, *14*, 1939–1947. [CrossRef] [PubMed]

59. Hu, F.B.; Rimm, E.B.; Stampfer, M.J.; Ascherio, A.; Spiegelman, D.; Willett, W.C. Prospective study of major dietary patterns and risk of coronary heart disease in men. *Am. J. Clin. Nutr.* **2000**, *72*, 912–921. [PubMed]

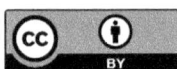

MDPI

Article

Adherence to a Healthy Nordic Food Index Is Associated with a Lower Risk of Type-2 Diabetes—The Danish Diet, Cancer and Health Cohort Study

Sandra Amalie Lacoppidan [1], Cecilie Kyrø [1,*], Steffen Loft [2], Anne Helnæs [1], Jane Christensen [1], Camilla Plambeck Hansen [3], Christina Catherine Dahm [3], Kim Overvad [3], Anne Tjønneland [1] and Anja Olsen [1]

[1] Danish Cancer Society Research Center, Strandboulevarden 49, 2100 Copenhagen, Denmark; sanlac@cancer.dk (S.A.L.) annhelh@cancer.dk (C.K.); akhj@cancer.dk (A.H.); jane@cancer.dk (J.C.); annet@cancer.dk (A.T.); anja@cancer.dk (A.O.)

[2] Department of Public Health, Section of Environmental Health, Faculty of Health and Medical Sciences, University of Copenhagen, Øster Farimagsgade 5, 1014 København K, Denmark; stl@sund.ku.dk

[3] Department of Public Health, Section for Epidemiology, Aarhus University, Bartholins Allé 2, 8000 Aarhus C, Denmark; cph@ph.au.dk (C.P.H.); ccd@ph.au.dk (C.C.D.); ko@ph.au.dk (K.O.)

* Correspondence: ceciliek@cancer.dk; Tel.: +45-35257915

Received: 28 August 2015 ; Accepted: 10 October 2015 ; Published: 20 October 2015

Abstract: Background: Type-2 diabetes (T2D) prevalence is rapidly increasing worldwide. Lifestyle factors, in particular obesity, diet, and physical activity play a significant role in the etiology of the disease. Of dietary patterns, particularly the Mediterranean diet has been studied, and generally a protective association has been identified. However, other regional diets are less explored. Objective: The aim of the present study was to investigate the association between adherence to a healthy Nordic food index and the risk of T2D. The index consists of six food items: fish, cabbage, rye bread, oatmeal, apples and pears, and root vegetables. Methods: Data was obtained from a prospective cohort study of 57,053 Danish men and women aged 50–64 years, at baseline, of whom 7366 developed T2D (median follow-up: 15.3 years). The Cox proportional hazards model was used to assess the association between the healthy Nordic food index and risk of T2D, adjusted for potential confounders. Results: Greater adherence to the healthy Nordic food index was significantly associated with lower risk of T2D after adjusting for potential confounders. An index score of 5–6 points (high adherence) was associated with a statistically significantly 25% lower T2D risk in women (HR: 0.75, 95%CI: 0.61–0.92) and 38% in men (HR: 0.62; 95%CI: 0.53–0.71) compared to those with an index score of 0 points (poor adherence). Conclusion: Adherence to a healthy Nordic food index was found to be inversely associated with risk of T2D, suggesting that regional diets other than the Mediterranean may also be recommended for prevention of T2D.

Keywords: Type-2 diabetes (T2D); Nordic diet; dietary pattern; prospective cohort

1. Introduction

Type-2 diabetes (T2D) is a chronic metabolic disease with an increasing global incidence and prevalence. Around 4 percent of the population worldwide were estimated to have diabetes in 2000, but the number is projected to increase to 4.4% or 366 million people by 2030 [1]. The majority of the cases are onset at age 40–59 and are expected be type 2 diabetes [1,2]. It is well established that lifestyle plays a significant role in the etiology of T2D [3,4]. Among lifestyle factors, overweight and obesity particularly increase the risk of T2D. Diet also plays a role in relation to T2D risk [3]. Several studies have investigated the effect of different dietary exposures in relation to development of T2D, and intakes of whole grains, dietary fibre, root vegetables, and green leafy vegetables have been suggested to be inversely associated with risk of T2D [5–7].

In nutrition research, focus has previously mainly been on single foods or nutrients. However, people consume meals consisting of combinations of numerous nutrients and foods. Hence, it is relevant to examine a combination of a variety of foods in relation to T2D. Different dietary indices, such as the Mediterranean diet, have been investigated in relation T2D, in Mediterranean, American as well as other European populations [8–12]. Compliance with this dietary pattern is low in non-Mediterranean countries, maybe because non-Mediterranean populations may find it difficult to comply with a diet which is foreign to them [6,13]. It might therefore be relevant to investigate health effects of other regional diets such as the Nordic diet within a Nordic population. It is possible that other regional diets also carry health benefits, and it might be easier for a population to comply with a diet that is familiar to them instead of adapting to a "foreign diet" [14]. Intervention studies have suggested that a healthy Nordic diet improves markers of T2D risk, such as body weight and insulin sensitivity [15–17]. A small prospective study found no association between adherence to a health Nordic diet and risk of T2D [18], but due to the small study size (total cohort $n < 7000$, cases = 541) results from larger prospective studies are needed. This aim of the study was to investigate the association between a healthy regional Nordic diet and risk of T2D in a large prospective cohort study.

2. Method and Material

2.1. Study Population

From December 1993 to May 1997, a total of 160,725 subjects (80,996 men and 79,729 women) were invited to participate in the Danish cohort study: the Diet, Cancer, and Health (DCH) cohort [19]. The criteria for invitation were: aged 50–64 years, born in Denmark, no diagnosis of cancer (registered in the Danish Cancer Registry), and living in greater Copenhagen and Aarhus areas at baseline. Unique personal identification numbers assigned to all Danish citizens from the Civil Registration System (CPR) were used to identify potential participants [20]. The DCH cohort had a 35% overall participation, comprising a total of 57,053 eligible subjects [19]. The cohort was approved by the regional ethical committees on human studies in Copenhagen and Aarhus and by the Danish Protection Agency. Moreover, written informed consent was obtained from all participants.

Of the 57,053 participants, 1766 were excluded, due to diagnosis of cancer and/or T2D before baseline. Furthermore, participants with missing information on the exposure variables of interest in this study ($n = 55$) or potential confounders ($n = 149$) were excluded. Finally, subjects diagnosed with diabetes before 1st January 1995 were excluded ($n = 15$) as well as persons that were included and deceased before this date ($n = 8$), because the National Diabetes Registry is only well defined for subjects entering after this date (see "*case ascertainment and selection*") [21]. Thus, leaving 55,060 eligible subjects (28,953 women and 26,107 men) for the present study.

2.2. Case Ascertainment and Selection

There were 7366 incident cases of diabetes (3269 women and 4097 men) identified from the National Diabetes Registry (NDR) [21]. The NDR was established in 2006 by the National Board of Health by linking nationwide registries. Because of different dates of initiation of the underlying registers and accumulation of prevalent cases, dates of inclusion into the NDR has been found to be well defined only for persons entering after 1st January 1995, even though inclusion of cases started at 1st January 1990) [21,22]. Subjects are registered in NDR if they are classified as having diabetes with a date of inclusion equal to the earliest of the dates where one of the following criteria were met: Diagnosis of diabetes in the National Patient Registry; Chiropody for diabetic patients; Five blood glucose measurements within one year; Two blood glucose measurements per year in five consecutive years; Second purchase of oral glucose-lowering drugs within six months; Second purchase of prescribed insulin. As the register is based on administrative records, the date of inclusion can only be taken as a proxy for the date of diagnosis. 56.6% of the cases included in the present study met more than one of the criteria.

NDR does not distinguish between cases of type-1 diabetes (T1D) and T2D. Since the present study is investigating a middle-aged population, and thus it is assumed that the entire incident cases of diabetes registered in NDR can be attributed T2D. Moreover lifestyle behaviour and diet habits are associated with T2D risk and not believed to influence T1D risk, the present study therefore exclusively focuses on T2D.

All 55,060 cohort participants were followed from baseline until censoring, which was the date of diagnosis of diabetes, date of death, date of emigration, or end of follow-up (31st December 2011), whichever came first. Date of death and date of emigration was identified from the CPR. Baseline was defined as the data of visiting the center, however, with the exception of participants who visited the center before 1st January 1995. For those, baseline was set to 1st January 1995.

2.3. Dietary Assessment

Prior to attendance in the study, the participants completed a 192-item FFQ, which has been validated previously [23,24]. In the questionnaire, the participants were asked to report their average intake within the last 12 months in twelve categories ranging from never to more than eight times a day. The intake of specific foods and nutrients was calculated for each participant by the software program FoodCalc [25], using specifically developed standardized recipes and portions sizes. The FFQs were processed by optical scanning and checked for missing values and reading errors. The errors were clarified and corrected by trained professionals before the participants left the study center [19].

Food items of the healthy Nordic diet index included in the study as exposure variables were: fish, cabbage, rye bread, oatmeal, apples and pears, and root vegetables. The index has previously been defined and the foods included in the index were chosen *a priori* based on the following criteria: (1) that they had to have an anticipated health benefit; (2) information on intake should be obtainable from the FFQ; (3) they had to originate from the Nordic nature, and (4) they should still hold a quantitative role the Nordic diet [26]. Information on intake of fish, cabbage, apples and pears, and root vegetables was derived from multiple questions in the FFQ, whereas information on oatmeal and rye bread originated from one question each. Fish intake was based on 23 questions regarding a variety of fish consumed as hot meals or in sandwiches, while cabbages intake was derived from six questions of different cabbage types (cauliflower, Brussels sprouts, broccoli, kale, white cabbage, and red cabbage). Information about apple and pear intake was collected from two questions: one on apple and one on pear intake. Intake of root vegetables was collected from several questions concerning intake of raw and cooked root vegetables separately, as well as part of recipes. In the DCH cohort, carrot was the main root vegetable consumed.

The healthy Nordic index is developed in accordance with the original Mediterranean Diet score constructed by Trichopoulou and colleagues [27,28]. Thus, for each of the six Nordic food items, one point was given for intake equal to or greater than the sex-specific median. As information on both oatmeal and rye bread intake was obtained from only one question each, it was not possible to use medians as cut-off values. Thus, the cut-off values for oatmeal and rye bread were defined using sex-specific spline curves with boundaries at predefined questionnaire categories. One point was given for an intake of the following: Men: fish $\geq$ 42 g/day, cabbage $\geq$ 14 g/day, oatmeal $\geq$ 21 g/day, rye bread $\geq$ 113 g/day, apples and pears $\geq$ 56 g/day, and root vegetables $\geq$ 16 g/day. Women: fish $\geq$ 35 g/day, cabbage $\geq$ 16 g/day, oatmeal $\geq$ 21 g/day, rye bread $>$ 63 g/day, apples and pears $>$ 71 g/day, and root vegetables $\geq$ 28 g/day. A score of either 0 or 1 was given for each item, allowing each participant to score between 0 (lowest adherence) and 6 (highest adherence).

2.4. Statistical Analysis

The association between the healthy Nordic food index and T2D was estimated using Cox proportional hazards models using age as the underlying time scale, and expressed as hazard ratios

(HR) with corresponding 95% confidence intervals (CI). Time under study was included as a linear spline with boundaries at one, two, and three years after entry into the study. All P-values were two-sided, and the statistical significance level was set to 0.05.

Interaction between the healthy Nordic food index and sex was investigated, and significant interaction was identified (p = 0.0186). Consequently, all analyses were stratified by sex.

The healthy Nordic food index was assessed as a linear variable (1-point unit) and as a categorical variable (0–6 points). The reference category comprised individuals with the poorest adherence to the index (0 points). The highest adherence categories, 5 and 6 points were combined to one category (5–6 points), due to few cases in the category rating "6 points".

All estimates are presented as both crude (model 1) and adjusted (models 2, 3, and 4). In model 2, adjustments were made for the following potential confounding lifestyle factors: alcohol (abstainers and drinkers with different boundaries set for men and women), smoking status (never, former, current), schooling level (low: ≤7 years, medium 8–10 years, and high: ≥10 years), participation in sports (yes/no), intake of meat (g/day of red and processed meat). In model 3, adjustment was additionally done for total energy intake (kJ/day) using the standard multivariate method [29]. Model 4 was additionally adjusted for two potential mediators: waist circumference (WC) and body mass index (BMI). In order to preserve statistical power, we adjusted for physical activity using the indicator variable "Participate in sports (yes/no)". We also had several other measures of physical activity, but adding them to the model did not change the results considerably.

Linearity of continuous variables were evaluated graphically by linear splines with three or nine knots placed at quartiles or deciles among cases. The healthy Nordic food index, BMI, WC, and intake of red and processed meat were found to be linearly associated with T2D, whereas alcohol intake was related to T2D risk with an apparently U-shaped pattern. To ensure proper adjustment accounting for this non-linear association, alcohol intake among drinkers was included as linear splines with boundaries: alcohol intake 12 g/day for women and 24 g/day for men, respectively.

For the analyses evaluating the individual association between T2D and each of the six food items included in the index, the same confounder adjustments were made, but further adjustments for the remaining five food items (mutually adjustment) were performed.

A sensitivity analysis was conducted including only "confirmed cases". It is possible that the register may have included some non-diabetics as cases. Two of the inclusion criteria in NDR: *five blood glucose measurements within one year* and *two blood glucose measurements per year for five consecutive years*, might have questionable validity [30], and thus a sensitivity analysis was conducted excluding these (n = 3113).

Possible multiplicative interactions between the healthy Nordic food index and BMI were investigated.

SAS® statistical software (release 9.3, SAS Institute, Inc., Cary, NC, USA) was used for all statistical analyses. The PHREG procedure was used for the Cox proportional hazards models and the UNIVARIATE and FREQ procedures for the descriptive statistics.

3. Results

During a median of 15 years of follow-up, 3269 women and 4097 men of the 55,060 cohort participants were diagnosed with T2D. Table 1 shows the baseline characteristics stratified by sex for all and according to the healthy Nordic food index score: lowest adherence (0–1 points), middle adherence (2–3 points), and highest adherence (4–6 points), respectively. A larger proportion of cases was present in the lowest adherence score category, compared to highest scores. Moreover, individuals with the highest scores also had the healthiest lifestyles for both men and women, *i.e.*, men and women with a high adherence score had more participation in sports and were less likely to be smokers compared to those with the poorest adherence to the index.

Table 1. Baseline characteristics of all participants in the Danish Diet, Cancer and Health cohort in relation to adherence to the healthy Nordic food index (n = 55,060).

	Women (n = 28,953)								Men (n = 26,107)							
	All		0-1		2-3		4-6		All		0-1		2-3		4-6	
Cases, n / total participants, n (% cases)	3,269/28,953 (11%)		679/5,332 (13%)		1,570/13,477 (12%)		1,020/10,144 (10%)		4,097/26,107 (16%)		706/4,346 (18%)		1,888/11,570 (16%)		1,039/8,191 (13%)	
Characteristic	Median or %	P5-P95 or n (50-64)	Median or %	P5-P95 or n (50-64)	Median or %	P5-P95 or n (50-64)	Median or %	P5-P95 or n (50-64)	Median or %	P5-P95 or n (50-64)	Median or %	P5-P95 or n (50-64)	Median or %	P5-P95 or n (50-64)	Median or %	P5-P95 or n (50-64)
Age (years)	56	(50-64)	55	(50-64)	56	(50-64)	56	(50-64)	55	(50-64)	55	(50-64)	56	(50-64)	55	(50-64)
School (%)																
Short (<7 years)	31%	(9025)	37%	(1,962)	34%	(4,250)	28%	(2,813)	35%	(9,040)	42%	(2,658)	35%	(4,130)	29%	(2,395)
Medium (8-10 years)	50%	(14,560)	49%	(2,607)	51%	(6,921)	50%	(5,033)	42%	(10,851)	42%	(2,646)	42%	(4,998)	40%	(3,304)
Long (≥11 years)	19%	(5368)	14%	(763)	17%	(2,307)	23%	(2,299)	24%	(6,216)	16%	(1,044)	23%	(2,646)	31%	(2,525)
Smoking (%)																
Never	44%	(12,617)	37%	(1,967)	42%	(5,718)	49%	(4,933)	26%	(6,740)	22%	(1,372)	25%	(2,911)	30%	(2,455)
Former	23%	(6,794)	19%	(999)	23%	(3,038)	27%	(2,757)	35%	(9,021)	28%	(1,803)	35%	(3,993)	39%	(3,227)
Current	33%	(9,542)	44%	(2,366)	35%	(4,722)	24%	(2,455)	40%	(10,346)	50%	(3,173)	40%	(4,670)	31%	(2,507)
Alcohol intake																
Abstainer (% = yes)	3%	(773)	4%	(195)	3%	(378)	2%	(200)	2%	(463)	2%	(148)	2%	(197)	1%	(118)
Alcohol * ≤12 g/day (women), ≤24 g/day (men)	58%	(16,856)	59%	(3,138)	57%	(7,736)	59%	(5,982)	56%	(14,567)	51%	(3,233)	56%	(6,436)	60%	(4,898)
Alcohol * >12 g/day (women), >24 g/day (men)	39%	(11,324)	37%	(1,999)	40%	(5363)	39%	(3,862)	42%	(11,077)	47%	(2,965)	42%	(4,937)	39%	(3175)
BMI (kg/m²)	24.8	(19.9-33.6)	24.8	(19.8-33.9)	24.8	(19.9-33.6)	24.6	(19.3-33.2)	26.1	(21.5-33.6)	26.5	(21.5-33.6)	26.2	(21.5-32.9)	25.8	(21.4-32.2)
Waist circumference (cm)	80	(67-103)	81	(67-104)	80	(67-103)	79	(67-102)	89	(81-113)	96	(82-115)	89	(82-113)	94	(81-111)
Participate in sports (% = yes)	59%	(16,960)	45%	(2,379)	57%	(7,637)	70%	(4,749)	49%	(12,766)	38%	(2379)	48%	(5567)	59%	(4821)
Total energy intake including alcohol (mJ/day)	8.5	(5.4-12.7)	7.1	(4.5-10.6)	8.2	(5.5-12.0)	9.6	(6.6-13.8)	10.7	(7.1-15.9)	9.4	(6.2-12.8)	11.6	(7.3-12.3)	11.9	(8.5-17.1)
Intake of red meat (g/day)	63	(27-120)	59	(27-111)	63	(27-118)	67	(26-128)	100	(46-190)	93	(44-175)	100	(47-188)	105	(47-200)
Intake of processed meat (g/day)	18	(4-50)	17	(4-48)	18	(4-51)	18	(3-1)	35	(9-89)	33	(10-87)	35	(9-90)	36	(9-89)

Abbreviation: P5: 5th percentile, P95: 95th percentile, d: day; * Among drinkers, Values are medians (for continuous variables) or percentages (for categorical variables). Values in brackets are 5–95 percentiles or numbers.

Adherence to the healthy Nordic food index was associated with a lower risk of T2D for both men and women (Table 2). In the model adjusted for potential confounding factors (model 2), a one-point higher in the index was associated with a 6% lower risk for women (HR, model 2: 0.94, 95%CI = 0.92–0.97) and a 9% lower risk for men (HR, model 2: 0.91; 95% CI: 0.89–0.93). When the index was assessed as a categorical variable, significant inverse associations were also found. Women with the highest adherence (5–6 points) had a 25% lower risk of T2D (HR, model 2: 0.75, 95%CI: 0.61–0.92) compared to women with the lowest adherence (0 points). For men, the association was even more pronounced with a 38% lower risk of T2D (HR, model 2: 0.62, 95%CI: 0.53–0.71) among men with the highest adherence (5–6 points).

The confounder-adjusted estimates were less strong than the crude estimates. In the energy-adjusted model (model 3), a significant inverse association was also found, however, it was not significant when assessed categorical for women. Adjusting for BMI and WC (considered mediators) additionally moved the association towards unity, and the resulted in insignificant results for women.

When evaluating associations between the single index food items and T2D (Table 3), intakes of oatmeal and root vegetables above the cut-off values were associated with lower risk of T2D for both sexes. Moreover, for men significant associations were also found for intake of rye bread and cabbage.

In the sensitivity analysis where only "confirmed" cases (women = 1821, men = 2432) were included (Supplementary Table 1), the association between the index and T2D risk appeared slightly stronger. No significant interactions were found between BMI and the index when assessed in men and women (results not shown).

Table 2. Hazard ratio for the association between adherence to the healthy Nordic food index and T2D risk (*n* = 55,060)—The Danish Diet, Cancer and Health cohort.

Women (*n* = 28,953)

	Cases (*n*)	Model 1 *		Model 2 **		Model 3 ***		Model 4 ****	
		HR	95% CI	HR	95% CI	HR	95% CI	HR	95% CI
Healthy Nordic food index *(linear, per 1-unit increase)*	3269	0.92	0.90–0.94	0.94	0.92–0.97	0.96	0.94–0.99	0.97	0.94–1.00
Healthy Nordic food index *(category)*									
0	126	1.00	Reference	1.00	Reference	1.00	Reference	1.00	Reference
1	553	1.00	0.83–1.26	0.99	0.82–1.20	1.02	0.84–1.23	1.01	0.83–1.23
2	792	0.93	0.77–1.12	0.94	0.78–1.14	0.99	0.82–1.12	1.02	0.85–1.24
3	778	0.85	0.70–1.03	0.89	0.73–1.07	0.95	0.78–1.15	0.97	0.80–1.18
4	627	0.80	0.66–0.94	0.86	0.71–1.04	0.94	0.77–1.15	0.96	0.79–1.17
5–6	393	0.68	0.56–0.84	0.75	0.61–0.92	0.85	0.85–1.05	0.89	0.72–1.10
P for trend (linear)		*p* < 0.0001		*p* < 0.0001		*p* = 0.0100		*p* = 0.0436	

Men (*n* = 26,107)

	Cases (*n*)	Model 1 *		Model 2 *		Model 3 ***		Model 4 ****	
		HR	95% CI	HR	95% CI	HR	95% CI	HR	95% CI
Healthy Nordic food index *(linear, per 1-unit increase)*	4397	0.89	0.87–0.90	0.91	0.8–0.93	0.93	0.91–0.95	0.95	0.93–0.98
Healthy Nordic food index *(category)*									
0	367	1.00	Reference	1.00	Reference	1.00	Reference	1.00	Reference
1	503	0.87	0.77–0.98	0.89	0.77–1.00	0.91	0.80–1.03	0.96	0.85–1.09
2	640	0.83	0.74–0.94	0.88	0.77–0.99	0.91	0.81–1.03	0.98	0.86–1.11
3	898	0.72	0.63–0.81	0.78	0.69–0.88	0.82	0.72–0.93	0.89	0.78–1.02
4	652	0.61	0.54–0.70	0.69	0.60–0.78	0.74	0.65–0.86	0.83	0.72–0.95
5–6	387	0.54	0.47–0.62	0.62	0.53–0.71	0.69	0.59–0.80	0.80	0.69–0.94
P for trend (linear)		*p* < 0.0001		*p* < 0.0001		*p* < 0.0001		*p* < 0.0001	

Note: All models are adjusted for age as underlying time scale and for "time under study"; *Abbreviations*: HR: Hazard Ratio. CI: Confidence intervals; * Crude; ** Adjusted for schooling level, participation in sports, smoking status, alcohol intake, red and processed meat; *** Additionally adjusted for total energy intake; **** Additionally adjusted for body mass index and waist circumference.

129

Nutrients 2015, 7, 8633–8644

Table 3. Hazard ratio for the association between adherence to the single food items in the healthy Nordic food index and T2D risk (n = 55,060)—The Danish Diet, Cancer and Health cohort.

	Women (n = 28,953)								Men (n = 26,107)							
	Model 1 *		Model 2 **		Model 3 ***		Model 4 ****		Model 1 *		Model 2 **		Model 3 ***		Model 4 ****	
	HR	95% CI	HR	95% CI	HR	95% CI	HR	95% CI	HR	95% CI	HR	95% CI	HR	95% CI	HR	95% CI
Healthy Nordic food items																
Fish																
<Median	1.00	Reference	1.00	Reference	1.00	Reference	1.00	Reference	1.00	Reference	1.00	Reference	1.00	Reference	1.00	Reference
≥Median	1.00	0.93–1.08	1.00	0.93–1.08	1.03	0.96–1.11	0.98	0.91–1.06	1.02	0.96–1.08	1.02	0.96–1.09	1.04	0.97–1.11	1.02	0.95–1.08
Cabbage																
<Median	1.00	Reference	1.00	Reference	1.00	Reference	1.00	Reference	1.00	Reference	1.00	Reference	1.00	Reference	1.00	Reference
≥Median	0.92	0.86–0.99	0.98	0.91–1.06	0.99	0.92–1.07	0.99	0.92–1.06	0.84	0.78–0.90	0.89	0.83–0.95	0.89	0.83–0.96	0.92	0.86–0.99
Rye bread																
<Median	1.00	Reference	1.00	Reference	1.00	Reference	1.00	Reference	1.00	Reference	1.00	Reference	1.00	Reference	1.00	Reference
≥Median	0.94	0.87–1.02	0.91	0.84–0.99	0.94	0.86–1.02	0.96	0.88–1.04	0.84	0.79–0.89	0.79	0.74–0.85	0.82	0.76–0.87	0.89	0.84–0.96
Oatmeal																
<Median	1.00	Reference	1.00	Reference	1.00	Reference	1.00	Reference	1.00	Reference	1.00	Reference	1.00	Reference	1.00	Reference
≥Median	0.74	0.67–0.81	0.79	0.71–0.87	0.81	0.73–0.90	0.90	0.81–0.99	0.71	0.65–0.77	0.75	0.69–0.82	0.77	0.71–0.84	0.88	0.81–0.96
Apples and pears																
<Median	1.00	Reference	1.00	Reference	1.00	Reference	1.00	Reference	1.00	Reference	1.00	Reference	1.00	Reference	1.00	Reference
≥Median	1.02	0.95–1.09	1.01	0.94–1.09	1.04	0.96–1.12	1.03	0.96–1.11	0.98	0.92–1.04	1.02	0.96–1.09	1.04	0.97–1.11	0.97	0.91–1.04
Root vegetables																
<Median	1.00	Reference	1.00	Reference	1.00	Reference	1.00	Reference	1.00	Reference	1.00	Reference	1.00	Reference	1.00	Reference
≥Median	0.84	0.78–0.90	0.89	0.82–0.96	0.91	0.84–0.98	0.94	0.87–1.02	0.78	0.73–0.83	0.93	0.86–0.99	0.94	0.87–1.01	0.98	0.91–1.05

Note: All models are adjusted for age as underlying time scale and for "time under study"; *Abbreviations:* HR: Hazard Ratio. CI: Confidence intervals; * Crude; ** Adjusted for schooling level, participation in sports, smoking status, alcohol intake, red and processed meat; *** Additionally adjusted for total energy intake; **** Additionally adjusted for body mass index and waist circumference.

4. Discussion

In the present study, adherence with a healthy Nordic food index was associated with a lower risk of T2D. More specifically, women had a 6% lower risk and men had a 9% lower risk per one-point increment on the index score. A healthy Nordic food index score of 5−6 points (high adherence) was associated with a statistically significant 25% lower T2D risk for women and 38% for men compared to those with an index score of 0 points (poor adherence), when adjusted for potential confounders.

The strengths of the present study include the prospective design, large number of cases, detailed information about potential confounding factors, and long follow-up time. Further, a validated FFQ was used to assess food intake [23]. The study does, however, also have limitations: even though we used a validated FFQ as exposure measurement, measurement errors are likely, and further the diet of the participants was only assessed at baseline and might have changed during the long follow-up period. Furthermore, other healthy Nordic foods in the index could have been relevant to include, such as rapeseed oil. In studies of the Mediterranean diet, olive oil has shown to be associated with lower T2D risk [31]. It is possible that rapeseed oil would have similar beneficial effects [32]. However, it was not possible to include rapeseed oil due to the design of the FFQ. Finally, even though potential confounders were thoroughly considered, we cannot rule out the risk of residual confounding.

The main hypothesis was that adherence to the healthy Nordic food index was associated with lower T2D risk, which was also the case in the present study. These findings might not be surprising given that each of the included food items are considered to carry health-enhancing effects [6,33,34]. Overall, none of the food items in the index seemed to be solely responsible for the association found, and thus this supports the idea that dietary patterns provides extra information compared to when studying individual foods [35]. The beneficial association found for *oatmeal, rye bread, root vegetables,* and *cabbages* might be explained by the high content of dietary fibre in these foods, as dietary fibers slow digestion and absorption, affecting the level of glucose as well as insulin sensitivity [36,37], which are markers related to development of T2D [5]. The lack of associations with *fish* and *apples/pears* in the present study is in congruence with the existing literature [38,39]. This may be that *fish* and *apples/pears* are not directly expected to have blood glucose-stabilizing effects, contrary to the other four food items in the index.

Our results are also supported by findings from other studies, where a healthy Nordic diet has been investigated in relation to disease makers including markers of T2D risk [15–17,40,41]. For instance in the Swedish intervention study "NORDIET" where 33 mildly hypercholesterolemia participants were randomized to follow the NORDIET or a control diet [15]. The investigators found that adherence to NORDIET improved blood lipid profile (in respect to cholesterol) and reduced body weight in hypercholesterolemia participants, although there was no effect on blood pressure, plasma glucose, plasma triglyceride, or the inflammation marker C-reactive protein [15].

We expected that part of the association could be explained by high fibre content and low energy contents of the foods included in the index, and thus a lower risk of overweight and obesity, which are main risk factors of T2D [3,42]. Thus, we regarded BMI and WC as mediators rather than confounders in the association between the index and risk of T2D. As analyses including BMI and WC as covariates yielded less strong associations, it could be that the association is partly mediated by these. As most studies on Mediterranean diet consider BMI as potential confounder rather than mediator [43], we presented results both adjusted and unadjusted for BMI and WC in the tables to facilitate comparison.

A small prospective study of less than 7000 participants with 541 incident T2D cases investigated the association between a healthy Nordic food index (The Baltic Sea Score) and risk of T2D. They found a tendency for an inverse association, but it was not statistically significant, probably due to the small study size [18]. To our knowledge, no previous large observational study has investigated a Nordic food in relation to incidence of T2D particularly. However, the regional Mediterranean diet has been related to lower risk of T2D in several observational studies [8,10,11]. Thus both a healthy Nordic diet and the Mediterranean diet seems to be related to lower risk of T2D. Previous studies have

Nutrients **2015**, *7*, 8633–8644

indicated that it might be difficult for people to comply with a "foreign" diet [13]. Therefore, it could be advocated that a more regional diet should be promoted. Thus, this could not only enhance compliance, but also help in conserving the environment and cultural diversity [6].

The result of the present study may not be entirely generalizable. The cohort included only people aged 50-64 and thus may represent a population with a higher T2D risk than the entire population. It is therefore likely that the associations found are stronger than expected for the entire population.

5. Conclusions

In conclusion, we found an inverse association between a healthy Nordic index and risk of T2D for both men and women. Thus, healthy aspects of the Nordic diet may play a role in the prevention of T2D. Promoting regional diets might be an effective and sustainable way of improving public health.

Supplementary Materials: Supplementary materials can be accessed at: http://www.mdpi.com/2073-4360/7/10/5418/s1.

Acknowledgments: We acknowledge Nick Martinussen and Katja Doll for their data management assistance. The present study was funded by NordForsk (Centre of Excellence programme HELGA (070015)) and the Danish Cancer Society.

Author Contributions: A.T., K.O., A.O., S.A.L., S.L., and C.K. designed and performed the study; J.C. and S.A.L. conducted the data analysis; S.A.L. drafted the manuscript, and C.K. and S.A.L. bear the primary responsibility for final contents. All authors were involved in data interpretation and manuscript preparation. All authors have read and approved the submitted manuscript.

Conflicts of Interest: The authors declare no conflicts of interest.

References

1. Wild, S.; Roglic, G.; Green, A.; Sicree, R.; King, H. Global prevalence of diabetes: Estimates for the year 2000 and projections for 2030. *Diabetes Care* **2004**, *27*, 1047–1053. [CrossRef] [PubMed]
2. Alberti, K.G.; Zimmet, P.Z. Definition, diagnosis and classification of diabetes mellitus and its complications. Part 1: Diagnosis and classification of diabetes mellitus provisional report of a who consultation. *Diabet. Med. J. Br. Diabet. Assoc.* **1998**, *15*, 539–553. [CrossRef]
3. Hu, F.B.; Manson, J.E.; Stampfer, M.J.; Colditz, G.; Liu, S.; Solomon, C.G.; Willett, W.C. Diet, lifestyle, and the risk of type 2 diabetes mellitus in women. *N. Engl. J. Med.* **2001**, *345*, 790–797. [CrossRef] [PubMed]
4. Tuomilehto, J.; Lindstrom, J.; Eriksson, J.G.; Valle, T.T.; Hamalainen, H.; Ilanne-Parikka, P.; Keinanen-Kiukaanniemi, S.; Laakso, M.; Louheranta, A.; Rastas, M.; *et al.* Prevention of type 2 diabetes mellitus by changes in lifestyle among subjects with impaired glucose tolerance. *N. Engl. J. Med.* **2001**, *344*, 1343–1350. [CrossRef] [PubMed]
5. Montonen, J.; Knekt, P.; Jarvinen, R.; Aromaa, A.; Reunanen, A. Whole-grain and fiber intake and the incidence of type 2 diabetes. *Am. J. Clin. Nutr.* **2003**, *77*, 622–629. [PubMed]
6. Bere, E.; Brug, J. Towards health-promoting and environmentally friendly regional diets—A nordic example. *Public Health Nutr.* **2009**, *12*, 91–96. [CrossRef] [PubMed]
7. Akesson, A.; Andersen, L.F.; Kristjansdottir, A.G.; Roos, E.; Trolle, E.; Voutilainen, E.; Wirfalt, E. Health effects associated with foods characteristic of the nordic diet: A systematic literature review. *Food Nutr. Res.* **2013**, *57*. [CrossRef] [PubMed]
8. Martinez-Gonzalez, M.A.; de la Fuente-Arrillaga, C.; Nunez-Cordoba, J.M.; Basterra-Gortari, F.J.; Beunza, J.J.; Vazquez, Z.; Benito, S.; Tortosa, A.; Bes-Rastrollo, M. Adherence to mediterranean diet and risk of developing diabetes: Prospective cohort study. *BMJ* **2008**, *336*, 1348–1351. [CrossRef] [PubMed]
9. Sofi, F.; Cesari, F.; Abbate, R.; Gensini, G.F.; Casini, A. Adherence to mediterranean diet and health status: Meta-analysis. *BMJ* **2008**, *337*, a1344. [CrossRef] [PubMed]
10. De Koning, L.; Chiuve, S.E.; Fung, T.T.; Willett, W.C.; Rimm, E.B.; Hu, F.B. Diet-quality scores and the risk of type 2 diabetes in men. *Diabetes Care* **2011**, *34*, 1150–1156. [CrossRef] [PubMed]

11. Romaguera, D.; Guevara, M.; Norat, T.; Langenberg, C.; Forouhi, N.G.; Sharp, S.; Slimani, N.; Schulze, M.B.; Buijsse, B.; Buckland, G.; *et al.* Mediterranean diet and type 2 diabetes risk in the european prospective investigation into cancer and nutrition (EPIC) study: The interact project. *Diabetes Care* **2011**, *34*, 1913–1918. [PubMed]

12. Sofi, F.; Macchi, C.; Abbate, R.; Gensini, G.F.; Casini, A. Mediterranean diet and health. *Biofactors* **2013**, *39*, 335–342. [CrossRef] [PubMed]

13. Da Silva, R.; Bach-Faig, A.; Raido, Q.B.; Buckland, G.; Vaz de Almeida, M.D.; Serra-Majem, L. Worldwide variation of adherence to the mediterranean diet, in 1961–1965 and 2000–2003. *Public Health Nutr.* **2009**, *12*, 1676–1684. [CrossRef] [PubMed]

14. Bere, E.; Brug, J. Is the term "mediterranean diet" a misnomer? *Public Health Nutr.* **2010**, *13*, 2127–2129. [CrossRef] [PubMed]

15. Adamsson, V.; Reumark, A.; Fredriksson, I.B.; Hammarstrom, E.; Vessby, B.; Johansson, G.; Riserus, U. Effects of a healthy nordic diet on cardiovascular risk factors in hypercholesterolaemic subjects: A randomized controlled trial (nordiet). *J. Intern. Med.* **2011**, *260*, 150–159. [CrossRef] [PubMed]

16. Kanerva, N.; Kaartinen, N.E.; Schwab, U.; Lahti-Koski, M.; Mannisto, S. Adherence to the baltic sea diet consumed in the nordic countries is associated with lower abdominal obesity. *Br. J. Nutr.* **2013**, *109*, 520–528. [CrossRef] [PubMed]

17. Poulsen, S.K.; Due, A.; Jordy, A.B.; Kiens, B.; Stark, K.D.; Stender, S.; Holst, C.; Astrup, A.; Larsen, T.M. Health effect of the new nordic diet in adults with increased waist circumference: A 6-mo randomized controlled trial. *Am. J. Clin. Nutr.* **2014**, *99*, 35–45. [CrossRef] [PubMed]

18. Kanerva, N.; Rissanen, H.; Knekt, P.; Havulinna, A.S.; Eriksson, J.G.; Mannisto, S. The healthy nordic diet and incidence of type 2 diabetes - 10-year follow-up. *Diabetes Res. Clin. Pract.* **2014**, *106*, e34–e37. [CrossRef] [PubMed]

19. Tjonneland, A.; Olsen, A.; Boll, K.; Stripp, C.; Christensen, J.; Engholm, G.; Overvad, K. Study design, exposure variables, and socioeconomic determinants of participation in diet, cancer and health: A population-based prospective cohort study of 57,053 men and women in denmark. *Scand. J. Public Health* **2007**, *35*, 432–441. [CrossRef] [PubMed]

20. Pedersen, C.B. The danish civil registration system. *Scand. J. Public Health* **2011**, *39*, 22–25. [CrossRef] [PubMed]

21. Carstensen, B.; Kristensen, J.K.; Marcussen, M.M.; Borch-Johnsen, K. The national diabetes register. *Scand. J. Public Health* **2011**, *39*, 58–61. [CrossRef] [PubMed]

22. Sorensen, M.; Andersen, Z.J.; Nordsborg, R.B.; Becker, T.; Tjonneland, A.; Overvad, K.; Raaschou-Nielsen, O. Long-term exposure to road traffic noise and incident diabetes: A cohort study. *Environ. Health Perspect.* **2013**, *121*, 217–222. [PubMed]

23. Tjonneland, A.; Overvad, K.; Haraldsdottir, J.; Bang, S.; Ewertz, M.; Jensen, O.M. Validation of a semiquantitative food frequency questionnaire developed in Denmark. *Int. J. Epidemiol.* **1991**, *20*, 906–912. [CrossRef] [PubMed]

24. Overvad, K.; Tjonneland, A.; Haraldsdottir, J.; Ewertz, M.; Jensen, O.M. Development of a semiquantitative food frequency questionnaire to assess food, energy and nutrient intake in Denmark. *Int. J. Epidemiol.* **1991**, *20*, 900–905. [CrossRef] [PubMed]

25. Lauritzen, J. Foodcalc. Available online: http://www.Ibt.Ku.Dk/jesper/foodcalc/default.Htm (accessed on 7 December 2014).

26. Olsen, A.; Egeberg, R.; Halkjaer, J.; Christensen, J.; Overvad, K.; Tjonneland, A. Healthy aspects of the nordic diet are related to lower total mortality. *J. Nutr.* **2011**, *141*, 639–644. [CrossRef] [PubMed]

27. Trichopoulou, A.; Kouris-Blazos, A.; Wahlqvist, M.L.; Gnardellis, C.; Lagiou, P.; Polychronopoulos, E.; Vassilakou, T.; Lipworth, L.; Trichopoulos, D. Diet and overall survival in elderly people. *BMJ* **1995**, *311*, 1457–1460. [CrossRef] [PubMed]

28. Trichopoulou, A.; Costacou, T.; Bamia, C.; Trichopoulos, D. Adherence to a mediterranean diet and survival in a greek population. *N. Engl. J. Med.* **2003**, *348*, 2599–2608. [CrossRef] [PubMed]

29. Willett, W.C.; Howe, G.R.; Kushi, L.H. Adjustment for total energy intake in epidemiologic studies. *Am. J. Clin. Nutr.* **1997**, *65*, 1220S–1228S. [PubMed]

30. Andersen, Z.J.; Raaschou-Nielsen, O.; Ketzel, M.; Jensen, S.S.; Hvidberg, M.; Loft, S.; Tjonneland, A.; Overvad, K.; Sorensen, M. Diabetes incidence and long-term exposure to air pollution: A cohort study. *Diabetes Care* **2012**, *35*, 92–98. [CrossRef] [PubMed]

31. Salas-Salvado, J.; Bullo, M.; Estruch, R.; Ros, E.; Covas, M.I.; Ibarrola-Jurado, N.; Corella, D.; Aros, F.; Gomez-Gracia, E.; Ruiz-Gutierrez, V.; *et al.* Prevention of diabetes with mediterranean diets: A subgroup analysis of a randomized trial. *Ann. Intern. Med.* **2014**, *160*, 1–10. [CrossRef] [PubMed]

32. Kruse, M.; von Loeffelholz, C.; Hoffmann, D.; Pohlmann, A.; Seltmann, A.C.; Osterhoff, M.; Hornemann, S.; Pivovarova, O.; Rohn, S.; Jahreis, G.; *et al.* Dietary rapeseed/canola-oil supplementation reduces serum lipids and liver enzymes and alters postprandial inflammatory responses in adipose tissue compared to olive-oil supplementation in obese men. *Mol. Nutr. Food Res.* **2015**, *59*, 507–519. [CrossRef] [PubMed]

33. Boyer, J.; Liu, R.H. Apple phytochemicals and their health benefits. *Nutr. J.* **2004**, *3*, 5. [CrossRef] [PubMed]

34. Sahlstrøm, S.; Knutsen, S.H. Oats and rye: Production and usage in nordic and baltic countires. *Cereal Foods World* **2010**, *55*, 12–14. [CrossRef]

35. Hu, F.B. Dietary pattern analysis: A new direction in nutritional epidemiology. *Curr. Opin. Lipidol.* **2002**, *13*, 3–9. [CrossRef] [PubMed]

36. McKeown, N.M. Whole grain intake and insulin sensitivity: Evidence from observational studies. *Nutr. Rev.* **2004**, *62*, 286–291. [PubMed]

37. Weickert, M.O.; Mohlig, M.; Schofl, C.; Arafat, A.M.; Otto, B.; Viehoff, H.; Koebnick, C.; Kohl, A.; Spranger, J.; Pfeiffer, A.F. Cereal fiber improves whole-body insulin sensitivity in overweight and obese women. *Diabetes Care* **2006**, *29*, 775–780. [CrossRef] [PubMed]

38. Knekt, P.; Kumpulainen, J.; Jarvinen, R.; Rissanen, H.; Heliovaara, M.; Reunanen, A.; Hakulinen, T.; Aromaa, A. Flavonoid intake and risk of chronic diseases. *Am. J. Clin. Nutr.* **2002**, *76*, 560–568. [PubMed]

39. Kaushik, M.; Mozaffarian, D.; Spiegelman, D.; Manson, J.E.; Willett, W.C.; Hu, F.B. Long-chain omega-3 fatty acids, fish intake, and the risk of type 2 diabetes mellitus. *Am. J. Clin. Nutr.* **2009**, *90*, 613–620. [CrossRef] [PubMed]

40. De Mello, V.D.; Schwab, U.; Kolehmainen, M.; Koenig, W.; Siloaho, M.; Poutanen, K.; Mykkanen, H.; Uusitupa, M. A diet high in fatty fish, bilberries and wholegrain products improves markers of endothelial function and inflammation in individuals with impaired glucose metabolism in a randomised controlled trial: The sysdimet study. *Diabetologia* **2011**, *54*, 2755–2767. [CrossRef] [PubMed]

41. Uusitupa, M.; Hermansen, K.; Savolainen, M.J.; Schwab, U.; Kolehmainen, M.; Brader, L.; Mortensen, L.S.; Cloetens, L.; Johansson-Persson, A.; Onning, G.; *et al.* Effects of an isocaloric healthy nordic diet on insulin sensitivity, lipid profile and inflammation markers in metabolic syndrome—A randomized study (sysdiet). *J. Intern. Med.* **2013**, *274*, 52–66. [CrossRef] [PubMed]

42. Fletcher, B.; Gulanick, M.; Lamendola, C. Risk factors for type 2 diabetes mellitus. *J. Cardiovasc. Nurs.* **2002**, *16*, 17–23. [CrossRef] [PubMed]

43. Dominguez, L.J.; Bes-Rastrollo, M.; de la Fuente-Arrillaga, C.; Toledo, E.; Beunza, J.J.; Barbagallo, M.; Martinez-Gonzalez, M.A. Similar prediction of total mortality, diabetes incidence and cardiovascular events using relative- and absolute-component mediterranean diet score: The sun cohort. *Nutr. Metab. Cardiovasc. Dis.* **2013**, *23*, 451–458. [CrossRef] [PubMed]

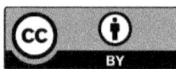

nutrients

MDPI

Article

Better Adherence to the Mediterranean Diet Could Mitigate the Adverse Consequences of Obesity on Cardiovascular Disease: The SUN Prospective Cohort

Sonia Eguaras [1,2], Estefanía Toledo [2,3], Aitor Hernández-Hernández [2,4], Sebastián Cervantes [2,5] and Miguel A. Martínez-González [2,3,*]

1   Servicio Navarro de Salud-Osasunbidea-IdiSNA, Navarra Institute for Health Research, 31002 Pamplona, Spain; seguaras@alumni.unav.es
2   Department of Preventive Medicine and Public Health, Navarra Institute for Health Research, University of Navarra-IdiSNA, 31008 Pamplona, Spain; etoledo@unav.es (E.T.); aitorhernandez86@gmail.com (A.H.-H); sebcervantes@gmail.com (S.C.)
3   Biomedical Research Center Network on Obesity and Nutrition (CIBERobn) Physiopathology of Obesity and Nutrition, Instituto de Salud Carlos III, 28029 Madrid, Spain
4   Department of Cardiology, Navarra Institute for Health Research, University Clinic of Navarra-IdiSNA, 31008 Pamplona, Spain
5   Department of Radiology, Hospital of Navarra, Servicio Navarro de Salud-Osasunbidea-IdiSNA, Navarra Institute for Health Research, 31008 Pamplona, Spain
*   Correspondence: mamartinez@unav.es; Tel.: +34-948-425-600 (ext. 806463); Fax: +34-048-425-649

Received: 22 August 2015 ; Accepted: 29 October 2015 ; Published: 5 November 2015

Abstract: Strong observational evidence supports the association between obesity and cardiovascular events. In elderly high-risk subjects, the Mediterranean diet (MedDiet) was reported to counteract the adverse cardiovascular effects of adiposity. Whether this same attenuation is also present in younger subjects is not known. We prospectively examined the association between obesity and cardiovascular clinical events (myocardial infarction, stroke or cardiovascular death) after 10.9 years follow-up in 19,065 middle-aged men and women (average age 38 year) according to their adherence to the MedDiet (<6 points or ⩾6 points in the Trichopoulou's Mediterranean Diet Score). We observed 152 incident cases of cardiovascular disease (CVD). An increased risk of CVD across categories of body mass index (BMI) was apparent if adherence to the MedDiet was low, with multivariable-adjusted hazard ratios (HRs): 1.44 (95% confidence interval: 0.93–2.25) for ⩾25 – <30 kg/m^2 of BMI and 2.00 (1.04–3.83) for ⩾30 kg/m^2 of BMI, compared to a BMI < 25 kg/m^2. In contrast, these estimates were 0.77 (0.35–1.67) and 1.15 (0.39–3.43) with good adherence to MedDiet. Better adherence to the MedDiet was associated with reduced CVD events (p for trend = 0.029). Our results suggest that the MedDiet could mitigate the harmful cardiovascular effect of overweight/obesity.

Keywords: obesity; Mediterranean diet; prospective cohort study; cardiovascular disease; SUN project

1. Introduction

The prevalence of obesity is increasing globally, and it is one of the major public health problems in most countries. According to WHO, in the last three decades the prevalence of obesity has doubled worldwide. As a result, the majority of world population currently live in countries where overweight and obesity cause more deaths than insufficient weight [1].

Excess body weight is likely to be associated with clinical cardiovascular disease (CVD) even at moderate levels of overweight and independently of traditional cardiovascular risk factors [2–5]. On the other hand, dietary habits play an important role as determinants of optimal health and—more importantly they may be especially useful for the prevention of CVD [6,7]. There is compelling evidence that the traditional Mediterranean diet (MedDiet) has beneficial effects against all-cause mortality and clinical cardiovascular events [8–10]. In the context of the current pandemic of overweight/obesity, it is likely that dietary habits in line with the traditional Mediterranean dietary pattern may attenuate the well-known detrimental effects of adiposity on cardiovascular risk. In this line of thought, a recent study conducted in elderly high-risk subjects suggested that the MedDiet could counteract the adverse cardiovascular effects of an increased body weight [11]. It is not known whether this attenuation by the MedDiet of the harmful cardiovascular effects of even a moderate degree of excess adiposity is also present in younger subjects at lower cardiovascular risk. We prospectively assessed the association between obesity and incidence of major clinical cardiovascular events within categories of adherence to the MedDiet in a sample of 19,065 highly educated men and women followed-up for a mean period of 10.9 years, with mean age of 38 years old and a low predicted risk of cardiovascular disease at baseline.

2. Experimental Section

2.1. Study Population

The SUN project is a multipurpose prospective Spanish cohort study entirely composed of university graduates. This cohort was designed to assess associations of diet or lifestyle with the incidence of several chronic diseases and mortality. The study protocol was approved by the Institutional Review Board of the University of Navarra. The design, methods and objectives of the SUN project have been described previously [12].

The recruitment of participants started in December 1999. It is a dynamic cohort permanently open to recruitment of new participants. Up to December 2014, 22,175 participants had answered the baseline questionnaire. Follow-up information is collected through self-administered questionnaires sent biennially by mail.

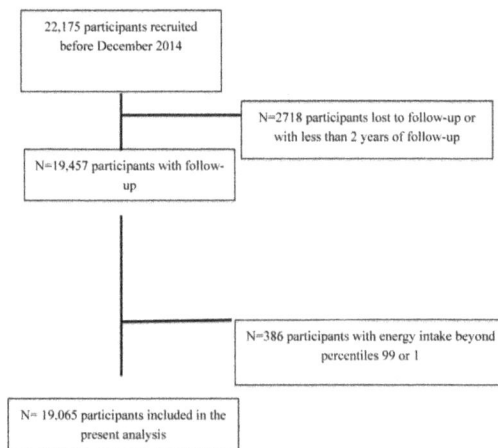

Figure 1. Flow-chart of participants in the SUN Project, 1999–2014.

For the present analysis, 2718 participants were lost to follow up or were recruited for the cohort only for a short period (less than 2 years) and were therefore excluded from our analyses; in addition, 386 participants with total daily energy intake beyond percentiles 1 or 99 were also excluded. Thus, our final sample included 19,065 participants (Figure 1).

2.2. Anthropometric Variables

Participants' weight was recorded at baseline. Reliability and validity of self-reported weight has been previously assessed in a subsample of the cohort, and has shown a high correlation with directly measured weight (r = 0.99; 95% CI: 0.99, 0.99) and a mean relative error of 1.45% [13]. Body mass index (BMI), defined as weight in kilograms divided by the square of height in meters, was computed in the baseline questionnaire. Reliability of self-reported weight and height used to calculate BMI has been previously assessed [13] (r = 0.94; 95% CI: 0.91, 0.97). Mean relative error in self-reported BMI was 2.64%.

2.3. Dietary Assessment

Usual diet was assessed at baseline with a validated semi-quantitative 136-item food-frequency questionnaire (FFQ) [14,15]. Each item included a typical portion size, and consumption frequencies were grouped in nine categories that ranged from "never or almost never" to "≥6 times/day." A trained team of dietitians updated the nutrient data bank using the latest available information included in food composition tables for Spain [16,17]. We used the Mediterranean Diet Score (ranging from 0 to 9 points) proposed by Trichopoulou *et al.* [18] to classify participants according to their baseline adherence to the Mediterranean diet [19]. One point was assigned to persons whose consumption was at or above the sex-specific median of components frequently consumed in the context of traditional Mediterranean diet (vegetables, fruits/nuts, legumes, fish/seafood, cereals, and monounsaturated/saturated (MUFA/SFA) fat ratio). The participant received also 1 point if her or his intake was below the median for the 2 components less frequently consumed in the context of traditional Mediterranean diet (meat and dairy products). For ethanol, 1 point was assigned only for moderate amounts of intake (5–25 g/day for women or 10–50 g/day for men.). We dichotomized adherence to MedDiet into 2 categories (<6 and ≥6 points in the Trichopoulou's score).

2.4. Other Covariates

We used standardized questionnaires included in the baseline questionnaire to gather information about socio-demographic parameters (sex, age), anthropometric measurements (weight, BMI) and health-related habits (smoking status, physical activity, sedentary lifestyle). Information on physical activity was collected at baseline through a previously validated questionnaire that contained time spent in 17 different activities. Physical activity was expressed in metabolic equivalent tasks (METs = time spent at each activity in hours/week multiplied by its typical energy expenditure) [20].

2.5. Outcome Assessment

Incidence of cardiovascular events, defined as non-fatal myocardial infarction, non-fatal stroke reported by participants on a follow-up questionnaire or deaths due to cardiovascular disease, was the primary endpoint. An expert panel of physicians, blinded to information on diet, anthropometric indexes and risk factors, reviewed medical records of participants and adjudicated events applying universal criteria for myocardial infarction and clinical criteria for the other outcomes. A non-fatal stroke was defined as a focal neurological deficit of sudden onset and vascular mechanism lasting >24 h. Cases of fatal stroke were documented if there was evidence of a cerebrovascular mechanism. Deaths were reported to our research team by the participants' next of kin, work associates and postal authorities. For participants lost to follow-up, we consulted the National Death Index every 6 months to identify deceased cohort members and to obtain their cause of death. Cases of fatal CHD or stroke reported by families or postal authorities were confirmed by a review of medical records with permission of the next of kin.

2.6. Statistical Analyses

Analyses were performed with STATA version 12.0 (StataCorp, College Station, TX 77840, USA). For descriptive purposes, we calculated means, standard deviations, proportions, medians, and percentiles of baseline characteristics across levels of adherence to the Mediterranean diet. We used Cox regression models to assess hazard ratios (HRs) and their 95% confidence intervals (CIs) for total CVD events across categories of BMI (cut off points: 25 and 30 kg/m^2). We used age as the underlying time variable and stratified all analyses for age groups. To assess attenuation by the MedDiet of the harmful effect of obesity, we stratified results for baseline adherence to the MedDiet (categorized into two groups: low adherence (<6 points) and high adherence (≥6 points)). We included as covariates potential confounders such as age (underlying time variable, plus stratification), sex, smoking status (3 categories), physical activity during leisure time, baseline hypertension status, baseline hypercholesterolemia status, diabetes, years of university education, and previous history of CVD (present in only 173 participants) in multivariable analyses.

We also assessed incidence of cardiovascular events according to four categories of adherence to MedDiet: low (2 points), low-moderate (3–4 points), moderate-high (5–6 points) and high (7–9 points). In addition, linear trend test were also conducted using Trichopoulou's score of adherence to MedDiet as a continuous variable.

3. Results

Table 1 shows the baseline characteristics of participants according to their baseline adherence to MedDiet and stratified by their baseline BMI. In addition to having a high level of education, SUN cohort participants were relatively young at baseline (mean age 38.4 years), more likely to be women (60.5%) and non-obese (average BMI = 23.5 kg/m^2; 95.3% of participants had a BMI < 30 kg/m^2). However, participants with better adherence to MedDiet were older, more physically active, more likely to be men and married and to follow special diets, and less likely to snacks between meals. They were also less likely to be current smokers but more prone to being former smokers. In addition, those participants with initial good adherence to the MedDiet were more likely to have a previous diagnosis of hypercholesterolemia, hypertriglyceridemia, diabetes or hypertension.

Table 1. Baseline characteristics of participants according to Mediterranean diet adherence and BMI.

	Low Adherence to MedDiet (<6/9)			High Adherence to MedDiet (≥6/9)		
	BMI <25	BMI 25–30	BMI >30	BMI <25	BMI 25–30	BMI >30
N	10,169	3396	663	3208	1396	233
Age (years)	35 (10)	43 (13)	45 (12)	39 (12)	48 (12)	48 (13)
Women (%)	74.3	30.4	32.0	71.7	28.2	23.6
BMI (kg/m^2)	21.6 (1.9)	26.9 (1.3)	32.5 (2.4)	21.9 (1.9)	26.9 (1.3)	32.7 (3.0)
Previous history of CVD (%)	0.4	1.3	1.5	0.8	3.0	4.3
Energy intake (kcal/day)	2479 (766)	2353 (756)	2386 (812)	2698 (786)	2633 (766)	2715 (800)
Leisure-time physical activity	20.6 (22.1)	20.4 (21.7)	15.2 (17.7)	26.8 (26.0)	24.6 (23.3)	19.7 (18.0)
Marital status						
Single	53.5	30.9	27.8	43.6	19.9	5.7
Married	42.4	63.9	65.6	50.7	74.4	70.4
Others	4.0	5.2	6.6	5.7	5.8	7.7
Smoking current smokers (%)	22.9	20.4	19.6	20.8	17.9	18.0
Former smokers (%)	22.6	34.9	39.5	30.5	44.4	48.1
Baseline hypercholesterolemia (%)	11.3	22.5	32.3	17.8	33.0	38.2
Baseline triglycerides (%)	2.9	12.1	23.5	4.4	16.3	30.9
Diabetes at baseline (%)	0.9	2.8	5.7	1.6	3.5	7.3
Hypertension at baseline (%)	3.0	12.5	25.9	5.2	19.3	32.6
Years of university education	5.0 (1.47)	5.2 (1.60)	5.0 (1.51)	5.0 (1.50)	5.3 (1.72)	5.1 (1.50)
Leisure-time spent sitting down, h/week.	3.8 (1.72)	3.8 (1.91)	3.8 (2.06)	3.9 (1.86)	4.0 (1.83)	4.1 (2.01)
TV watching, h/week.	1.6 (1.23)	1.7 (1.14)	1.8 (1.18)	1.6 (1.16)	1.7 (1.09)	1.8 (1.17)
Between-meal snacking (%)	35.2	34.7	51.3	27.9	29.3	40.8
Following special diets (%)	5.6	9.6	15.1	9.2	12.8	19.3

BMI: body mass index; SD: standard deviation; CVD: cardiovascular disease (acute coronary syndromes or stroke).

We observed 152 incident cases of CVD (56 non-fatal myocardial infarctions, 30 non-fatal strokes and 66 cardiovascular deaths) after a mean of 10.9 years of follow–up. As shown in Table 2, we assessed the relationship between classical categories of BMI and risk of CVD clinical events according to categories of baseline adherence to MedDiet (<6 and ⩾6 points in the Trichopoulou's score). An increased risk of CVD events across categories of BMI was apparent in the low adherence to MedDiet group. Within each group of BMI, the group with lesser conformity to MedDiet had higher rates of age-adjusted CVD than the group with good adherence to MedDiet.

Table 2. Relative risk (hazard ratios and 95% confidence intervals) of incident cardiovascular disease (myocardial infarction, stroke or cardiovascular death) according to baseline body mass index and adherence to MedDiet. The SUN project 1999–2014.

Body mass index	Low Adherence to MedDiet (<6/9)			High Adherence to MedDiet (⩾6/9)		
	<25	25–30	>30	<25	25–30	⩾30
n	10,169	3396	663	3208	1396	233
Median body mass index	21.6	26.9	32.5	21.9	26.9	32.7
events	38	59	15	15	19	6
Person-years	95,620	30,961	5814	28,260	11,917	1789
Age-adjusted rate/10^5 (95% CI)	40 (28–55)	74 (49–113)	97 (53–177)	31 (17–57)	43 (25–76)	86 (36–206)
Sex-, age-adjusted HR	1 (ref.)	1.52 (0.99–2.35)	2.14 (1.14–4.00)	1 (ref.)	0.97 (0.48–1.95)	1.77 (0.61–5.17)
Multivariable-adjusted HR *	1 (ref.)	1.44 (0.93–2.25)	2.00 (1.04–3.83)	1 (ref.)	0.77 (0.35–1.67)	1.15 (0.39–3.43)

* Adjusted for age (underline time variable plus stratification), sex, smoking, baseline hypercholesterolemia, hypertension, leisure-time physical activity, hypertension, diabetes and previous history of cardiovascular disease. Robust standard errors were used. *p* for interaction (BMI × MedDiet) = 0.10.

Among participants with low adherence to the MedDiet and compared to participants with a BMI < 25 kg/m^2, multivariable-adjusted hazard ratios (95% confidence intervals) of CVD were 1.44 (0.93–2.25) for participants with a BMI ⩾25 – <30 kg/m^2, and 2.00 (1.04–3.83) for participants with BMI > 30 kg/m^2. On the other hand, in the group with good adherence to the MedDiet, multivariable-adjusted hazard ratios (HRs) were 0.77 (0.35–1.67) and 1.15 (0.39–3.43), respectively. Therefore, there was a trend towards an attenuation of the harmful effects of obesity by the MedDiet. However, the *p* value for the multiplicative interaction (to test for an effect beyond the multiplication of both independent effects) was not statistically significant (*p* = 0.10).

We also confirmed an inverse association between adherence to MedDiet and CVD events (Table 3), which was previously reported when the accrual in this cohort, measured as person-years, was smaller [21]. In this updated analysis, participants with the highest adherence (score >7) showed a 53% lower risk of cardiovascular events as compared to participants in the lowest adherence category (score <2), after adjustment for potential confounders. The inverse linear trend for the association between adherence to the MedDiet and CVD was statistically significant (*p* = 0.029). A two-point increment in the Mediterranean-diet score was associated with a 7% relative reduction in CVD risk.

Table 3. Relative risk (Hazard Ratios and 95% confidence intervals) of incident cardiovascular disease (myocardial infarction, stroke or cardiovascular death) according to baseline adherence to the MedDiet. The SUN project 1999–2014.

Adherence to the Mediterranean Diet	Low 0–2	Low-Moderate 3–4	Moderate-High 5–6	High 7–9	*p* for Trend	For Each +2 Points
n	3334	7160	6431	2140		
Incident cases of CVD	23	57	51	21		
Person-years	32,001	66,900	57,120	18,341		
Sex-, age-adjusted HR	1 (ref.)	0.88 (0.53–1.46)	0.68 (0.40–1.15)	0.58 (0.31–1.09)	0.097	0.95 (0.91–0.99)
Multivariable-adjusted HR *	1 (ref.)	0.81 (0.48–1.38)	0.58 (0.34–1.00)	0.47 (0.25–0.89)	0.029	0.93 (0.89–0.98)

* Adjusted for age (underline time variable plus stratification), sex, smoking, baseline hypercholesterolemia, hypertension, leisure-time physical activity, hypertension, diabetes and previous history of cardiovascular disease. Robust standard errors were used. *p* for interaction (BMI × MedDiet) = 0.10.

Figure 2 presents multivariable-adjusted hazard ratios for the joint classification according to both values of BMI (3 groups with the following 2 cut-off points: 25 and 30 kg/m^2) and adherence to MedDiet (two categories: low adherence (<6 points) and high adherence (≥6 points)). The reference category was the group with low BMI (<25) and high adherence to MedDiet (score ≥6). In the group with better adherence to MedDiet, the risk of CVD was lower than in the poor adherence group across all BMI categories.

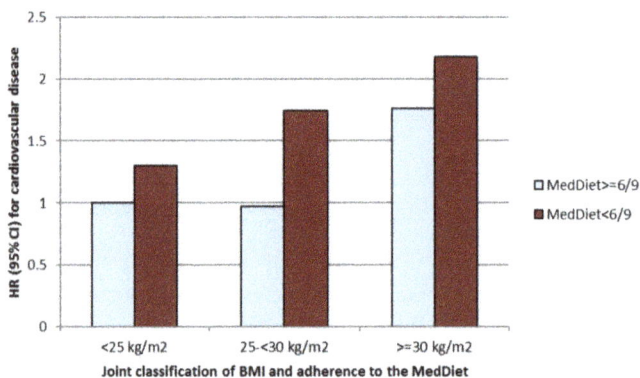

Figure 2. Relative risk of cardiovascular disease (HR and 95% confidence intervals) in the SUN project according to baseline body mass index and adherence to MedDiet.

4. Discussion

This study contributes to support the evidence that closer adherence to the MedDiet could counteract some of the adverse cardiovascular effects of overweight/obesity, not only in elderly persons at high cardiovascular risk but also in young, healthier and highly-educated persons. Though we did not find a statistically significant interaction and the *p* value for the product-term only approached statistical significance, a biological interaction was suggested by our results. In fact, the effect of increased adiposity was mitigated in subjects with high adherence to MedDiet.

There is evidence that excess body weight is associated with an increased risk of CVD [22,23]. Excess weight is associated with both subclinical metabolic and vascular dysfunction that, with the passage of time, lead to an increased risk of CV events, due to a state of low-grade inflammation that increases cardiovascular risk [24–26]. Therefore, it seems biologically plausible that the MedDiet's anti-inflammatory effects [27] could counter-balance the detrimental effects of obesity-associated low-grade inflammation.

The association between overweight and CVD is not as universally acknowledged as that between obesity and CVD. For instance, a recently published meta-analysis suggested that overweight subjects (defined as those with a BMI of 25 to 30 kg/m^2) have lower all-cause mortality as compared to normal weight subjects. In addition, persons with grade I obesity (BMI between 30 and 35 kg/m^2) had a significantly lower risk of mortality [28]. In contrast, in our study an increased risk of CVD was observed both in obese and overweight subjects. A possible explanation for this discrepancy lies in the presence of potential biases that may have attenuated the association between obesity and CVD risk in previous studies conducted with older participants, such as higher rate of tobacco use and presence of preclinical diseases. We were able to avoid this problem as our examined sample was composed of healthy and young individuals with a low prevalence of pre-existing disease.

We used BMI to measure excess of body weight, as it is the most widely used and accepted index for assessing obesity. However, anthropometric indexes such as the waist-to-height (WHtR) or waist circumference (WC) have been shown to have advantages as predictors of CVD [29,30]. Nevertheless, weight and height are objective and reproducible measures that have been accurately reported by our participants in a validation study of self-reported measurements [13].

Previous studies have suggested the beneficial metabolic effects of the MedDiet, regardless of abdominal adiposity [31–34]. Our results support a previous study that suggested a beneficial effect from the MedDiet in obese subjects [11]. In addition, we have found evidence that extends this benefit to overweight subjects.

There are several strengths in our research that deserve to be mentioned. We used a large sample of participants with a high retention rate. The prospective nature of our study with its long follow-up period allowed us to detect CVD events and avoid reverse causation bias in the reported associations. In addition, multiple-adjusted models enabled us to control for a wide array of potential confounders.

We find that our study has a strong internal validity thanks to a high retention rate and reliable self-reported measures reported by highly educated participants. In addition, internal validity is reinforced by restriction to subjects with high educational levels so that the risk for confounding by education or socio-economic levels is minimized. On the other hand, we acknowledge some limitations of our study. First, the information on several variables was collected through self-reporting. However, parameters such as self-reported usual diet, weight or BMI have been previously validated [13], therefore decreasing risk of residual misclassification. In addition, outcomes were confirmed by a panel of physicians after blindly reviewing participants' medical records. Second, the product-term in the fully adjusted model showed a non-significant interaction. The relatively small number of events observed in our cohort could explain the lack of statistical significance of this interaction product-term. However, this low number of cardiovascular events should not be surprising given the young age and healthy characteristics of our participants.

5. Conclusions

Our study suggests benefits from the MedDiet as an effective tool for counteracting the detrimental effects of obesity on cardiovascular health.

Acknowledgments: The authors thank the SUN project participants for their enthusiastic collaboration and participation. The authors also thank the other members of the SUN study group: Álvaro Alonso, Silvia Benito, Maira Bes-Rastrollo, Juan José Beunza, Jokin de Irala, Carmen De la Fuente, Miguel Delgado-Rodríguez, Francisco Guillén Grima, Jan Krafka, Javier Llorca, Cristina López del Burgo, Amelia Martí, Jose Alfredo Martínez, Jorge María Núñez-Córdoba, Adriano Pimenta, Miguel Ruiz-Canela, David Sánchez, Manuel Serrano-Martínez, and Zenaida Vázquez, as well as the members of the Department of Nutrition, Harvard School of Public Health (Alberto Ascherio, Walter Willett, and Frank B. Hu), who helped us to design the SUN project.

Author Contributions: Conceived and designed: Miguel A. Martínez-González; Performed the research: Sonia Eguaras; Analyzed data: Sonia Eguaras and Miguel A. Martínez-González; Wrote the paper: Sonia Eguaras and Miguel A. Martínez-González; Critical review: all authors; Approval of the final version: all authors.

Conflicts of Interest: The authors declare no conflict of interest.

Acknowledgments: The SUN project has received funding from the Instituto de Salud Carlos III, Official Agency of the Spanish Government for biomedical research (grants no. PI01/0619, PI030678, PI040233, PI042241, OI050976, PI070240, PI070312, PI081943, PI080819, PI1002293, PI1002658, RD06/0045, and G03/140); the Ministerio de Sanidad, Política Social e Igualdad through the Plan Nacional de Drogas (2010/087); the Navarra Regional Government (36/2001, 43/2002, 41/2005, 36/2008, 45/2011); and the University of Navarra.

References

1. World Health Organization. *World Health Statistics*; World Health Organization: Geneva, Switzerland, 2015.
2. Prospective Studies Collaboration; Whitlock, G.; Lewington, S.; Sherliker, P.; Clarke, R.; Emberson, J.; Halsey, J.; Qizilbash, N.; Collins, R.; Peto, R. Body-mass index and cause-specific mortality in 900,000 adults: Collaborative analyses of 57 prospective studies. *Lancet* **2009**, *373*, 1083–1096. [CrossRef] [PubMed]
3. Chen, Z.; Yang, G.; Zhou, M.; Smith, M.; Offer, A.; Ma, J.; Wang, L.; Pan, H.; Whitlock, G.; Collins, R.; et al. Body mass index and mortality from ischaemic heart disease in a lean population: 10 year prospective study of 220,000 adult men. *Int. J. Epidemiol.* **2006**, *35*, 141–150. [CrossRef] [PubMed]
4. Berrington de Gonzalez, A.; Hartge, P.; Cerhan, J.R.; Flint, A.J.; Hannan, L.; Macinnis, R.J.; Moore, S.C.; Tobias, G.S.; Anton-Culver, H.; Freeman, L.B.; et al. Body-mass index and mortality among 1.46 million white adults. *N. Engl. J. Med.* **2010**, *363*, 2211–2219. [CrossRef] [PubMed]
5. Bogers, R.P.; Bemelmans, W.J.; Hoogenveen, R.T.; Boshuizen, H.C.; Woodward, M.; Knekt, P.; van Dam, R.M.; Hu, F.B.; Visscher, T.L.; Menotti, A.; et al. Association of overweight with increased risk of coronary heart disease partly independent of blood pressure and cholesterol levels: A meta-analysis of 21 cohort studies including more than 300,000 persons. *Arch. Intern. Med.* **2007**, *167*, 1720–1728. [CrossRef] [PubMed]
6. Hu, F.B.; Willett, W.C. Optimal diets for prevention of coronary heart. *JAMA* **2002**, *288*, 2569–2578. [CrossRef] [PubMed]
7. Mozaffarian, D.; Appel, L.J.; van Horn, L. Components of a cardioprotective diet: New insights. *Circulation* **2011**, *123*, 2870–2891. [CrossRef] [PubMed]
8. Martinez-Gonzalez, M.A.; Bes-Rastrollo, M. Dietary patterns, Mediterranean diet, and cardiovascular disease. *Curr. Opin. Lipidol.* **2014**, *25*, 20–26. [CrossRef] [PubMed]
9. Martínez-González, M.A.; Salas-Salvadó, J.; Estruch, R.; Corella, D.; Fitó, M.; Ros, E. Benefits of the Mediterranean Diet: Insights from the PREDIMED Study. *Prog. Cardiovasc. Dis.* **2015**, *58*, 50–60. [CrossRef] [PubMed]
10. Sofi, F.; Macchi, C.; Abbate, R.; Gensini, G.F.; Casini, A. Mediterranean diet and health status: An updated meta-analysis and a proposal for a literature-based adherence score. *Public Health Nutr.* **2014**, *17*, 2769–2782. [CrossRef] [PubMed]
11. Eguaras, S.; Toledo, E.; Buil-Cosiales, P.; Salas-Salvadó, J.; Corella, D.; Gutierrez-Bedmar, M.; Santos-Lozano, J.M.; Arós, F.; Fiol, M.; Fitó, M.; et al. Does the Mediterranean diet counteract the adverse effects of abdominal adiposity? *Nutr. Metab. Cardiovasc. Dis.* **2015**, *25*, 569–574. [CrossRef] [PubMed]
12. Martínez-González, M.A.; Sanchez-Villegas, A.; de Irala, J.; Marti, A.; Martínez, J.A. Mediterranean diet and stroke: Objectives and design of the SUN project. Seguimiento Universidad de Navarra. *Nutr. Neurosci.* **2002**, *5*, 65–73. [PubMed]
13. Bes-Rastrollo, M.; Perez Valdivieso, J.R.; Sanchez-Villegas, A.; Alonso, A.; Martínez-González, M.A. Validation of the self-reported weight and body mass index of the participants in a cohort of university graduates. *Rev. Esp. Obes.* **2005**, *3*, 352–358, (In Spanish).
14. Martínez-González, M.A.; de la Fuente-Arrillaga, C.; Nunez-Córdoba, J.M.; Basterra-Gortari, F.J.; Beunza, J.J.; Vazquez, Z.; Benito, S.; Tortosa, A.; Bes-Rastrollo, M. Adherence to Mediterranean diet and risk of developing diabetes: Prospective cohort study. *BMJ* **2008**, *336*, 1348–1351. [CrossRef] [PubMed]
15. De la Fuente-Arrillaga, C.; Vazquez Ruiz, Z.; Bes-Rastrollo, M.; Sampson, L.; Martínez-González, M.A. Reproducibility of an FFQ validated in Spain. *Public Health Nutr.* **2010**, *13*, 1364–1372. [CrossRef] [PubMed]
16. Mataix, J. *Tabla de Composición de Alimentos (Food Composition Tables)*, 4th ed.; Universidad de Granada: Granada, Spain, 2003.
17. Moreiras, O. *Tablas de Composición de Alimentos (Food Composition Tables)*, 5th ed.; Ediciones Pirámide: Madrid, Spain, 2003.
18. Trichopoulou, A.; Costacou, T.; Bamia, C.; Trichopoulos, D. Adherence to a Mediterranean diet and survival in a Greek population. *N. Engl. J. Med.* **2003**, *348*, 2599–2608. [CrossRef] [PubMed]

Nutrients **2015**, *7*, 9154–9162

19. Trichopoulou, A.; Kouris-Blazos, A.; Wahlqvist, M.L.; Gnardellis, C.; Lagiou, P.; Polychronopoulos, E.; Vassilakou, T.; Lipworth, L.; Trichopoulous, D. Diet and overall survival in elderly people. *BMJ* 1995, *311*, 1457–1460. [CrossRef] [PubMed]
20. Martínez-González, M.A.; López-Fontana, C.; Varo, J.J.; Sánchez-Villegas, A.; Martinez, J.A. Validation of the Spanish version of the physical activity questionnaire used in the Nurses' Health Study and the Health Professionals' Follow-up Study. *Public Health Nutr.* 2005, *8*, 920–927. [CrossRef] [PubMed]
21. Martínez-González, M.A.; García-López, M.; Bes-Rastrollo, M.; Toledo, E.; Martínez-Lapiscina, E.H.; Delgado-Rodriguez, M.; Vazquez, Z.; Benito, S.; Beunza, J.J. Mediterranean diet and the incidence of cardiovascular disease: A Spanish cohort. *Nutr. Metab. Cardiovasc. Dis.* 2011, *21*, 237–244. [CrossRef] [PubMed]
22. Kwagyan, J.; Retta, T.M.; Ketete, M.; Bettencourt, C.N.; Maqbool, A.R.; Xu, S.; Randall, O.S. Obesity and cardiovascular diseases in a high-risk population: Evidence-based approach to CHD risk reduction. *Ethn. Dis.* 2015, *25*, 208–213. [PubMed]
23. Masi, S.; Khan, T.; Johnson, W.; Wong, A.; Whincup, P.; Kuh, D.; Hughes, A.; Richards, M.; Hardy, R.; Deanfield, J. 4C.01: Lifetime obesity, cardiovascular disease and cognitive function: A longitudinal study from the 1946 birth cohort. *J. Hypertens.* 2015, *33* (Suppl. 1), e56. [CrossRef]
24. Peters, A.; McEwen, B.S. Stress habituation, body shape and cardiovascular mortality. *Neurosci. Biobehav. Rev.* 2015, *56*, 139–150. [CrossRef] [PubMed]
25. Esser, N.; Legrand-Poels, S.; Piette, J.; Scheen, A.J.; Paquot, N. Inflammation as a link between obesity, metabolic síndrome and type 2 diabetes. *Diabetes. Res. Clin. Pract.* 2014, *105*, 141–150. [CrossRef] [PubMed]
26. Oliver, E.; McGillicuddy, F.; Philips, C.; Toomey, S.; Roche, H.M. The role of inflammation and macrophage accumulation in the development of obesity-induced type 2 diabetes mellitus and the possible therapeutic effects of long-chain n 3 PUFA. *Proc. Nutr. Soc.* 2010, *69*, 232–243. [CrossRef] [PubMed]
27. Schwingshackl, L.; Hoffmann, G. Mediterranean dietary pattern, inflammation and endothelial function: A systematic review and meta-analysis of intervention trials. *Nutr. Metab. Cardiovasc. Dis.* 2014, *24*, 929–939. [CrossRef] [PubMed]
28. Flegal, K.M.; Kit, B.K.; Orpana, H.; Graubard, B.I. Association of all-cause mortality with overweight and obesity using standard body mass index categories: A systematic review and meta-analysis. *JAMA* 2013, *309*, 71–82. [CrossRef] [PubMed]
29. Gelber, R.P.; Gaziano, J.M.; Orav, E.J.; Manson, J.E.; Buring, J.E.; Kurth, T. Measures of obesity and cardiovascular risk among men and women. *J. Am. Coll. Cardiol.* 2008, *52*, 605–615. [CrossRef] [PubMed]
30. De Hollander, E.L.; Bemelmans, W.J.; Boshuizen, H.C.; Friedrich, N.; Wallaschofski, H.; Guallar-Castillón, P.; Walter, S.; Zillikens, M.C.; Rosengren, A.; Lissner, L.; *et al.* The association between waist circumference and risk of mortality considering body mass index in 65-to 74-years-olds: A meta-analysis of 29 cohorts involving more than 58,000 elderly persons. *Int. J. Epidemiol.* 2012, *41*, 805–817. [CrossRef] [PubMed]
31. Guallar-Castillón, P.; Rodríguez-Artalejo, F.; Tormo, M.J.; Sánchez, M.J.; Rodríguez, L.; Quirós, J.R.; Navarro, C.; Molina, E.; Martínez, C.; Marín, P.; *et al.* Major dietary patterns and risk of coronary heart disease in middle-aged persons from a Mediterranean country: The EPIC-Spain cohort study. *Nutr. Metab. Cardiovasc. Dis.* 2012, *22*, 192–199. [CrossRef] [PubMed]
32. Sánchez-Taínta, A.; Estruch, R.; Bulló, M.; Corella, D.; Gómez-Gracia, E.; Fiol, M.; Algorta, J.; Covas, M.I.; Lapetra, J.; Zazpe, I.; *et al.* Adherence to a Mediterranean-type diet and reduced prevalence of clustered cardiovascular risk factors in a cohort of 3204 high-risk patients. *Eur. J. Cardiovasc. Prev. Rehabil.* 2008, *15*, 589–593. [CrossRef] [PubMed]
33. García-Férnandez, E.; Rico-Cabanas, L.; Rosgaard, N.; Estruch, R.; Bach-Faig, A. Mediterranean diet and cardiodiabesity: A review. *Nutrients* 2014, *6*, 3474–3500. [CrossRef] [PubMed]
34. Aljefree, N.; Ahmed, F. Association between dietary pattern and risk of cardiovascular disease among adults in the Middle East and North Africa region: A systematic review. *Food Nutr. Res.* 2015, *59*, 27486. [CrossRef] [PubMed]

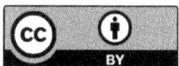

nutrients

MDPI

Article

Diet Quality Scores and Risk of Nasopharyngeal Carcinoma in Chinese Adults: A Case-Control Study

Cheng Wang [1,†], Xiao-Ling Lin [2,†], Yu-Ying Fan [3], Yuan-Ting Liu [4], Xing-Lan Zhang [5], Yun-Kai Lu [3], Chun-Hua Xu [6] and Yu-Ming Chen [1,*]

[1] Guangdong Provincial Key Laboratory of Food, Nutrition and Health, School of Public Health, Sun Yat-sen University, Guangzhou 510080, China; wangch28@mail2.sysu.edu.cn
[2] Department of Gynecologic Oncology, Sun Yat-sen University Cancer Center, Guangzhou 510060, China; Linxiaol@sysucc.org.cn
[3] Sun Yat-sen University Ophthalmic Center, Guangzhou 510060, China; Fanyy@sysucc.org.cn (Y.-Y.F.); luyunkai@mail.sysu.edu.cn (Y.-K.L.)
[4] Information Section, Central Hospital of Panyu District, Guangzhou 511400, China; tingty@126.com
[5] Department of Radiotherapy, Sun Yat-sen University Cancer Center, Guangzhou 510060, China; Zhangxingl@sysucc.org.cn
[6] Clinical laboratory section of the office outpatient Department public security board, Guangdong 510050, China; ladychun@126.com
* Correspondence: chenyum@mail.sysu.edu.cn; Tel.: +86-20-87330605; Fax: +86-20-87330446
† These authors contributed equally to this article.

Received: 4 January 2016; Accepted: 3 February 2016; Published: 25 February 2016

Abstract: Many studies show that dietary factors may affect the risk of nasopharyngeal carcinoma (NPC). We examined the association between overall diet quality and NPC risk in a Chinese population. This case-control study included 600 NPC patients and 600 matched controls between 2009 and 2011 in Guangzhou, China. Habitual dietary intake and various covariates were assessed via face-to-face interviews. Diet quality scores were calculated according to the Healthy Eating Index-2005 (HEI-2005), the alternate Healthy Eating Index (aHEI), the Diet Quality Index-International (DQI-I), and the alternate Mediterranean Diet Score (aMed). After adjustment for various lifestyle and dietary factors, greater diet quality scores on the HEI-2005, aHEI, and DQI-I—but not on the aMed—showed a significant association with a lower risk of NPC (p-trends, <0.001–0.001). The odds ratios (95% confidence interval) comparing the extreme quartiles of the three significant scores were 0.47 (0.32–0.68) (HEI-2005), 0.48 (0.33–0.70) (aHEI), and 0.43 (0.30–0.62) (DQI-I). In gender-stratified analyses, the favorable association remained significant in men but not in women. We found that adherence to the predefined dietary patterns represented by the HEI-2005, aHEI, and DQI-I scales predicted a lower risk of NPC in adults from south China, especially in men.

Keywords: nasopharyngeal carcinoma; diet quality; dietary pattern; case-control study; Chinese; adults

1. Introduction

Nasopharyngeal carcinoma (NPC), which originates in the epithelial cells lining the nasopharynx, is a rare type of neoplasm worldwide. The Global Cancer estimation project for 2012 indicated an age-standardized incidence of 1.2 and mortality rate of 0.7 per 10^5 [1]. However, much higher incidences have been observed in southern China, especially in the province of Guangdong (incidence, 10.5×10^{-5}; mortality rate, 5.3×10^{-5}) in 2011 [2]. More efforts are needed to explore the risk factors of NPC to allow more effective prevention in the Guangdong population.

NPC is believed to result from a combination of genetic susceptibility, Epstein–Barr virus infection, and a variety of environmental factors (e.g., carcinogens and dietary factors) [3,4]. An increasing body of evidence has shown that dietary factors may have an enigmatic effect on the initiation and promotion of NPC [4–6]. Studies have consistently reported a positive association between the risk of NPC and the consumption of salt-preserved fish [7,8], salted vegetables, and preserved meat [9,10], and favorable associations have been observed between the intake of fresh fruit and vegetables and the risk of NPC in Chinese adults [4,11]. However, data on the role of overall dietary quality in the risk of NPC are scarce.

A larger number of scores have been developed to assess overall dietary quality according to various dietary guidelines, such as the Healthy Eating Index-2005 (HEI-2005) [12], the alternate Healthy Eating Index (aHEI) [13], the Diet Quality Index-International (DQI-I) [14], and other beneficial dietary patterns (e.g., the alternate Mediterranean Diet (aMed) [15]). Many studies have shown associations between higher overall diet scores and a lower risk of various cancers, including head and neck cancer [16], gastric cancer [17], esophageal cancer [18], rectal cancer [19], and breast cancer [20]. Moreover, different dietary scales have different predictive values on the risk of individual cancers. However, to our knowledge, no study has yet reported associations between overall diet quality scores and the risk of NPC.

This study was performed to determine the association between four widely used diet quality scores (HEI-2005, aHEI, DQI-I, and aMed) and the risk of NPC and to assess which scores may best predict the risk of NPC in a high-incidence population in southern China.

2. Methods

2.1. Study Population

This matched case-control study was conducted between July 2009 and March 2011 in Guangzhou, Guangdong Province, China. The design of the study was described previously [11]. The patients and control subjects were matched in a 1:1 ratio by gender, age ($\pm$3 years), and household type (urban *vs.* rural in the past 10 years). The detailed inclusion and exclusion criteria for patients and control subjects are shown in Supplemental Table S1. The ethics committee of the School of Public Health of Sun Yat-sen University approved the study, and written informed consent was obtained from all participants.

2.2. Data Collection

Face-to-face interviews were conducted by experienced interviewers with relevant medical knowledge using a structured questionnaire that included information on (1) sociodemographic characteristics; (2) occupational and domestic exposure to toxic substances; (3) lifestyle habits (e.g., smoking and alcohol consumption); (4) habitual dietary consumption over the year before diagnosis (patients) or before the interview (control subjects); (5) all physical activities, including occupational and leisure activities, over the past month before admission to hospital (or interview); and (6) history of chronic diseases. Each interviewer completed an equal proportion of questionnaire interviews between the patient and control groups.

2.3. Assessment of Dietary Intake

A semiquantitative 78-item food frequency questionnaire (FFQ) was used to assess dietary consumption [11,21]. The mean intake of food per day, week, month, or year was reported for each food item on the FFQ. For seasonal foods, the participants were asked to report how many months of the year they consumed each item. Food photographs were provided as visual aids to assess portion sizes. The average daily intake of nutrients and total energy were calculated according to the Chinese Food Composition Table, 2002 [22]. We adjusted grams per day to servings per day according to the serving size definitions of the U.S. Food Guide Pyramid (2005) and Chinese dietary guidelines (2007) when appropriate [23].

2.4. Calculation of Diet Quality Scores

We calculated the diet quality scores of HEI-2005, aHEI, DQI-I, and aMed on the basis of the data from the FFQ interview. The calculations for the HEI-2005, aHEI, and DQI-I were mainly based on the distribution of intake of foods, nutrients, energy, and/or ratios of the relevant items, or the median values for aMed, as described in detail in previous reports [24].

The 100-point HEI-2005 scale includes 14 items [12]. Fruits, vegetables, grains, milk, meat and beans, and oils were measured as servings per 1000 kcal, and solid fat, alcohol, and added sugar were expressed as the percentage of total calories. For sodium, we only asked whether the subject's taste was light, moderate, or heavy, and each corresponding choice was valued 0, 5, or 10 points, respectively.

The nine-item aHEI score was developed by McCullough *et al.* [13] based on foods and nutrients (e.g., nut and soy protein, cereal fiber, *trans*fate, and the ratio of polyunsaturated to saturated fat) that are associated with a risk of chronic disease. Each component is worth 0 to 10 points except for the multivitamin item, which was either 2.5 or 7.5. We excluded *trans*fats because they are consumed at a very low level in the middle-aged and elderly Chinese population [25]. Therefore, the aHEI scores contained eight components for a total of 77.5 points in our study.

The DQI-I score was calculated on the basis of the methods developed by Kim *et al.* [14]. Briefly, the DQI-I assesses four categories (variety, adequacy, moderation, and overall balance) and contains six food items and 11 nutrient items. The maximum possible score for each item ranges from 4 to 15 points, for a total score of 100 points.

The aMed score was modified by Fung *et al.* [15] from the original Mediterranean diet score [26] to evaluate nine components with a maximum score of 9. One point for each item is assigned to subjects with high intake of whole grains, vegetables, fruit, legumes, nuts, fish, ratio of monounsaturated to saturated fat, a moderate intake of alcohol, and a low intake of red and processed meats, respectively, based upon the sex-specific median in the control subjects.

2.5. Statistical Analysis

Common characteristics between the patients and the control subjects were compared using paired *t*-tests for continuous variables and paired chi-square tests for categorical variables. Logarithmic transformation was used for energy intake, and square root transformation was applied to the other dietary factors. Dietary intakes were adjusted for total energy intake using the residual method. The diet quality scores on the HEI-2005, aHEI, DQI-I, and aMED were categorized into four quartiles (Q1 to Q4) on the basis of the sex-specific quartile cutoffs among the control subjects. Odds ratios and 95% confidence intervals (CIs) for NPC were estimated with the use of univariate and multivariate conditional logistic regression models for each score using the lowest quartile (Q1) as the referent. *p* values for the between quartiles were also calculated using quartile 2 and 3 as the referent, respectively. The *p* values for linear trends were estimated by modeling the quartiles of diet quality scores as continuous variables. In the multivariate model, we adjusted for age, body mass index, occupation, marital status, education level, household income, current smoking status, current drinking status, exposure to potential toxic substances, history of chronic rhinitis, physical activity, energy intake, intake of preserved vegetables and animal food, and multivitamin supplements, except for the aHEI score analysis. Stratified analyses were performed by gender. The interaction significance was evaluated with the Wald χ^2 test with a multiplicative interaction term ($\alpha = 0.05$ divided by the number of tests). Statistical significance was inferred for two-tailed *p* values of less than 0.05. All statistical analyses were performed with SPSS software (version 17.0, SPSS, Chicago, IL, USA).

3. Results

We screened 653 eligible patients from all 851 inpatients in the hospital during the study period. We excluded those with an incomplete questionnaire (20 patients), those who refused to participate (31 patients), and those who had implausible daily energy intakes (700 to 4200 kcal for men and 500 to 3500 kcal for women) (2 patients). The final analysis included 600 patients and 600 matched control subjects.

The patients with NPC and the control subjects had similar distributions of age, gender, and household type. There were three times as many men (74.7%) as women. The patients with NPC were more likely than the control subjects to have a history of chronic rhinitis ($p < 0.001$), a higher body mass index ($p < 0.002$), less intense occupational activity ($p < 0.001$) and physical activity ($p = 0.013$), and lower total energy intake ($p = 0.029$). No significant differences were observed for current drinking status, current smoking status, and exposure to toxic substances (Table 1).

Table 1. Participants' characteristics in nasopharyngeal carcinoma cases and controls [a].

	Cases (*n* = 600)	Controls (*n* = 600)	*p*-Value
Age, year	47.4 ± 9.0	47.4 ± 9.0	0.992
Gender (Male/Female)	448/152	448/152	
Body mass index, kg/m²	23.2 ± 3.1	22.7 ± 2.8	0.002
Marital status			0.007
Married	590 (98.3)	574 (95.7)	
Single	10 (1.7)	26 (4.3)	
Household type, *n* (%)			
Urban	399 (66.5)	399 (66.5)	
Rural	201 (33.5)	201 (33.5)	
Education, *n* (%)			0.001
Primary school or below	109 (18.2)	130 (21.7)	
Secondary school	190 (31.7)	229 (38.2)	
High school	170 (28.3)	158 (26.3)	
College or above	131 (21.8)	83 (13.8)	
Family monthly income, Yuan/person			0.007
<1500	256 (42.7)	304 (50.7)	
1500–3000	158 (26.3)	153 (25.5)	
>3000	186 (31.0)	143 (23.8)	
Occupation, *n* (%)			<0.001
Light intensity of activity	228 (38.0)	192 (32.0)	
Moderate intensity of activity	188 (31.3)	158 (26.3)	
Heavy intensity of activity	184 (30.7)	250 (41.7)	
Chronic rhinitis history, *n* (%)	164 (27.3)	108 (18.0)	<0.001
Exposure to toxic substances, *n* (%) [b]	274 (45.7)	269 (44.8)	0.814
Current drinking, *n* (%) [c]	132 (22.0)	121 (20.2)	0.489
Current smoking, *n* (%) [d]	294 (49.0)	277 (46.2)	0.343
Physical activities, MET h/day [e]	38.2 ± 8.9	39.7 ± 12.2	0.013
Dietary energy intake, kcal/day	1873 ± 600	1953 ± 642	0.029
Multivitamin use, *n* (%)	32 (5.3)	35 (5.8)	0.711

[a] Continuous values are described by means ± SD. Categorical variables are described by numbers (%); [b] Exposure to potential toxic substances or detrimental environment included exposuring to one of the following factors over one year: heat, organic solvents, pesticides, heavy metals, smoke from burning incense, anti-mosquito coils, new furniture or decoration and radiation; [c] Current drinking was defined as having had alcohol drinks at least once weekly for at least six consecutive months; [d] Current smoking was defined as having smoked at least one cigarette daily for at least six consecutive months; [e] Physical activities included daily occupational, leisure-time and household-chores, evaluated by metabolic equivalent (MET) hours per day.

The median scores for patients and control subjects were 71 (range, 35 to 86) and 72 (32 to 87) for the HEI-2005, 39.5 (13.5 to 62.5) and 41.5 (11.5 to 62.5) for the aHEI, 52 (22 to 74) and 54 (27 to 74) for the DQI-I, and 4 (0 to 8) and 4 (0 to 9) for the aMed. The diet quality scores all had significant correlations (all $p < 0.01$) to each other (Supplemental Table S2).

The univariate analyses showed that subjects with higher scores on the HEI-2005, aHEI, and DQI-I—but not the aMed—had a significantly lower risk of NPC (*p* trends, <0.001 to 0.006). Similar associations remained after adjustment for multiple covariates (*p* trends, <0.001 to 0.001) (Table 2). The odds ratios (95% CI) of NPC risk for the extreme quartiles (Q4 *vs.* Q1) of the diet quality scores were 0.47 (0.32 to 0.68) for the HEI-2005 score, 0.48 (0.33 to 0.70) for the aHEI score, and 0.43 (0.30 to 0.62) for the DQI-I score, respectively (Table 2).

Table 2. ORs (95% CIs) of nasopharyngeal carcinoma for quartiles of diet-quality scores (*n* = 600 pairs) [a].

| | ORs (95% CI) by Quartiles of Each Scores | | | | *p*-Trend |
	Q1	Q2	Q3	Q4 (Highest)	
HEI-2005					
N (case/control)	189/175	165/146	168/144	78/135	
Score [b]	62	69	75	80	
Crude OR	1.00	1.02 (0.76,1.38)	1.01 (0.75,1.36)	0.54 (0.38,0.77) **,##,&&	0.006
Adjusted OR [c]	1.00	0.95 (0.69,1.31)	0.90 (0.65,1.24)	0.47 (0.32,0.68) **,##,&&	0.001
aHEI					
N (case/control)	196/158	180/149	128/153	96/140	
Score	31.5	39.5	44.5	50.5	
Crude OR	1.00	0.93 (0.69,1.24)	0.64 (0.46,0.89) **,#	0.54 (0.39,0.76) **,##	<0.001
Adjusted OR	1.00	0.93 (0.67,1.28)	0.50 (0.34,0.73) **,#	0.48 (0.33,0.70) **,#	<0.001
DQI-I					
N (case/control)	229/164	115/151	163/142	93/143	
Score	44	52	57	63	
Crude OR	1.00	0.53 (0.38,0.73) **	0.81 (0.60,1.11) #	0.45 (0.32,0.64) **,&&	<0.001
Adjusted OR	1.00	0.45 (0.31,0.64) **	0.75 (0.53,1.05) #	0.43 (0.30,0.62) **,&&	<0.001
aMed					
N (case/control)	137/136	122/103	185/181	156/180	
Score	2	3	4	6	
Crude OR	1.00	1.17 (0.82,1.66)	1.01 (0.73,1.38)	0.86 (0.62,1.18)	0.240
Adjusted OR	1.00	1.06 (0.72,1.56)	0.98 (0.69,1.37)	0.85 (0.59,1.22)	0.319

[a] Abbreviations: aHEI: alternate Healthy Eating Index; aMed: alternate Mediterranean Diet Score; DASH: Dietary approach to stop hypertension; DQI-I: Diet Quality Index–International; HEI-2005: Healthy Eating Index—2005; ORs (95% CI): Odds ratios (95% confidence interval); **: Compared with Quartile 1, *p* < 0.01; #,##: Compared with Quartile 2, *p* < 0.05, *p* < 0.01; &&: Compared with Quartile 3, *p* < 0.01; [b] Median score in controls; [c] Crude and adjusted ORs (95% CI) from conditional logistic regression models. For the adjusted ORs, covariates include age, body mass index, occupation, marital status, educational level, household income, current smoking, current drinking, exposure to potential toxic substances, multivitamin supplements, chronic rhinitis history, physical activity, daily energy intake, preserved vegetables and animal food, and multivitamin supplements except for the aHEI score analysis.

In gender-stratified analyses, significant associations between the HEI-2005, aHEI, and DQI-I scores, and the risk of NPC were observed only in men but not in women. The corresponding odds ratios (Q4 *vs.* Q1) ranged from 0.36 to 0.40 in men and 0.55 to 0.72 in women for the three scores (*p* interactions: 0.048 to 0.212) (Table 3).

Table 3. Adjusted ORs (95% CIs) of nasopharyngeal carcinoma for quartiles of diet-quality scores by gender [a].

| | ORs (95% CI) [b] by Quartiles of Each Score | | | | *p*-Trend | *p*-Inter-Action |
	Q1	Q2	Q3	Q4 (Highest)		
HEI-2005						
Gender						0.055
Men	1.00	0.90 (0.61,1.33)	0.79 (0.53,1.19)	0.40 (0.25,0.65) **,##,&	0.001	
Women	1.00	1.13 (0.56,2.28)	1.54 (0.83,2.86)	0.71 (0.32,1.57)	0.934	

Table 3. *Cont.*

	ORs (95% CI) [b] by Quartiles of Each Score				*p*-Trend	*p*-Inter-Action
	Q1	Q2	Q3	Q4 (Highest)		
aHEI						
Gender						0.212
Men	1.00	0.90 (0.61,1.32)	0.47 (0.31,0.74) **	0.40 (0.26,0.62) **	<0.001	
Women	1.00	1.07 (0.58,1.97)	0.66 (0.30,1.42)	0.72 (0.35,1.47)	0.221	
DQI-I						
Gender						0.048
Men	1.00	0.41 (0.27,0.64) **	0.61 (0.41,0.92) *,#	0.36 (0.23,0.55) **,&&	<0.001	
Women	1.00	0.55 (0.26,1.16)	1.25 (0.62,2.49)	0.55 (0.25,1.22)	0.644	
aMed						
Gender						0.199
Men	1.00	1.10 (0.70,1.72)	0.99 (0.67,1.46)	0.74 (0.48,1.15)	0.170	
Women	1.00	1.64 (0.74,3.63)	0.79 (0.35,1.76)	1.26 (0.65,2.44)	0.797	

[a] Abbreviations: see Table 2; *n*: men 448 pairs, women 152 pairs; *,**: Compared with Quartile 1, *p* < 0.05, *p* < 0.01; #,##: Compared with Quartile 2, *p* < 0.05, *p* < 0.01; &,&&: Compared with Quartile 3, *p* < 0.05, *p* < 0.01; [b] Odds ratios (95% CI): from multivariate conditional logistic regression models after adjustments for the covariates as indicated in Table 2. α for interactions = 0.05/4 tests = 0.0125.

4. Discussion

This case-control study with 600 patients and 600 control subjects showed that three diet quality scores (HEI-2005, aHEI, and DQI-I) had approximate favorable associations with the risk of NPC, but the aMed score had no such association. These results suggest that adherence to these three indices could play a role in the prevention of NPC. Although these three scores had similar associations with the risk of NPC, public health messages should pay more attention to the aHEI score for the prediction of NPC because it has fewer scoring items and the simplest scoring method.

Up to date, no study has yet reported the relationship between diet quality scores and the risk of NPC. However, significant inverse associations have been shown between diet quality scores and the risks of many other cancers in most [18,19,27–30], but not all [31,32], previous studies. In the National Institutes of Health–AARP Diet and Health Study with 537,218 men and women (followed-up for 10.5 years), the consumption of a diet with a high HEI-2005 and aHEI score may reduce the risk of pancreatic [27], prostate [28], esophageal [18], and colorectal [19] cancers, with multivariable adjusted hazard ratios ranging from 0.51 to 0.92 when comparing the highest and lowest quintiles. Data from the Health Professional's Follow-up Study and Nurses' Health Study showed that the HEI-2005 and aHEI-2010, which are strongly correlated with the aHEI, had an inverse association with the overall risk of cancer among women and men (*p* trend, 0.003 and 0.001, respectively) [29]. Similar findings were seen in a recent systematic review and meta-analysis of cohort studies, in which diets of the highest quality, as assessed by the HEI, aHEI, and DASH (Dietary approach to stop hypertension) score, resulted in a significant reduction in the incidence and mortality risk of cancer (relative risk, 0.85; 95% CI, 0.82 to 0.88) [30]. Few studies have examined the association between cancer risk and the DQI-I, although a higher DQI-I score was shown to be associated with a reduced risk of other chronic diseases, such as non-alcoholic fatty liver disease and diabetes, that may promote cancer risk [33,34]. We found that subjects with scores in the highest (*vs.* lowest) quartile of the HEI-2005, aHEI, and DQI-I had 52% to 57% lower risks of NPC (*p* trend, <0.001 to 0.001); these findings are consistent with those in other cancers in previous studies. Our results may provide new evidence for overall dietary quality in the prevention of NPC. Further studies are needed to address whether the favorable association is site specific, as null associations are likely to be observed in some hormone-related cancers, such as endometrial cancer [31], ovarian cancer [32] and estrogen-receptor–positive breast cancer [20].

The beneficial effects of high-quality dietary scores may reflect the synergistic effects of diverse foods and numerous nutrients characterized in higher vegetables, fruit, total grains, and nuts consumption. Previous studies suggested that greater consumption of vegetables and fruit may lower the risk of NPC [11,35]. In the individual component analyses, we found significant inverse associations between vegetables, fruit, fiber, and vitamin C components and the incidence of NPC (Supplemental Table S3). Many ingredients of vegetables and fruit may contribute to a reduction in NPC risk, including dietary fiber, antioxidants, and other phytochemicals [36]. Antioxidants, such as vitamin A, C, and E and carotenoids, contribute to the prevention of nasopharyngeal oncogenesis via regulation of the progress of cell differentiation and proliferation, reduction of oxidative DNA fragmentation in nasal epithelial cells, and inhibition of the early antigen expression of the Epstein–Barr virus [37–39]. Moreover, inflammation is a major feature in carcinogenesis, and the overexpression of inflammation cytokine has been a promoter for NPC progression [40]. Higher diet quality scores have been related to lower concentrations of inflammatory biomarkers, which may help prevent the development of NPC [41].

Although the various dietary quality scores all emphasized greater intake of fruits and vegetables and less intake of saturated fat, only the aMed showed no significant association with NPC in our study, which is inconsistent with several reports in which the aMed showed an inverse relationship to the risk of other cancers [26,42,43]. A partial reason for the null association may be the differences in the numbers of score items and scoring criteria. The aMed has a much narrower possible score range, and its significant components had relatively lower weight (Supplemental Table S3) compared to those in the HEI-2005, aHEI, and DQI-I. Thus, the aMed score may not be able to finely discriminate dietary healthfulness in terms of NPC risk in our population. In addition, Davis *et al.* [44] recently found that the average nutrients and bioactive contents of the diet was relatively consistent in the food groups among previous studies in which the Mediterranean diet showed a positive effect on chronic disease. More studies are needed to confirm our findings with regard to NPC.

In gender-stratified analyses, the favorable association between the HEI-2005, aHEI, and DQI-I scores and NPC remained significant in men but not in women, although no significant gender interactions were observed (p interaction, 0.055 to 0.212, >0.05/4 tests). These differences might be partly a result of genetic variations in NPC susceptibility, with almost twofold incidence in men than in women and stronger acceleration of dietary risk factors on the relevant biomarkers of inflammation in men [45,46]. Posteriorly, the relatively small sample size for women (case-control pairs, men *vs.* women: 448 *vs.* 152) might contribute to the gender differences.

Our study has several strengths. To our knowledge, this was the first study to systematically test the associations between diet quality scores derived from various dietary guidelines and the risk of NPC using a well-constructed FFQ with satisfactory reproducibility and validity [21]. The interviewers were well-trained, and each interviewer surveyed the same proportion of patients and control subjects. A 1:1 matched study was designed to minimize the influence of age, gender, and household types. In addition, adjustments were made in the multivariate analysis for a number of potential covariates, including socioeconomic status, body mass index, and some dietary factors (such as intake of preserved vegetables and animal foods).

This study also has several limitations that should be considered. First, inverse causality could not be fully excluded in a case-control study because the diet information was collected after the diagnosis of NPC. To minimize this possibility, only new cases (within three months of diagnosis) were included in our study, and both the patients and the control subjects were confined to those without a substantial change in dietary habits over the previous five years. Moreover, patients were more likely to change their dietary habits in a favorable direction, which might underestimate the protective effect of dietary patterns. Second, recall bias of one's habitual diet is unavoidable in retrospective data collection, but differential report bias between patients and control subjects was unlikely to be present in this study because NPC is considered to be a major genetic and virus-related cancer, and there was little public awareness of a potential dietary influence except for salted or preserved foods. Finally, the patients with NPC and the control subjects were recruited from two different hospitals, which might have resulted in a selection bias. However, both hospitals were top-ranking specialized institutions with comparable reputations and coverage areas. The distributions of the major demographic characteristics (for example, age and sex) in our study matched those in a population-based epidemiological survey of NPC [47].

5. Conclusions

In summary, our results first suggest that the dietary patterns represented by the HEI-2005, AHEI and DQI-I scores predict a lower risk of NPC in adults in southern China, especially in men. Our findings provide evidence for adherence to the general dietary guidelines for the prevention of NPC. We found no association between the aMED score and NPC, which differs from studies about many other chronic diseases. Further prospective studies are merited to confirm our findings.

Supplementary Materials: The following are available online at http://www.mdpi.com/2072-6643/8/3/112/s1, Table S1: Inclusion and exclusion criteria for NPC cases and controls, Table S2. Spearman's rank correlation coefficients for NPC cases ($n = 600$) and controls ($n = 600$) among total summary scores for the HEI-2005, aHEI, DQI-I, and aMed scores, Table S3. Odds ratio (95% CIs) of nasopharyngeal carcinoma for the highest (*vs.* lowest) quartile of the individual components of the selected diet-quality scores.

Acknowledgments: This study was supported by the 5010 Program for Clinical Researches of Sun Yat-sen University, Guangzhou, China (2007032). The funding sources had no role in the design, implementation, or interpretation of this work or in the manuscript preparation.

Author Contributions: Yu-Ming Chen conceived and designed the study, and critically revised the manuscript; Cheng Wang analyzed the data and wrote the paper. Xiao-Ling Lin, Yu-Ying Fan, Yuan-Ting Liu, Xing-Lan Zhang, Yun-Kai Lu and Chun-Hua Xu, carried out the study and participated in paper writing. All authors read and approved the final manuscript.

Conflicts of Interest: The authors declare no conflict of interest.

Abbreviations

aHEI: alternate Healthy Eating Index; aMed: alternate Mediterranean Diet Score; DASH: Dietary approach to stop hypertension; DQI-I: Diet Quality Index–International; HEI-2005: Healthy Eating Index–2005; NPC: nasopharyngeal carcinoma.

References

1. Globocan 2012: Estimated Cancer Incidence and Mortality and Prevalence Worldwide in 2012. International Agency for Research on Cancer. Available online: http://globocan.iarc.fr (accessed on 3 August 2015).
2. Li, K.; Lin, G.Z.; Shen, J.C.; Zhou, Q. Time trends of nasopharyngeal carcinoma in urban Guangzhou over a 12-year period (2000–2011): Declines in both incidence and mortality. *Asian Pac. J. Cancer Prev.* **2014**, *15*, 9899–9903. [CrossRef] [PubMed]
3. Lee, A.W.M.; Foo, W.; Mang, O.; Sze, W.M.; Chappell, R.; Lau, W.H.; Ko, W.M. Changing epidemiology of nasopharyngeal carcinoma in hongkong over a 20-year period (1980–1999): An encouraging reduction in both incidence and mortality. *Int. J. Cancer* **2003**, *103*, 680–685. [CrossRef] [PubMed]
4. Jia, W.H.; Luo, X.Y.; Feng, B.J.; Ruan, H.L.; Bei, J.X.; Liu, W.S.; Qin, H.D.; Feng, Q.S.; Chen, L.Z.; Yao, S.Y.; *et al.* Traditional cantonese diet and nasopharyngeal carcinoma risk: A large-scale case-control study in Guangdong, china. *BMC Cancer* **2010**, *10*, 446. [CrossRef] [PubMed]
5. Chang, E.T.; Adami, H.O. The enigmatic epidemiology of nasopharyngeal carcinoma. *Cancer Epidemiol. Biomarkers Prev.* **2006**, *15*, 1765–1777. [CrossRef] [PubMed]
6. Feng, B.J.; Jalbout, M.; Ayoub, W.B.; Khyatti, M.; Dahmoul, S.; Ayad, M.; Maachi, F.; Bedadra, W.; Abdoun, M.; Mesli, S.; *et al.* Dietary risk factors for nasopharyngeal carcinoma in maghrebian countries. *Int. J. Cancer* **2007**, *121*, 1550–1555. [CrossRef] [PubMed]
7. Ho, J.H.; Huang, D.P.; Fong, Y.Y. Salted fish and nasopharyngeal carcinoma in southern Chinese. *Lancet* **1978**, *2*, 626. [CrossRef]
8. Guo, X.; Johnson, R.C.; Deng, H.; Liao, J.; Guan, L.; Nelson, G.W.; Tang, M.; Zheng, Y.; de The, G.; O'Brien, S.J.; *et al.* Evaluation of nonviral risk factors for nasopharyngeal carcinoma in a high-risk population of southern china. *Int. J. Cancer* **2009**, *124*, 2942–2947. [CrossRef] [PubMed]

9. Yu, M.C.; Huang, T.B.; Henderson, B.E. Diet and nasopharyngeal carcinoma: A case-control study in Guangzhou, china. *Int. J. Cancer* **1989**, *43*, 1077–1082. [CrossRef] [PubMed]
10. Chen, D.L.; Huang, T.B. A case-control study of risk factors of nasopharyngeal carcinoma. *Cancer Lett.* **1997**, *117*, 17–22. [CrossRef]
11. Liu, Y.-T.; Dai, J.-J.; Xu, C.-H.; Lu, Y.-K.; Fan, Y.-Y.; Zhang, X.-L.; Zhang, C.-X.; Chen, Y.-M. Greater intake of fruit and vegetables is associated with lower risk of nasopharyngeal carcinoma in Chinese adults: A case-control study. *Cancer Causes Control* **2012**, *23*, 589–599. [CrossRef] [PubMed]
12. Guenther, P.M.; Reedy, J.; Krebs-Smith, S.M. Development of the healthy eating index-2005. *J. Am. Diet Assoc.* **2008**, *108*, 1896–1901. [CrossRef] [PubMed]
13. McCullough, M.L.; Feskanich, D.; Stampfer, M.J.; Giovannucci, E.L.; Rimm, E.B.; Hu, F.B.; Spiegelman, D.; Hunter, D.J.; Colditz, G.A.; Willett, W.C. Diet quality and major chronic disease risk in men and women: Moving toward improved dietary guidance. *Am. J. Clin. Nutr.* **2002**, *76*, 1261–1271. [PubMed]
14. Kim, S.; Haines, P.S.; Siega-Riz, A.M.; Popkin, B.M. The diet quality index-international (DQI-I) provides an effective tool for cross-national comparison of diet quality as illustrated by China and the United States. *J. Nutr.* **2003**, *133*, 3476–3484. [PubMed]
15. Fung, T.T.; Rexrode, K.M.; Mantzoros, C.S.; Manson, J.E.; Willett, W.C.; Hu, F.B. Mediterranean diet and incidence of and mortality from coronary heart disease and stroke in women. *Circulation* **2009**, *119*, 1093–1100. [CrossRef] [PubMed]
16. Li, W.Q.; Park, Y.; Wu, J.W.; Goldstein, A.M.; Taylor, P.R.; Hollenbeck, A.R.; Freedman, N.D.; Abnet, C.C. Index-based dietary patterns and risk of head and neck cancer in a large prospective study. *Am. J. Clin. Nutr.* **2014**, *99*, 559–566. [CrossRef] [PubMed]
17. Buckland, G.; Travier, N.; Huerta, J.M.; Bueno-de-Mesquita, H.B.; Siersema, P.D.; Skeie, G.; Weiderpass, E.; Engeset, D.; Ericson, U.; Ohlsson, B.; *et al.* Healthy lifestyle index and risk of gastric adenocarcinoma in the epic cohort study. *Int. J. Cancer* **2015**, *137*, 598–606. [CrossRef] [PubMed]
18. Li, W.Q.; Park, Y.; Wu, J.W.; Ren, J.S.; Goldstein, A.M.; Taylor, P.R.; Hollenbeck, A.R.; Freedman, N.D.; Abnet, C.C. Index-based dietary patterns and risk of esophageal and gastric cancer in a large cohort study. *Clin. Gastroenterol. Hepatol.* **2013**, *11*, 1130–1136. [CrossRef] [PubMed]
19. Reedy, J.; Mitrou, P.N.; Krebs-Smith, S.M.; Wirfalt, E.; Flood, A.; Kipnis, V.; Leitzmann, M.; Mouw, T.; Hollenbeck, A.; Schatzkin, A.; *et al.* Index-based dietary patterns and risk of colorectal cancer: The nih-aarp diet and health study. *Am. J. Epidemiol.* **2008**, *168*, 38–48. [CrossRef] [PubMed]
20. Fung, T.T.; Hu, F.B.; McCullough, M.L.; Newby, P.K.; Willett, W.C.; Holmes, M.D. Diet quality is associated with the risk of estrogen receptor-negative breast cancer in postmenopausal women. *J. Nutr.* **2006**, *136*, 466–472. [PubMed]
21. Zhang, C.X.; Ho, S.C. Validity and reproducibility of a food frequency questionnaire among Chinese women in Guangdong province. *Asian Pac. J. Clin. Nutr.* **2009**, *18*, 240–250.
22. Yang, Y.X.; Wang, G.Y.; Pan, X.C. *China Food Composition Table*; Peking University Medical Press: Beijing, China, 2002.
23. Department of Health and Human Services and Department of Agriculture. *Dietary Guidelines for Americans 2005*, 6th ed.; Government Printing Office: Washington, DC, USA, 2005.
24. Zeng, F.F.; Xue, W.Q.; Cao, W.T.; Wu, B.H.; Xie, H.L.; Fan, F.; Zhu, H.L.; Chen, Y.M. Diet-quality scores and risk of hip fractures in elderly urban Chinese in Guangdong, China: A case-control study. *Osteoporos. Int.* **2014**, *25*, 2131–2141. [CrossRef] [PubMed]
25. Astrup, A.; Dyerberg, J.; Selleck, M.; Stender, S. Nutrition transition and its relationship to the development of obesity and related chronic diseases. *Obes. Rev.* **2008**, *9* (Suppl. 1), 48–52. [CrossRef] [PubMed]
26. Trichopoulou, A.; Costacou, T.; Bamia, C.; Trichopoulos, D. Adherence to a mediterranean diet and survival in a Greek population. *N. Engl. J. Med.* **2003**, *348*, 2599–2608. [CrossRef] [PubMed]
27. Arem, H.; Reedy, J.; Sampson, J.; Jiao, L.; Hollenbeck, A.R.; Risch, H.; Mayne, S.T.; Stolzenberg-Solomon, R.Z. The healthy eating index 2005 and risk for pancreatic cancer in the nih-aarp study. *J. Natl. Cancer Inst.* **2013**, *105*, 1298–1305. [CrossRef] [PubMed]
28. Bosire, C.; Stampfer, M.J.; Subar, A.F.; Park, Y.; Kirkpatrick, S.I.; Chiuve, S.E.; Hollenbeck, A.R.; Reedy, J. Index-based dietary patterns and the risk of prostate cancer in the nih-aarp diet and health study. *Am. J. Epidemiol.* **2013**, *177*, 504–513. [CrossRef] [PubMed]

29. Chiuve, S.E.; Fung, T.T.; Rimm, E.B.; Hu, F.B.; McCullough, M.L.; Wang, M.L.; Stampfer, M.J.; Willett, W.C. Alternative dietary indices both strongly predict risk of chronic disease. *J. Nutr.* **2012**, *142*, 1009–1018. [CrossRef] [PubMed]

30. Schwingshackl, L.; Hoffmann, G. Diet quality as assessed by the healthy eating index, the alternate healthy eating index, the dietary approaches to stop hypertension score, and health outcomes: A systematic review and meta-analysis of cohort studies. *J. Acad. Nutr. Diet.* **2015**, *115*, 780–800. [CrossRef] [PubMed]

31. Chandran, U.; Bandera, E.V.; Williams-King, M.G.; Sima, C.; Bayuga, S.; Pulick, K.; Wilcox, H.; Zauber, A.G.; Olson, S.H. Adherence to the dietary guidelines for americans and endometrial cancer risk. *Cancer Causes Control* **2010**, *21*, 1895–1904. [CrossRef] [PubMed]

32. Xie, J.; Poole, E.M.; Terry, K.L.; Fung, T.T.; Rosner, B.A.; Willett, W.C.; Tworoger, S.S. A prospective cohort study of dietary indices and incidence of epithelial ovarian cancer. *J. Ovarian Res.* **2014**, *7*, 112. [CrossRef] [PubMed]

33. Chan, R.; Wong, V.W.; Chu, W.C.; Wong, G.L.; Li, L.S.; Leung, J.; Chim, A.M.; Yeung, D.K.; Sea, M.M.; Woo, J.; *et al.* Diet-quality scores and prevalence of nonalcoholic fatty liver disease: A population study using proton-magnetic resonance spectroscopy. *PLoS ONE* **2015**, *10*, e0139310. [CrossRef] [PubMed]

34. Kim, J.; Cho, Y.; Park, Y.; Sohn, C.; Rha, M.; Lee, M.K.; Jang, H.C. Association of dietary quality indices with glycemic status in korean patients with type 2 diabetes. *Clin. Nutr. Res.* **2013**, *2*, 100–106. [CrossRef] [PubMed]

35. Polesel, J.; Serraino, D.; Negri, E.; Barzan, L.; Vaccher, E.; Montella, M.; Zucchetto, A.; Garavello, W.; Franceschi, S.; La Vecchia, C.; *et al.* Consumption of fruit, vegetables, and other food groups and the risk of nasopharyngeal carcinoma. *Cancer Causes Control* **2013**, *24*, 1157–1165. [CrossRef] [PubMed]

36. Wiseman, M. The second world cancer research fund/American institute for cancer research expert report. Food, nutrition, physical activity, and the prevention of cancer: A global perspective. *Proc. Nutr. Soc.* **2008**, *67*, 253–256. [CrossRef] [PubMed]

37. Million, K.; Tournier, F.; Houcine, O.; Ancian, P.; Reichert, U.; Marano, F. Effects of retinoic acid receptor-selective agonists on human nasal epithelial cell differentiation. *Am. J. Respir. Cell Mol. Biol.* **2001**, *25*, 744–750. [CrossRef] [PubMed]

38. Ben Chaaben, A.; Mariaselvam, C.; Salah, S.; Busson, M.; Dulphy, N.; Douik, H.; Ghanem, A.; Boukaouci, W.; Al Daccak, R.; Mamoghli, T.; *et al.* Polymorphisms in oxidative stress-related genes are associated with nasopharyngeal carcinoma susceptibility. *Immunobiology* **2015**, *220*, 20–25. [CrossRef] [PubMed]

39. Jian, S.W.; Mei, C.E.; Liang, Y.N.; Li, D.; Chen, Q.L.; Luo, H.L.; Li, Y.Q.; Cai, T.Y. Influence of selenium-rich rice on transformation of umbilical blood B lymphocytes by Epstein-Barr virus and Epstein-Barr virus early antigen expression. *Ai Zheng* **2003**, *22*, 26–29. [PubMed]

40. Song, Q.; Wang, G.; Chu, Y.; Zhou, L.; Jiang, M.; He, Q.; Liu, M.; Qin, J.; Hu, J. TNF-α up-regulates cellular inhibitor of apoptosis protein 2 (c-IAP2) via c-Jun N-terminal kinase (JNK) pathway in nasopharyngeal carcinoma. *Int. Immunopharmacol.* **2013**, *16*, 148–153. [CrossRef]

41. Fung, T.T.; McCullough, M.L.; Newby, P.K.; Manson, J.E.; Meigs, J.B.; Rifai, N.; Willett, W.C.; Hu, F.B. Diet-quality scores and plasma concentrations of markers of inflammation and endothelial dysfunction. *Am. J. Clin. Nutr.* **2005**, *82*, 163–173. [PubMed]

42. Buckland, G.; Agudo, A.; Lujan, L.; Jakszyn, P.; Bueno-de-Mesquita, H.B.; Palli, D.; Boeing, H.; Carneiro, F.; Krogh, V.; Sacerdote, C.; *et al.* Adherence to a mediterranean diet and risk of gastric adenocarcinoma within the european prospective investigation into cancer and nutrition (EPIC) cohort study. *Am. J. Clin. Nutr.* **2010**, *91*, 381–390. [CrossRef] [PubMed]

43. Harmon, B.E.; Boushey, C.J.; Shvetsov, Y.B.; Ettienne, R.; Reedy, J.; Wilkens, L.R.; Le Marchand, L.; Henderson, B.E.; Kolonel, L.N. Associations of key diet-quality indexes with mortality in the multiethnic cohort: The dietary patterns methods project. *Am. J. Clin. Nutr.* **2015**, *101*, 587–597. [CrossRef] [PubMed]

44. Davis, C.; Bryan, J.; Hodgson, J.; Murphy, K. Definition of the mediterranean diet; a literature review. *Nutrients* **2015**, *7*, 9139–9153. [CrossRef] [PubMed]

45. Ganz, M.; Csak, T.; Szabo, G. High fat diet feeding results in gender specific steatohepatitis and inflammasome activation. *World J. Gastroenterol.* **2014**, *20*, 8525–8534. [CrossRef] [PubMed]

46. Al-Attas, O.S.; Al-Daghri, N.M.; Alokail, M.S.; Alkharfy, K.M.; Khan, N.; Alfawaz, H.A.; Aiswaidan, I.A.; Al-Ajlan, A.S.; Chrousos, G.P. Association of dietary fatty acids intake with pro-coagulation and inflammation in saudi adults. *Asian Pac. J. Clin. Nutr.* **2014**, *23*, 55–64.

47. Jia, W.H.; Huang, Q.H.; Liao, J.; Ye, W.M.; Shugart, Y.Y.; Liu, Q.; Chen, L.Z.; Li, Y.H.; Lin, X.; Wen, F.L.; *et al.* Trends in incidence and mortality of nasopharyngeal carcinoma over a 20–25 years period (1978/1983–2002) in sihui and cangwu counties in southern china. *BMC Cancer* **2006**, *6*. [CrossRef] [PubMed]

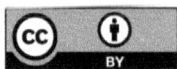

nutrients

MDPI

Article

Is Healthier Nutrition Behaviour Associated with Better Self-Reported Health and Less Health Complaints? Evidence from Turku, Finland

Walid El Ansari [1],*, Sakari Suominen [2,3,4] and Gabriele Berg-Beckhoff [5]

[1] Faculty of Applied Sciences, University of Gloucestershire, Gloucester GL2-9HW, UK
[2] Department of Public Health, University of Turku, Turku FIN-20014, Finland; suominen@utu.fi
[3] Department of Public Health, University of Skövde, Skövde S-54128, Sweden
[4] Folkhälsan Research Center, FIN-00251 Helsinki, Finland
[5] Unit for Health Promotion Research, Institute of Public Health, University of Southern Denmark, 6700 Esbjerg, Denmark; gbergbeckhoff@health.sdu.dk
* Correspondence: walidansari@glos.ac.uk; Tel.: +44-1242-715274; Fax: +44-1242-715222

Received: 24 July 2015 ; Accepted: 5 October 2015 ; Published: 14 October 2015

Abstract: We examined nutrition behaviour, self-reported health and 20 health complaints of undergraduates in Finland. Students at the University of Turku in Finland participated in a cross-sectional online survey ($N = 1189$). For nutrition behaviour, we computed two composite food intake pattern scores (sweets, cakes and snacks; and fruits and vegetables), a dietary guideline adherence index and the subjective importance of healthy eating. Multinomial logistic regression assessed the association of students' nutrition behaviour with three levels of self-reported health, controlling for many potential confounders (age, sex, living with partner, economic situation, moderate physical activity, Faculty and BMI). Factor analysis of the 20 health complaints revealed three components (psychological, pains/aches and circulatory/breathing symptoms). Multiple linear regression tested the association of students' eating habits with the three components of health complaints, controlling for the same confounders. Fruits and raw and cooked vegetable consumption, dietary guideline adherence index and subjective importance of healthy eating were highest among students with excellent/very good self-reported health, exhibiting a decreasing trend for those individuals with poor/fair self-reported health. High levels of psychological symptoms were associated with decreased consumption of fruits and vegetables, less dietary guideline adherence and less subjective importance of healthy eating. Pain/aches symptoms were associated with a higher consumption of sweets, cookies and snacks and a lower adherence to dietary guidelines. More healthy nutrition behaviour was consistently associated with better self-reported health and less health complaints. Of the four nutrition behaviour indicators we employed, the dietary guideline adherence index was the best indicator and exhibited the most consistent associations with self-reported health and health complaints.

Keywords: Finland; food intake; health complaints; gender; student health; eating healthy; dietary guidelines adherence

1. Introduction

Healthy nutrition behaviour is an important component that is required to maintain health. However, there is only limited research examining this relationship, as many studies focused on the associations between nutrition behaviour/eating habits and disease (rather than health), e.g., [1–3]. As regards health, some research examined the associations between nutritional status and quality of life; a population-based cohort study found that adherence to a Mediterranean diet (MD) pattern was associated with better health-related quality of life and that the association was stronger with mental health than with physical health [4]. In addition, two systematic reviews on the associations between nutritional status and quality of life concluded that few studies were available that explored the relationships between nutrition and quality of life or health [5,6]. The scarcity of such research on the links between nutrition habits and health is further demonstrated by an older review [5], which found only three studies that reported a positive association between nutritional status and quality of life. Whereas the more recent review [6] was based on a larger sample of published papers (13 relevant studies), unfortunately, the authors only evaluated the tools (questionnaires) that were used to determine the association between dietary habits and quality of life, and therefore, no results on the links between nutrition behaviour and health were presented.

Such a paucity of research on the relationships between nutrition behaviour and health exists despite that the health behaviour patterns throughout life are largely established in the young adulthood period and that certain foods/nutrients can moderately influence several health outcomes. In France, compliance with nutrition guidelines was positively associated with mental health [7]. Similarly, in Chile, the importance of healthy eating was one of five factors that characterised the students according to their different eating habits and explained the greater satisfaction with life [8]. Students with higher levels of life satisfaction and satisfaction with food-related life reported fewer health problems, had healthful eating habits and considered food very important for their well-being [9].

In addition to the general scarcity of studies globally on the links between nutrition behaviour and health, very few studies on eating habits have been undertaken in Finland among university students and across a range of food groups in order to examine the multiple aspects of healthy eating behaviours, adherence to dietary guidelines, subjective importance of healthy eating and their two-pronged relationships to: (1) health features (e.g., self-reported health); and (2) unhealthy symptoms (e.g., health complaints). Some dietary research in Finland was population based [10], among adolescents [11] and elementary school pupils [12], or explored the intake of isolated food groups, e.g., daily vegetables [10] or bread [13]. Hence, Finnish studies on students' nutrition behaviour and adherence to dietary guidelines are extremely lacking. The present study bridges these knowledge gaps, thus attaching high importance to the findings of the current research.

Several approaches are employed in order to estimate healthy nutrition behaviour/eating habits, particularly when examining many food groups rather than isolated individual foods. In a simple manner, the extent of consumption of the different kinds of healthy food groups (e.g., fruits and vegetables) has been used to estimate healthy nutrition behaviour [14–16]. Conversely, an alternative approach assessed healthy nutrition behaviour by the extent of omission (non-consumption) of the less healthy foods (e.g., sweets and snacks) [17–19]. In addition, the appraisal of the extent of compliance/adherence with general nutritional guidelines allows an overall view of healthy nutrition behaviour [7,15,18]. Likewise, studies [8] have shown that an individual's own perception of the importance of healthy eating is critical with regards to a healthy life style; and research has similarly employed such subjective importance of healthy nutrition behaviour in examining the links between food and mood [15,18].

University students are the future of families, communities and countries and are an important population of young adults that face the challenges of, e.g., trying to achieve academic success despite financial constraints, and stressors that include personal expectations, peer competition, having to attain good grades or fear of failing/repeating their course. They are expected to be competitive, and the university period is one of responsibility for choices and lifestyle practices, where students are exposed to the challenges of young adulthood and also tackle the mental and social issues of student life. They confront changes in living conditions and (health promoting/damaging) adjustments to lifestyle and the environment, where a key concern is the food consumption patterns and associated nutritional risks specific to college students.

Given the knowledge gaps highlighted above, the aim of the current analysis is to assess the different aspects of healthy eating behaviours on health features (self-reported health) and unhealthy symptoms (health complaints). We assessed students' two food intake pattern scores (health and unhealthy food groups), a dietary guidelines adherence index and the objective importance of healthy eating and their relationships with self-reported health and three groups of health complaints.

2. Methods

2.1. Sample, Ethics and Procedures

The research and ethics committee at the University of Turku in Turku, Finland, approved the study. Data were collected using a secure online survey in the English language (academic year 2013–2014). An invitation email with the research aims and objectives was sent in September 2013 to all ($n = 4387$) first, second and third year undergraduates at all faculties at the University, inviting students to participate by completing the online survey. We employed universal sampling, where all students were invited to participate in the study, with no inclusion/exclusion criteria. Participation was voluntary and anonymous, and data were confidential and protected. Students received contact information in case they had questions and were informed that by completing the survey, they agree to participate in the study. Two weeks later, a follow-up reminder email was sent again to the same undergraduate sample. Respondents completed the online survey and submitted their electronic responses that were automatically saved and sent to the Student Management Office at the University of Turku. The total number of responses was 1189 (response rate: 27.1%). For the current analysis, we excluded participants with missing data in nutrition intake and health complaints, reducing the number to 1027 students; 302 males (29.4%) and 725 females (70.6%). Participating students were enrolled at the seven faculties of the University: Humanity (31.3%), Mathematics and Natural Science (21.2%), Medicine (12.8%), Law (6.5%), Social Science (8.4%), Education (8.1%) and Economics (12.0%). The questionnaire collected general self-reported health data: socio-demographic information (gender, age, year of study, Faculty, living arrangements during university terms); lifestyle behaviours and a short food frequency questionnaire; the questionnaire has been used and field-tested across many student populations [20–22].

2.2. Questionnaire

Self-reported health was assessed with the question "How would you describe your general health" Responses were coded in a five-point scale from excellent to poor. For the analysis, three categories were built: (1) excellent and very good; (2) good; (3) fair and poor.

Assessment of self-reported health complaints (22 items): Students were asked how often they have had health complaints in the last year. Responses were coded in a four-point scale from never to very often. The following symptoms were asked about: depressive mode, nervousness/anxiety, mood swings, difficulties to concentrate, fear/phobia, sleep disorders/insomnia, nightmares, fatigue, lack of appetite, stomach trouble/heartburn, abdominal problems, neck and shoulder pain, back pain, diarrhoea, constipation, headaches, trembling hands, trembling, rapid heartbeat/circulatory problems, breathing difficulties, weight gain/weight loss and speech impediment. The last two symptoms were dropped from further analysis, because of unclear precision (weight gain/weight loss) and too many missing responses (e.g., item on speech impediment). Given the result from the factor analysis, three components were developed with nine variables for psychosomatic complaints (Cronbach's alpha = 0.86), seven variables for pain and aches (Cronbach's alpha = 0.73) and, finally, four variables for cardiovascular symptoms (Cronbach's alpha = 0.74).

Assessment of food consumption habits (12 items): Students self-reported their nutritional behaviour in a food frequency questionnaire (FFQ) comprising 12 variables that measured their consumption of sweets, cakes/cookies, snacks and fast/canned food, fresh fruits, raw and cooked vegetables and salads, meat and fish, milk products and cereals. The introductory question, "How often do you eat the following foods?" queried students about the frequency of their usual consumption of each food group individually (5-point scale: "several times a day", "daily", "several times a week", "1–4 times a month" and "never"). The question was asked generally to get information about the food consumption during a whole year. The instrument was based on pre-existing food frequency questionnaires, adapted for the study. Both the face and content validity of the instrument were ascertained by grounding the questionnaire on a literature review. No formal test of validity was performed, but the questionnaire was very similar to other food frequency questionnaires that had been validated, e.g., [23,24]. For descriptive purposes, the categories "several times a week" and "daily" were collapsed together. Then, in order to bring together (bundle) each of the healthy and less healthy food groups, two composite food intake pattern scores were developed (*a posteriori*-derived). The first was for the less healthy options, sweets, cake/cookies and snacks, where their relevant 5-point scales (see above) were added (summed up); and the second food intake pattern score was for the healthier options, fruits, raw and cooked vegetables, where their relevant 5-point scales were added (summed up).

The dietary guideline adherence index was computed using the FFQ. For sweets, cake/cookies, snacks, fast food/canned food and lemonade/soft drinks, no specific guidelines exist; hence, we employed "1–4 times a month" and "never", as recommended. To consider all sweets, cake/cookies and snacks together, we used the above composite food intake pattern score (sweets, cookies and snacks score), and healthy eating was considered present if this score was ⩽6 corresponding, to 3-times the intake of these items of "less often than 1–4 times a month". Each of the fast food/canned food and lemonade/soft drinks were included as individual items in computing the objective guideline adherence index. For the remaining food groups, we used the WHO dietary guidelines recommendations for the European region [25]. Consequently, for the number of daily fruit, raw and cooked vegetable servings, the cut-off was "daily" or "several times a day". For meat, the cut-off was "less than daily"; and for fish, "several times per week" was the cut-off. Milk and cereals were not included in the computing of the dietary guideline adherence index, as the information about milk and cereals was generally too unspecific in order to categorize as healthy or unhealthy nutrition. The dietary guideline adherence index has a maximum of 8 points (8 guidelines) calculated from 8 food group recommendations: (1) sweets, cookies, snacks; (2) fast food/canned food; (3) lemonade/soft drinks; (4) fruits; (5) salad, raw vegetables; (6) cooked vegetables; (7) meat; and (8) fish.

Importance of eating healthy (1 item): "How important is for you to eat healthy?" on a 5-point scale (1 = "Not at all important" to 5 = "very important").

Socio-demographic and lifestyle variables (potential confounders): Due to their possible associations with eating behaviour, other variables employed in the analysis (potential confounders that were controlled for in the regression analysis) included: (1) age; (2) gender; (3) economic situation ("How sufficient is your income?", coded into sufficient *vs.* not sufficient); (4) living situation/arrangements during university terms ("Where do you live during university term time?", coded into living with partner *vs.* not living with partner); (5) moderate physical activity (PA) ("On how many of the past 7 days did you participate in moderate exercise for at least 30 minutes?"); participants answered with 0–7 days; we used a cut-off of ⩾5 days/week as adherence to PA guidelines [26]; and, (6) BMI was calculated (kg/m^2) and categorized into underweight (BMI < 18.5 kg/m^2), normal weight (18.5–25 kg/m^2) and overweight (>25 kg/m^2) [27]. The overweight category also included the obese students (BMI > 30 $kg/^2$). In addition, Faculty was also included as a potential confounder.

2.3. Statistical Analysis

Analysis was conducted in SAS Version 9.4 (SAS Institute, Cary, NC, USA) (p < 0.05). Factor analysis was employed in order to reduce the scale of health complaints to the main factors. Due to similar studies [17,22] and to facilitate the interpretation of the findings, a three-factor solution was selected with good factor loadings. The associations between food pattern and self-reported health were analysed using multinomial logistic regression, employing students who rated their health as excellent or very good as the reference group. Analyses were adjusted for age, sex, living situation, economic situation, moderate physical activity, faculty and BMI. The associations between food pattern and three different health complaints' scores were analysed employing multiple linear regression models. Standardized beta-coefficients were additionally presented in order to allow the comparison of results between the three different health complaint scores. Data were also adjusted for age, sex, living situation, economic situation, moderate PA, faculty and BMI. Model assumptions were graphically tested and were fulfilled for the psychological complaint score and also for the pains/aches complaint score, but not for the circulatory/breathing complaint score (residuals were not normally distributed). Hence, the multiple linear regression analysis with the outcome of circulatory/breathing complaints results should therefore be interpreted with caution.

3. Results

Table 1 shows the socio-demographic characteristics and intake of 12 food groups for the whole sample and by gender. For both genders, the age ranged from 17–65 years (median = 21 years). Less than a third of students lived with their partners, and ≈40% felt they had sufficient money. Thirteen percent of women and 30% of men were overweight (BMI > 25 kg/m^2). Both genders rarely ate sweets, cakes and cookies, did not commonly eat fast food and did not drink soft drinks on a daily basis. Both genders ate fruits and vegetables regularly (daily/several times a day).

Table 1. Socio-demographic and lifestyle characteristics and intake of 12 food groups by gender among undergraduates, University of Turku, Finland, 2013–2014.

	Males	Females	p **
	N (%)	N (%)	
	302 (29.4)	725 (70.6)	
Age group (years)			0.04
<20	78 (25.8)	232 (32.0)	
20–25	183 (60.6)	376 (51.9)	
⩾25	41 (13.6)	116 (16.0)	
Living situation			0.02
Living with partner	71 (23.7)	220 (30.5)	
Economic situation			0.41
Always/mostly sufficient	120 (40.3)	309 (43.1)	
Moderate physical activity			0.64
Adherence to guideline	45 (15.0)	116 (16.1)	
BMI (reported)			<0.0001
Underweight (⩽18.5 kg/m^2)	10 (3.3)	49 (6.8)	
Normal (18.5–25 kg/m^2)	201 (65.6)	581 (80.1)	
Overweight (>25 kg/m^2)	91 (30.1)	95 (13.1)	
Food frequency questionnaire (FFQ) *			
Sweets	7 (2.3)	58 (8.0)	0.0007
Cake, cookies	1 (0.3)	11 (1.5)	0.11
Snacks	1 (0.3)	4 (0.5)	0.64
Fresh fruits	108 (35.8)	429 (59.1)	<0.0001
Salad, raw vegetables	173 (57.3)	525 (72.4)	<0.0001
Cooked vegetables	60 (19.9)	233 (32.1)	<0.0001
Fast food, canned food	3 (1.0)	1 (0.1)	<0.0001
Lemonade, soft drinks	19 (6.3)	21 (2.9)	0.01
Meat, sausages	165 (54.6)	215 (29.6)	<0.0001
Fish, sea food	19 (6.3)	15 (2.1)	0.0006
Milk, milk products	232 (76.8)	560 (77.2)	0.88
Cereals, cereal products	133 (44.0)	429 (59.2)	<0.0001

Table 1. *Cont.*

Self-reported health			0.001
Excellent/very good	178 (58.9)	330 (52.4)	
Good	94 (31.1)	303 (41.8)	
Fair/poor	30 (9.9)	42 (5.7)	
Faculty			<0.0001
Humanity	61 (20.3)	257 (35.7)	
Mathematics Natural Science	95 (31.5)	120 (16.7)	
Medicine	50 (16.6)	86 (12.0)	
Law	8 (2.7)	54 (7.5)	
Social Science	24 (7.8)	63 (8.8)	
Education	15 (5.0)	65 (9.0)	
Economics	48 (16.0)	74 (10.3)	

* Percentages calculated for intake of "several times per day" or "daily"; ** chi-square test.

Table 2 depicts the factor analysis of students' health complaints into three components and their factor loadings. The first component included psychological symptoms, e.g., depressive mood, nervousness/anxiety, mood swings, difficulties to concentrate, fear/phobia, sleep disorders/insomnia, nightmares, fatigue and lack of appetite. The second component comprised pain and ache symptoms, e.g., stomach trouble/heartburn, abdominal problems, neck and shoulder pain, back pain, diarrhoea, constipation and headaches. Finally, the third component encompassed circulatory/breathing symptoms, e.g., trembling hands, trembling, rapid heartbeat/circulatory problems and breathing difficulties.

Table 2. Factor analysis of 20 health complaints into three components.

Health Complaint	Component		
	1 Psychological (9 items)	2 Pains/aches (7 items)	3 Circulatory/breathing (4 items)
Depressive mood	0.76		
Nervousness/anxiety	0.67		
Mood swings	0.66		
Difficulties to concentrate	0.57		
Fear/phobia	0.54		
Sleep disorders/insomnia	0.47		
Nightmares	0.44		
Fatigue	0.43		
Lack of appetite	0.41		
Stomach trouble/heartburn		0.62	
Abdominal problems		0.55	
Neck and shoulder pain		0.52	
Back pain		0.44	
Diarrhoea		0.44	
Constipation		0.42	
Headaches		0.38	
Trembling hands			0.74
Trembling			0.64
Rapid heartbeat/circulatory problems			0.51
Breathing difficulties			0.38

Note: Varimax rotation.

Table 3 depicts students' health complaints, two food intake pattern scores, dietary guideline adherence index and the subjective importance of healthy eating by gender and by self-reported health categories. Women reported more health complaints than men and also ate more sweets, cookies, snacks and more fruits and vegetables than men. Additionally, women adhered more often to dietary guidelines and regarded healthy eating as important more than men. The three health complaint scores (psychological, pains/aches, and circulatory/breathing symptoms) were worse (*i.e.*, higher scores) for students who reported worse self-reported health, exhibiting a distinct and consistent stepladder appearance. Students' consumption of sweets, cookies and snacks did not differ by the self-reported health categories. In contrast, fruits and raw and cooked vegetable consumption, dietary guideline adherence index, as well as the subjective importance of healthy eating were highest among students who reported excellent/very good self-reported health and exhibited in all three scores a decreasing trend (stepladder appearance) compared to those individuals with poor/fair self-reported health.

The association between healthy eating habits and self-reported health is shown in the multinomial logistic regression model adjusted for many potential confounders (Table 4). The sweets, cookies and snack score was not associated with self-reported health. High fruit and vegetables consumption, good dietary guideline adherence and subjective importance of health eating were all less strongly associated with poor/fair self-reported health and increased in a linear manner with better self-reported health. This trend was most pronounced with the subjective importance of healthy eating, followed by fruits and vegetable consumption. The trend was less pronounced with the dietary guideline adherence.

Table 3. Health complaints and eating habits of undergraduates by gender and self-reported health, University of Turku, Finland, 2013–2014.

	Gender		Self-Reported Health		
	Male N = 302	Female N = 725	Excellent/Very Good N = 558	Good N = 397	Fair/Poor N = 72
	M(SD)	M(SD)	M(SD)	M(SD)	M(SD)
Health complaints					
Psychological symptoms score *[1]	16.39(5.18)	19.74(5.28)	16.77(4.57)	20.43(5.26)	24.82(5.50)
Pains/aches symptoms score *[2]	12.86(3.03)	15.81(3.52)	13.73(3.34)	16.21(3.54)	17.36(3.82)
Circulatory/breathing symptoms score *[3]	5.58(1.97)	6.12(2.22)	5.34(1.68)	6.45(2.26)	7.96(2.91)
Food intake pattern score					
Sweets, cookies, and snacks **	6.32(1.27)	6.66(1.17)	6.52(1.21)	6.64(1.21)	6.44(1.19)
Fruit, and raw and cooked vegetable **	9.49(1.93)	10.74(1.93)	10.61(1.97)	10.21(1.91)	9.42(2.45)
Dietary guideline adherence index [†]	4.03(1.68)	4.93(1.63)	4.81(1.68)	4.59(1.66)	3.94(1.86)
Subjective importance of healthy eating [††]	3.78(0.92)	4.10(0.77)	4.16(0.78)	3.88(0.82)	3.56(0.98)

M: mean; SD: standard deviation; *[1] range: 4–36, higher values correspond to more perceived psychological symptoms; *[2] range: 4–28, higher values correspond to more perceived pains/aches symptoms; *[3] range: 4–16, higher values correspond to more perceived cardiovascular/breathing symptoms; ** range: 3–15, each score increases as more is eaten; [†] range: 1–8, each point increase represents an additional food group that shows adherence to dietary guidelines; [††] range: 1–5, higher values indicate higher importance.

Table 4. Multinomial logistic regression of nutrition behaviours on self-reported health among undergraduates by gender, University of Turku, Finland, 2013–2014.

	Self-Reported Health		
	Excellent/Very Good	Good	Fair/Poor
	OR	OR (95% CI)	OR (95% CI)
Food intake pattern score			
Sweets, cookies, and snacks	1 (reference)	1.03 (0.92–1.15)	0.91 (0.73–1.13)
Fruits, and raw and cooked vegetables	1 (reference)	**0.92 (0.85–0.99)**	**0.80 (0.70–0.92)**
Dietary guideline adherence index	1 (reference)	0.94 (0.86–1.01)	**0.82 (0.70–0.96)**
Subjective importance of healthy eating	1 (reference)	**0.69 (0.57–0.82)**	**0.51 (0.38–0.69)**

OR: odds ratio; CI: confidence interval; models adjusted for age, sex, living with partner, economic situation, moderate physical activity, faculty and BMI; bolded cells indicate statistical significance ($p < 0.05$).

Table 5 shows the association between healthy eating habits and health complaints. In this multiple linear regression model (adjusted for age, sex, living with partner, economic situation, moderate physical activity, Faculty and BMI), high levels of psychological symptoms were associated with decreased consumption of fruits and vegetables, less dietary guideline adherence and less subjective importance of healthy eating. Pain/aches symptoms were associated with a higher consumption of sweets, cookies and snacks and a lower adherence to dietary guidelines. Finally, circulatory/breathing symptoms were not explained well by this multiple linear regression model on eating habits, as the model fit was poor; despite this, we observed that students with circulatory/breathing symptoms less often viewed healthy eating as important and also adhered to dietary guidelines less often.

Table 6 summarises the utility of employing such different nutritional behaviour (variables) indicators for health (different levels of self-reported health) and "unhealthy" (*i.e.*, different health complaints).

Table 5. Multiple linear regression of nutrition behaviours on health complaints among undergraduates by gender, University of Turku, Finland, 2013–2014.

	Health Complaints					
	Psychological		Pains/Aches		Circulatory/Breathing	
	Std-ß	β (95% CI)	Std-ß	β (95% CI)	Std-ß	β (95% CI)
Food intake pattern score						
Sweets, cookies, snacks	0.02	0.08 (−0.18; 0.34)	**0.10**	**0.30 (0.12; 0.47)**	0.03	0.05 (−0.06; 0.16)
Fruits, raw and cooked vegetables	−0.05	−0.13 (−0.30; 0.04)	0.01	0.01 (−0.09; 0.13)	−0.04	−0.04 (−0.10; 0.03)
Dietary guideline adherence index	**−0.06**	**−0.20 (−0.40; −0.01)**	**−0.09**	**−0.20 (−0.33; −0.06)**	−0.03	−0.04 (−0.12; 0.04)
Subjective importance of healthy eating	**−0.08**	**−0.50 (−0.89; −0.11)**	−0.01	−0.04 (−0.30; 0.23)	**−0.07**	**−0.19 (−0.35; −0.02)**

Std-ß: standardized beta coefficient; ß: beta coefficient; CI: confidence interval; models adjusted for age, sex, living with partner, economic situation, moderate physical activity, faculty and BMI; bolded cells indicate statistical significance ($p < 0.05$).

Table 6. Utility of different nutritional behaviour indicators for different levels of self-reported health and different health complaints.

Nutritional Behaviour Indicator Used	Outcome Used				
	Self-Reported Health		Health Complaints		
	Good *	Fair/Poor *	Psychological	Pains/Aches	Circulatory/Breathing
Food intake pattern score					
Sweets, cookies and snacks	No	No	No	Yes	No
Fruits, and raw and cooked vegetables	Yes	Yes	No	No	No
Dietary guideline adherence index	No	Yes	Yes	Yes	No
Subjective importance of healthy eating	Yes	Yes	Yes	No	Yes

* As compared to "excellent/very good" self-reported health.

4. Discussion

We observed that less healthy nutrition behaviour was consistently associated with worse self-reported health and more health complaints. Of the four nutrition behaviour indicators we employed, the dietary guideline adherence index revealed the most consistent association with self-reported health and more health complaints. For a better understanding, self-reported health and health complaints are discussed separately.

4.1. Nutritional Behaviour Indicators and Self-Reported Health

For the aspects of self-reported health, we observed that two nutrition behaviour indicators (fruits, and raw and cooked vegetables intake score and subjective importance of healthy eating) were more sensitive to various levels of self-reported health than the dietary guideline adherence index, a point to note for nutrition intervention programs in selecting appropriate indicators in order to track their success. In addition to the above, we observed that the sweets, cookies and snacks score (unhealthy food score) was not associated with self-reported health. This finding suggested: (1) such an unhealthy food score might not be suitable for nutrition campaigns that tackle the composition of unhealthy foods and simultaneously use self-reported health as a measure to trace their own progress; and (2) individuals seem not to view sweets, cookie and snack consumption as having much to do with their health, a very erroneous point that needs to be addressed by health nutrition intervention initiatives.

Despite the difficulty of locating published studies that are directly comparable to the current research, our findings that, generally, better nutritional behaviour was associated with better (excellent/very good) self-reported health agree with parallel literature. At the population level, in Spain, adherence to the Mediterranean diet (MD) was associated with a higher self-perceived health score [28]; and across university students in 21 countries, a healthful diet was positively related to greater life satisfaction [29]. Likewise, we found that only the consumption of fruits and raw and cooked vegetables (as opposed to sweets, cookies and snacks) were associated with better (excellent/very good) self-reported health, in support of the fact that life satisfaction was positively associated with eating fruit in students aged 17–30 [29]; and in agreement with university students in Chile, where only fruit consumption was linked to a higher satisfaction with life [9]. Similarly, on the population level, in Italy, adherence to an MD pattern (primarily plant-based foods, e.g., fruits and vegetables) was associated with better health-related quality of life, which is the subjective evaluation of one's own health (i.e., self-reported health) and well-being [4,30].

4.2. Nutritional Behaviour Indicators and Health Complaints

In terms of the different health complaints, we observed selectivity in the associations between nutrition behaviour (different food groups) and different health complaints. Hence, the consumption of more fruits and raw and cooked vegetables was more associated with less psychological health complaints; whereas conversely, regularly eating sweets, cookies and snacks was more associated with more pains and aches symptoms. These selectivity findings suggested direct implications for prevention programs among university student populations. Strategies and policies aimed at promoting healthy nutrition behaviours (food) are likely to simultaneously have beneficial effects on mental health (mood). Likewise, regularly eating fruits and raw and cooked vegetables was associated with better psychological health. Because of the cross-sectional design of the current study, we are unable to make solid conclusions about the direction of any of the associations we observed. The relationships could also be bi-directional; whether worse psychological health influences eating less fruits and vegetables or more pain and aches influences consuming more sweets, snacks and cookies, or conversely, does nutrition behaviour influence health complains? In our opinion, it might be more plausible that nutrition behaviour is influenced by health complaints. Further research would help with understanding these relationships.

Our finding that consumption of more fruits and raw and cooked vegetables was more associated with less psychological health complaints supports other research. At the level of adolescents, in Greece, good adherence to the MD (better diet quality) was associated with better psychological health [31]; and for university graduates, in Spain, multivariate-adjusted models revealed a significant direct association between MD adherence (high in fruits/vegetables) and most mental health domains (vitality, social functioning and role emotional) [32]. Our finding also agrees with the inverse relationship between fruits and vegetable consumption and psychological health (e.g., perceived stress and depressive symptoms) demonstrated across university students of both genders in the United Kingdom [17], among female undergraduates in Germany, Poland and Bulgaria [33] and among college students in China [34].

Another feature of selectivity in terms of the relationships between nutrition behaviour and health complaints) was between the different health complaints and the various nutrition behaviour indicators. Psychological health complaints were more consistently associated with three of the four nutrition behaviour indicators; as opposed to the pains/aches complaints and the circulatory/breathing complaints, where each was associated with only two of the nutrition behaviour indicators we used. Hence mood (psychological symptoms) might be more sensitive to healthy nutrition behaviour indicators than other health complaints and would be better employed as an outcome measure to calibrate the effectiveness of prevention polices and nutritional (food) campaigns that foster healthful eating in university populations. Future research would assist in uncovering the details of these associations.

A further aspect of selectivity in terms of the aspects of health complaints was between the various indicators we employed and the different health complaints. Of the four indicators that were employed, the dietary guideline adherence index exhibited the most sensitivity to health complaints (associated with all three different groups of health complaints that were examined). This was followed by the subjective importance of healthy eating indicator (associated with only two of the three groups of health complaints). The least sensitive indicators were the food intake pattern scores, where each was only associated with only one of the three groups of health complaints. Such findings suggested that: (1) dietary guideline adherence indices or similar measures would be more preferable over other nutrition behaviour indicators when examining the relationships between food and health complaints/symptoms; (2) using individual food groups in isolation (e.g., either "healthy" and "unhealthy" food intake pattern scores) might be unhelpful when examining the relationships between food and health complaints; and (3) for prevention strategies/intervention programs that target students' psychosomatic complaints and self-reported symptoms, highlighting the importance of adhering to nutritional guidelines and recommendations should be an important component of such efforts. Future research would assist in unearthing more features of these associations.

The paucity of research of such relationships rendered it challenging to compare our findings to other published work. However, our finding of the sensitivity of the dietary guideline adherence index supports some of the studies across the globe that used adherence levels to a particular diet (e.g., MD) [4,7,27,31], compliance with international nutritional guidelines [15,18] or the adequacy in following national nutritional recommendations [35] when examining the relationships between nutrition behaviour and a variety of outcomes. Nevertheless, whilst most of these studies used only an adherence index (perhaps blindly or for convenience), the current study undertook the arduous task of employing four different nutritional behaviour indicators to explore their utility in research and practice, as highlighted in Table 6.

This study has some limitations. We undertook the study at one university in Finland, and the response rate was not very high; hence, generalizations need to be cautious. Self-reports are prone to sociability/social desirability with the implication that the current findings could represent an underestimation of less healthy nutritional habits (e.g., sweets, cakes and cookies); no objective food consumption was undertaken; self-reporting was used to estimate the frequency of symptoms, and clinical validations were not undertaken. For some food groups, we did not assess serving sizes. As this survey was cross-sectional, the direction of the association (temporal relationship) between food intake and health complaints cannot be ascertained. Students with higher health complaints, worse self-reported health, or those with more unhealthy patterns of eating might have chosen not to participate in the study, and selection bias cannot be ruled out. Therefore, the reported prevalence of symptoms in the current study may under-estimate the true morbidity in this population. It would have also been useful to assess whether any systematic differences existed between students who participated in the survey and those who did, but we were unable to undertake this task, as we had no data about those who did not participate in the survey. We did not control for participants' co-morbidities that could affect subjects' health practices and dietary behaviour. However, university populations traditionally represent young and healthy adults with minimal comorbidities. Future research should consider such limitations. Despite these limitations, the current research also has strengths. For data collection, our sample comprised students across seven faculties and many scientific disciplines. The sample comprised more females than males (a reality at higher education institutions across the globe), which could be associated with an increased likelihood of social desirability; hence, we analysed the relationships controlling for gender and other confounders to avoid potential confounding gender effects. For the analysis, we used WHO dietary guidelines that are appropriate for Finland. Recommendations for Nordic countries, as well as the recent Baltic Sea diet do exist [36,37], but they differ from WHO recommendations only in terms of food items within food groups (e.g., fruit and vegetables found in Nordic countries are different than the ones recommended by the Mediterranean diet), but not in terms of portions and frequency. There were very few missing values in the students' responses (most students answered all of the food frequency questions), thus avoiding any potential effects of missing values on the observed adherence estimates and associations. No previous studies in Finland of university students undertook such tasks of the links between eating habits, diet quality and dietary guidelines adherence and health complaints.

5. Conclusions

Despite the scarce research available, in the current study, healthier nutrition behaviour was consistently associated with better self-reported health and less health complaints. Of the four nutrition behaviour indicators we employed, the dietary guideline adherence index was the best indicator and exhibited the most consistent associations with self-reported health and more health complaints. Prevention and intervention efforts that aim at improving awareness and compliance with dietary guidelines might also be associated with decreased health complaints and improved health of university students.

Acknowledgments: The authors acknowledge the University, the faculties and students who participated in this study. The authors also acknowledge and thank the Student Management Office at the University of Turku for their assistance with the online survey and for their inputs in data collection. There was no external financial support/funding for this study.

Author Contributions: Walid El Ansari: study concept and design, analysis and interpretation of the data and manuscript preparation. Sakari Suominen: acquisition of the data, review of the manuscript. Gabriele Berg-Beckhoff: statistical analysis and interpretation of the data, review of the manuscript.

Conflicts of Interest: The authors declare no conflict of interest.

References

1. Guasch-Ferré, M.; Hruby, A.; Salas-Salvadó, J.; Martínez-González, M.A.; Sun, Q.; Willett, W.C.; Hu, F.B. Olive oil consumption and risk of type 2 diabetes in US women. *Am. J. Clin. Nutr.* **2015**, *102*, 479–486. [CrossRef] [PubMed]
2. Aljefree, N.; Ahmed, F. Association between dietary pattern and risk of cardiovascular disease among adults in the Middle East and North Africa region: A systematic review. *Food Nutr. Res.* **2015**, *59*, 27486. [CrossRef] [PubMed]
3. Lachance, L.; Ramsey, D. Food, mood, and brain health: Implications for the modern clinician. *Mo Med.* **2015**, *112*, 111–115. [PubMed]
4. Bonaccio, M.; di Castelnuovo, A.; Bonanni, A.; Costanzo, S.; de Lucia, F.; Pounis, G.; Zito, F.; Donati, M.B.; de Gaetano, G.; Iacoviello, L.; *et al.* Adherence to a Mediterranean diet is associated with a better health-related quality of life: A possible role of high dietary antioxidant content. *BMJ Open* **2013**, *3*. [CrossRef] [PubMed]
5. Wanden-Berghe, C.; Sanz-Valero, J.; Escribà-Agüir, V.; Castelló-Botia, I.; Guardiola-Wanden-Berghe, R. Evaluation of quality of life related to nutritional status. *Br. J. Nutr.* **2009**, *101*, 950–960. [CrossRef] [PubMed]
6. Ruano-Rodríguez, C.; Serra-Majem, L.; Dubois, D. Assessing the impact of dietary habits on health-related quality of life requires contextual measurement tools. *Front Pharmacol.* **2015**, *6*, 101. [CrossRef] [PubMed]
7. Germain, L.; Latarche, C.; Kesse-Guyot, E.; Galan, P.; Hercberg, S.; Briançon, S. Does compliance with nutrition guidelines lead to healthy aging? A quality-of-life approach. *J. Acad. Nutr. Diet.* **2013**, *113*. [CrossRef]
8. Schnettler, B.; Denegri, M.; Miranda, H.; Sepúlveda, J.; Orellana, L.; Paiva, G.; Grunert, K.G. Eating habits and subjective well-being among university students in southern Chile. *Nutr. Hosp.* **2013**, *28*, 2221–2228. [PubMed]
9. Schnettler, B.; Miranda, H.; Lobos, G.; Orellana, L.; Sepúlveda, J.; Denegri, M.; Etchebarne, S.; Mora, M.; Grunert, K.G. Eating habits and subjective well-being. A typology of students in Chilean state universities. *Appetite* **2015**, *89*, 203–214. [CrossRef] [PubMed]
10. Roos, E.; Talala, K.; Laaksonen, M.; Helakorpi, S.; Rahkonen, O.; Uutela, A.; Prättälä, R. Trends of socioeconomic differences in daily vegetable consumption, 1979–2002. *Eur. J. Clin. Nutr.* **2008**, *62*, 823–833. [CrossRef] [PubMed]
11. Pohjanheimo, T.; Luomala, H.; Tahvonen, R. Finnish adolescents' attitudes towards wholegrain bread and healthiness. *J. Sci. Food Agric.* **2010**, *90*, 1538–1544. [CrossRef] [PubMed]
12. Laitinen, P.; Nissinen, A.; Myllykangas, M. Fat consumption of first-grade students in elementary school. Quality and quantity of fats used at home and at school. *Hoitotiede* **1993**, *5*, 50–55. [PubMed]
13. Prättälä, R.; Helasoja, V.; Mykkänen, H. The consumption of rye bread and white bread as dimensions of health lifestyles in Finland. *Public Health Nutr.* **2001**, *4*, 813–819. [CrossRef] [PubMed]
14. El Ansari, W.; Clausen, S.V.; Mabhala, A.; Stock, C. How do I look? Body image perceptions among university students from England and Denmark. *Int. J. Environ. Res. Public Health* **2010**, *7*, 583–595. [CrossRef] [PubMed]
15. El Ansari, W.; Suominen, S.; Berg-Beckhoff, G. Mood and Food at the University of Turku in Finland: Nutritional correlates of perceived stress are most pronounced among overweight students. *Int. J. Public Health* **2015**, *60*, 707–716. [CrossRef] [PubMed]
16. El Ansari, W. Health and well-being of students at higher education institutions—Time for urgent action? *Cent. Eur. J. Public Health* **2014**, *22*, 67. [PubMed]

17. El Ansari, W.; Adetunji, H.; Oskrochi, R. Food and mental health: Relationship between food and perceived stress and depressive symptoms among university students in the United Kingdom. *Cent. Eur. J. Public Health* **2014**, *22*, 90–97. [PubMed]

18. El Ansari, W.; Suominen, S.; Samara, A. Eating Habits and Dietary Intake: Is Adherence to Dietary Guidelines Associated with Importance of Healthy Eating among Undergraduate University Students in Finland? *Cent. Eur. J. Public Health* **2015**, in press.

19. El Ansari, W.; Dibba, E.; Stock, C. Body image concerns: Levels, correlates and gender differences among students in the United Kingdom. *Cent. Eur. J. Public Health* **2014**, *22*, 106–117. [PubMed]

20. El Ansari, W.; Stock, C. Is the health and wellbeing of university students associated with their academic performance? Cross sectional findings from the United Kingdom. *Int. J. Environ. Res. Public Health* **2010**, *7*, 509–527. [CrossRef] [PubMed]

21. El Ansari, W.; Stock, C.; Mikolajczyk, R.T. Relationships between food consumption and living arrangements among university students in four European countries a cross sectional study. *Nutr. J.* **2012**, *11*, 28. [CrossRef] [PubMed]

22. El Ansari, W.; Oskrochi, R.; Haghgoo, G. Are students' symptoms and health complaints associated with perceived stress at university? Perspectives from the United Kingdom and Egypt. *Int. J. Environ. Res. Public Health* **2014**, *11*, 9981–10002. [CrossRef] [PubMed]

23. Osler, M.; Heitmann, B.L. The validity of a short food frequency questionnaire and its ability to measure changes in food intake: A longitudinal study. *Int. J. Epidemiol.* **1996**, *25*, 1023–1029. [CrossRef] [PubMed]

24. Roddam, A.W.; Spencer, E.; Banks, E.; Beral, V.; Reeves, G.; Appleby, P.; Barnes, I.; Whiteman, D.C.; Key, T.J. Reproducibility of a short semi- quantitative food group questionnaire and its performance in estimating nutrient intake compared with a 7-day diet diary in the Million Women Study. *Public Health Nutr.* **2005**, *8*, 201–213. [CrossRef] [PubMed]

25. WHO. *Food Based Dietary Guidelines in the WHO European Region*; World Health Organization Regional Office: Copenhagen, Denmark, 2003.

26. Haskell, W.L.; Lee, I.M.; Pate, R.R.; Powell, K.E.; Blair, S.N.; Franklin, B.A.; Macera, C.A.; Heath, G.W.; Thompson, P.D.; Bauman, A. Physical activity and public health: Updated recommendation for adults from the American College of Sports Medicine and the American Heart Association. *Circulation* **2007**, *116*, 1081–1093. [CrossRef] [PubMed]

27. WHO. *Obesity: Preventing and Managing the Global Epidemic*; World Health Organization: Geneva, Switzerland, 2000.

28. Muñoz, M.A.; Fíto, M.; Marrugat, J.; Covas, M.I.; Schröder, H.; REGICOR and HERMES investigators. Adherence to the Mediterranean diet is associated with better mental and physical health. *Br. J. Nutr.* **2009**, *101*, 1821–1827. [CrossRef] [PubMed]

29. Grant, N.; Wardle, J.; Steptoe, A. The relationship between life satisfaction and health behavior. A cross-cultural analysis of young adults. *Int. J. Behav. Med.* **2009**, *16*, 259–268. [CrossRef] [PubMed]

30. Baumann, C.; Erpelding, M.L.; Perret-Guillaume, C.; Gautier, A.; Régat, S.; Collin, J.F.; Guillemin, F.; Briançon, S. Health-related quality of life in French adolescents and adults: Norms for the DUKE Health Profile. *BMC Public Health* **2011**, *11*, 401. [CrossRef] [PubMed]

31. Costarelli, V.; Koretsi, E.; Georgitsogianni, E. Health-related quality of life of Greek adolescents: The role of the Mediterranean diet. *Qual. Life Res.* **2013**, *22*, 951–956. [CrossRef] [PubMed]

32. Henríquez Sánchez, P.; Ruano, C.; de Irala, J.; Ruiz-Canela, M.; Martínez-González, M.A.; Sánchez-Villegas, A. Adherence to the Mediterranean diet and quality of life in the SUN Project. *Eur. J. Clin. Nutr.* **2012**, *66*, 360–368. [CrossRef] [PubMed]

33. Mikolajczyk, R.T.; el Ansari, W.; Maxwell, A.E. Food consumption frequency and perceived stress and depressive symptoms among students in three European countries. *Nutr. J.* **2009**, *8*, 31. [CrossRef] [PubMed]

34. Liu, C.; Xie, B.; Chou, C.P.; Koprowski, C.; Zhou, D.; Palmer, P.; Sun, P.; Guo, Q.; Duan, L.; Sun, X.; *et al.* Perceived stress, depression and food consumption frequency in the college students of China Seven Cities. *Physiol. Behav.* **2007**, *92*, 748–754. [CrossRef] [PubMed]

35. Estaquio, C.; Kesse-Guyot, E.; Deschamps, V.; Bertrais, S.; Dauchet, L.; Galan, P.; Hercberg, S.; Castetbon, K. Adherence to the French Programme National Nutrition Sante Guideline Score is associated with better nutrient intake and nutritional status. *J. Am. Diet. Assoc.* **2009**, *109*, 1031–1041. [CrossRef] [PubMed]

36. Kanerva, N.; Kaartinen, N.E.; Schwab, U.; Lahti-Koski, M.; Mannisto, S. Adherence to the Balti Sea diet consumed in the Nordic countries is associated with lower abdominal obesity. *Br. J. Nutr.* **2013**, *109*, 520–528. [CrossRef] [PubMed]
37. Uusitupa, M.; Hermansen, K.; Savolainen, M.J.; Schwab, U.; Kolehmainen, M.; Brader, L.; Mortensen, L.S.; Cloetens, L.; Johansson-Persson, A.; Onning, G.; *et al.* Effects of an isocaloric healthy Nordic diet on insulin sensitivity, lipid profile and inflammation markers in metabolic syndrome—a randomized study (SYSDIET). *J. Intern. Med.* **2013**, *274*, 52–66. [CrossRef] [PubMed]

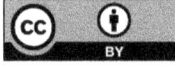

MDPI

Article

Adherence to Guidelines for Cancer Survivors and Health-Related Quality of Life among Korean Breast Cancer Survivors

Sihan Song [1], Eunkyung Hwang [2], Hyeong-Gon Moon [2,3], Dong-Young Noh [2,3] and
Jung Eun Lee [1,*]

[1] Department of Food and Nutrition, Sookmyung Women's University, Cheonpa-ro 47-gil 100, Yongsan-gu, Seoul 140-742, Korea; songsihan@sm.ac.kr

[2] Breast Care Center, Seoul National University Hospital, 103 Daehak-ro, Jongno-gu, Seoul 110-744, Korea; gogh001@hanmail.net (E.H.); moonhg74@snu.ac.kr (H.-G.M.); dynoh@snu.ac.kr (D.-Y.M.)

[3] Department of Surgery and Cancer Research Institute, Seoul National University College of Medicine, 103 Daehak-ro, Jongno-gu, Seoul 110-744, Korea

* Correspondence: junglee@sm.ac.kr; Tel.: +82-2-2077-7560; Fax: +82-2-710-9479

Received: 6 September 2015; Accepted: 30 November 2015; Published: 9 December 2015

Abstract: There is limited evidence on the association between adherence to guidelines for cancer survivors and health-related quality of life (HRQoL). In a cross-sectional study of Korean breast cancer survivors, we examined whether adherence to the guidelines of the American Cancer Society (ACS) and World Cancer Research Fund/American Institute for Cancer Research (WCRF/AICR) for cancer survivors was related to levels of HRQoL, assessed by the Korean version of Core 30 (C30) and Breast cancer module 23 (BR23) of the European Organization for Research and Treatment of Cancer-Quality of Life Questionnaire (EORTC-QLQ). We included a total of 160 women aged 21 to 79 years who had been diagnosed with breast cancer according to American Joint Committee on Cancer (AJCC) stages I to III and had breast cancer surgery at least six months before the interview. Increasing adherence to ACS guidelines was associated with higher scores of social functioning (p for trend = 0.05), whereas increasing adherence to WCRF/AICR recommendations was associated with higher scores of arm symptoms (p for trend = 0.01). These associations were limited to those with stage II or III cancer. Diet may be an important factor in relation to quality of life among Korean breast cancer survivors, however our findings warrant further prospective studies to evaluate whether healthy diet improves survivors' quality of life.

Keywords: breast cancer survivors; cancer survivor guidelines; health-related quality of life

1. Introduction

Breast cancer is the most frequent cancer among women worldwide [1]; nonetheless, early detection and advances in breast cancer treatment have continued to contribute to a decline in breast cancer mortality [2,3]. In Korea, the age-standardized incidence rate of breast cancer was 10.7 per 100,000 in 1999, which increased to 22.6 per 100,000 in 2012, with a 6.0% average annual percentage change and becoming the second most commonly diagnosed cancer among women [4]. From 2008 to 2012, the five-year survival rate of breast cancer patients was 91.3% [4]. This dramatic increase in breast cancer incidence and the high survival rate among Korean breast cancer patients indicates the importance of health-related quality of life (HRQoL) and its relationship with lifestyle, including diet and exercise [5].

Evidence regarding how breast cancer survivors try to improve their prognosis is limited to date. In 2007, the World Cancer Research Fund/American Institute for Cancer Research (WCRF/AICR) advised that cancer survivors should follow recommendations for cancer prevention [6]. For breast cancer survivors, in 2014, the Continuous Update Project of the World Cancer Research Fund concluded that there was limited evidence for the specific recommendations for breast cancer survivors and its advice was to follow WCRF/AICR cancer prevention recommendations [7]. In 2012, the American Cancer Society (ACS) released "Nutrition and Physical Activity Guidelines for Cancer Survivors", providing guidelines on body weight, physical activity and diet, in which the dietary guideline was based on the ACS guidelines for the prevention of cancer [8].

A recent review of epidemiological studies on breast cancer survivorship reported that high body fat and most likely low physical activity increase the risk of breast cancer mortality; however, the association of dietary factors with cancer survivorship was unclear [9]. Several prospective cohort studies have suggested the potential link between adherence to guidelines for cancer prevention and breast cancer incidence among the cancer-free population [10–14]. However, only a few studies have explored whether adherence to these guidelines improves quality of life or prognosis among breast cancer survivors. The ACS's Study of Cancer Survivors-II showed that cancer survivors, including breast cancer survivors, who followed the recommendations for physical activity, fruit and vegetable consumption and smoking, had significantly higher HRQoL scores [15]. For cancer survivors in general, some studies reported that adherence to WCRF/AICR guidelines for cancer prevention was associated with a lower risk of death [16] and higher levels of HRQoL [17] among female cancer survivors.

Although healthy lifestyle may benefit Korean breast cancer survivors, evidence is limited. Therefore, we examined whether adherence to lifestyle behavior recommendations was associated with HRQoL levels among Korean breast cancer survivors.

2. Materials and Methods

2.1. Study Population

Study participants who had been diagnosed with breast cancer according to the American Joint Committee on Cancer (AJCC) Cancer Staging Manual were enrolled at University Hospital in Seoul between September 2012 and July 2014. Two-hundred and nineteen women aged 21 to 79 years signed an informed consent form. We included participants who had been diagnosed with invasive primary breast cancer at AJCC stages I to III and had breast cancer surgery at least 6 months before the interview. We excluded the following respondents: women who had breast cancer surgery less than 6 months before the interview ($n = 9$), women who had been diagnosed with stage 0 breast cancer ($n = 6$), women who had metastasis ($n = 14$), women who had been diagnosed with other cancers before the interview of our study ($n = 16$), of whom medical records were missing ($n = 17$) or women who did not appropriately complete dietary records ($n = 5$). As a result, a total of 160 women were eligible for this study. The institutional review board at Seoul National University Hospital, Seoul, Korea, approved this study.

2.2. Data Collection

Participants were surveyed by well-trained nurses using a structured questionnaire. Data on height and weight, socio-demographic status, smoking status, alcohol intake, physical activity, HRQoL, reproductive history, and use of dietary supplements were collected. Clinical features including T stage (tumor), N stage (node), M stage (metastasis), and hormone receptor status were obtained from hospital medical records. The participants recorded their food intake for 2 weekdays and 1 weekend day. Body mass index was calculated as weight (kg) divided by the square of height (m^2). We obtained information about the duration and frequency of post-diagnosis physical activity and calculated the scores for metabolic equivalent task (MET) hours per week by multiplying the hours per week engaged in that activity by the activity's corresponding MET value [18,19]. The scores of MET-hours per week for each activity were summed to calculate a total MET-hours per week score. We calculated the energy and nutrient intake of the participants using the Computer-Aided Nutritional Analysis Program (CAN-Pro) 4.0 (Korean Nutrition Information Center, Seoul, Korea).

2.3. Operationalization of ACS Guidelines

The ACS guidelines for cancer survivors are as follows: (1) achieving and maintaining a healthy body weight; (2) adopting regular physical activity; and (3) achieving a dietary pattern that is high in vegetables, fruits, and whole grains [8]. The scoring criteria of the ACS guidelines are presented in Table 1. For BMI classification of the Asia-Pacific region [20], we assigned 0, 1 and 2 to <18.5 or >25, 23 to 25, and 18.5 to 22.9 kg/m^2 of BMI, respectively. We grouped participants into three groups based on tertiles of adherence levels for physical activity (MET-hour/week), fruit and vegetable intake (g/day), proportion of whole grain to total grain intake (%), and red and processed meat intake (g/day). The highest adherence levels were given a score of 2, middle levels were given a score of 1, and the lowest levels were given a score of 0. Because the third guideline includes three sub-guidelines, in order to treat the three guidelines the same, we regrouped the participants into three categories of 0, 1, and 2 based on tertiles of the sum of the three adherence scores of the sub-guidelines. We calculated the overall adherence scores by summing the three scores of adherence to the ACS guidelines (range 0–6).

Table 1. Operationalization of adherence to ACS guidelines.

ACS Guidelines for Cancer Survivors	Sub-Guidelines		Operationalization	Scoring
1. Achieve and maintain a healthy weight.	If overweight or obese, limit consumption of high-calorie foods and beverages and increase physical activity to promote weight loss.		BMI (kg/m^2)	
			18.5–22.9	2
			23-25	1
			<18.5 or >25	0
2. Engage in regular physical activity.	Avoid inactivity and return to normal daily activities as soon as possible following diagnosis. Aim to exercise at least 150 min per week. Include strength training exercises at least 2 days per week.		METs (h/week)	
			Tertile 3 (>40.3)	2
			Tertile 2 (19.6–43.3)	1
			Tertile 1 (<19.6)	0
3. Achieve a dietary pattern that is high in vegetables, fruits, and whole grains.	(3a) Eat 5 or more servings of a variety of vegetables and fruits each day.		Fruits and vegetables intake (g/day)	
			Tertile 3 (>659.2)	2
			Tertile 2 (443.1–659.2)	1
			Tertile 1 (<443.1)	0
	(3b) Choose whole grains in preference to processed (refined) grains.		Percentage of grains consumed as whole grains (%)	Tertiles High 2 Middle 1 Low 0
			Tertile 3 (90–100)	2
			Tertile 2 (64.3–90)	1
			Tertile 1 (0–64.3)	0
	(3c) Limit consumption of processed and red meats.		Red and processed meat intake (g/day)	
			Tertile 1 (<5)	2
			Tertile 2 (5–60.7)	1
			Tertile 3 (>60.7)	0

Abbreviations: ACS, American Cancer Society; BMI, Body Mass Index; MET, metabolic equivalent task.

2.4. Operationalization of WCRF/AICR Recommendations

The WCRF/AICR has released 10 recommendations including 2 special recommendations for cancer prevention [6]. We constructed adherence scores using the following 6 recommendations: (1) be as lean as possible within the normal range of body weight; (2) be physically active as part of everyday life; (3) limit consumption of energy-dense foods and avoid sugary drinks; (4) eat mostly foods of plant origin; (5) limit intake of red meat and avoid processed meat; and (6) limit consumption of salt and avoid moldy cereals (grains) or pulses (legumes). We excluded the parts on alcohol consumption and dietary supplement use because of mixed findings for the association between alcohol drinking [21–24] or supplement use [25,26] and breast cancer recurrence or death among breast cancer survivors. We did not include the breastfeeding recommendation because previous studies on breast cancer mortality have reported inconsistent results [27–29].

171

The scoring criteria of the WCRF/AICR recommendations are presented in Table 2. For BMI classification of the Asia-Pacific region [20], we assigned 0, 1 and 2 to <18.5 or >25, 23 to 25, and 18.5 to 22.9 kg/m^2 of BMI, respectively. We grouped the participants into three groups based on tertiles of adherence levels for physical activity (MET-hour/week), energy-dense food intake (kcal/100 g), non-starchy vegetable and fruit intake (g/day), refined grain intake (g/day), red and processed meat intake (g/day), and sodium intake (mg/day). The highest adherence levels were given a score of 2, middle levels were given a score of 1, and the lowest levels were given a score of 0. We assigned 0, 1 and 2 to >50, 0–50, and 0 g/day of sugary drinks, respectively. Because the third and fourth guidelines include two sub-guidelines, to treat the scoring the same, we regrouped the participants into three categories of 0, 1, and 2 based on tertiles of the sum of two adherence scores of the sub-guidelines of the third or fourth guidelines. We calculated the overall adherence scores by summing the six scores of adherence to the WCRF/AICR guidelines (range 0–12).

Table 2. Operationalization of adherence to WCRF/AICR recommendations.

WCRF/AICR Recommendations for Cancer Survivors		Sub-Recommendations	Operationalization	Scoring	
1. Body fatness: Be as lean as possible without becoming underweight	(1a)	Ensure that body weight throughout childhood and adolescent growth projects toward the lower end of the normal BMI range at age 21 years	BMI (kg/m^2)		
			18.5–22.9	2	
	(1b)	Maintain body weight within the normal range from age 21 years	23-25	1	
	(1c)	Avoid weight gain and increases in waist circumference throughout adulthood	<18.5 or >25	0	
2. Physical activity: Be physically active as part of your everyday life	(2a)	Be moderately physically active, equivalent to brisk walking, for ⩾30 min every day	Physical activity (MET-hour/week)		
			Tertile 3 (>40.3)	2	
	(2b)	As fitness improves, aim for ⩾60 min of moderate, or for ⩾30 min of vigorous physical activity every day	Tertile 2 (19.6–43.3)	1	
	(2c)	Limit sedentary habits such as watching television	Tertile 1 (<19.6)	0	
3. Foods and drinks that promote weight gain: Limit consumption of energy-dense foods; avoid sugary drinks	(3a)	Consume energy-dense foods (225–275 kcal/100 g) sparingly	Energy dense diet [1] (kcal/100 g)		Tertiles
			Tertile 1 (<154.2)	2	High 2
			Tertile 2 (132–154.2)	1	Middle 1
	(3b)	Avoid sugary drinks (servings/week)	Tertile 3 (>132)	0	Low 0
			Sugary drinks (g/day)		
	(3c)	Consume fast foods sparingly, if at all	None	2	
			⩽50	1	
			>50	0	
4. Plant foods: Eat mostly foods of plant origin	(4a)	Eat ⩾5 portions/servings (>400 g) of a variety of non-starchy vegetables and of fruits every day	Non-starchy vegetable and fruit intake (g/day)		
			Tertile 3 (>586.2)	2	Tertiles
	(4b)	Eat relatively unprocessed cereals (grains) and/or pulses (legumes) with every meal	Tertile 2 (371.5–586.2)	1	High 2
	(4c)	Limit refined starchy foods	Tertile 1 (<371.5)	0	Middle 1
	(4d)	People who consume starchy roots or tubers as staples should also ensure sufficient intake of non-starchy vegetables, fruit, and pulses (legumes)	Refined grains (g/day)		Low 0
			Tertile 1 (<15)	2	
			Tertile 2 (15–45)	1	
			Tertile 3 (>45)	0	
5. Animal foods: Limit intake of red meat (beef, pork, lamb, and goat) and avoid processed meat	(5a)	People who eat red meat should consume <500 g/week, very little if any to be processed meats	Red meat and processed meat intake (g/day)		
			Tertile 1 (<5)	2	
			Tertile 2 (5–60.5)	1	
			Tertile 3 (>60.5)	0	
6. Preservation, processing, preparation: Limit consumption of salt. Avoid moldy cereals (grains) or pulses (legumes)	(6a)	Avoid salt-preserved, salted, or salty foods; preserve foods without using salt	Sodium intake (mg/day)		
			Tertile 1 (<3521.7)	2	
	(6b)	Limit consumption of processed foods with added salt to ensure an intake of<6 g (2.4 g sodium)/day	Tertile 2 (3521.7–4602.2)	1	
			Tertile 3 (>4602.2)	0	
	(6c)	Do not eat moldy cereals (grains) or pulses (legumes)			

Abbreviations: WCRF/AICR, World Cancer Research Fund/American Institute for Cancer Research; BMI, Body Mass Index; MET, metabolic equivalent task; [1] Energy dense diet denotes energy intake per amount of total food intake (kcal per 100 g).

2.5. Health-Related Quality of Life Measurement

We assessed HRQoL in breast cancer survivors using a validated Korean version of European Organization for Research and Treatment of Cancer Quality of Life Questionnaire Core 30 (EORTC QLQ-C30) version 3.0 and Quality of Life Questionnaire Breast Cancer Module 23 (QLQ-BR23) [30,31]. The QLQ-C30, developed for assessing cancer survivors HRQoL in international clinical trials, is composed of 30 items, with subcategories of global health status/quality of life (QoL) scale, functional scales (physical, role, emotional, cognitive, and social) and symptom scales (fatigue, nausea and vomiting, pain, dyspnea, insomnia, appetite loss, constipation, diarrhea, and financial difficulty). The QLQ-BR23 is a questionnaire for breast cancer survivors with regard to disease stage and treatment modality. The breast cancer module incorporates four functional scales (body image, sexual functioning, sexual enjoyment, and future perspective) and four symptom scales (systemic therapy side effects, breast symptoms, arm symptoms, and upset by hair loss) [32]. Sexual enjoyment was not included in this analysis because 70% of the participants did not respond to this domain. According to the EORTC scoring manual, we transformed raw scores, including 4-point or 7-point scales, to a 0 to 100 scale [33]. A higher score represents a higher ("better") level of functioning and global health status /QoL or a higher ("worse") level of symptoms or problems.

2.6. Statistical Analyses

Socio-demographic, lifestyle and clinical characteristics of the study participants are presented as the mean or frequency according to quartiles of adherence scores to ACS or WCRF/AICR guidelines. To examine the association between adherence scores to ACS or WCRF/AICR guidelines and HRQoL levels, we calculated the least square means (LS means) and 95% confidence intervals (95% CIs) using generalized linear models (GLMs).

We log-transformed variables and exponentiated them if they did not meet normality. To test for trends, we assigned the median values of the quartiles of adherence scores and treated the variable as a continuous variable. In the multivariate-adjusted models, we adjusted for age (year), energy intake (kcal/day), dietary supplement use (yes, no), marital status (married or cohabitation, unmarried or divorced or widowed), education level (high school or below, college or above), stage at diagnosis (I, II, and III), and time since surgery (6 months to 1 year, 1 year to 5 years, 5 years or more). We also conducted subgroup analyses to examine the associations by breast cancer stage at diagnosis (I, II or III) or time since surgery (<1.9 or ⩾1.9 years, median). We grouped stage II and III because of the small number of breast cancer survivors (*n* = 17) with stage III. The statistical tests were two-sided, and *p* < 0.05 was considered statistically significant. All analyses were conducted using the SAS software 9.3.

3. Results

A total of 160 breast cancer survivors were included in our study. The ACS guideline score ranged from zero to six, and the WCRF/AICR recommendation score ranged from one to 12. The mean (SD) age of the study participants was 50.96 (8.72) years (range, 21–79 years). Of the study participants, 83.75% had undergone breast cancer surgery less than five years before the interview. The mean (SD) of physical activity level was 37.88 (37.78) METs-hour/week, and the mean (SD) of BMI was 22.58 (2.84) kg/m^2. In total, 42.50% of the participants had graduated from college or an education above. Most of them were married (84.38%), and never smokers (86.88%). The prevalences of breast cancer stages I, II, and III were 45.63%, 43.75%, and 10.63%, respectively (Table 3). Breast cancer survivors in the highest quartile of ACS guideline scores or WCRF/AICR recommendation scores had lower BMI, and higher physical activity compared to those in the lowest quartile (Table 3).

Breast cancer survivors who had high adherence to ACS guidelines tended to have higher social functioning scores (*p* for trend = 0.05) compared to those with lower adherence to ACS guidelines (Table 4). When we analyzed according to the breast cancer stage at diagnosis (stages I and II–III), social functioning scores tended to rise with increasing scores of adherence to ACS guidelines (*p* for trend = 0.05), and sexual functioning scores significantly increased with increasing scores of adherence to ACS guidelines (*p* for trend = 0.01) among those with stages II or III (Table S2). Among 73 breast cancer survivors who had been diagnosed with stage I breast cancer, physical functioning was significantly associated with increasing scores of adherence to ACS guidelines (*p* for trend = 0.01) (Table S1).

Table 3. Characteristics of study participants according to adherence score of ACS or WCRF/AICR guidelines.

Characteristic	All (*n* = 160)	ACS Guidelines Score		WCRF/AICR Recommendation Score	
		Q1 (*n* = 50)	Q4 (*n* = 48)	Q1 (*n* = 40)	Q4 (*n* = 33)
Age, mean ± SD (year)	50.96 ± 8.72	51.78 ± 6.84	52.75 ± 8.45	50.50 ± 9.09	50.76 ± 8.54
Body mass index, mean ± SD (kg/m^2)	22.58 ± 2.84	24.19 ± 3.57	21.25 ± 1.39	24.36 ± 3.44	21.41 ± 1.50
Physical activity, mean ± SD (MET-hour/week)	37.88 ± 37.78	16.19 ± 22.74	58.07 ± 40.16	15.26 ± 11.59	52.56 ± 34.67
Education level, *n* (%) [1]					
High school or below	90 (56.25)	25 (50.00)	29 (60.42)	20 (50.00)	17 (51.52)
College or above	68 (42.50)	25 (50.00)	18 (37.50)	20 (50.00)	15 (45.45)
Marital status, *n* (%) [1]					
Married or cohabitation	135 (84.38)	41 (82.00)	40 (83.33)	30 (75.00)	29 (87.88)
Unmarried or divorced or widowed	24 (15.00)	9 (18.00)	8 (16.67)	10 (25.00)	4 (12.12)
Current menopausal status, *n* (%) [1]					
Premenopausal	16 (10.00)	5 (10.00)	1 (2.08)	5 (12.50)	3 (9.09)
Postmenopausal	137 (85.63)	43 (86.00)	44 (91.67)	35 (87.50)	29 (87.88)
Time since surgery, *n* (%)					
6 month–<1 year	26 (16.25)	8 (16.00)	8 (16.67)	7 (17.50)	3 (9.09)
1 year–<2 years	65 (40.63)	17 (34.00)	24 (50.00)	15 (37.50)	18 (54.55)
2 years–<5 years	43 (26.88)	14 (28.00)	11 (22.92)	9 (22.50)	8 (24.24)
⩾5 years	26 (16.25)	11 (22.00)	5 (10.42)	9 (22.50)	4 (12.12)
AJCC stage at diagnosis, *n* (%)					
I	73 (45.63)	21 (42.00)	24 (50.00)	20 (50.00)	16 (48.48)
II	70 (43.75)	22 (44.00)	19 (39.58)	14 (35.00)	15 (45.45)
III	17 (10.63)	7 (14.00)	5 (10.42)	6 (15.00)	2 (6.06)
Estrogen receptor status, *n* (%) [1]					
Negative	49 (30.63)	14 (28.00)	17 (35.42)	8 (20.00)	12 (36.36)
Positive	108 (67.50)	34 (68.00)	30 (62.50)	31 (77.50)	21 (63.64)
Progesterone receptor status, *n* (%) [1]					
Negative	70 (43.75)	19 (38.00)	21 (43.75)	17 (42.50)	16 (48.48)
Positive	87 (54.38)	29 (58.00)	26 (54.17)	22 (55.00)	17 (51.52)
Energy intake, mean ± SD (kcal/day)	1749.59 ± 380.37	1676.96 ± 319.93	1871.90 ± 413.24	1779.77 ± 375.23	1796.31 ± 435.29
Dietary supplement use, *n* (%)					
No	56 (35.00)	17 (34.00)	12 (25.00)	17 (42.50)	8 (24.24)
Yes	104 (65.00)	33 (66.00)	36 (75.00)	23 (57.50)	25 (75.76)
Alcohol intake, *n* (%) [1]					
Never drinker	76 (47.50)	28 (56.00)	24 (50.00)	19 (47.50)	15 (45.45)
Ever drinker	83 (51.88)	22 (44.00)	23 (47.92)	21 (52.50)	18 (54.55)
Smoking status, *n* (%) [1]					
Never smoker	139 (86.88)	45 (90.00)	36 (75.00)	36 (90.00)	26 (78.79)
Ever smoker	5 (3.13)	1 (2.00)	2 (4.17)	2 (5.00)	1 (3.03)

Abbreviations: ACS, American Cancer Society; WCRF/AICR, World Cancer Research Fund/American Institute for Cancer Research; SD, standard deviation; MET, metabolic equivalent task; AJCC, American Joint Committee on Cancer; [1] Number of participants was less than 160 because some participants did not provide relevant information.

Table 4. Health-related quality of life (HRQoL) scores according to ACS guidelines adherence score among breast cancer survivors with stage I to III (*n* = 160) [1].

HRQOL Items	*n*	Q1 (*n* = 50)	Q2 (*n* = 32)	Q3 (*n* = 30)	Q4 (*n* = 48)	*p* for Trend [2]
		ACS Guidelines Score				
ACS score, range	160	0–2	3	4	5–6	
EORTC QLQ-C30, LS means (95% CI)						
Global health status/QoL	134	23.36 (15.32–35.62)	30.73 (18.74–50.39)	33.10 (19.08–57.44)	25.19 (16.00–39.67)	0.68
Functioning						
Physical Functioning	158	75.67 (65.17–87.87)	77.87 (65.48–92.59)	83.99 (69.25–101.86)	76.60 (65.13–90.09)	0.74
Role Functioning	160	63.64 (48.26–83.92)	79.45 (56.88–110.98)	105.76 (72.86–153.52)	81.32 (59.63–110.89)	0.07
Emotional Functioning	160	71.80 (58.30–88.43)	73.83 (57.41–94.96)	60.06 (45.36–79.51)	79.72 (63.11–100.70)	0.67
Cognitive Functioning	160	72.15 (61.40–84.79)	71.48 (58.82–86.86)	88.74 (71.40–110.29)	66.52 (55.51–79.72)	0.77
Social Functioning	160	57.16 (46.21–70.69)	64.57 (49.95–83.48)	77.86 (58.47–103.67)	71.06 (55.99–90.19)	0.05
Symptom						
Fatigue	159	27.30 (20.25–36.79)	25.76 (18.12–36.62)	19.77 (13.35–29.28)	24.65 (17.74–34.24)	0.37
Nausea and vomiting	160	2.71 (1.59–4.62)	2.93 (1.54–5.57)	2.35 (1.15–4.82)	2.60 (1.43–4.73)	0.79
Pain	159	10.26 (5.74–18.35)	15.99 (8.06–31.72)	6.79 (3.16–14.59)	8.38 (4.42–15.89)	0.28
Dyspnea	158	4.04 (2.53–9.24)	4.53 (2.11–9.71)	4.20 (1.80–9.84)	3.32 (1.63–6.78)	0.32
Insomnia	158	12.66 (6.94–23.09)	17.57 (8.65–35.69)	18.25 (8.27–40.28)	21.30 (10.95–41.44)	0.14
Loss of appetite	158	2.48 (1.34–4.59)	2.27 (1.10–4.68)	3.08 (1.37–6.93)	1.89 (0.96–3.73)	0.59
Constipation	158	6.92 (3.62–13.21)	5.00 (2.34–10.65)	6.96 (2.99–16.20)	6.48 (3.19–13.14)	0.99
Diarrhea	160	3.83 (2.14–6.84)	2.73 (1.35–5.50)	2.76 (1.26–6.03)	2.93 (1.53–5.62)	0.45
Financial impact	160	9.73 (5.17–18.29)	7.18 (3.35–15.40)	9.18 (3.92–21.49)	5.70 (2.81–11.57)	0.22
EORTC QLQ-BR23, LS means (95% CI)						
Functioning						
Body image	160	42.54 (27.15–66.64)	32.57 (18.94–56.01)	48.20 (26.33–88.24)	29.92 (18.08–49.50)	0.35
Sexual functioning	153	1.91 (1.03–3.55)	2.70 (1.28–5.67)	2.36 (1.05–5.30)	4.01 (2.00–8.03)	0.06
Future perspective	160	36.99 (21.71–63.02)	27.65 (14.53–52.64)	43.67 (21.30–89.53)	32.90 (18.10–59.82)	0.95
Symptom						
Systematic therapy side effects	160	21.95 (16.30–29.55)	25.72 (17.95–36.84)	19.12 (12.80–28.54)	18.89 (13.53–26.36)	0.26
Breast symptoms	160	14.19 (8.71–23.11)	12.32 (6.83–22.21)	10.31 (5.35–19.89)	11.08 (6.41–19.14)	0.34
Arm symptoms	160	19.25 (12.92–28.68)	25.87 (15.99–41.87)	20.03 (11.71–34.26)	28.65 (18.32–44.79)	0.17
Upset by hair loss	101	23.78 (11.61–48.74)	19.30 (8.45–44.07)	18.83 (6.41–55.36)	42.87 (18.83–97.59)	0.20

Abbreviations: ACS, American Cancer Society; LS means, least-squares means; 95% CI, 95% confidence interval; EORTC QLQ-C30, European Organization for Research and Treatment of Cancer Quality of Life Questionnaire Core 30; BR23, breast cancer module 23; [1] Models were adjusted for age (year; continuous), energy intake (kcal/day; continuous), dietary supplement use (yes, no), education level (high school or below, college or above), marital status (married or cohabitation, unmarried or divorced or widowed), breast cancer stage (I, II, III), and time since surgery (6 month-1, 1–5, ⩾5 years); [2] *p* for trend was calculated using the median value of each quartile category as a continuous variable.

Breast cancer survivors who had higher adherence to WCRF/AICR recommendations had significantly higher scores of arm symptoms (*p* for trend = 0.01) and tended to have higher scores of insomnia (*p* for trend = 0.05) compared to those with lower adherence to WCRF/AICR recommendations

(Table 5). When we examined the relationship between WCRF/AICR recommendation adherence and HRQoL according to the stage at diagnosis (stages I and II-III), significant associations were not observed between HRQoL scores and the level of adherence to WCRF/AICR recommendations among stage I breast cancer survivors (Table S1). Breast cancer survivors at breast cancer stage II or III with higher adherence to WCRF/AICR recommendations had significantly higher arm symptom scores (*p* for trend = 0.01) and higher scores for upset by hair loss (*p* for trend = 0.03) compared to those with lower adherence to WCRF/AICR recommendations (Table S2).

Table 5. Health-related quality of life (HRQoL) scores according to WCRF/AICR recommendation adherence score among breast cancer survivors with stage I to III (*n* = 160) [1].

HRQOL Items	n	WCRF/AICR Recommendation Score				*p* for Trend [2]
		Q1 (*n* = 40)	Q2 (*n* = 46)	Q3 (*n* = 41)	Q4 (*n* = 33)	
WCRF/AICR score, range	160	1–4	5–6	7–8	9–12	
EORTC QLQ-C30, LS means (95% CI)						
Functioning						
Global health status/QoL	134	28.10 (18.45–42.79)	24.41 (14.76–40.38)	24.46 (15.37–38.92)	30.15 (17.70–51.35)	0.90
Functioning						
Physical Functioning	158	76.29 (65.68–88.62)	82.08 (69.05–97.58)	78.00 (66.15–91.98)	73.95 (61.33–89.16)	0.63
Role Functioning	160	68.05 (50.95–90.89)	84.26 (60.64–117.08)	77.20 (56.02–106.39)	84.76 (58.87–122.05)	0.44
Emotional Functioning	160	70.61 (57.00–87.47)	80.71 (63.27–102.94)	75.44 (59.50–95.63)	62.86 (48.00–82.32)	0.41
Cognitive Functioning	160	70.72 (59.80–83.63)	77.45 (64.01–93.71)	74.37 (61.76–89.56)	64.81 (52.46–80.05)	0.46
Social Functioning	160	54.17 (43.64–67.25)	77.34 (60.49–98.89)	68.10 (53.59–86.54)	76.71 (58.42–100.73)	0.09
Symptom						
Fatigue	159	24.81 (18.36–33.52)	22.30 (15.67–31.74)	27.73 (19.81–38.80)	25.92 (17.69–37.97)	0.45
Nausea and vomiting	160	2.67 (1.55–4.62)	2.41 (1.29–4.48)	2.76 (1.51–5.05)	3.09 (1.55–6.14)	0.61
Pain	159	11.07 (6.13–19.99)	8.51 (4.25–17.02)	11.01 (5.69–21.30)	8.50 (4.02–18.00)	0.81
Dyspnea	158	4.86 (2.55–9.29)	3.62 (1.69–7.73)	4.63 (2.25–9.54)	2.65 (1.17–6.03)	0.39
Insomnia	158	11.98 (6.59–21.78)	18.84 (9.34–38.00)	18.97 (9.73–36.99)	29.80 (13.87–64.04)	0.05
Loss of appetite	158	2.12 (1.15–3.92)	2.78 (1.36–5.71)	2.94 (1.48–5.83)	1.49 (0.68–3.27)	0.61
Constipation	158	6.99 (3.67–13.31)	3.64 (1.72–7.69)	7.45 (3.65–15.19)	6.33 (2.82–14.22)	0.52
Diarrhea	160	4.35 (2.41–7.86)	2.31 (1.18–4.53)	2.39 (1.24–4.59)	3.52 (1.67–7.42)	0.57
Financial impact	160	9.56 (5.00–18.26)	5.68 (2.72–11.86)	8.70 (4.24–17.83)	5.44 (2.40–12.30)	0.54
EORTC QLQ-BR23, LS means (95% CI)						
Functioning						
Body image	160	37.58 (23.91–59.07)	41.99 (25.12–70.21)	44.50 (26.96–73.45)	19.70 (11.15–34.83)	0.13
Sexual functioning	153	1.74 (0.92–3.27)	3.57 (1.73–7.37)	3.86 (1.93–7.71)	2.23 (1.03–4.84)	0.42
Future perspective	160	39.37 (22.84–67.85)	40.48 (21.80–75.15)	28.91 (15.81–52.86)	23.83 (12.00–47.31)	0.10
Symptom						
Systematic therapy side effects	160	24.14 (17.78–32.77)	17.69 (12.50–25.04)	20.63 (14.70–28.95)	21.59 (14.69–31.73)	0.86
Breast symptoms	160	13.62 (8.26–22.47)	11.63 (6.59–20.55)	10.44 (6.00–18.18)	15.16 (8.07–28.48)	0.99
Arm symptoms	160	18.09 (12.07–27.13)	22.70 (14.32–35.98)	27.16 (17.34–42.55)	35.55 (21.34–59.23)	0.01
Upset by hair loss	101	24.21 (11.96–48.97)	11.95 (4.80–29.77)	29.39 (12.72–67.89)	39.41 (16.07–96.68)	0.10

Abbreviations: WCRF/AICR, World Cancer Research Fund/American Institute for Cancer Research; LS means, least-squares means; 95% CI, 95% confidence interval; EORTC QLQ-C30, European Organization for Research and Treatment of Cancer Quality of Life Questionnaire Core 30; BR23, breast cancer module 23; [1] Models were adjusted for age (year; continuous), energy intake (kcal/day; continuous), dietary supplement use (yes, no), education level (high school or below, college or above), marital status (married or cohabitation, unmarried or divorced or widowed), breast cancer stage (I, II, III), and time since surgery (6 month-1, 1–5, ⩾5 years); [2] *p* for trend was calculated using the median value of each quartile category as a continuous variable.

When we examined the association between adherence to ACS or WCRF/AIR guidelines and HRQoL levels according to the time since surgery (<1.9 or ⩾1.9 years, median), social functioning scores tended to increase with increasing scores of adherence to ACS guidelines (p for trend = 0.05) or increasing scores of adherence to WCRF/AICR recommendations (p for trend = 0.04) among those who had 1.9 or more years since surgery. Among breast cancer survivors who had less than 1.9 years since surgery, those who had higher adherence to WCRF/AICR recommendations tended to have higher arm symptoms scores (p for trend = 0.05) compared to those who had lower adherence to WCRF/AICR recommendations (Data not shown).

4. Discussion

We examined the association between adherence to guidelines for cancer survivors and HRQoL among 160 Korean breast cancer survivors. High adherence to ACS guidelines was associated with increasing scores of social functioning, whereas adherence to WCRF/AICR recommendations was significantly associated with the higher scores of arm symptoms. Our findings may suggest that breast cancer survivors who had healthy dietary habits could have favorable social functioning once they manage to cope with cancer, but those with worse symptoms could try to have healthy diet partly because of some emotional anxiety. More apparent associations for social functioning among breast cancer survivors with a longer time since surgery and for arm symptoms among those with a short time since surgery may partly support our explanations. It warrants further prospective study, where a clear temporal relationship can be assessed. When we examined whether our findings differed by the stage at diagnosis, the associations for social functioning and arm symptoms were more pronounced in breast cancer survivors at stage II or III. For breast cancer survivors diagnosed with breast cancer stage I, increasing adherence to ACS guidelines was associated with enhanced physical functioning scores. It is possible that physical functioning could be an indicator of quality of life among those with early stage, and social functioning and arm symptoms may be important factors related to or trigger healthy diet among those with stage II or III.

Our finding of the association between social functioning and healthy diet corresponded to findings of a previous cross-sectional study nested in a breast cancer survivorship cohort, the Health, Eating, Activity, and Lifestyle (HEAL) study [34]. That study examined the association between HRQoL and diet quality using the Diet Quality index and found better scores of physical functioning, bodily pain, social functioning, role-emotional, and mental health subscales with higher diet quality compared to the those with poor diet quality among breast cancer survivors [34]. Several epidemiologic studies that examined overall or sub-scaled HRQoL found significant better HRQoL scores with increasing adherence to guidelines. Among the participants of ACS's Study of Cancer Survivors-II, breast cancer survivors who met the recommendations, (1) accumulated at least 150 min of moderate-to-strenuous or 60 min of strenuous physical activity per week; (2) consumed at least five servings of fruits and vegetables each day (5-A-Day); and (3) did not smoke, had significantly better overall HRQoL scores compared to those who did not follow the recommendations [15]. The Iowa Women's Health Study (IWHS) examined the relationship between adherence to WCRF/AICR recommendations and summary scores of the physical and mental components of SF-36 among elderly female cancer survivors and found that higher adherence scores to the recommendations were significantly associated with higher physical or mental summary scores among breast cancer survivors [17]. Another cross-sectional study found that breast, prostate, and colorectal cancer survivors with healthier diet quality had better scores of physical quality of life [35].

Our study found that those who had higher adherence to WCRF/AICR recommendations had higher scores of arm symptoms compared to those with lower adherence, however, four cross-sectional studies aforementioned did not find positive association between pain and adherence to guidelines. Differences between our study and previous studies may be partly because time since diagnosis was relatively shorter in our population than other study populations. We found that this association existed among only breast cancer survivors with a short time since surgery, but not among those with a relatively longer time since surgery. It is possible that emotional anxiety, which could be stimulated by pain or symptoms, promoted adherence to healthy diet among those who had a relatively short time since diagnosis. There is a report that breast cancer survivors who initiated dietary changes after diagnosis were more likely to have psychological distress than those who did not [36]. Further larger studies are needed to examine differences in the association between diet and HRQoL levels by time since diagnosis or levels of emotional anxiety.

For body mass index and physical activity, there is evidence that maintaining healthy weight and being physically active improved quality of life. A recent meta-analysis of 25 physical exercise intervention trials on quality of life of breast cancer survivors reported increased overall quality of life in the intervention group compared to control group [37]. Short-term intervention studies of breast cancer survivors have reported improvements in HRQoL levels with exercise and dietary intervention [38–40]. The Lifestyle Intervention in Adjuvant Treatment of Early Breast Cancer (LISA) study found that individualized lifestyle intervention groups had significantly higher improvement in physical HRQoL compared to the mail-based intervention group [41]. Although we cannot infer a causal relationship in this cross-sectional study, our findings may suggest the potential benefit of healthy lifestyle, involving normal body weight, physical activity and healthy diet for Korean breast cancer survivors. Further investigation with larger number of Korean breast cancer survivors is needed to provide evidence-based lifestyle guidelines for breast cancer survivors.

This is the first study to examine the association between the AICR guideline or WCRF/AICR recommendation adherence and HRQoL among Korean breast cancer survivors. Other strengths of our study include dietary assessment by three-day dietary records, which is regarded as the gold standard, and good medical information related to breast cancer diagnosis and treatment. However, we do not have information on the comorbidity status at diagnosis, which has been suggested as a predictor of impaired overall quality of life as well as functional status [42,43], and we could not determine the causal relationship between the ACS guideline and WCRF/AICR recommendation adherence and HRQoL because this is a cross-sectional study. Our findings may not be generalizable to all Korean breast cancer survivors because of the small sample size and their comparably higher level of education. Although the ACS and WCRF/AICR guidelines are widely used to estimate the overall lifestyle of the general population and cancer survivors, its scoring methods can involve arbitrary decisions, especially with regard to diet adherence scores.

5. Conclusions

In conclusion, we identified that adherence to ACS guidelines was associated with better social functioning scales, and this association was more pronounced among survivors with stage II or III cancer. We found that adherence to WCRF/AIRCR recommendations was associated with worse arm symptoms scales. Our results suggest that although ACS and WCRF/AICR guideline adherence by cancer survivors is associated with the status of health-related quality of life among breast cancer survivors, it may differ according to the breast cancer stage or the time since surgery. Although our study does not directly infer a causal relationship, significant association between lifestyle factors and quality of life observed in our study emphasizes the need of Korean breast cancer survivorship studies that examine the role of diet, physical activity, and other lifestyle factors in the progression of breast cancer.

Supplementary Materials: Supplementary materials can be accessed at: http://www.mdpi.com/2072-6643/7/12/5532/s1.

Acknowledgments: This research was supported by the Basic Science Research Program through the National Research Foundation of Korea (NRF) funded by the Ministry of Science, ICT & Future Planning (NRF-2014R1A2A2A01007794), and by the Korean Breast Cancer Foundation (2014).

Author Contributions: Jung Eun Lee designed the study and drafted the manuscript. Sihan Song conducted statistical analyses and drafted the manuscript. Eunkyung Hwang, Hyeong-Gon Moon, and Dong-Young Noh collected the data and reviewed the manuscript.

Nutrients **2015**, *7*, 10307–10319

Conflicts of Interest: The authors declare no conflict of interest.

References

1. Ferlay, J.; Soerjomataram, I.; Dikshit, R.; Eser, S.; Mathers, C.; Rebelo, M.; Parkin, D.M.; Forman, D.; Bray, F. Cancer incidence and mortality worldwide: Sources, methods and major patterns in globocan 2012. *Int. J. Cancer* **2015**, *136*, E359–E386. [CrossRef] [PubMed]
2. American Cancer Society. *Breast Cancer Facts & Figures 2013–2014*; American Cancer Society, Inc.. Atlanta, GA, USA, 2013.
3. Berry, D.A.; Cronin, K.A.; Plevritis, S.K.; Fryback, D.G.; Clarke, L.; Zelen, M.; Mandelblatt, J.S.; Yakovlev, A.Y.; Habbema, J.D.; Feuer, E.J.; *et al.* Effect of screening and adjuvant therapy on mortality from breast cancer. *N. Engl. J. Med.* **2005**, *353*, 1784–1792. [CrossRef] [PubMed]
4. Jung, K.W.; Won, Y.J.; Kong, H.J.; Oh, C.M.; Cho, H.; Lee, D.H.; Lee, K.H. Cancer statistics in Korea: Incidence, mortality, survival, and prevalence in 2012. *Cancer Res. Treat.* **2015**, *47*, 127–141. [CrossRef] [PubMed]
5. Demark-Wahnefried, W.; Aziz, N.M.; Rowland, J.H.; Pinto, B.M. Riding the crest of the teachable moment: Promoting long-term health after the diagnosis of cancer. *J. Clin. Oncol.* **2005**, *23*, 5814–5830. [CrossRef] [PubMed]
6. World Cancer Research Fund/American Institute for Cancer Research. *Food, Nutrition, Physical Activity, and the Prevention of Cancer: A Global Perspective*; AICR: Washington, DC, USA, 2007.
7. World Cancer Research Fund. *Diet, Nutrition, Physical Activity and Breast Cancer Survivors*; World Cancer Research Fund International: London, UK, 2014.
8. Rock, C.L.; Doyle, C.; Demark-Wahnefried, W.; Meyerhardt, J.; Courneya, K.S.; Schwartz, A.L.; Bandera, E.V.; Hamilton, K.K.; Grant, B.; McCullough, M.; *et al.* Nutrition and physical activity guidelines for cancer survivors. *Cancer J. Clin.* **2012**, *62*, 243–274. [CrossRef] [PubMed]
9. Patterson, R.E.; Cadmus, L.A.; Emond, J.A.; Pierce, J.P. Physical activity, diet, adiposity and female breast cancer prognosis: A review of the epidemiologic literature. *Maturitas* **2010**, *66*, 5–15. [CrossRef] [PubMed]
10. Hastert, T.A.; Beresford, S.A.; Patterson, R.E.; Kristal, A.R.; White, E. Adherence to WCRF/AICR cancer prevention recommendations and risk of postmenopausal breast cancer. *Cancer Epidemiol. Biomark. Prev.* **2013**, *22*, 1498–1508. [CrossRef] [PubMed]
11. Romaguera, D.; Vergnaud, A.C.; Peeters, P.H.; van Gils, C.H.; Chan, D.S.; Ferrari, P.; Romieu, I.; Jenab, M.; Slimani, N.; Clavel-Chapelon, F.; *et al.* Is concordance with world cancer research fund/american institute for cancer research guidelines for cancer prevention related to subsequent risk of cancer? Results from the epic study. *Am. J. Clin. Nutr.* **2012**, *96*, 150–163. [CrossRef] [PubMed]
12. Thomson, C.A.; McCullough, M.L.; Wertheim, B.C.; Chlebowski, R.T.; Martinez, M.E.; Stefanick, M.L.; Rohan, T.E.; Manson, J.E.; Tindle, H.A.; Ockene, J.; *et al.* Nutrition and physical activity cancer prevention guidelines, cancer risk, and mortality in the women's health initiative. *Cancer Prev. Res.* **2014**, *7*, 42–53. [CrossRef] [PubMed]
13. Catsburg, C.; Miller, A.B.; Rohan, T.E. Adherence to cancer prevention guidelines and risk of breast cancer. *Int. J. Cancer* **2014**, *135*, 2444–2452. [CrossRef] [PubMed]
14. Kabat, G.C.; Matthews, C.E.; Kamensky, V.; Hollenbeck, A.R.; Rohan, T.E. Adherence to cancer prevention guidelines and cancer incidence, cancer mortality, and total mortality: A prospective cohort study. *Am. J. Clin. Nutr.* **2015**, *101*, 558–569. [CrossRef] [PubMed]
15. Blanchard, C.M.; Courneya, K.S.; Stein, K. Cancer survivors' adherence to lifestyle behavior recommendations and associations with health-related quality of life: Results from the american cancer society's scs-II. *J. Clin. Oncol.* **2008**, *26*, 2198–2204. [CrossRef] [PubMed]
16. Inoue-Choi, M.; Robien, K.; Lazovich, D. Adherence to the WCRF/AICR guidelines for cancer prevention is associated with lower mortality among older female cancer survivors. *Cancer Epidemiol. Biomark. Prev.* **2013**, *22*, 792–802. [CrossRef] [PubMed]
17. Inoue-Choi, M.; Lazovich, D.; Prizment, A.E.; Robien, K. Adherence to the world cancer research fund/american institute for cancer research recommendations for cancer prevention is associated with better health-related quality of life among elderly female cancer survivors. *J. Clin. Oncol.* **2013**, *31*, 1758–1766. [CrossRef] [PubMed]

18. Ainsworth, B.E.; Haskell, W.L.; Herrmann, S.D.; Meckes, N.; Bassett, D.R., Jr.; Tudor-Locke, C.; Greer, J.L.; Vezina, J.; Whitt-Glover, M.C.; Leon, A.S. 2011 compendium of physical activities: A second update of codes and met values. *Med. Sci. Sports Exerc.* **2011**, *43*, 1575–1581. [CrossRef] [PubMed]

19. Ainsworth, B.E.; Herrmann, S.D.; Meckes, N.; Bassett, D.R., Jr.; Tudor-Locke, C.; Greer, J.L.; Vezina, J.; Whitt-Glover, M.C.; Leon, A.S. The Compendium of Physical Activities Tracking Guide. Availavble online: https://sites.google.com/site/compendiumofphysicalactivities/ (accessed on 1 May 2015).

20. WHO/IASO/IOTF. *The Asia-Pacific Perspective: Redefining Obesity and Its Treatment*; Health Communications Australia: Melbourne, Australia, 2000.

21. Flatt, S.W.; Thomson, C.A.; Gold, E.B.; Natarajan, L.; Rock, C.L.; Al-Delaimy, W.K.; Patterson, R.E.; Saquib, N.; Caan, B.J.; Pierce, J.P. Low to moderate alcohol intake is not associated with increased mortality after breast cancer. *Cancer Epidemiol. Biomark. Prev.* **2010**, *19*, 681–688. [CrossRef] [PubMed]

22. Li, C.I.; Daling, J.R.; Porter, P.L.; Tang, M.T.C.; Malone, K.E. Relationship between potentially modifiable lifestyle factors and risk of second primary contralateral breast cancer among women diagnosed with estrogen receptor-positive invasive breast cancer. *J. Clin. Oncol.* **2009**, *27*, 5312–5318. [CrossRef] [PubMed]

23. Trentham-Dietz, A.; Newcomb, P.A.; Nichols, H.B.; Hampton, J.M. Breast cancer risk factors and second primary malignancies among women with breast cancer. *Breast Cancer Res. Treat.* **2007**, *105*, 195–207. [CrossRef] [PubMed]

24. Kwan, M.L.; Kushi, L.H.; Weltzien, E.; Tam, E.K.; Castillo, A.; Sweeney, C.; Caan, B.J. Alcohol consumption and breast cancer recurrence and survival among women with early-stage breast cancer: The life after cancer epidemiology study. *J. Clin. Oncol.* **2010**, *28*, 4410–4416. [CrossRef] [PubMed]

25. Saquib, J.; Rock, C.L.; Natarajan, L.; Saquib, N.; Newman, V.A.; Patterson, R.E.; Thomson, C.A.; al-Delaimy, W.K.; Pierce, J.P. Dietary intake, supplement use, and survival among women diagnosed with early-stage breast cancer. *Nutr. Cancer* **2011**, *63*, 327–333. [CrossRef] [PubMed]

26. Fleischauer, A.T.; Simonsen, N.; Arab, L. Antioxidant supplements and risk of breast cancer recurrence and breast cancer-related mortality among postmenopausal women. *Nutr. Cancer* **2003**, *46*, 15–22. [CrossRef] [PubMed]

27. Phillips, K.A.; Milne, R.L.; West, D.W.; Goodwin, P.J.; Giles, G.G.; Chang, E.T.; Figueiredo, J.C.; Friedlander, M.L.; Keegan, T.H.; Glendon, G.; et al. Prediagnosis reproductive factors and all-cause mortality for women with breast cancer in the breast cancer family registry. *Cancer Epidemiol. Biomark. Prev.* **2009**, *18*, 1792–1797. [CrossRef] [PubMed]

28. Trivers, K.F.; Gammon, M.D.; Abrahamson, P.E.; Lund, M.J.; Flagg, E.W.; Kaufman, J.S.; Moorman, P.G.; Cai, J.; Olshan, A.F.; Porter, P.L.; et al. Association between reproductive factors and breast cancer survival in younger women. *Breast Cancer Res. Treat.* **2007**, *103*, 93–102. [CrossRef] [PubMed]

29. Alsaker, M.D.; Opdahl, S.; Asvold, B.O.; Romundstad, P.R.; Vatten, L.J. The association of reproductive factors and breastfeeding with long term survival from breast cancer. *Breast Cancer Res. Treat.* **2011**, *130*, 175–182. [CrossRef] [PubMed]

30. Yun, Y.H.; Park, Y.S.; Lee, E.S.; Bang, S.M.; Heo, D.S.; Park, S.Y.; You, C.H.; West, K. Validation of the korean version of the EORTC QLQ-C30. *Qual. Life Res.* **2004**, *13*, 863–868. [CrossRef] [PubMed]

31. Yun, Y.H.; Bae, S.H.; Kang, I.O.; Shin, K.H.; Lee, R.; Kwon, S.I.; Park, Y.S.; Lee, E.S. Cross-cultural application of the korean version of the european organization for research and treatment of cancer (EORTC) breast-cancer-specific quality of life questionnaire (EORTC QLQ-BR23). *Support. Care Cancer* **2004**, *12*, 441–445. [PubMed]

32. Aaronson, N.K.; Bergman, B.; Bullinger, M.; Cull, A.; Duez, N.J.; Filiberti, A.; Flechtner, H.; Fleishman, S.B.; de Haes, J.C.J.M.; Kaasa, S.; et al. The european organisation for research and treatment of cancer QLQ-C30: A quality-of-life instrument for use in international clinical trials in oncology. *J. Natl. Cancer Inst.* **1993**, *85*, 365–376. [CrossRef] [PubMed]

33. Fayers PM, A.N.; Bjordal, K.; Groenvold, M.; Curran, D.; Bottomley, A.; on behalf of the EORTC Quality of Life Group. *The Eortc QLQ-C30 Scoring Manual*, 3rd ed.; European Organisation for Research and Treatment of Cancer: Brussels, Belgium, 2001; pp. 55–58.

34. Wayne, S.J.; Baumgartner, K.; Baumgartner, R.N.; Bernstein, L.; Bowen, D.J.; Ballard-Barbash, R. Diet quality is directly associated with quality of life in breast cancer survivors. *Breast Cancer Res. Treat.* **2006**, *96*, 227–232. [CrossRef] [PubMed]

35. Mosher, C.E.; Sloane, R.; Morey, M.C.; Snyder, D.C.; Cohen, H.J.; Miller, P.E.; Demark-Wahnefried, W. Associations between lifestyle factors and quality of life among older long-term breast, prostate, and colorectal cancer survivors. *Cancer* **2009**, *115*, 4001–4009. [CrossRef] [PubMed]

36. Maunsell, E.; Drolet, M.; Brisson, J.; Robert, J.; Deschenes, L. Dietary change after breast cancer: Extent, predictors, and relation with psychological distress. *J. Clin. Oncol.* **2002**, *20*, 1017–1025. [CrossRef] [PubMed]

37. Zeng, Y.; Huang, M.; Cheng, A.S.; Zhou, Y.; So, W.K. Meta-analysis of the effects of exercise intervention on quality of life in breast cancer survivors. *Breast Cancer* **2014**, *21*, 262–274. [CrossRef] [PubMed]

38. Travier, N.; Fonseca-Nunes, A.; Javierre, C.; Guillamo, E.; Arribas, L.; Peiro, I.; Buckland, G.; Moreno, F.; Urruticoechea, A.; Oviedo, G.R.; *et al.* Effect of a diet and physical activity intervention on body weight and nutritional patterns in overweight and obese breast cancer survivors. *Med. Oncol.* **2014**, *31*, 783. [CrossRef] [PubMed]

39. Swisher, A.K.; Abraham, J.; Bonner, D.; Gilleland, D.; Hobbs, G.; Kurian, S.; Yanosik, M.A.; Vona-Davis, L. Exercise and dietary advice intervention for survivors of triple-negative breast cancer: Effects on body fat, physical function, quality of life, and adipokine profile. *Support. Care Cancer* **2015**, *23*, 2995–3003. [CrossRef] [PubMed]

40. Lee, M.K.; Yun, Y.H.; Park, H.A.; Lee, E.S.; Jung, K.H.; Noh, D.Y. A web-based self-management exercise and diet intervention for breast cancer survivors: Pilot randomized controlled trial. *Int. J. Nurs. Stud.* **2014**, *51*, 1557–1567. [CrossRef] [PubMed]

41. Goodwin, P.J.; Segal, R.J.; Vallis, M.; Ligibel, J.A.; Pond, G.R.; Robidoux, A.; Blackburn, G.L.; Findlay, B.; Gralow, J.R.; Mukherjee, S.; *et al.* Randomized trial of a telephone-based weight loss intervention in postmenopausal women with breast cancer receiving letrozole: The lisa trial. *J. Clin. Oncol.* **2014**, *32*, 2231–2239. [CrossRef] [PubMed]

42. Mols, F.; Vingerhoets, A.J.J.M.; Coebergh, J.W.; van de Poll-Franse, L.V. Quality of life among long-term breast cancer survivors: A systematic review. *Eur. J. Epidemiol.* **2005**, *41*, 2613–2619. [CrossRef] [PubMed]

43. Howard-Anderson, J.; Ganz, P.A.; Bower, J.E.; Stanton, A.L. Quality of life, fertility concerns, and behavioral health outcomes in younger breast cancer survivors: A systematic review. *J. Natl. Cancer Inst.* **2012**, *104*, 386–405. [CrossRef] [PubMed]

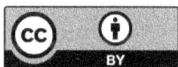

![nutrients logo]

nutrients

Article

Impact of Weight Loss on Plasma Leptin and Adiponectin in Overweight-to-Obese Post Menopausal Breast Cancer Survivors

Henry J. Thompson [1,†,*], **Scot M. Sedlacek** [1,2,†], **Pamela Wolfe** [3], **Devchand Paul** [2], **Susan G. Lakoski** [4], **Mary C. Playdon** [1,5], **John N. McGinley** [1] and **Shawna B. Matthews** [1]

1   Cancer Prevention Laboratory, Colorado State University, Fort Collins, CO 80523-1173, USA; john.mcginley@colostate.edu (J.N.M.); scomer@rams.colostate.edu (S.B.M.)
2   Rocky Mountain Cancer Centers, Denver, CO 80220, USA; scot.sedlacek@usoncology.com (S.M.S.); devchand.paul@usoncology.com (D.P.)
3   Colorado Biostatistics Consortium, University of Colorado, Denver, CO 80045, USA; pamela.wolfe@ucdenver.edu
4   Department of Internal Medicine, University of Vermont, Burlington, VT 05405, USA; susan.lakoski@med.uvm.edu
5   Department of Chronic Disease Epidemiology, Yale University, New Haven, CT 06520, USA; mary.playdon@yale.edu
*   Author to whom correspondence should be addressed; henry.thompson@colostate.edu; Tel.: +1-970-491-7748; Fax: +1-970-491-3542.
†   These authors contributed equally to this work.

Received: 27 April 2015; Accepted: 18 June 2015; Published: 26 June 2015

Abstract: Women who are obese at the time of breast cancer diagnosis have higher overall mortality than normal weight women and some evidence implicates adiponectin and leptin as contributing to prognostic disadvantage. While intentional weight loss is thought to improve prognosis, its impact on these adipokines is unclear. This study compared the pattern of change in plasma leptin and adiponectin in overweight-to-obese post-menopausal breast cancer survivors during weight loss. Given the controversies about what dietary pattern is most appropriate for breast cancer control and regulation of adipokine metabolism, the effect of a low fat *versus* a low carbohydrate pattern was evaluated using a non-randomized, controlled study design. Anthropometric data and fasted plasma were obtained monthly during the six-month weight loss intervention. While leptin was associated with fat mass, adiponectin was not, and the lack of correlation between leptin and adiponectin concentrations throughout weight loss implies independent mechanisms of regulation. The temporal pattern of change in leptin but not adiponectin was affected by magnitude of weight loss. Dietary pattern was without effect on either adipokine. Mechanisms not directly related to dietary pattern, weight loss, or fat mass appear to play dominant roles in the regulation of circulating levels of these adipokines.

Keywords: adiponectin; body composition; breast cancer survivors; dietary pattern; leptin; weight loss

1. Introduction

Prognosis for long-term survival following treatment for breast cancer is poorer in overweight or obese women with either pre- or postmenopausal breast cancer [1]. The prognostic disadvantage is accounted for by a higher risk of recurrence with subsequent metastatic progression and by the occurrence of cardiovascular disease and type-2 diabetes, which are common co-morbidities of breast cancer survivors [2]. Among women who were obese at the time of diagnosis as compared to normal weight women, a 33% higher risk for overall mortality has been reported in a meta-analysis of 43 studies [3]. A number of mechanisms have been proposed to mediate prognostic disadvantage, including those involving two adipokines, adiponectin and leptin [4–8]. However, the clinical significance of these findings remains controversial; many studies were conducted using cross-sectional designs that failed to establish temporal relationships for causality and results have been inconsistent.

The primary intervention used to treat obesity-associated diseases is weight loss via lifestyle modifications involving energy intake and expenditure [9]. In post-menopausal women, limiting caloric intake rather than increasing energy expenditure via physical activity is the key to achieving weight loss [10]. Of the dietary patterns used for weight loss, those that have received the most attention, low carbohydrate or low fat, are the same patterns that are at the center of a controversy about dietary approaches for breast cancer prevention and control [11–24]. In both weight control and cancer control, many studies have focused on low-fat diets; however, proponents of low carbohydrate diets report that high carbohydrate intake results in higher plasma insulin levels and promotes lipogenesis [25]; hence the popularity of low-carbohydrate diets for weight loss among the general population. Clearly, the same characteristics associated with low fat weight loss diets, *i.e.*, higher insulin and promotion of lipogenesis, would be considered to be a prognostic disadvantage in the breast cancer survivor population [6,26].

This paper focuses on the effects of intentional weight loss achieved using two different dietary patterns on circulating concentrations of leptin and adiponectin. These adipokines are the most abundant proteins synthesized and secreted by adipocytes. Adiponectin and leptin have been reported to play roles in obesity as well as obesity-associated diseases such as cardiovascular disease, type-2 diabetes, and cancer, including breast cancer [27–31]. Adiponectin is 1000 times more abundant in plasma than is leptin. Leptin has been reported to be positively associated with fat mass; whereas, plasma adiponectin has been reported to increase as fat mass decreases. The mechanisms that regulate synthesis and secretion of these adipokines *in vivo* are not well understood. In general, both proteins appear to act via binding to their cognate receptors. Adiponectin has been reported to be insulin sensitizing and to antagonize the effects of leptin on the carcinogenic process in the breast [32–35]. Leptin is associated with eating behavior and has been reported to promote breast carcinogenesis and tumor progression via effects on multiple regulatory nodes that drive mitogenesis while blocking apoptosis and enhancing angiogenesis [29,36,37].

This study, referred to as CHOICE, was designed to investigate how weight loss induced using two dietary patterns, low fat or low carbohydrate, affected biomarkers that have been reported to impact breast cancer recurrence and other common comorbidities of breast cancer survivors, *i.e.*, type 2 diabetes and cardiovascular disease. Herein we report on adiponectin and leptin. We hypothesized that adiponectin would increase and leptin would decrease in a manner directly proportional to weight loss and decrease in fat mass and a low carbohydrate dietary pattern would induce a more favorable response. Unlike most other studies of weight loss, anthropometric data were collected monthly so that changes in the rate of weight loss and body fat mass could be computed and provide insight into patterns of change in circulating concentrations of leptin and adiponectin and whether the dietary approach to weight loss had any impact on the outcomes observed.

We report that while leptin was strongly associated with fat mass at baseline, adiponectin was not, and the lack of correlation between changes in leptin and adiponectin implies independent mechanisms of regulation. The temporal pattern of change in leptin and adiponectin varied markedly and was not directly related to change in fat mass. Dietary pattern was without effect on plasma concentrations of either adipokine. Since adiponectin and leptin have been reported to have opposing activities on breast cancer progression, we also assessed whether their ratio might provide an index of intervention effectiveness but found that the variability of the ratio makes it problematic in this regard.

2. Experimental Section

2.1. Study Design

This study, referred to as CHOICE, compared two weight loss interventions that differed only in the dietary pattern that was investigated, *i.e.*, low carbohydrate *versus* low fat with dietary protein content equivalent in both interventions. The details of the CHOICE research protocol have been published [38]. Briefly, participants were followed for 6 months. Demographic and anthropometric data were collected at baseline and we continued to measure weight, waist and hip circumference, body mass index, and body composition via Bod Pod® (Life Measurement, Inc., Concord, CA, USA) at 4-week intervals thereafter up to six months. The clinical protocol was approved by the Colorado State University Institutional Review Board for the Protection of Human Subjects. Written consent was obtained before enrolling participants.

2.2. Participants

Women recruited for participation were from a single oncology practice and were at least 4 months post chemotherapy, radiation and surgical treatment for breast cancer and were considered clinically free of cancer. Accrual occurred from 2008 to 2012. Participants were referred by their medical oncologist and had a body mass index in the overweight or obese class I range (BMI 25.0–34.9Kg/m^2). Eligibility criteria have been reported elsewhere [38]. A total 249 participants were assigned to the study (Supplementary Figure S1). Clinical characteristics and demographic data across groups at baseline are shown in Supplementary Table S1. Participants were predominately non-Hispanic whites (89%) with a mean age of 54.9 ± 9.2 years, a mean BMI of 29.0 ± 2.6 kg/m^2 and an average of 43 ± 5% body fat. There were no differences among study arms in clinical or demographic characteristics, including disease stage or treatment regime. During the course of the study, dropout rate was similar in the low carbohydrate (15%) and the low fat (18%) study arms, although it was higher in the non-intervention control (26%); the differences were not statistically significant ($p = 0.22$). Demographics for those lost to follow up were not different from those who completed the study, with the exception of time since end of treatment ($p = 0.01$). Overall compliance with the menu and recipe defined dietary patterns was determined using the daily food logs kept by each participant and that were reviewed at each monthly clinic visit. The mean compliance for the 6-month intervention was 73% (monthly range: 65%–81%) and was not different by intervention arm ($p = 0.80$).

2.3. Adverse Events

One participant was treated for a pulmonary embolism, one participant was treated at an emergency room for stomach pain, two participants were treated for falls, one of which resulted in a hairline hip fracture, and one individual experienced an allergic reaction to an antibiotic. The adverse events were not attributed to the weight loss intervention.

2.4. Non Intervention Control

Individuals not interested in joining the weight loss arms of the study but who wished to participate were assigned to the non-intervention control group.

2.5. Intervention

Two interventions were developed and were comprised of a structured diet and physical activity program with daily recording of body weight and activity. Each program was designed to create a weekly negative energy balance equivalent to 3500 kcal, after adjustments for metabolic adaptations that occur during extended periods of weight loss; however, participants were not limited in the amount of weight they lost and individuals who lost more than the target weight were considered compliant if they followed their prescribed dietary pattern. The diet plan for each intervention arm was comprised of a 42-day cycle of menus and recipes that were designed for five calorie levels in each intervention arm (Supplementary Table S2). The meal plans included interchangeable meal options (home-prepared recipes and meal instructions; eating out and convenience meal options), educational material and a program incorporating weight loss strategies based on a systematic review of the literature. The intervention was designed as a feeding study but was conducted in free living individuals, where strict dietary structure is presented in a format that also offers enough flexibility to be adopted into daily living and by the families and social support networks of participants.

2.6. Laboratory Analyses

For measurement of leptin and adiponectin, EDTA plasma samples were assayed with solid phase quantitative sandwich ELISA (R&D systems, Minneapolis, MN, USA) according to standard protocol. All assays were carried out blinded to intervention arm assignment. Leptin and adiponectin interassay coefficients of variation ranged from 4.9% to 8.1% and from 10.0% to 11.3%, respectively.

2.7. Statistical Methods

Analysis was restricted to the subjects who completed the study, as the effects of 6 months of weight loss were of primary interest in these analyses. Correlations at baseline and 6 months were estimated using spearman's rank statistic. Six-month changes in weight and body composition for each diet group *vs.* control were evaluated in an ANCOVA model. All other inference was done on longitudinal data using a maximum likelihood model for repeated measures. The correlation structure was assumed to be autoregressive, except in the analysis of leptin and adiponectin, where compound symmetry was used due to lack of convergence. Because diet group was not assigned at random, baseline body mass index, resting metabolic rate and elapsed time since the end of cancer treatment were added to all regressions; the time varying covariate steps was also included. Differences across visit and between diet group were estimated using linear contrasts. For the question of whether fat loss or time on study was more important, change in fat mass was added to the regression model. All analyses were done in SAS 9.3, SAS Inc., Cary, NC, USA. GraphPad Prism 5.0 (GraphPad Software, Inc., La Jolla, CA, USA) was used to visualize the data.

3. Results

3.1. Anthropometric Determinates

Body weight and fat mass decreased in each of the six-month weight loss interventions (Table 1). Body weight and fat mass were lower at the end of the six-month intervention in each intervention arm compared to the control group ($p < 0.001$). Percent body fat was lower in the low fat than the low carbohydrate intervention arm at all time points; however, the slope of the regression lines describing the rate of change in percent body fat over time did not differ between intervention arms.

Table 1. Anthropometric measurements over time [1].

Variable	Group	Baseline	Month 1	Month 2	Month 3	Month 4	Month 5	Month 6
Body Weight (kg)	CTRL	53, 79.7 ± 9.3 (11.7)						53, 79.4 ± 10.1 (12.7)
	LC	65, 79.8 ± 8.7 (10.9)	65, 76.0 ± 8.4 (11.1)	65, 74.0 ± 8.4 (11.4)	64, 72.3 ± 8.4 (11.7)	62, 71.2 ± 8.7 (12.2)	61, 70.2 ± 8.9 (12.6)	65, 69.4 ± 9.0 (13.0)
	LF	73, 77.6 ± 7.7 (9.9)	73, 74.2 ± 7.4 (10.0)	71, 72.3 ± 7.5 (10.3)	69, 71.1 ± 7.5 (10.5)	69, 70.0 ± 7.4 (10.6)	67, 69.0 ± 7.6 (11.0)	73, 68.3 ± 7.5 (11.0)
Fat Mass (kg)	CTRL	53, 34.9 ± 7.3 (20.9)						53, 34.9 ± 8.2 (23.4)
	LC	65, 35.0 ± 6.1 (17.4)	65, 31.9 ± 5.7 (18.0)	65, 30.2 ± 5.6 (18.7)	64, 28.5 ± 5.8 (20.5)	62, 27.4 ± 6.2 (22.5)	61, 26.1 ± 6.4 (24.5)	65, 25.4 ± 6.6 (26.1)
	LF	73, 33.0 ± 5.8 (17.6)	73, 29.8 ± 5.7 (19.2)	71, 28.1 ± 5.6 (19.8)	69, 26.7 ± 5.8 (21.6)	69, 25.7 ± 5.6 (21.8)	67, 24.8 ± 5.9 (23.9)	73, 24.1 ± 5.7 (23.7)
Waist (cm)	CTRL	53, 94.9 ± 8.3 (8.7)						53, 94.8 ± 8.8 (9.3)
	LC	65, 94.3 ± 6.9 (7.4)	65, 91.6 ± 7.5 (8.2)	65, 89.8 ± 7.6 (8.4)	64, 87.8 ± 7.6 (8.6)	62, 87.1 ± 7.7 (8.9)	61, 86.0 ± 7.7 (8.9)	65, 85.0 ± 7.5 (8.8)
	LF	73, 91.6 ± 7.2 (7.9)	73, 89.0 ± 6.8 (7.6)	71, 86.7 ± 7.0 (8.1)	69, 85.6 ± 7.8 (9.1)	69, 84.4 ± 7.0 (8.3)	67, 83.5 ± 7.3 (8.7)	73, 83.1 ± 7.4 (8.9)
Hip (cm)	CTRL	53, 110.5 ± 7.4 (6.7)						53, 111.0 ± 9.2 (8.3)
	LC	65, 112.0 ± 7.2 (6.4)	65, 109.3 ± 6.9 (6.3)	65, 107.4 ± 6.9 (6.5)	64, 106.1 ± 7.3 (6.9)	62, 104.7 ± 7.3 (7.0)	61, 103.9 ± 8.2 (7.9)	65, 103.2 ± 7.3 (7.1)
	LF	73, 110.7 ± 5.8 (5.2)	73, 107.6 ± 5.8 (5.3)	71, 105.9 ± 6.2 (5.8)	69, 105.1 ± 5.4 (5.1)	69, 103.7 ± 5.3 (5.1)	67, 102.8 ± 6.1 (6.0)	73, 102.2 ± 5.6 (5.5)
WHR	CTRL	53, 0.9 ± 0.1 (8.2)						53, 0.9 ± 0.1 (9.1)
	LC	65, 0.8 ± 0.1 (7.9)	65, 0.8 ± 0.1 (7.9)	65, 0.8 ± 0.1 (9.0)	64, 0.8 ± 0.1 (8.1)	62, 0.8 ± 0.1 (7.6)	61, 0.8 ± 0.1 (8.5)	65, 0.8 ± 0.1 (7.5)
	LF	73, 0.8 ± 0.1 (6.4)	73, 0.8 ± 0.1 (6.4)	71, 0.8 ± 0.1 (6.7)	69, 0.8 ± 0.1 (7.5)	69, 0.8 ± 0.1 (6.7)	67, 0.8 ± 0.1 (6.7)	73, 0.8 ± 0.1 (6.8)

[1] Values are n, means ± SD (CV); CTRL, control; LC, low carbohydrate; LF, low fat; and WHR, waist hip ratio.

There are two primary sites of lipid storage, central (abdominal) and peripheral (subcutaneous), and storage of fat in these depots is estimated by measuring waist and hip circumference, respectively. Both measures decreased progressively with fat loss, and there was only a slight but statistically significant change in the WH ratio ($p = 0.04$), indicating that waist circumference decreased slightly more than hip circumference (Table 1). Total fat lost, change in percent body fat, and change in the WH ratio were unaffected by the dietary pattern used to induce weight loss.

3.2. Fat Mass and Plasma Concentrations of Leptin and Adiponectin

Because leptin and adiponectin are synthesized primarily by adipocytes and secreted into blood, we next used baseline data to determine the pre-intervention relationship between fat mass and plasma concentrations of leptin and adiponectin (Figure 1). Fat mass explained 35% of the variability in leptin ($r^2 = 0.41$); whereas, fat mass explained only 1% of the variability in plasma adiponectin ($r^2 = 0.008$). Given these findings it was not surprising that regression analysis showed no association between plasma leptin and adiponectin ($r^2 = 0.025$). The same analyses were done at end of study, after an overall decrease in fat mass of 27.3%, and very similar r^2 values were found (Supplementary Figure S2).

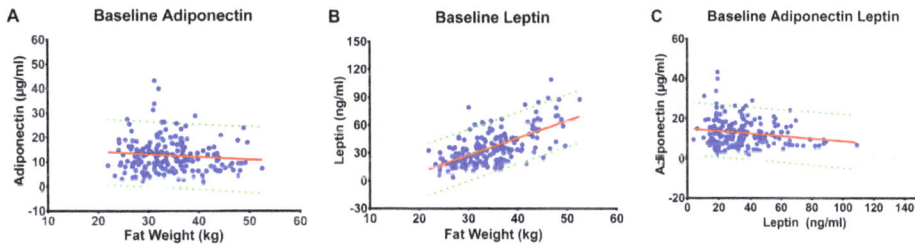

Figure 1. Regression Analyses of Baseline data: (**a**) Regression of plasma adiponectin on fat mass (kg) with 95% confidence intervals; $r^2 = 0.008$, $p = 0.210$. (**b**) Regression of plasma leptin on fat mass (kg) with 95% confidence intervals; $r^2 = 0.41$, $p < 0.001$. (**c**) Regression of plasma adiponectin on plasma leptin with 95% confidence intervals; $r^2 = 0.025$, $p = 0.028$.

3.3. Pattern of Change

We examined the temporal pattern of change in leptin and adiponectin (Figure 2 and Table 2). Given the strong correlation between fat mass and plasma leptin at baseline and end of study, we expected that leptin would decrease as fat mass decreased, but it did not. Rather, there was a large decrease in leptin over the first month of weight loss (81% of the six-month decrease) with relatively small decreases thereafter, while fat mass decreased only 34% of the six-month total reduction during the first month of the intervention. This pattern of change in leptin was observed in both intervention arms and the decrease in leptin was unaffected by dietary pattern.

Despite the very low correlation with fat mass at baseline, we expected plasma levels of adiponectin to increase throughout weight loss based on published reports [39,40]. Thus the marked decrease in plasma adiponectin observed after the first month of weight loss (6%, $p < 0.001$ relative to baseline) was unexpected and was observed in both intervention arms. Thereafter, plasma adiponectin increased ($p = 0.004$), but was not different from the control in either intervention group by end of study. Although adiponectin levels were greater in the low fat group, the rate of increase in adiponectin from intervention months 1 to 6 in the two diet groups were approximately the same ($p = 0.85$); the increase in the last month of the intervention was somewhat greater in the low fat group than the low carbohydrate group ($p = 0.03$).

Because computation of the ratio of adiponectin to leptin has been suggested as an index for assessing net effects of these adipokines on diseases like breast cancer, the ratio was also evaluated. However, we found that the coefficient of variation (CV) for the ratio was extremely high (92%), whereas the CVs for leptin, adiponectin and fat mass were 51%, 53%, and 18%, respectively. Similar values were found at end of study. The high variability in the ratio suggests it would not be a sensitive marker for meaningfully assessing biological effects.

Table 2. Adiponectin and leptin with change relative to baseline [1].

Variable	Group	Baseline	Month 1	Month 2	Month 3	Month 4	Month 5	Month 6
Adiponectin (μg/mL)	CTRL	53, 12.1 ± 7.2 (59.8)						52, 12.5 ± 6.8 (54.0)
	LC	65, 11.9 ± 7.3 (61.3)	65, 11.4 ± 6.3 (59.6)	65, 11.6 ± 6.1 (52.6)	63, 12.1 ± 6.3 (52.3)	62, 12.3 ± 6.2 (50.7)	61, 13.0 ± 6.4 (49.4)	65, 12.7 ± 6.7 (52.9)
	LF	72, 14.0 ± 5.7 (41.0)	73, 12.5 ± 5.4 (43.1)	71, 12.8 ± 5.4 (42.4)	69, 13.6 ± 5.6 (40.8)	69, 13.7 ± 5.4 (39.2)	66, 13.9 ± 5.9 (42.2)	72, 15.0 ± 6.3 (42.1)
Adiponectin (%) Δ from baseline	CTRL							52, 10.6 ± 38.7 (363)
	LC		65, −3.4 ± 20.7 (−615)	65, 2.5 ± 23.2 (925)	63, 6.8 ± 27.7 (381)	62, 10.5 ± 32.3 (309)	61, 14.1 ± 32.7 (231)	65, 13.0 ± 25.7 (198)
	LF		72, −7.8 ± 21.8 (−279)	71, −6.0 ± 25.1 (−420)	69, 1.1 ± 23.3 (2093)	69, 2.9 ± 27.7 (961)	66, 2.7 ± 24.5 (918)	71, 12.1 ± 27.0 (223)
Leptin (ng/mL)	CTRL	53, 34.6 ± 17.7 (51.2)						52, 35.1 ± 19.4 (55.3)
	LC	65, 36.5 ± 16.2 (44.5)	65, 20.0 ± 9.7 (48.5)	65, 18.4 ± 10.5 (57.2)	63, 17.3 ± 10.4 (60.0)	62, 16.5 ± 10.6 (64.4)	61, 16.4 ± 11.1 (68.1)	65, 16.4 ± 11.8 (71.8)
	LF	72, 35.1 ± 20.7 (59.1)	73, 18.9 ± 11.2 (59.0)	71, 17.7 ± 11.7 (66.4)	69, 17.6 ± 11.3 (63.9)	69, 15.8 ± 9.0 (57.2)	66, 15.0 ± 10.5 (69.7)	72, 15.3 ± 9.8 (64.0)
Leptin (%) Δ from baseline	CTRL							52, 6.5 ± 41.7 (643)
	LC		65, −43 ± 20.1 (−47)	65, −46 ± 25.9 (−56)	63, −50 ± 23.3 (−47)	62, −53 ± 24.5 (−46)	61, −53 ± 26.2 (−49)	65, −52 ± 30.6 (−59)
	LF		72, −44 ± 17.6 (−40)	71, −48 ± 20.5 (−42)	69, −48 ± 24.0 (−50)	69, −53 ± 18.6 (−35)	66, −54 ± 24.2 (−45)	71, −51 ± 31.9 (−62)
Ratio Adiponectin/leptin	CTRL	53, 0.5 ± 0.4 (87.0)						52, 0.5 ± 0.4 (78.0)
	LC	65, 0.4 ± 0.5 (119)	65, 0.8 ± 1.0 (123)	65, 0.9 ± 1.0 (112)	63, 1.1 ± 1.3 (121)	62, 1.2 ± 1.3 (114)	61, 1.4 ± 2.5 (175)	65, 1.4 ± 2.1 (144)
	LF	72, 0.6 ± 0.4 (75.1)	73, 0.9 ± 0.6 (68.5)	71, 1.1 ± 0.9 (83.5)	69, 1.2 ± 1.0 (57.0)	69, 1.3 ± 1.1 (85.4)	66, 1.4 ± 1.4 (96.7)	72, 1.6 ± 1.7 (108)

[1] Values are *n*, means ± SD (CV). CTRL, control; LC, low carbohydrate; LF, low fat.

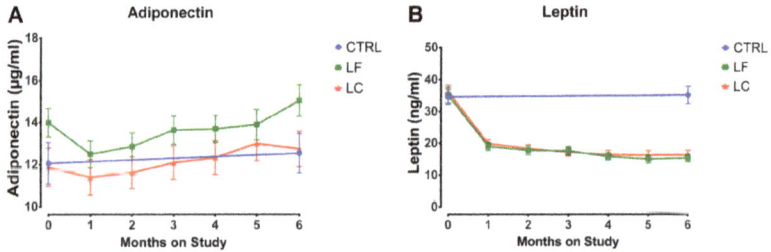

Figure 2. Plasma adipokine concentrations duration weight loss. Groups are non intervention control, CTRL; low fat dietary pattern weight loss intervention arm, LF; and low carbohydrate dietary pattern weight loss intervention arm, LC. Values are means ± SD. (**a**) Plasma adiponectin (μg/mL) as a function of months on weight loss intervention. The decrease in plasma adiponectin observed after the first month of weight loss (6%, $p < 0.001$ relative to baseline) was observed in both intervention arms. Thereafter, plasma adiponectin increased ($p = 0.004$), but was not different from the control in either intervention group by end of study. Although adiponectin levels were greater in the low fat group, the rate of increase in adiponectin from intervention months 1 to 6 in the two diet groups were approximately the same ($p = 0.85$); the increase in the last month of the intervention was somewhat greater in the low fat group than the low carbohydrate group ($p = 0.03$). (**b**) Plasma leptin (ng/mL) as a function of months on weight loss intervention. There was a large decrease in leptin over the first month of weight loss (81% of the six-month decrease) with relatively small decreases thereafter. This pattern of change in leptin was observed in both intervention arms and the decrease in leptin was unaffected by dietary pattern.

3.4. Impact of Weight Loss Magnitude

The analyses performed to this point indicated that 35% of the variation in leptin and only 1% of the variation in plasma adiponectin could be accounted for by fat mass at baseline and that change in leptin was far more pronounced in the first month of the intervention, while loss of fat mass continued throughout. An alternative hypothesis to explain change in the plasma concentrations of these adipokines is that magnitude of energy restriction was exerting effects on circulating leptin and adiponectin independent of body composition. To evaluate this possibility, the subset of individuals who lost at least 5% of initial body weight (92% of all individuals who completed the study), a level that is considered clinically meaningful [2], were divided into tertiles of weight loss, which corresponded to >5%, >10%, and >15% of initial body weight. Plasma leptin and adiponectin concentrations were plotted over time by weight loss tertile (Figure 3). It is clear that with weight loss >10%, leptin decreased progressively over time, and the decrease was significant with weight loss >15% ($p = 0.007$); whereas, there was no significant effect of weight loss magnitude on circulating levels of adiponectin.

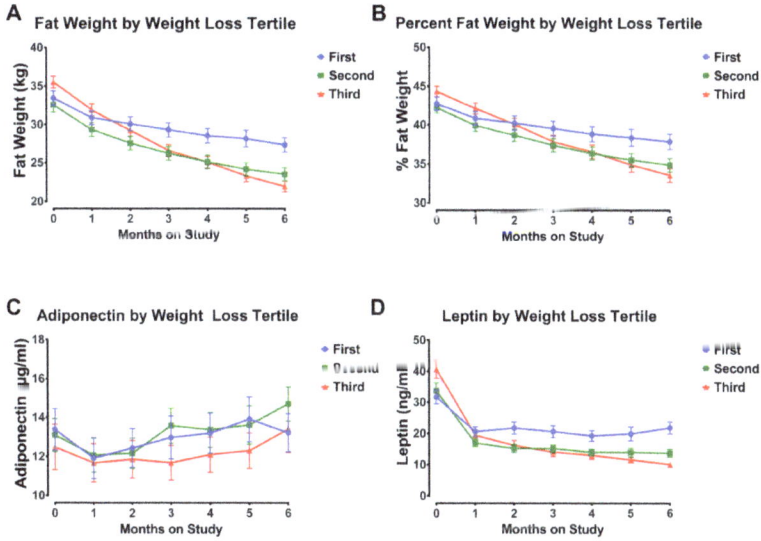

Figure 3. Body fat mass and plasma adipokines by weight loss tertile. The subset of individuals who lost at least 5% of initial body weight (92% of all individuals who completed the study) were divided into tertiles of weight loss, which corresponded to >5%, tertile 1; >10%, tertile 2; and >15%, tertile 3 of initial body weight. (**a**) Fat mass in kg over successive months of the weight loss intervention. (**b**) Body fat expressed as a (%) over successive months of the weight loss intervention. (**c**) Adiponectin (µg/mL) over successive months of the weight loss intervention. (**d**) Leptin (ng/mL) over successive months of the weight loss intervention. Values are means ± SEM. With weight loss >10%, leptin decreased progressively over time, and the decrease was significant with weight loss >15% ($p = 0.007$); whereas, there was no significant effect of weight loss magnitude on circulating levels of adiponectin.

3.5. Clinical Relevance of Changes in Plasma Adipokines

A concentration of 5 to 10 ng leptin per mL is typically observed in normal weight individuals [41]. In this study, the mean leptin concentration at baseline was 36.0 ± 18.5 ng/mL and in the intervention arms decreased to 15.8 ± 10.8 by end of study (Figure 4); however, only in the highest tertile of weight loss did plasma levels reach the normal range of plasma concentrations (baseline 40.6 ± 19.6 down to 10.0 ± 5.7 ng/mL). The distribution of change (baseline to end of study) in plasma leptin in the CHOICE cohort (Figure 4) indicates that 92% of participants in the weight loss intervention experienced a decrease in plasma leptin.

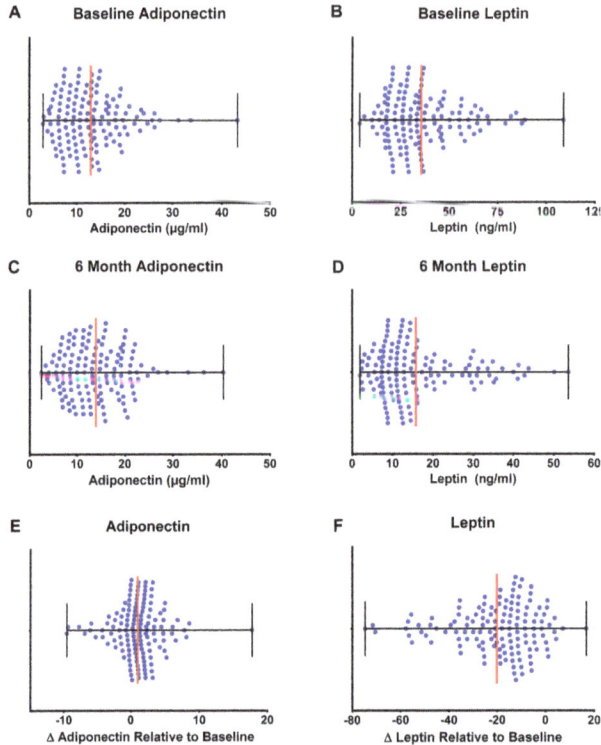

Figure 4. Distribution of plasma adipokines at baseline and end of study. (**a**) Scatterplot showing the mean and range for plasma adiponectin and leptin at baseline. The plasma concentration of adiponectin that is observed in normal weight individuals is 7–5 µg/mL. Greater than 50% of participants in CHOICE were within this range at baseline. A concentration of 5 to 10 ng leptin per mL is typically observed in normal weight individuals. In this study, the mean leptin concentration at baseline was 36.0 ± 18.5 ng/mL. (**b**) Scatterplot showing the mean and range for plasma adiponectin and leptin at end of study. The plasma concentration of adiponectin that is observed in normal weight individuals is 7–15 µg/mL and 47% remained within this range by end of study and those percentages were not significantly affected by weight loss tertile or dietary pattern. Plasma leptin decreased to 15.8 ± 10.8 ng/mL by end of study; however, only in the highest tertile of weight loss did plasma levels reach the normal range of plasma concentrations (baseline 40.6 ±19.6 down to 10.0 + 5.7 ng/mL). (**c**) Scatterplot showing the mean and range for the change (end of study-baseline) in plasma adiponectin (µg/mL) and leptin (ng/mL) at end of study relative to baseline. The distribution of change in plasma adiponectin indicates that 32% of the individuals in the intervention arms experienced a six-month decrease in adiponectin; whereas, the remainder increased somewhat. The distribution of change in plasma leptin indicates that 92% of participants in the weight loss intervention experienced a decrease in plasma leptin.

The plasma concentration of adiponectin that is observed in normal weight individuals is 7–15 µg/mL [42]. Greater than 50% of participants in CHOICE were within this range at baseline and 47% remained within this range by end of study and those percentages were not significantly affected by weight loss tertile or dietary pattern (Figure 4). Plasma adiponectin in the highest weight loss tertile was 12.7 ± 7.7 at baseline and 13.7 ± 8.0 at end of study. The distribution of change in plasma adiponectin indicates that 32% of the individuals in the intervention arms experienced a six-month decrease in adiponectin; whereas, the remainder increased somewhat (Figure 4).

4. Discussion

Reports on the relationship of circulating levels of adiponectin and leptin to incident post-menopausal breast cancer are contradictory [27,43–48], and the association of breast cancer recurrence and survival with circulating concentrations of these adipokines is equally mixed [4–8]. This study was not designed to directly answer questions about effects of intentional weight loss on recurrence or survival or whether adiponectin or leptin play a causal role in this regard. Rather, the goal was to define how leptin and adiponectin are affected by weight loss and dietary pattern as a first step in establishing whether those changes support the biological plausibility for these adipokines to play a causal role in weight loss mediated effects. Because of the monthly assessment of anthropometric endpoints and collection of plasma in CHOICE, our results shed light on how circulating levels of leptin and adiponectin change in relation to changes in body weight, body fat, and weight loss dietary pattern. The expectations that we had from the preclinical and clinical literature were: (1) that leptin would decrease and adiponectin would increase in a manner proportional to weight loss; (2) that there would be a strong relationship between plasma leptin and adiponectin and both fat mass and changes in fat mass; (3) that there would be a strong relationship between leptin and adiponectin as well as changes in leptin and adiponectin throughout the weight loss intervention; and (4) that changes in leptin and adiponectin would be influenced by dietary pattern. The extent to which these expectations were supported by our findings forms the basis for the remainder of the discussion.

4.1. Leptin

Leptin decreased during the six-month weight loss intervention (Figure 2) and the 52% reduction observed between baseline and end of study is consistent with other reports [39,40,49,50]. By assessing weight loss and plasma leptin concentrations monthly, it became clear that the changes in leptin were not directly proportional to the amount of weight loss or to loss of fat mass *per se*. Rather, most change in leptin occurred during the first month of the intervention with limited reductions thereafter (Figure 2). Given the dramatic decrease in leptin during this timeframe and that significant remodeling of adipose tissue is reported to accompany weight loss [51], the manner in which leptin synthesis and secretion are affected by tissue remodeling merits consideration. We also observed that weight loss greater than 15% resulted in significant additional decreases in plasma leptin between one and six months (Figure 3) but that dietary pattern was without effect (Figure 2). These findings are consistent with reports that energy restriction decreases leptin gene expression in white fat adipocytes and that magnitude of energy restriction plays a role [52]. The same dietary patterns that were used in CHOICE were also found to be without effect on leptin gene expression in the weight loss context [52]. Thus, despite a mixture of reports about the effects of dietary patterns on circulating concentrations of leptin [49,53–63], our findings are very clear-cut and also in agreement with another study in a population of breast cancer survivors in which effects of weight loss and dietary pattern have been reported [49]. Given that the manner in which leptin gene expression is regulated remains poorly understood [64], these findings indicate the need to look beyond linkages of leptin to fat mass or body weight *per se* in efforts to identify new approaches to modulating the secretion of leptin from adipose tissue. In terms of a potential causal role of leptin as a driver of breast carcinogenesis, preclinical data show that leptin regulates JAK2/STAT3 and inflammatory cytokine related signaling, which is altered by obesity and reregulated via weight loss [65,66]. However, two clinical reports fail to link circulating leptin with breast cancer recurrence [4,5], although another has shown leptin to be associated with distant recurrence and death even when statistical models were adjusted for BMI and body weight [6]. Plasma leptin data have to be interpreted with caution since leptin and the two main isoforms of its receptor have been reported to be expressed in 84% of breast cancers suggesting that cells within tumors can respond to leptin via autocrine as well as paracrine and endocrine pathways [67].

4.2. Adiponectin

If the focus of CHOICE was simply on assessing the plasma concentration of adiponectin at baseline and end of study, we would have concluded that there was no effect of weight loss on this adipokine, which is consistent with one report [49] but at odds with others [39,40]. However, the monthly collection of data provided clear evidence that after an initial fall in adiponectin, which was consistent with another report [42], there was a small but progressive increase observed over the remaining five months of the study. Moreover, our findings show that changes in adiponectin were not significantly linked to either loss in body weight or fat mass, or the magnitude of weight loss (Tables 1 and 2). These findings fail to support commonly stated perceptions about the relationship of adiponectin to body mass, body composition or weight control. Similarly, and consistent with [49], CHOICE data indicate that neither the low carbohydrate or low fat dietary patterns had an effect on changes in plasma adiponectin concentration in the weight loss context, despite many reports indicating dietary composition would impact circulating concentrations of this adipokine [56,58,59,61,63,68–71]. Collectively, the CHOICE results support an earlier study that reported that weight loss using either a low fat or a low carbohydrate pattern had no effect on adiponectin gene expression in white adipose tissue [52].

Of particular interest to us was the dichotomous nature of the change in adiponectin that was observed in the CHOICE cohort, which differed markedly from the predominant decrease observed in plasma leptin (Figure 4). While the net effect of weight loss on plasma adiponectin was null, about 32% of the population experienced a net decrease; and the remainder a net increase. The factors that account for the differences in response in these two subpopulations are unclear, but could relate to polymorphisms in the adiponectin gene or to differences among individuals that determine whether synthesized adiponectin is secreted into the circulatory system or retained within the cell and degraded via lysosomal metabolism [42]. Nonetheless, the normal range for plasma adiponectin is 7–15 μg/mL and most of the CHOICE population remained within this range throughout the intervention.

Preclinical data provide a clear set of pathways that are impacted by adiponectin and that are linked to tumorigenesis, particularly tumor progression. Prominent among these are the activation of AMP-activated protein kinase, and deactivation of acetyl CoA carboxylase, effects that are considered to protective against cancer [72]. However, as with leptin, evidence linking adiponectin to recurrence or survival is mixed [4–7], and adiponectin and its receptors have been detected in breast cancer tissue indicating that autocrine as well as paracrine and endocrine pathways are operative [27]. Thus circulating adipokine data alone are unlikely to be sufficient to determine causal relationships. In line with this observation, it is worth noting that interpretation of plasma adiponectin data relative to health benefits is complex. Some reports indicate that vascular health and the predisposition to diabetes are negatively affected by adiponectin levels below 6 μg/mL, and that increased risk of all cause and cardiovascular mortality is observed above 12.2 μg/mL [73]. When these values are juxtaposed to the 15.5 μg/mL plasma concentration of adiponectin below which breast cancer survival has been reported to be adversely affected (above the median: 15.5 μg/mL, longer breast cancer survival, HR, 0.39; 95% CI, 0.15 to 0.95, [74]), it would seem premature to consider adiponectin of value in assessing prognosis for survival benefit, particularly in the weight loss setting.

4.3. Adiponectin to Leptin Ratio and Causal Mechanisms

There have been many reports suggesting the use of the ratio of adiponectin to leptin to infer cancer risk [30,31,40,75]. In support of that concept is our finding that neither plasma concentration of adiponectin or leptin nor change in adiponectin and leptin were statistically correlated indicating that each adipokine is providing independent information. Similarly, there are several recent reviews detailing candidate mechanisms by which leptin and adiponectin could be impacting various aspects in the development of cancer in an integrated manner [65,66,72]. However, across the CHOICE cohort, the coefficient of variation in the adiponectin to leptin ratio at any time point assessed was between 90% and 120%. Moreover, when we determined whether the ratio increased monotonically within an individual during progressive weight loss, it did so in less than 10% of the cohort (data not shown). Thus, while the ratio might have some value in risk assessment in cross sectional studies, its use for individual risk assessment is likely to require a more complex approach to algorithm development.

4.4. Strengths and Limitations

The strengths of this study included the highly effective weight loss intervention, the menu and recipe defined approach to defining and delivering the low fat and low carbohydrate dietary pattern-based interventions and the monthly collection of anthropometric data and biospecimens. While a non-randomized design is subject to potential confounding, the value of such designs in research on dietary patterns has also been advocated [76].

We report compliance in terms of adherence to the menu and recipe defined dietary patterns that each participant was asked to follow. An alternative approach is to consider compliance in terms of whether the total amount of dietary carbohydrate and fat consumed daily, when adjusted for differences in body size and body composition, was the same among participants within a dietary pattern group. Since total amounts of these macronutrients varied due to the differences that were observed in amount of weight lost among participants, the contribution of total daily amounts of dietary fat and carbohydrate consumed to study results was not determined.

5. Conclusions

CHOICE permitted us to look closely at general conclusions from many studies that were either cross sectional or that collected data only at the beginning and end of weight loss. Thus, while leptin is generally stated to be strongly related to fat mass, adiposity fails to explain the majority of the variation in circulating levels of leptin and there are clearly factors unrelated to fat mass *per se* that account for marked changes in plasma leptin during weight loss. CHOICE also revealed unexpected changes in circulating adiponectin and raised questions about how to interpret plasma data relative to the competing factors that determine prognosis in the breast cancer survivor population. Finally, despite many reports about the potential value of the ratio of adiponectin to leptin as an index of effect, we found so much variability within and among individuals who were assessed monthly that we raise a cautionary note about the usefulness of the ratio. The fact that the dietary patterns evaluated failed to alter adipokines during weight loss should not be used to rule out the possibility that dietary pattern effects could be exerted during weight maintenance and/or the possibility that other dietary patterns might exert effects during weight loss/weight maintenance in specific individuals. In designing additional studies, it would be useful to focus on gaps in understanding of the regulation of both adiponectin and leptin gene expression. If weight loss is shown to favorably affect survival prognosis among breast cancer patients, CHOICE findings fail to provide strong support for investigating a causal linkage between adiponectin or leptin and changes in prognosis mediated by weight loss. Mechanisms not directly related to dietary pattern, weight loss, or fat mass appear to play dominant roles in the regulation of circulating levels of these adipokines.

Acknowledgments: In memory of Catherine Glendorn. This work was supported in part by a gift from the Glendorn Foundation and by United States Public Health Service Grant CA125243 from the National Cancer Institute. The authors thank Elizabeth Daeninck, Sara Bartels, Laura Ulfers, Zongjian Zhu, and Weiqin Jiang for their excellent technical assistance in the conduct of this study.

Author Contributions: H.J.T., S.M.S., P.W. participated in the design, data evaluation and interpretation, and implementation of the study. All authors participated in implementation of the study, data evaluation and interpretation, and preparation of the manuscript.

Conflicts of Interest: The authors declare no conflict of interest.

References

1. Ewertz, M.; Jensen, M.B.; Gunnarsdottir, K.A.; Hojris, I.; Jakobsen, E.H.; Nielsen, D.; Stenbygaard, L.E.; Tange, U.B.; Cold, S. Effect of obesity on prognosis after early-stage breast cancer. *J. Clin. Oncol.* **2011**, *29*, 25–31.

2. Demark-Wahnefried, W.; Platz, E.A.; Ligibel, J.A.; Blair, C.K.; Courneya, K.S.; Meyerhardt, J.A.; Ganz, P.A.; Rock, C.L.; Schmitz, K.H.; Wadden, T.; *et al.* The role of obesity in cancer survival and recurrence. *Cancer Epidemiol. Biomarkers Prev.* **2012**, *21*, 1244–1259.

3. Protani, M.; Coory, M.; Martin, J.H. Effect of obesity on survival of women with breast cancer: Systematic review and meta-analysis. *Breast Cancer Res. Treat.* **2010**, *123*, 627–635.

4. Al-Delaimy, W.K.; Flatt, S.W.; Natarajan, L.; Laughlin, G.A.; Rock, C.L.; Gold, E.B.; Caan, B.J.; Parker, B.A.; Pierce, J.P. IGF1 and risk of additional breast cancer in the WHEL study. *Endocr. Relat. Cancer* **2011**, *18*, 235–244.

5. Oh, S.W.; Park, C.Y.; Lee, E.S.; Yoon, Y.S.; Lee, E.S.; Park, S.S.; Kim, Y.; Sung, N.J.; Yun, Y.H.; Lee, K.S.; *et al.* Adipokines, insulin resistance, metabolic syndrome, and breast cancer recurrence: A cohort study. *Breast Cancer Res.* **2011**, *13*, R34.

6. Goodwin, P.J.; Ennis, M.; Pritchard, K.I.; Trudeau, M.E.; Koo, J.; Taylor, S.K.; Hood, N. Insulin- and obesity-related variables in early-stage breast cancer: Correlations and time course of prognostic associations. *J. Clin. Oncol.* **2012**, *30*, 164–171.

7. Macis, D.; Gandini, S.; Guerrieri-Gonzaga, A.; Johansson, H.; Magni, P.; Ruscica, M.; Lazzeroni, M.; Serrano, D.; Cazzaniga, M.; Mora, S.; *et al.* Prognostic effect of circulating adiponectin in a randomized 2 × 2 trial of low-dose tamoxifen and fenretinide in premenopausal women at risk for breast cancer. *J. Clin. Oncol.* **2012**, *30*, 151–157.

8. Cho, Y.A.; Sung, M.K.; Yeon, J.Y.; Ro, J.; Kim, J. Prognostic role of interleukin-6, interleukin-8, and leptin levels according to breast cancer subtype. *Cancer Res. Treat.* **2013**, *45*, 210–219.

9. Wadden, T.A.; Butryn, M.L.; Wilson, C. Lifestyle modification for the management of obesity. *Gastroenterology* **2007**, *132*, 2226–2238.

10. Foster-Schubert, K.E.; Alfano, C.M.; Duggan, C.R.; Xiao, L.; Campbell, K.L.; Kong, A.; Bain, C.E.; Wang, C.Y.; Blackburn, G.L.; McTiernan, A. Effect of diet and exercise, alone or combined, on weight and body composition in overweight-to-obese postmenopausal women. *Obesity* **2012**, *20*, 1628–1638.

11. Thomson, C.A.; Thompson, P.A. Dietary patterns, risk and prognosis of breast cancer. *Future Oncol.* **2009**, *5*, 1257–1269.

12. Gold, E.B.; Pierce, J.P.; Natarajan, L.; Stefanick, M.L.; Laughlin, G.A.; Caan, B.J.; Flatt, S.W.; Emond, J.A.; Saquib, N.; Madlensky, L.; *et al.* Dietary pattern influences breast cancer prognosis in women without hot flashes: The women's healthy eating and living trial. *J. Clin. Oncol.* **2009**, *27*, 352–359.

13. Prentice, R.L.; Anderson, G.L. The women's health initiative: Lessons learned. *Annu. Rev. Public Health* **2008**, *29*, 131–150.

14. Prentice, R.L. Observational studies, clinical trials, and the women's health initiative. *Lifetime Data Anal.* **2007**, *13*, 449–462.

15. Pierce, J.P.; Faerber, S.; Wright, F.A.; Rock, C.L.; Newman, V.; Flatt, S.W.; Kealey, S.; Jones, V.E.; Caan, B.J.; Gold, E.B.; *et al.* A randomized trial of the effect of a plant-based dietary pattern on additional breast cancer events and survival: The Women's Healthy Eating and Living (WHEL) Study. *Control Clin. Trials* **2002**, *23*, 728–756.

16. Ho, V.W.; Hamilton, M.J.; Dang, N.H.; Hsu, B.E.; Adomat, H.H.; Guns, E.S.; Weljie, A.; Samudio, I.; Bennewith, K.L.; Krystal, G. A low carbohydrate, high protein diet combined with celecoxib markedly reduces metastasis. *Carcinogenesis* **2014**, *35*, 2291–2299.

17. Liebman, M. When and why carbohydrate restriction can be a viable option. *Nutrition* **2014**, *30*, 748–754.

18. Huebner, J.; Marienfeld, S.; Abbenhardt, C.; Ulrich, C.; Muenstedt, K.; Micke, O.; Muecke, R.; Loeser, C. Counseling patients on cancer diets: A review of the literature and recommendations for clinical practice. *Anticancer Res.* **2014**, *34*, 39–48.

19. Paoli, A.; Rubini, A.; Volek, J.S.; Grimaldi, K.A. Beyond weight loss: A review of the therapeutic uses of very-low-carbohydrate (ketogenic) diets. *Eur. J. Clin. Nutr.* **2013**, *67*, 789–796.

20. Nilsson, L.M.; Winkvist, A.; Johansson, I.; Lindahl, B.; Hallmans, G.; Lenner, P.; Van, G.B. Low-carbohydrate, high-protein diet score and risk of incident cancer; a prospective cohort study. *Nutr. J.* **2013**, *12*, 58.

21. Busetto, L.; Marangon, M.; De, S.F. High-protein low-carbohydrate diets: What is the rationale? *Diabetes Metab. Res. Rev.* **2011**, *27*, 230–232.

22. Thomson, C.A.; Stopeck, A.T.; Bea, J.W.; Cussler, E.; Nardi, E.; Frey, G.; Thompson, P.A. Changes in body weight and metabolic indexes in overweight breast cancer survivors enrolled in a randomized trial of low-fat *vs.* reduced carbohydrate diets. *Nutr. Cancer* **2010**, *62*, 1142–1152.

23. Boeke, C.E.; Eliassen, A.H.; Chen, W.Y.; Cho, E.; Holmes, M.D.; Rosner, B.; Willett, W.C.; Tamimi, R.M. Dietary fat intake in relation to lethal breast cancer in two large prospective cohort studies. *Breast Cancer Res. Treat.* **2014**, *146*, 383–392.

24. Michels, K.B.; Willett, W.C. The women's health initiative randomized controlled dietary modification trial: A post-mortem. *Breast Cancer Res. Treat.* **2009**, *114*, 1–6.

25. Bilsborough, S.A.; Crowe, T.C. Low-carbohydrate diets: What are the potential short and long-term health implications? *Asia Pac. J. Clin. Nutr.* **2003**, *12*, 396–404.

26. McTiernan, A. Obesity and cancer: The risks, science, and potential management strategies. *Oncology* **2005**, *19*, 871–881.

27. Chen, X.; Wang, Y. Adiponectin and breast cancer. *Med. Oncol.* **2011**, *28*, 1288–1295.

28. Garofalo, C.; Koda, M.; Cascio, S.; Sulkowska, M.; Kanczuga-Koda, L.; Golaszewska, J.; Russo, A.; Sulkowski, S.; Surmacz, E. Increased expression of leptin and the leptin receptor as a marker of breast cancer progression: Possible role of obesity-related stimuli. *Clin. Cancer Res.* **2006**, *12*, 1447–1453.

29. Gaudet, M.M.; Falk, R.T.; Gierach, G.L.; Lacey, J.V., Jr.; Graubard, B.I.; Dorgan, J.F.; Brinton, L.A. Do adipokines underlie the association between known risk factors and breast cancer among a cohort of United States women? *Cancer Epidemiol.* **2010**, *34*, 580–586.

30. Grossmann, M.E.; Ray, A.; Nkhata, K.J.; Malakhov, D.A.; Rogozina, O.P.; Dogan, S.; Cleary, M.P. Obesity and breast cancer: Status of leptin and adiponectin in pathological processes. *Cancer Metastasis Rev.* **2010**, *29*, 641–653.

31. Grossmann, M.E.; Cleary, M.P. The balance between leptin and adiponectin in the control of carcinogenesis—Focus on mammary tumorigenesis. *Biochimie* **2012**, *94*, 2164–2171.

32. Havel, P.J. Control of energy homeostasis and insulin action by adipocyte hormones: Leptin, acylation stimulating protein, and adiponectin. *Curr. Opin. Lipidol.* **2002**, *13*, 51–59.

33. Rose, D.P.; Komninou, D.; Stephenson, G.D. Obesity, adipocytokines, and insulin resistance in breast cancer. *Obes. Rev.* **2004**, *5*, 153–165.

34. Forsblom, C.; Thomas, M.C.; Moran, J.; Saraheimo, M.; Thorn, L.; Waden, J.; Gordin, D.; Frystyk, J.; Flyvbjerg, A.; Groop, P.H. Serum adiponectin concentration is a positive predictor of all-cause and cardiovascular mortality in type 1 diabetes. *J. Intern. Med.* **2011**, *270*, 346–355.

35. Trujillo, M.E.; Scherer, P.E. Adiponectin—Journey from an adipocyte secretory protein to biomarker of the metabolic syndrome. *J. Intern. Med.* **2005**, *257*, 167–175.

36. Gautron, L.; Elmquist, J.K. Sixteen years and counting: An update on leptin in energy balance. *J. Clin. Investig.* **2011**, *121*, 2087–2093.

37. Harwood, H.J., Jr. The adipocyte as an endocrine organ in the regulation of metabolic homeostasis. *Neuropharmacology* **2012**, *63*, 57–75.

38. Sedlacek, S.M.; Playdon, M.C.; Wolfe, P.; McGinley, J.N.; Wisthoff, M.R.; Daeninck, E.A.; Jiang, W.; Zhu, Z.; Thompson, H.J. Effect of a low fat *versus* a low carbohydrate weight loss dietary intervention on biomarkers of long term survival in breast cancer patients ("CHOICE"): Study protocol. *BMC Cancer* **2011**, *11*, 287.

39. Abbenhardt, C.; McTiernan, A.; Alfano, C.M.; Wener, M.H.; Campbell, K.L.; Duggan, C.; Foster-Schubert, K.E.; Kong, A.; Toriola, A.T.; Potter, J.D.; *et al.* Effects of individual and combined dietary weight loss and exercise interventions in postmenopausal women on adiponectin and leptin levels. *J. Intern. Med.* **2013**, *274*, 163–175.

40. Fabian, C.J.; Kimler, B.F.; Donnelly, J.E.; Sullivan, D.K.; Klemp, J.R.; Petroff, B.K.; Phillips, T.A.; Metheny, T.; Aversman, S.; Yeh, H.W.; *et al.* Favorable modulation of benign breast tissue and serum risk biomarkers is associated with >10% weight loss in postmenopausal women. *Breast Cancer Res. Treat.* **2013**, *142*, 119–132.

41. Considine, R.V.; Sinha, M.K.; Heiman, M.L.; Kriauciunas, A.; Stephens, T.W.; Nyce, M.R.; Ohannesian, J.P.; Marco, C.C.; McKee, L.J.; Bauer, T.L. Serum immunoreactive-leptin concentrations in normal-weight and obese humans. *N. Engl. J. Med.* **1996**, *334*, 292–295.

42. Swarbrick, M.M.; Havel, P.J. Physiological, pharmacological, and nutritional regulation of circulating adiponectin concentrations in humans. *Metab. Syndr. Relat. Disord.* **2008**, *6*, 87–102.
43. Harris, H.R.; Tworoger, S.S.; Hankinson, S.E.; Rosner, B.A.; Michels, K.B. Plasma leptin levels and risk of breast cancer in premenopausal women. *Cancer Prev. Res.* **2011**, *4*, 1449–1456.
44. Tian, Y.F.; Chu, C.H.; Wu, M.H.; Chang, C.L.; Yang, T.; Chou, Y.C.; Hsu, G.C.; Yu, C.P.; Yu, J.C.; Sun, C.A. Anthropometric measures, plasma adiponectin, and breast cancer risk. *Endocr. Relat. Cancer* **2007**, *14*, 669–677.
45. Tworoger, S.S.; Eliassen, A.H.; Kelesidis, T.; Colditz, G.A.; Willett, W.C.; Mantzoros, C.S.; Hankinson, S.E. Plasma adiponectin concentrations and risk of incident breast cancer. *J. Clin. Endocrinol. Metab.* **2007**, *92*, 1510–1516.
46. Woo, H.Y.; Park, H.; Ki, C.S.; Park, Y.L.; Bae, W.G. Relationships among serum leptin, leptin receptor gene polymorphisms, and breast cancer in Korea. *Cancer Lett.* **2006**, *237*, 137–142.
47. Wu, M.H.; Chou, Y.C.; Chou, W.Y.; Hsu, G.C.; Chu, C.H.; Yu, C.P.; Yu, J.C.; Sun, C.A. Circulating levels of leptin, adiposity and breast cancer risk. *Br. J. Cancer* **2009**, *100*, 578–582.
48. Ye, J.; Jia, J.; Dong, S.; Zhang, C.; Yu, S.; Li, L.; Mao, C.; Wang, D.; Chen, J.; Yuan, G. Circulating adiponectin levels and the risk of breast cancer: A meta-analysis. *Eur. J. Cancer Prev.* **2014**, *23*, 158–165.
49. Llanos, A.A.; Krok, J.L.; Peng, J.; Pennell, M.L.; Olivo-Marston, S.; Vitolins, M.Z.; Degraffinreid, C.R.; Paskett, E.D. Favorable effects of low-fat and low-carbohydrate dietary patterns on serum leptin, but not adiponectin, among overweight and obese premenopausal women: A randomized trial. *Springerplus* **2014**, *3*, 175.
50. Rock, C.L.; Pande, C.; Flatt, S.W.; Ying, C.; Pakiz, B.; Parker, B.A.; Williams, K.; Bardwell, W.A.; Heath, D.D.; Nichols, J.F. Favorable changes in serum estrogens and other biologic factors after weight loss in breast cancer survivors who are overweight or obese. *Clin. Breast Cancer* **2013**, *13*, 188–195.
51. Sun, K.; Kusminski, C.M.; Scherer, P.E. Adipose tissue remodeling and obesity. *J. Clin. Investig.* **2011**, *121*, 2094–2101.
52. Viguerie, N.; Vidal, H.; Arner, P.; Holst, C.; Verdich, C.; Avizou, S.; Astrup, A.; Saris, W.H.; Macdonald, I.A.; Klimcakova, E.; *et al.* Adipose tissue gene expression in obese subjects during low-fat and high-fat hypocaloric diets. *Diabetologia* **2005**, *48*, 123–131.
53. Beasley, J.M.; Ange, B.A.; Anderson, C.A.; Miller, E.R., III; Erlinger, T.P.; Holbrook, J.T.; Sacks, F.M.; Appel, L.J. Associations between macronutrient intake and self-reported appetite and fasting levels of appetite hormones: Results from the Optimal Macronutrient Intake Trial to Prevent Heart Disease. *Am. J. Epidemiol.* **2009**, *169*, 893–900.
54. Bluher, M.; Rudich, A.; Kloting, N.; Golan, R.; Henkin, Y.; Rubin, E.; Schwarzfuchs, D.; Gepner, Y.; Stampfer, M.J.; Fiedler, M.; *et al.* Two patterns of adipokine and other biomarker dynamics in a long-term weight loss intervention. *Diabetes Care* **2012**, *35*, 342–349.
55. Ebbeling, C.B.; Swain, J.F.; Feldman, H.A.; Wong, W.W.; Hachey, D.L.; Garcia-Lago, E.; Ludwig, D.S. Effects of dietary composition on energy expenditure during weight-loss maintenance. *JAMA* **2012**, *307*, 2627–2634.
56. Esposito, K.; Di, P.C.; Maiorino, M.I.; Petrizzo, M.; Bellastella, G.; Siniscalchi, I.; Giugliano, D. Long-term effect of mediterranean-style diet and calorie restriction on biomarkers of longevity and oxidative stress in overweight men. *Cardiol. Res. Pract.* **2011**, *2011*, 293916.
57. Ganji, V.; Kafai, M.R.; McCarthy, E. Serum leptin concentrations are not related to dietary patterns but are related to sex, age, body mass index, serum triacylglycerol, serum insulin, and plasma glucose in the US population. *Nutr. Metab.* **2009**, *6*, 3.
58. Hatami, Z.Z.; Salehi, M.; Heydari, S.T.; Babajafari, S. The effects of 6 isocaloric meals on body weight, lipid profiles, leptin, and adiponectin in overweight subjects (BMI > 25). *Int. Cardiovasc. Res. J.* **2014**, *8*, 52–56.
59. Jacobs, D.R., Jr.; Sluik, D.; Rokling-Andersen, M.H.; Anderssen, S.A.; Drevon, C.A. Association of 1-y changes in diet pattern with cardiovascular disease risk factors and adipokines: Results from the 1-y randomized Oslo Diet and Exercise Study. *Am. J. Clin. Nutr.* **2009**, *89*, 509–517.
60. Jafari-Vayghan, H.; Tarighat-Esfanjani, A.; Jafarabadi, M.A.; Ebrahimi-Mameghani, M.; Ghadimi, S.S.; Lalezadeh, Z. Association between dietary patterns and serum leptin-to-adiponectin ratio in apparently healthy adults. *J. Am. Coll. Nutr.* **2015**, *34*, 49–55.

Nutrients **2015**, *7*, 5156–5176

61. Saneei, P.; Hashemipour, M.; Kelishadi, R.; Esmaillzadeh, A. The Dietary Approaches to Stop Hypertension (DASH) diet affects inflammation in childhood metabolic syndrome: A randomized cross-over clinical trial. *Ann. Nutr. Metab.* **2014**, *64*, 20–27.

62. Schoeller, D.A.; Buchholz, A.C. Energetics of obesity and weight control: Does diet composition matter? *J. Am. Diet. Assoc.* **2005**, *105*, 24–28.

63. Sofer, S.; Eliraz, A.; Kaplan, S.; Voet, H.; Fink, G.; Kima, T.; Madar, Z. Changes in daily leptin, ghrelin and adiponectin profiles following a diet with carbohydrates eaten at dinner in obese subjects. *Nutr. Metab. Cardiovasc. Dis.* **2013**, *23*, 744–750.

64. Friedman, J.M.; Mantzoros, C.S. 20 years of leptin: From the discovery of the leptin gene to leptin in our therapeutic armamentarium. *Metabolism* **2015**, *64*, 1–4.

65. Newman, G.; Gonzalez-Perez, R.R. LeptinGÇôcytokine crosstalk in breast cancer. *Mol. Cell. Endocrinol.* **2014**, *382*, 570–582.

66. Khan, S.; Shukla, S.; Sinha, S.; Meeran, S.M. Role of adipokines and cytokines in obesity-associated breast cancer: Therapeutic targets. *Cytokine Growth Factor Rev.* **2013**, *24*, 503–513.

67. Revillion, F.; Charlier, M.; Lhotellier, V.; Hornez, L.; Giard, S.; Baranzelli, M.C.; Djiane, J.; Peyrat, J.P. Messenger RNA expression of leptin and leptin receptors and their prognostic value in 322 human primary breast cancers. *Clin. Cancer Res.* **2006**, *12*, 2088–2094.

68. Fargnoli, J.L.; Fung, T.T.; Olenczuk, D.M.; Chamberland, J.P.; Hu, F.B.; Mantzoros, C.S. Adherence to healthy eating patterns is associated with higher circulating total and high-molecular-weight adiponectin and lower resistin concentrations in women from the Nurses' Health Study. *Am. J. Clin. Nutr.* **2008**, *88*, 1213–1224.

69. Yannakoulia, M.; Yiannakouris, N.; Melistas, L.; Kontogianni, M.D.; Malagaris, I.; Mantzoros, C.S. A dietary pattern characterized by high consumption of whole-grain cereals and low-fat dairy products and low consumption of refined cereals is positively associated with plasma adiponectin levels in healthy women. *Metabolism* **2008**, *57*, 824–830.

70. Mantzoros, C.S.; Williams, C.J.; Manson, J.E.; Meigs, J.D.; Hu, F.B. Adherence to the Mediterranean dietary pattern is positively associated with plasma adiponectin concentrations in diabetic women. *Am. J. Clin. Nutr.* **2006**, *84*, 328–335.

71. Heidemann, C.; Hoffmann, K.; Spranger, J.; Klipstein-Grobusch, K.; Mohlig, M.; Pfeiffer, A.F.; Boeing, H. A dietary pattern protective against type 2 diabetes in the European Prospective Investigation into Cancer and Nutrition (EPIC)—Potsdam Study cohort. *Diabetologia* **2005**, *48*, 1126–1134.

72. Van Saun, M.N. Molecular pathways: Adiponectin and leptin signaling in cancer. *Clin. Cancer Res.* **2013**, *19*, 1926–1932.

73. Kizer, J.R.; Benkeser, D.; Arnold, A.M.; Mukamal, K.J.; Ix, J.H.; Zieman, S.J.; Siscovick, D.S.; Tracy, R.P.; Mantzoros, C.S.; Defilippi, C.R.; *et al.* Associations of total and high-molecular-weight adiponectin with all-cause and cardiovascular mortality in older persons: The Cardiovascular Health Study. *Circulation* **2012**, *126*, 2951–2961.

74. Duggan, C.; Irwin, M.L.; Xiao, L.; Henderson, K.D.; Smith, A.W.; Baumgartner, R.N.; Baumgartner, K.B.; Bernstein, L.; Ballard-Barbash, R.; McTiernan, A. Associations of insulin resistance and adiponectin with mortality in women with breast cancer. *J. Clin. Oncol.* **2011**, *29*, 32–39.

75. Cleary, M.P.; Ray, A.; Rogozina, O.P.; Dogan, S.; Grossmann, M.E. Targeting the adiponectin:Leptin ratio for postmenopausal breast cancer prevention. *Front. Biosci.* **2009**, *1*, 329–357.

76. Satija, A.; Yu, E.; Willett, W.C.; Hu, F.B. Understanding nutritional epidemiology and its role in policy. *Adv. Nutr.* **2015**, *6*, 5–18. [CrossRef] [PubMed]

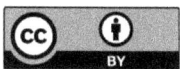

nutrients

MDPI

Article

Sex Differences in the Impact of the Mediterranean Diet on LDL Particle Size Distribution and Oxidation

Alexandra Bédard [1,2], Louise Corneau [1], Benoît Lamarche [1,2], Sylvie Dodin [1,3] and Simone Lemieux [1,2,*]

[1] Institute of Nutrition and Functional Foods (INAF), 2440 Hochelaga Boulevard, Laval University, Québec, QC G1V 0A6, Canada; alexandra.bedard.1@ulaval.ca (A.B.); louise.corneau@fsaa.ulaval.ca (L.C.); benoit.lamarche@fsaa.ulaval.ca (B.L.); sylvie.dodin@fmed.ulaval.ca (S.D.)
[2] School of Nutrition, Pavillon Paul-Comtois, 2425 rue de l'Agriculture, Laval University, Québec, QC G1V 0A6, Canada
[3] Department of Obstetrics and Gynaecology, Pavillon Ferdinand-Vandry, 1050 Medicine Avenue, Laval University, Québec, QC G1V 0A6, Canada
*   Author to whom correspondence should be addressed; simone.lemieux@fsaa.ulaval.ca; Tel.: +1-418-656-2131 (ext. 3637); Fax: +1-418-656-5877.

Received: 24 March 2015; Accepted: 5 May 2015; Published: 15 May 2015

Abstract: Sex differences have been previously highlighted in the cardioprotective effects of the Mediterranean diet (MedDiet). The objective of this study was to investigate whether sex differences also exist with regard to LDL particle size distribution and oxidation. Participants were 37 men and 32 premenopausal women (24–53 years) with slightly elevated LDL-C concentrations (3.4–4.9 mmol/L) or total cholesterol/HDL-C $\geq$5.0. Variables were measured before and after a four-week isoenergetic MedDiet. Sex differences were found in response to the MedDiet for the proportion of medium LDL (255–260 Å) (p for sex-by-time interaction = 0.01) and small, dense LDL (sdLDL; <255 Å) (trend; p for sex-by-time interaction = 0.06), men experiencing an increase in the proportion of medium LDL with a concomitant reduction in the proportion of sdLDL, while an opposite trend was observed in women. A sex difference was also noted for estimated cholesterol concentrations among sdLDL (p for sex-by-time interaction = 0.03), with only men experiencing a reduction in response to the MedDiet. The MedDiet marginally reduced oxidized LDL (oxLDL) concentrations (p = 0.07), with no sex difference. Results suggest that short-termconsumption of the MedDiet leads to a favorable redistribution of LDL subclasses from smaller to larger LDL only in men. These results highlight the importance of considering sex issues in cardiovascular benefits of the MedDiet.

Keywords: Mediterranean diet; LDL size; oxidized LDL; men; women

1. Introduction

Lowering LDL-C concentration is the primary target of therapy for the prevention of cardiovascular disease (CVD) [1–3]. However, in addition to LDL-C concentrations, it has been shown that a more detailed analysis of LDL physico-chemical properties (e.g., size and oxidation) provides further insight into individual cardiovascular risk [4–6]. Individuals characterized by a predominance of small, dense LDL particles (sdLDL) are at increased risk of coronary heart disease compared to those with larger, buoyant LDL particles [7–9]. Compared with large LDL, sdLDL possess a lower affinity for the LDL receptor and a longer half-life in plasma [10], bind more tightly to arterial proteoglycans [11], penetrate the arterial subendothelial space more easily [12] and are more susceptible to oxidation [13]. LDL oxidation is another process through which LDL contribute to atherosclerotic plaque formation by favoring endothelial dysfunction, the release of inflammatory cytokines and macrophage transformation into foam cells [6]. Accordingly, oxidized LDL (oxLDL) concentrations have been identified as an important marker of atherosclerotic lesions [5,6].

Sex disparities have been previously reported for LDL physico-chemical properties, men being characterized by a higher proportion of sdLDL and greater concentrations of oxLDL than premenopausal women [14–19]. Given that the presence of both sdLDL and oxLDL are predictive of an increased cardiovascular risk, such sex differences could contribute in part to the higher risk of coronary heart disease found in men compared with premenopausal women.

Adopting the traditional Mediterranean diet (MedDiet) has been identified as a useful strategy in the prevention of cardiovascular events. The Prevención con Dieta Mediterránea (PREDIMED) study, consisting of a nutritional intervention among 7447 high-risk individuals, indicates that the adherence to an energy-unrestricted MedDiet supplemented with extra-virgin olive oil or mixed nuts for 4.8 years reduces by approximately 30% the incidence of myocardial infarction, stroke and cardiovascular death compared with a low-fat diet [20]. Different mechanisms of action have been proposed for the beneficial cardioprotective effects of the MedDiet, one largely documented being its LDL-C lowering effects [21]. Nevertheless, strong evidence suggests beneficial effects of the MedDiet beyond its impact on LDL-C and other traditional risk factors [22].

A shift toward larger LDL particles and a reduction in oxLDL concentrations have been previously observed with the consumption of the MedDiet in some [23–27], but not all studies [28], suggesting that some factors, such as the characteristics of participants (e.g., sex, age, genetic predisposition, usual dietary intakes) may modulate these effects. In this sense, previous results suggest that men have greater cardiometabolic changes in response to the MedDiet than premenopausal women [29–31]. However, no study has examined whether sex differences exist in the effects of this food pattern on LDL physico-chemical properties. One could speculate that, because of the higher proportion of sdLDL habitually found in men compared with premenopausal women [14–17], men may experience a more important shift toward larger LDL particles than women in response to the MedDiet. Consequently, since larger, less dense LDL particles are less susceptible to oxidation than sdLDL [13], men may have greater reduction in oxLDL concentrations than women. As estrogens exert beneficial effects on LDL size and oxidation [18,32–35] and the MedDiet has been previously shown to reduce estrogen concentrations in women [36], these facts further support the hypothesis that men may benefit more than premenopausal women from this food pattern.

The aim of the present study was to verify whether the impact of the MedDiet on LDL size distribution, as well as on oxLDL concentrations differs between men and women. Results presented in this paper suggest that adhering to the MedDiet, in addition to a clinically-relevant reduction in LDL-C concentrations, also has additional positive effects on LDL particle size phenotype, leading to a favorable redistribution from smaller to larger LDL in men, but not in women. This study provides new and useful clinical information in order to improve our understanding of the variability in the response to the MedDiet and, ultimately, to further individualize dietary recommendations in the prevention of cardiovascular disease.

2. Experimental Section

2.1. Subjects

Thirty-eight men and 32 premenopausal women took part to this study. However, one man was excluded from analyses, because of a lack of dietary compliance due to illness during several days just before the end of the controlled MedDiet phase. Analyses were therefore conducted in a sample of 37 men and 32 premenopausal women, aged between 24 and 53 years, who participated in a study that was initially designed to directly document sex differences in the impact of a MedDiet on LDL-C concentrations [29]. The main inclusion criteria were to have slightly elevated LDL-C concentrations (between 3.4 and 4.9 mmol/L) or a total cholesterol to HDL-C ratio ≥ 5.0, as well as at least one of the four following CVD risk factors: waist circumference >94 cm in men and >80 cm in women [37]; TG $\geq$1.7 mmol/L; fasting glycemia between 6.1 and 6.9 mmol/L and/or blood pressure levels $\geq$130/85 mm Hg. No participant had a history of cardiovascular events, and none were taking medication that could affect the dependent variables under study (e.g., lipid-lowering medication). Smokers and pregnant women or those using systemic hormonal contraceptives were excluded from this study. The present study was conducted according to the guidelines laid down in the Declaration of Helsinki, and all procedures involving human subjects were approved by the Laval University Ethics Committee (#2007-180, 4 October 2007). This clinical trial was registered at www.clinicaltrials.govasNCT01293344.

Before the intervention (*i.e.*, at screening), no difference between men and women was found for age (mean (SD): men 42.5 (7.3) years; women 41.1 (7.4) years, *p* for sex difference = 0.45) and BMI (mean (SD): men 28.8 (3.1) kg/m^2; women 29.2 (5.6) kg/m^2, *p* for sex difference = 0.92). However, men had higher mean values than women for body weight (mean (SD): men 90.7 (13.7) kg; women 77.4 (14.7) kg, *p* for sex difference <0.001) and waist circumference (mean (SD): men 102.1 (9.9) cm; women 94.3 (10.3) cm, *p* for sex difference = 0.001).

Power analyses for repeated measures and within-between interactions showed that a total sample size of *n* = 69 is sufficient to detect significant differences in all outcomes measured with a small effect size estimate (Cohen's d of 0.20 [38]) and with an α = 0.05 and a power of 0.8 (G*Power Version 3.0.10, Franz Faul, Universität Kiel, Germany).

2.2. Study Design

The study protocol consisted of a 4-week run-in period, immediately followed by a 4-week fully-controlled MedDiet phase [29]. During the run-in period, subjects received personalized recommendations by a registered dietitian in order to follow the healthy recommendations of Canada's Food Guide [39]. Briefly, Canada's Food Guide is an educational tool that promotes healthy eating for Canadians in order to reduce the risk of chronic diseases and to achieve overall health. It indicates the recommended number of food guide servings per day for each of the four food groups (vegetables and fruits, grain products, milk and alternatives and meat and alternatives) according to the age and sex of individuals. In addition, more specific recommendations are provided for each food groups (e.g., eat at least one dark green and one orange vegetable each day, make at least half of your grain products whole grain each day, select lower fat milk and alternatives, have meat alternatives, such as beans, lentils and tofu, often and eat at least two servings of fish each week). The 4-week run-in period allowed comparing the effects of the MedDiet between men and women having similar baseline dietary intakes, as reported previously [29]. Moreover, the concordance of men's and women's diet with the traditional MedDiet was similar at the end of the run-in period, as suggested by a Mediterranean score (MedScore; from 0–44 points: 24.8 (5.9) points in men and 24.6 (4.4) points in women, *p* for sex difference = 0.87) [40]. This MedScore has been previously shown to be a valid indicator of MedDiet adherence [40,41]. A MedScore of forty-four would imply a food pattern that is perfectly concordant with the traditional MedDiet. No change in body weight was found during the run-in period (+0.02 (0.19) kg in men and −0.01 (0.16) kg in women, respectively *p* = 0.93 and *p* = 0.84).

During the 4-week fully-controlled feeding phase, subjects consumed an experimental MedDiet formulated to be concordant with the characteristics of the traditional MedDiet [42]. More precisely, the experimental MedDiet included an abundance of fruits, vegetables, whole grain cereals, nuts and legumes, moderate amounts of fish, poultry, eggs and low-fat dairy products and low amounts of red meat and sweets. Olive oil was the main source of fat, and wine accompanied meals with moderation. The percentages of energy derived from lipids, carbohydrates, proteins and alcohol were respectively 32% (7.2% SFA, 17.9% MUFA and 4.6% PUFA), 46%, 17% and 5%. Details about the composition of the MedDiet have been already reported [29].

A 4-week controlled phase has been demonstrated as sufficient to induce significant changes in LDL particle size features [43,44] and oxLDL concentrations [45,46]. All foods for the MedDiet phase were prepared in a standardized manner in the Clinical Investigation Unit (CIU). Subjects were instructed to consume only the foods and beverages provided to them, which corresponded to 100% of their estimated energy needs. Energy needs were established by averaging energy requirements estimated by a validated food frequency questionnaire (FFQ) [47] administered at the beginning of the run-in period and energy needs as determined by the Harris–Benedict formula. Participant's body weight was monitored daily before the consumption of the lunch at the CIU, and energy intake was increased or decreased by 250 kcal/day if a subject lost or gained greater than 1 kg and maintained that body weight for at least 3 days. Participants completed a daily checklist confirming the consumption of provided foods and beverages and, if needed, the amount of foods not consumed. Participants were instructed to maintain their usual physical activity level. However, in order to verify whether participants followed this instruction, daily energy expenditure from physical activity participation was evaluated using a validated 3-day activity diary record developed by Bouchard *et al.* [48] administered during the fourth week of both the run-in period and the MedDiet phase. Since some studies have suggested that fluctuations in female hormones influence the lipid lipoprotein profile [49], women's feeding was shortened or prolonged if needed in order to be able to carry out all tests in the early follicular phase of their menstrual cycle (from the third to the ninth day of the menstrual cycle; mean duration of the feeding period in women (SD): 28.8 (4.3) days).

2.3. Laboratory Analyses

Blood samples were collected from an antecubital vein into vacutainer tubes after a 12-h overnight fast. Total plasma cholesterol, TG and HDL-C concentrations were measured using commercial reagents on a Modular P chemistry analyzer (Roche Diagnostics, Mannheim, Germany). Apo B was measured by immunoturbidimetry (Roche Diagnostics, Mannheim, Germany). LDL-C was obtained by the equation of Friedewald [50]. Plasma apo A-1 and apo A-2 concentrations were measured by immunonephelometry. For the measurements of LDL particle size features and oxLDL concentrations, analyses were performed using plasma stored at −80 °C. Non-denaturing 2%–16% polyacrylamide gradient gel electrophoreses were used to characterize LDL particle size distribution, as previously described [51]. LDL particle size was computed on the basis of the relative migration of plasma standards of known diameter [52]. The LDL peak particle size was computed as the estimated diameter for the major peak of each scan. An integrated (or mean) LDL size, corresponding to the weighed mean size of all LDL subclasses in each individual, was also determined. As revealed by the analysis of pooled plasma standards, measurements of LDL peak particle size and LDL integrated particle size were highly reproducible, considering an inter-assay coefficient of variation of <2%. The relative proportion of sdLDL, characterized by a diameter <255 Å ($LDL_{<255Å}$), was obtained by computing the relative area of the densitometric scan <255 Å. The absolute concentration of cholesterol in sdLDL particles was estimated by multiplying the total plasma LDL-C concentrations by the relative proportion of $LDL_{<255Å}$. Similar approaches were used to estimate the relative proportion of medium and large LDL particles and their specific estimated cholesterol concentration, using respectively a diameter between 255 and 260 Å ($LDL_{255-260Å}$) and >260 Å ($LDL_{>260Å}$). LDL subclass Pattern A was characterized by an LDL peak particle size ≥255 Å, whereas LDL subclass Pattern B by a LDL peak particle size <255 Å. The measurements of the proportion of medium LDL and large LDL had a coefficient of variation of 12% and 9.3% respectively. oxLDL concentrations were measured using a commercial enzyme-linked immune-sorbent assay (ELISA) kit (Alpco, Salem, NH), with an intra-assay coefficient of variation of 3.9%–5.7% and inter-assay coefficient of variation of 9%–11%.

2.4. Statistical Analyses

Statistical analyses were performed using SAS statistical package Version 9.4 (SAS Institute Inc., Cary, NC, USA). All statistical tests were two-sided. $p \leq 0.05$ was considered as significant. Data were collected before (*i.e.*, immediately after the run-in period, referred as baseline values) and after the controlled MedDiet phase. Differences in baseline characteristics between men and women were assessed using Student's *t*-test. Mixed procedures for repeated measurements were used to assess the main effects of time, sex and sex-by-time interaction on LDL particle size features and oxLDL concentrations. When a significant main effect was found, Tukey-Kramer adjusted *p*-values were used to identify the precise location of differences. Associations between variables were assessed by Pearson's correlation analyses. One woman was excluded from analyses of oxLDL concentrations due to a baseline extreme value (*i.e.*, 3027.8 ng/mL *vs.* group's mean (SD) of 166.4 (200.6) ng/mL).

Although the MedDiet phase aimed at being isoenergetic, both men and women experienced a small, but significant body weight change (mean (SD): -1.19 (1.23) kg in men, $p < 0.001$ and -0.55 (0.98) kg in women, $p = 0.01$). Given that changes in body weight may influence LDL physico-chemical properties (both size and oxidation) [5,53], all analyses presented here were adjusted for this small change in body weight. Waist circumference did not statistically change during the MedDiet phase in both men and women (mean (SD): -0.29 (2.68) cm in men, $p = 0.56$; -0.80 (2.56) cm in women, $p = 0.09$).

3. Results

Even if there were no difference between men and women for LDL-C concentrations before the MedDiet (*i.e.*, immediately after the run-in period; $p = 0.36$), some sex differences were observed in LDL physico-chemical properties (Table 1). In fact, men had a lower proportion of medium LDL$_{(255-260 \text{ Å})}$ ($p = 0.02$) and a higher proportion of sdLDL$_{(<255 \text{ Å})}$ ($p = 0.01$) than women. Moreover, men had higher estimated cholesterol concentrations among sdLDL$_{(<255 \text{ Å})}$ than women ($p = 0.01$). Finally, men were characterized by smaller LDL peak particle size ($p = 0.04$) and LDL integrated size ($p = 0.04$) than women. No difference was found between men and women for all of the other variables related to LDL particle size features ($p > 0.08$). Men and women had similar oxLDL concentrations prior to the controlled MedDiet intervention ($p = 0.86$).

3.1. Plasma Lipids and Lipoproteins

As reported previously [29], reductions in total cholesterol, LDL-C, HDL-C, total cholesterol to HDL-C ratio and apo B were observed in response to the MedDiet, and no difference was found between men and women (*p* for sex-by-time interaction ≥ 0.16; Table 1). More precisely, reductions in LDL-C concentrations of 10.4% in men and 7.3% in women were noted (respectively, $p = 0.003$ and $p = 0.04$).

Table 1. Effects of the four-week Mediterranean diet (MedDiet) on the lipid-lipoprotein profile and LDL physical properties in men and women.

Variables	Men (n = 37)					Women (n = 22)					p-value [a]	
	Baseline [b]		After MedDiet		Change	Baseline [b]		After MedDiet		Change	Time	Sex * time
	Mean	SEM	Mean	SEM	%	Mean	SEM	Mean	SEM	%		
TG (mmol/L) [c,d]	1.86	0.19	1.59	0.10	−14.6	1.36	0.11	1.26	0.08	−7.7	0.06	0.53
Total cholesterol (mmol/L) [c]	5.56	0.15	5.01	0.13	−9.9	5.40	0.11	5.06	0.10	−6.2	<0.001	0.16
LDL-C (mmol/L) [c]	3.61	0.12	3.23	0.11	−10.4	3.47	0.09	3.22	0.09	−7.3	<0.001	0.34
HDL-C (mmol/L) [c,d]	1.09	0.05	1.05	0.04	−4.4	1.30	0.05	1.27	0.04	−2.6	0.02	0.57
Total cholesterol/HDL-C ratio [c]	5.30	0.17	4.97	0.17	−6.1	4.26	0.14	4.08	0.12	−4.3	0.001	0.36
Apo B (g/L) [c]	1.14	0.04	1.03	0.04	−9.5	1.04	0.03	0.95	0.03	−9.0	<0.001	0.69
LDL physical properties												
LDL peak particle diameter (Å) [d]	253.2	0.5	253.3	0.4	0.0	254.7	0.6	254.4	0.5	−0.1	0.79	0.42
LDL integrated size (Å) [d]	254.2	0.4	254.4	0.3	0.1	255.5	0.5	255.4	0.4	−0.1	0.70	0.25
Relative distribution among LDL subclasses												
Large LDL$_{>260Å}$ (%) [d]	17.0	2.0	16.5	1.6	−0.5	22.3	2.7	20.8	2.8	−1.5	0.41	0.57
Medium LDL$_{255-260Å}$ (%)	26.9	1.5	29.9	1.4	3.0	32.7	2.1	31.5	1.7	−1.2	0.25	0.01
Small LDL$_{<255Å}$ (%)	56.2	2.9	53.6	2.6	−2.5	45.0	3.4	47.7	3.0	2.6	0.97	0.06
Absolute concentration of cholesterol in LDL subclasses												
Large LDL-C$_{>260Å}$ (mmol/L) [d]	0.64	0.08	0.56	0.06	−12.6	0.77	0.09	0.71	0.11	−8.9	0.03	0.54
Medium LDL-C$_{255-260Å}$ (mmol/L) [d]	0.99	0.07	0.97	0.06	−1.2	1.14	0.08	1.01	0.06	−11.5	0.06	0.12
Small LDL-C$_{<255Å}$ (mmol/L) [d]	1.99	0.10	1.70	0.09	−14.3	1.55	0.12	1.49	0.09	−3.5	0.001	0.03
oxLDL (ng/mL) [d]	167.2	28.7	160.6	25.8	−4.0	165.5	41.5	152.6	32.5	−7.8	0.07	0.85

TG, triglycerides; LDL-C, low-density lipoprotein-cholesterol; HDL-C, high-density lipoprotein-cholesterol; Apo, apolipoprotein; oxLDL, oxidized LDL. [a] All analyses are adjusted for the body weight change during the MedDiet phase; [b] baseline values represent those collected after the run-in period, immediately before the 4-week MedDiet; [c] these data have been previously reported [3]; [d] since these variables were not normally distributed, a transformation was performed in order to obtain a normal distribution. TG, HDL-C and oxLDL were log-transformed; LDL peak particle diameter, LDL integrated size and small LDL-C$_{<255Å}$ were inversed transformed; and large LDL$_{>260Å}$ was square transformed.

3.2. LDL Size Distribution

Sex differences were observed in changes in LDL size distribution in response to the MedDiet and more precisely for the proportion of medium LDL$_{(255–260 Å)}$ (p for sex-by-time interaction = 0.01) and sdLDL$_{(<255 Å)}$ (trend; p for sex-by-time interaction = 0.06) (Table 1). Specifically, men experienced an increase in the proportion of medium LDL with a concomitant non-significant decrease in the proportion of sdLDL (respectively, p = 0.03 and p = 0.50), while an opposite non-significant trend was observed in women (respectively, p = 0.74 and p = 0.54). No change was observed for the proportion of large LDL$_{(>260 Å)}$ in both men and women (Table 1). These results suggest that short-term consumption of the MedDiet leads to a favorable redistribution of LDL subclasses from smaller to larger LDL only in men.

A similar LDL size distribution was found in men and in women after the MedDiet (p for sex difference for each proportion of LDL subclass ≥0.14), suggesting that sex differences at baseline were no longer present after the short term consumption of the MedDiet.

3.3. Estimated Cholesterol Concentration among Each LDL Subclass

A sex difference was noted for cholesterol concentrations among sdLDL$_{(<255 Å)}$ (p for sex-by-time interaction = 0.03), with only men experiencing a reduction in response to the MedDiet (p < 0.001 in men and p = 0.88 in women; Table 1). In men, the reduction in cholesterol concentration among sdLDL correlated with concomitant reductions in TG (r = 0.38, p = 0.02), LDL-C (r = 0.41, p = 0.01) and apo B (r = 0.57, p < 0.001). The sex difference in cholesterol concentrations among sdLDL observed at baseline was no longer present after the short-term consumption of the MedDiet (p for sex difference ≥0.11).

Significant reductions in cholesterol concentration among large LDL$_{(>260Å)}$ and a tendency for a decrease in cholesterol concentration among medium LDL$_{(255–260Å)}$ were found, and no sex differences were observed for these variables (Table 1).

3.4. LDL Peak and Integrated (Mean) Size

Consumption of the MedDiet did not affect LDL peak particle size or the LDL integrated size in both men and women (Table 1).

However, a three-way sex-by-time-by-LDL subclass pattern (A or B) interaction was found for LDL peak particle size (p for interaction = 0.01). Subgroup analysis indicated that, among men and women with LDL Pattern A at baseline (LDL peak particle size ≥255 Å), only men experienced a decrease in LDL peak particle size in response to the MedDiet (p = 0.03 for men and p = 0.54 for women; p for time effect = 0.004; p for sex-by-time interaction = 0.12) (Figure 1). Moreover, among those with LDL Pattern B at baseline (LDL peak particle size <255 Å), LDL peak particle size was increased in men only (p = 0.003 for men and p = 0.90 for women; p for time effect = 0.007; p for sex-by-time interaction = 0.08). Among each subgroup, no difference between men and women was found for baseline LDL peak particle size (p for sex difference at baseline > 0.99 for Pattern A subgroup and 0.94 for Pattern B subgroup). These results suggest that LDL subclass pattern at baseline influences the LDL peak particle size response to the MedDiet, but only in men. No three-way interaction was found for the LDL integrated size.

Pattern A

Pattern B

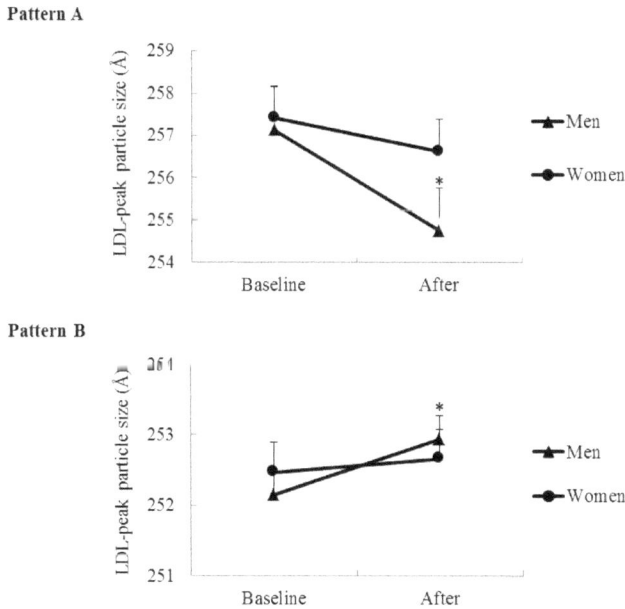

Figure 1. LDL peak particle size at baseline (*i.e.*, immediately before the MedDiet) and after the four-week MedDiet in men and women according to their initial LDL subclass pattern (Pattern A: LDL peak particle diameter $\geq$255 Å, men n = 8 and women n = 14, p for sex-by-time interaction = 0.12; Pattern B: LDL peak particle diameter <255 Å, men n = 29 and women n = 18, p for sex-by-time interaction = 0.08). Data are means (SEM). * Different from baseline in men, $p < 0.05$ by mixed procedure followed by the Tukey-Kramer test.

Since TG concentrations are the main determinant of LDL size [4] and TG reduction in men was twice the reduction in women in response to the MedDiet (respectively −14.6% and −7.7%; Table 1), we thereafter adjusted the analyses for changes in TG concentrations. Sex differences in changes in LDL particle size features in response to the MedDiet were still observed after these adjustments (not shown).

Adjustments for waist circumference at baseline did not influence the results obtained (not shown), suggesting that differences between men and women in abdominal obesity do not explain sex differences observed in LDL size response to the MedDiet.

3.5. Oxidized LDL

A trend for a reduction in oxLDL concentrations was found in response to the MedDiet, and no difference was observed between men and women (p for time effect = 0.07; p for sex-by-time interaction = 0.85; Table 1).

Diet-induced changes in oxLDL concentrations were not associated with oxLDL concentrations at baseline in either men or women (respectively r = −0.06, p = 0.71 and r = −0.16, p = 0.40). There was no association between changes in oxLDL concentrations and changes in LDL-C concentrations (respectively r = 0.20, p = 0.25 for men and r = 0.13, p = 0.50 for women) and changes in cholesterol concentration among sdLDL$_{(<255 Å)}$ (r = 0.11, p = 0.54 for men and r = 0.08, p = 0.67 for women).

Although participants were instructed to maintain their usual physical activity level, a similar decrease in daily energy expenditure from physical activity participation was observed during the MedDiet phase in men and women (−27.8% in men and −27.6% in women, p for sex-by-time interaction = 0.25). Adjustment for changes in physical activity participation did not influence the results obtained (not shown).

4. Discussion

Elevated LDL-C concentration has been established as a major risk factor for CVD [1–3]. However, a more detailed analysis of LDL physico-chemical properties is highly relevant given the important atherogenicity of sdLDL particles and of oxLDL [4–6]. Accordingly, results from the present study highlight sex-specific cardiovascular benefits of the MedDiet, which would not have been observed if only LDL-C concentrations had been measured. Indeed, despite the fact that men and women have similar reductions in LDL-C concentrations in response to the MedDiet, different responses in LDL particle size features to this food pattern are observed. More precisely, men experienced an increase in the proportion of medium LDL particles with a concomitant reduction in the proportion of sdLDL, while an opposite non-significant trend was observed in women. Moreover, a reduction in cholesterol concentrations among sdLDL with MedDiet was noted in men, but not in women. Finally, results showed that the more deteriorated LDL particle size features found in men compared with premenopausal women at baseline were no longer present after the short-term consumption of the MedDiet.

Even if a favorable LDL size redistribution and a reduction in cholesterol concentration among sdLDL were observed in men, one might question the clinical relevance of these changes, since the MedDiet had no global impact on LDL peak particle size, a widely-used surrogate marker of sdLDL. However, a prospective study including 2,034 middle-aged men suggested that LDL peak particle size is a weak predictor of ischemic heart disease risk compared with the proportion and the cholesterol content of sdLDL, which were identified as very powerful and independent risk predictors, even after adjustments for non-lipid and other lipid CVD risk factors, including LDL-C, HDL-C, TG and lipoprotein(a) (Lp(a)) concentrations [51]. Therefore, one mechanism behind the reduction in cardiovascular events with the consumption of the MedDiet could be a reduction of sdLDL in dyslipidemic men.

As previously found in the literature, our results highlight that, compared with premenopausal women, age-matched men have a greater proportion of sdLDL [14–17]. Given their greater proportion of sdLDL at baseline, men had more room for improvement, which may explain at least partly why they benefited more from the MedDiet than premenopausal women. Indeed, in previous studies, those including subjects with metabolic syndrome, which is a cluster of metabolic abnormalities characterized by a predominance of sdLDL, found increases in LDL size and/or a favorable redistribution of cholesterol among each LDL subclass with the MedDiet [23–25], while one studying the impact of the MedDiet in healthy individuals has observed no effect [28]. In line with these previous studies, strong negative correlations were found in the present study between the proportion and the cholesterol content of sdLDL at baseline and changes in these specific variables in response to the MedDiet, meaning that individuals who were characterized by a higher proportion and cholesterol content of sdLDL benefited more from the MedDiet (respectively, $r < -0.50$ and $r < -0.61$, $p < 0.001$). Additional analyses also showed that, when men and women were individually matched for the proportion of sdLDL at baseline (23 men and 23 women), differences between men and women in changes in cholesterol concentration among sdLDL were considerably smaller than the one found with the whole sample (-10.4% in men and -7.9% in women, p for sex-by-time interaction = 0.68 in subjects paired for the proportion of sdLDL at baseline; *vs.* -14.3% in men and -3.5% in women when the whole sample was considered).

In addition to the difference between men and women in LDL particle size features at baseline, other factors related to sex seem to influence the impact of the MedDiet on LDL size. In fact, in the present study, subjects characterized by the LDL Pattern B phenotype (*i.e.*, predominance of sdLDL) experienced a favorable increase in LDL peak particle size, whereas a reduction was found in those characterized by the LDL Pattern A phenotype (*i.e.*, predominance of large LDL particles).

However, this pattern of changes was observed only in men, while women experienced no change, regardless of their baseline LDL peak particle size phenotype. Since these sub-analyses are based on small numbers of subjects in each group, they need to be confirmed.

Although not significant from a statistical perspective, men experienced nearly a two-fold greater reduction in TG concentrations compared with women (14.6% *vs.* 7.7%), and such a difference could be clinically significant. High concentrations of TG favor the production of large, TG-rich, very low density lipoprotein (VLDL), a precursor of TG-rich LDL. In turn, lipolysis of TG in TG-enriched LDL by hepatic lipase leads to the formation of sdLDL [4]. One could therefore assume that the greater reduction in the concentrations of sdLDL found in men compared with women in response to the MedDiet could also be explained by this greater reduction in TG concentrations in men. In the present study, a strong association between changes in sdLDL and concomitant changes in TG concentrations was found in men. However, sex differences in LDL particle size feature responses to the MedDiet were still observed after adjustments for changes in TG concentrations, suggesting that sex differences observed in the present study were not due only to a greater reduction in TG concentrations in men compared with women.

The reduction in oxLDL concentrations was not associated with decreases in LDL-C concentrations in response to the MedDiet in both men and women, suggesting that oxLDL reduction does not simply reflect the LDL-lowering effects of the MedDiet, but is likely to be due to the antioxidant properties of this food pattern. Since men reduced their proportion and cholesterol content of sdLDL more than women in response to the MedDiet and sdLDL is more susceptible to oxidation compared with larger particles [13], it could be expected that men may have reduced their oxLDL concentrations to a greater extent compared with women. However, this was not the case. In fact, no sex difference was found in response to the MedDiet, with a modest reduction in oxLDL concentrations observed in both men and women. One possible explanation is that the consumption of a diet rich in oleic acid, the more abundant fatty acid in the olive oil, may reduce the susceptibility of sdLDL to oxidation [54], leading to a reduction in oxLDL, which is independent of the one found in sdLDL. This disassociation between changes in sdLDL and changes in oxLDL concentrations was observed in both men and women. Moreover, the MedDiet is rich in antioxidants, such as carotenoids, tocopherols and phenolic compounds, mainly contained in vegetables, fruits, olive oil and red wine [55], which may provide an important protection for sdLDL to oxidation. Therefore, these results suggest that the high oleic acid content of the MedDiet, along with its important antioxidant properties, may overshadow the link between sdLDL and LDL oxidation.

One of the strengths of our study is a design that included a highly-controlled dietary phase, which permitted precisely investigating sex differences in response to the MedDiet with a maximum control of possible confounding variables. Moreover, this study included a large number of subjects for a strictly controlled feeding study. However, results should not be generalized, and additional studies are needed. The duration of the controlled phase was appropriate, considering that previous studies of equal or shorter lengths showed significant effects of diet on LDL particle size [43,44] and oxLDL concentrations [45,46]. Among the limitations, the study's 'single strand before and after' design does not allow comparisons to a control diet, and therefore, non-specific treatment effects that are not attributable to the MedDiet cannot be ruled out. However, we consider that the absence of a control diet is not a major limitation, since the main objective of this study was to directly compare men's and women's response to the MedDiet.

5. Conclusions

In conclusion, data from this strictly-controlled feeding study indicated for the first time the existence of sex differences in the response of the LDL particle size features to the MedDiet in dyslipidemic men and premenopausal women. Our results suggest that adhering to the MedDiet, in addition to a clinically-relevant reduction in LDL-C concentrations (−10.4% in men and −7.3% in women), also has additional positive effects on LDL particle size phenotype, leading to a favorable redistribution from smaller to larger LDL in men, but not in women. Moreover, men, but not women, with smaller LDL peak particle size at baseline (<255 Å) increase LDL peak particle size in response to the MedDiet. Since sdLDL has been suggested as a strong predictor of the progression of atherosclerosis and CVD events [7–9], such findings have implications, both for improved understanding of sex-specific mechanisms behind the beneficial cardiovascular effects of the MedDiet and for the clinical management of dyslipidemic men.

Acknowledgments: The authors would like to thank Johanne Marin for her valuable contribution in the laboratory. This research was supported by the Canadian Institutes of Health Research (Grant Number MOP 84568) and the Heart and Stroke Foundation of Quebec (Grant Number 2007-180). Alexandra Bédard is a recipient of a studentship from Canadian Institutes of Health Research.

Author Contributions: Simone Lemieux designed the research. Alexandra Bédard and Louise Corneau conducted the research. Sylvie Dodin supervised the medical condition of participants. Alexandra Bédard analyzed the data and wrote the paper. All authors participated to the analysis and interpretation of the data, revised the manuscript critically and approved the final manuscript.

Conflicts of Interest: The authors declare no conflict of interest. The Canadian Institutes of Health Research and the Heart and Stroke Foundation of Quebec had no role in the design of the study; in the collection, analyses or interpretation of data; in the writing of the manuscript; nor in the decision to publish the results.

References

1. Anderson, T.J.; Gregoire, J.; Hegele, R.A.; Couture, P.; Mancini, G.B.; McPherson, R.; Francis, G.A.; Poirier, P.; Lau, D.C.; Grover, S.; *et al.* 2012 update of the canadian cardiovascular society guidelines for the diagnosis and treatment of dyslipidemia for the prevention of cardiovascular disease in the adult. *Can. J. Cardiol.* **2013**, *29*, 151–167. Available online: http://www.ncbi.nlm.nih.gov/pubmed/23351925 (accessed on 23 March 2015). [CrossRef]
2. European Association for Cardiovascular Prevention and Rehabilitation; Reiner, Z.; Catapano, A.L.; de Backer, G.; Graham, I.; Taskinen, M.R.; Wiklund, O.; Agewall, S.; Alegria, E.; *et al.* ESC/EAS guidelines for the management of dyslipidaemias: The task force for the management of dyslipidaemias of the european society of cardiology (ESC) and the european atherosclerosis society (EAS). *Eur. Heart J.* **2011**, *32*, 1769–1818. Available online: http://www.ncbi.nlm.nih.gov/pubmed/21712404 (accessed on 23 March 2015). [CrossRef]
3. National Cholesterol Education Program (NCEP) Expert Panel on Detection, Evaluation, and Treatment of High Blood Cholesterol in Adults (Adult Treatment Panel III). Third report of the national cholesterol education program (NCEP) expert panel on detection, evaluation, and treatment of high blood cholesterol in adults (Adult Treatment Panel III) final report. *Circulation* **2002**, *106*, 3143–3421. Available online: http://www.ncbi.nlm.nih.gov/pubmed/12485966 (accessed on 23 March 2015).
4. Mikhailidis, D.P.; Elisaf, M.; Rizzo, M.; Berneis, K.; Griffin, B.; Zambon, A.; Athyros, V.; de Graaf, J.; Marz, W.; Parhofer, K.G.; *et al.* "European panel on low density lipoprotein (LDL) subclasses": A statement on the pathophysiology, atherogenicity and clinical significance of LDL subclasses. *Curr. Vasc. Pharmacol.* **2011**, *9*, 533–571. Available online: http://www.ncbi.nlm.nih.gov/pubmed/21595628 (accessed on 23 March 2015). [CrossRef]
5. Ishigaki, Y.; Oka, Y.; Katagiri, H. Circulating oxidized LDL: A biomarker and a pathogenic factor. *Curr. Opin. Lipidol.* **2009**, *20*, 363–369. Available online: http://www.ncbi.nlm.nih.gov/pubmed/19625960 (accessed on 23 March 2015). [CrossRef]
6. Mitra, S.; Goyal, T.; Mehta, J.L. Oxidized ldl, lox-1 and atherosclerosis. *Cardiovasc. Drugs Ther.* **2011**, *25*, 419–429. Available online: http://www.ncbi.nlm.nih.gov.acces.bibl.ulaval.ca/pubmed/21947818 (accessed on 29 April 2015). [CrossRef]
7. Hoogeveen, R.C.; Gaubatz, J.W.; Sun, W.; Dodge, R.C.; Crosby, J.R.; Jiang, J.; Couper, D.; Virani, S.S.; Kathiresan, S.; Boerwinkle, E.; *et al.* Small dense low-density lipoprotein-cholesterol concentrations predict risk for coronary heart disease: The atherosclerosis risk in communities (ARIC) study. *Arterioscler. Thromb. Vasc. Biol.* **2014**, *34*, 1069–1077. Available online: http://www.ncbi.nlm.nih.gov/pubmed/24558110 (accessed on 23 March 2015). [CrossRef]

8. Lamarche, B.; St-Pierre, A.C.; Ruel, I.L.; Cantin, B.; Dagenais, G.R.; Despres, J.P. A prospective, population-based study of low density lipoprotein particle size as a risk factor for ischemic heart disease in men. *Can. J. Cardiol.* **2001**, *17*, 859–865. Available online: http://www.ncbi.nlm.nih.gov/pubmed/11521128 (accessed on 23 March 2015).

9. Lamarche, B.; Tchernof, A.; Moorjani, S.; Cantin, B.; Dagenais, G.R.; Lupien, P.J.; Despres, J.P. Small, dense low-density lipoprotein particles as a predictor of the risk of ischemic heart disease in men. Prospective results from the quebec cardiovascular study. *Circulation* **1997**, *95*, 69–75. Available online: http://www.ncbi.nlm.nih.gov/pubmed/8994419 (accessed on 23 March 2015).

10. Nigon, F.; Lesnik, P.; Rouis, M.; Chapman, M.J. Discrete subspecies of human low density lipoproteins are heterogeneous in their interaction with the cellular LDL receptor. *J. Lipid Res.* **1991**, *32*, 1741–1753. Available online: http://www.ncbi.nlm.nih.gov/pubmed/1770294 (accessed on 23 March 2015).

11. Camejo, G.; Hurt-Camejo, E.; Wiklund, O.; Bondjers, G. Association of apo B lipoproteins with arterial proteoglycans: Pathological significance and molecular basis. *Atherosclerosis* **1998**, *139*, 205–222. Available online: http://www.ncbi.nlm.nih.gov/pubmed/9712326 (accessed on 23 March 2015). [CrossRef]

12. Bjornheden, T.; Babyi, A.; Bondjers, G.; Wiklund, O. Accumulation of lipoprotein fractions and subfractions in the arterial wall, determined in an *in vitro* perfusion system. *Atherosclerosis* **1996**, *123*, 43–56. Available online: http://www.ncbi.nlm.nih.gov/pubmed/8782836 (accessed on 23 March 2015).

13. De Graaf, J.; Hak-Lemmers, H.L.; Hectors, M.P.; Demacker, P.N.; Hendriks, J.C.; Stalenhoef, A.F. Enhanced susceptibility to *in vitro* oxidation of the dense low density lipoprotein subfraction in healthy subjects. *Arterioscler. Thromb.* **1991**, *11*, 298–306. Available online: http://www.ncbi.nlm.nih.gov/pubmed/1998647 (accessed on 23 March 2015). [CrossRef]

14. Vekic, J.; Zeljkovic, A.; Jelic-Ivanovic, Z.; Spasojevic-Kalimanovska, V.; Bogavac-Stanojevic, N.; Memon, L.; Spasic, S. Small, dense LDL cholesterol and apolipoprotein B: Relationship with serum lipids and LDL size. *Atherosclerosis* **2009**, *207*, 496–501. Available online: http://www.ncbi.nlm.nih.gov/pubmed/19632678 (accessed on 23 March 2015). [CrossRef]

15. Lemieux, I.; Pascot, A.; Lamarche, B.; Prud'homme, D.; Nadeau, A.; Bergeron, J.; Despres, J.P. Is the gender difference in LDL size explained by the metabolic complications of visceral obesity? *Eur. J. Clin. Investig.* **2002**, *32*, 909–917. Available online: http://www.ncbi.nlm.nih.gov/pubmed/12534450 (accessed on 23 March 2015). [CrossRef]

16. Li, Z.; McNamara, J.R.; Fruchart, J.C.; Luc, G.; Bard, J.M.; Ordovas, J.M.; Wilson, P.W.; Schaefer, E.J. Effects of gender and menopausal status on plasma lipoprotein subspecies and particle sizes. *J. Lipid Res.* **1996**, *37*, 1886–1896. Available online: http://www.ncbi.nlm.nih.gov/pubmed/8895054 (accessed on 23 March 2015).

17. Nikkila, M.; Pitkajarvi, T.; Koivula, T.; Solakivi, T.; Lehtimaki, T.; Laippala, P.; Jokela, H.; Lehtomaki, E.; Seppa, K.; Sillanaukee, P. Women have a larger and less atherogenic low density lipoprotein particle size than men. *Atherosclerosis* **1996**, *119*, 181–190. Available online: http://www.ncbi.nlm.nih.gov/pubmed/8808495 (accessed on 23 March 2015). [CrossRef]

18. Miller, A.A.; de Silva, T.M.; Jackman, K.A.; Sobey, C.G. Effect of gender and sex hormones on vascular oxidative stress. *Clin. Exp. Pharmacol. Physiol.* **2007**, *34*, 1037–1043. Available online: http://www.ncbi.nlm.nih.gov/pubmed/17714091 (accessed on 23 March 2015). [CrossRef]

19. Wu, T.; Willett, W.C.; Rifai, N.; Shai, I.; Manson, J.E.; Rimm, E.B. Is plasma oxidized low-density lipoprotein, measured with the widely used antibody 4E6, an independent predictor of coronary heart disease among U.S. Men and women? *J. Am. Coll. Cardiol.* **2006**, *48*, 973–979. Available online: http://www.ncbi.nlm.nih.gov/pubmed/16949489 (accessed on 23 March 2015). [CrossRef]

20. Estruch, R.; Ros, E.; Martinez-Gonzalez, M.A. Mediterranean diet for primary prevention of cardiovascular disease. *N. Eng. J. Med.* **2013**, *369*, 676–677. Available online: http://www.ncbi.nlm.nih.gov/pubmed/23944307 (accessed on 23 March 2015). [CrossRef]

21. Serra Majem, L.; Roman, B.; Estruch, R. Scientific evidence of interventions using the mediterranean diet: A systematic review. *Nutr. Rev.* **2006**, *64*, S27–S47. Available online: http://www.ncbi.nlm.nih.gov/pubmed/16532897 (accessed on 23 March 2015).

22. Delgado-Lista, J.; Perez-Martinez, P.; Garcia-Rios, A.; Perez-Caballero, A.I.; Perez-Jimenez, F.; Lopez-Miranda, J. Mediterranean diet and cardiovascular risk: Beyond traditional risk factors. *Crit. Rev. Food Sci. Nutr.* **2014**, in press. Available online: http://www.ncbi.nlm.nih.gov/pubmed/25118147 (accessed on 23 March 2015). [CrossRef]

23. Richard, C.; Couture, P.; Ooi, E.M.; Tremblay, A.J.; Desroches, S.; Charest, A.; Lichtenstein, A.H.; Lamarche, B. Effect of mediterranean diet with and without weight loss on apolipoprotein B100 metabolism in men with metabolic syndrome. *Arterioscler. Thromb. Vasc. Biol.* **2014**, *34*, 433–438. Available online: http://www.ncbi.nlm.nih.gov/pubmed/24265415 (accessed on 23 March 2015). [CrossRef]

24. Damasceno, N.R.; Sala-Vila, A.; Cofan, M.; Perez-Heras, A.M.; Fito, M.; Ruiz-Gutierrez, V.; Martinez-Gonzalez, M.A.; Corella, D.; Aros, F.; Estruch, R.; *et al.* Mediterranean diet supplemented with nuts reduces waist circumference and shifts lipoprotein subfractions to a less atherogenic pattern in subjects at high cardiovascular risk. *Atherosclerosis* **2013**, *230*, 347–353. Available online: http://www.ncbi.nlm.nih.gov/pubmed/24075767 (accessed on 23 March 2015). [CrossRef]

25. Jones, J.L.; Comperatore, M.; Barona, J.; Calle, M.C.; Andersen, C.; McIntosh, M.; Najm, W.; Lerman, R.H.; Fernandez, M.L. A mediterranean-style, low-glycemic-load diet decreases atherogenic lipoproteins and reduces lipoprotein (a) and oxidized low-density lipoprotein in women with metabolic syndrome. *Metabolism* **2012**, *61*, 366–372. Available online: http://www.ncbi.nlm.nih.gov/pubmed/21944261 (accessed on 23 March 2015). [CrossRef]

26. Lapointe, A.; Goulet, J.; Couillard, C.; Lamarche, B.; Lemieux, S. A nutritional intervention promoting the mediterranean food pattern is associated with a decrease in circulating oxidized LDL particles in healthy women from the quebec city metropolitan area. *J. Nutr.* **2005**, *135*, 410–415. Available online: http://www.ncbi.nlm.nih.gov/pubmed/15735071 (accessed on 23 March 2015).

27. Fito, M.; Guxens, M.; Corella, D.; Saez, G.; Estruch, R.; de la, T.R.; Frances, F.; Cabezas, C.; Lopez-Sabater, M.C.; Marrugat, J.; *et al.* Effect of a traditional mediterranean diet on lipoprotein oxidation: A randomized controlled trial. *Arch. Intern. Med.* **2007**, *167*, 1195–1203. Available online: http://www.ncbi.nlm.nih.gov/pubmed/17563030 (accessed on 23 March 2015). [CrossRef]

28. Goulet, J.; Lamarche, B.; Charest, A.; Nadeau, G.; Lapointe, A.; Desroches, S.; Lemieux, S. Effect of a nutritional intervention promoting the mediterranean food pattern on electrophoretic characteristics of low-density lipoprotein particles in healthy women from the quebec city metropolitan area. *Br. J. Nutr.* **2004**, *92*, 285–293. Available online: http://www.ncbi.nlm.nih.gov/pubmed/15333160 (accessed on 23 March 2015). [CrossRef]

29. Bedard, A.; Riverin, M.; Dodin, S.; Corneau, L.; Lemieux, S. Sex differences in the impact of the mediterranean diet on cardiovascular risk profile. *Br. J. Nutr.* **2012**, *108*, 1428–1434. Available online: http://www.ncbi.nlm.nih.gov/pubmed/22221517 (accessed on 23 March 2015). [CrossRef]

30. Bedard, A.; Corneau, L.; Lamarche, B.; Dodin, S.; Lemieux, S. Sex-related differences in the effects of the mediterranean diet on glucose and insulin homeostasis. *J. Nutr. Metab.* **2014**, *2014*, 424130. Available online: http://www.ncbi.nlm.nih.gov/pubmed/25371817 (accessed on 23 March 2015). [CrossRef]

31. Bedard, A.; Tchernof, A.; Lamarche, B.; Corneau, L.; Dodin, S.; Lemieux, S. Effects of the traditional mediterranean diet on adiponectin and leptin concentrations in men and premenopausal women: Do sex differences exist? *Eur. J. Clin. Nutr.* **2014**, *68*, 561–566. Available online: http://www.ncbi.nlm.nih.gov/pubmed/24595221 (accessed on 23 March 2015). [CrossRef]

32. Packard, C.; Caslake, M.; Shepherd, J. The role of small, dense low density lipoprotein (LDL): A new look. *Int. J. Cardiol.* **2000**, *74* (Suppl. 1), S17–S22. Available online: http://www.ncbi.nlm.nih.gov/pubmed/10856769 (accessed on 23 March 2015). [CrossRef]

33. Schaefer, E.J.; Foster, D.M.; Zech, L.A.; Lindgren, F.T.; Brewer, H.B., Jr.; Levy, R.I. The effects of estrogen administration on plasma lipoprotein metabolism in premenopausal females. *J. Clin. Endocrinol. Metab.* **1983**, *57*, 262–267. Available online: http://www.ncbi.nlm.nih.gov/pubmed/6408108 (accessed on 23 March 2015). [CrossRef]

34. Law, J.; Bloor, I.; Budge, H.; Symonds, M.E. The influence of sex steroids on adipose tissue growth and function. *Horm. Mol. Biol. Clin. Investig.* **2014**, *19*, 13–24. Available online: http://www.ncbi.nlm.nih.gov/pubmed/25390013 (accessed on 23 March 2015). [CrossRef]

35. Arias-Loza, P.A.; Muehlfelder, M.; Pelzer, T. Estrogen and estrogen receptors in cardiovascular oxidative stress. *Pflug. Arch.* **2013**, *465*, 739–746. Available online: http://www.ncbi.nlm.nih.gov/pubmed/23417608 (accessed on 23 March 2015). [CrossRef]

36. Carruba, G.; Granata, O.M.; Pala, V.; Campisi, I.; Agostara, B.; Cusimano, R.; Ravazzolo, B.; Traina, A. A traditional mediterranean diet decreases endogenous estrogens in healthy postmenopausal women. *Nutr. Cancer* **2006**, *56*, 253–259. Available online: http://www.ncbi.nlm.nih.gov/pubmed/17474873 (accessed on 23 March 2015). [CrossRef]

37. International Diabetes Federation. IDF Worldwide Definition of the Metabolic Syndrome. 2010. Available online: http://www.idf.org/webdata/docs/MetS_def_update2006.pdf (accessed on 23 March 2015).

38. Bird, K.D. Confidence intervals for effect sizes in analysis of variance. *Educ. Psychol. Meas.* 2002, 62, pp. 197–226. Available online: http://epm.sagepub.com/content/62/2/197.abstract (accessed on 23 March 2015). [CrossRef]

39. Health Canada. Eating Well with Canada's Food Guide. Available online: http://www.hc-sc.gc.ca/fn-an/food-guide-aliment/index-eng.php (accessed on 23 March 2015).

40. Goulet, J.; Lamarche, B.; Nadeau, G.; Lemieux, S. Effect of a nutritional intervention promoting the mediterranean food pattern on plasma lipids lipoproteins and body weight in healthy french-canadian women. *Atherosclerosis* 2003, 170, 115–124. Available online: http://www.ncbi.nlm.nih.gov/pubmed/12957689 (accessed on 23 March 2015). [CrossRef]

41. Leblanc, V.; Begin, C.; Hudon, A.M.; Royer, M.M.; Corneau, L.; Dodin, S.; Lemieux, S. Gender differences in the long-term effects of a nutritional intervention program promoting the mediterranean diet: Changes in dietary intakes, eating behaviors, anthropometric and metabolic variables. *Nutr. J.* **2014**, *13*, 107. Available online: http://www.ncbi.nlm.nih.gov.acces.bibl.ulaval.ca/pubmed/25416917 (accessed on 29 April 2015). [CrossRef]

42. Willett, W.C.; Sacks, F.; Trichopoulou, A.; Drescher, G.; Ferro-Luzzi, A.; Helsing, E.; Trichopoulos, D. Mediterranean diet pyramid: A cultural model for healthy eating. *Am. J. Clin. Nutr.* **1995**, *61*, 1402S–1406S. Available online: http://www.ncbi.nlm.nih.gov/pubmed/7754995 (accessed on 23 March 2015).

43. Kratz, M.; Gulbahce, E.; von Eckardstein, A.; Cullen, P.; Cignarella, A.; Assmann, G.; Wahrburg, U. Dietary mono- and polyunsaturated fatty acids similarly affect LDL size in healthy men and women. *J. Nutr.* **2002**, *132*, 715–718. Available online: http://www.ncbi.nlm.nih.gov/pubmed/11925466 (accessed on 23 March 2015).

44. Lamarche, B.; Desroches, S.; Jenkins, D.J.; Kendall, C.W.; Marchie, A.; Faulkner, D.; Vidgen, E.; Lapsley, K.G.; Trautwein, E.A.; Parker, T.L.; *et al.* Combined effects of a dietary portfolio of plant sterols, vegetable protein, viscous fibre and almonds on ldl particle size. *Br. J. Nutr.* **2004**, *92*, 657–663. Available online: http://www.ncbi.nlm.nih.gov/pubmed/15522135 (accessed on 23 March 2015). [CrossRef]

45. Kay, C.D.; Gebauer, S.K.; West, S.G.; Kris-Etherton, P.M. Pistachios increase serum antioxidants and lower serum oxidized-LDL in hypercholesterolemic adults. *J. Nutr.* **2010**, *140*, 1093–1098. Available online: http://www.ncbi.nlm.nih.gov/pubmed/20357077 (accessed on 23 March 2015). [CrossRef]

46. Avellone, G.; Di Garbo, V.; Campisi, D.; de Simone, R.; Raneli, G.; Scaglione, R.; Licata, G. Effects of moderate sicilian red wine consumption on inflammatory biomarkers of atherosclerosis. *Eur. J. Clin. Nutr.* **2006**, *60*, 41–47. Available online: http://www.ncbi.nlm.nih.gov/pubmed/16132058 (accessed on 23 March 2015). [CrossRef]

47. Goulet, J.; Nadeau, G.; Lapointe, A.; Lamarche, B.; Lemieux, S. Validity and reproducibility of an interviewer-administered food frequency questionnaire for healthy french-canadian men and women. *Nutr. J.* **2004**, *3*, 13. Available online: http://www.ncbi.nlm.nih.gov/pubmed/15363100 (accessed on 23 March 2015). [CrossRef]

48. Bouchard, C.; Tremblay, A.; Leblanc, C.; Lortie, G.; Savard, R.; Theriault, G. A method to assess energy expenditure in children and adults. *Am. J. Clin. Nutr.* **1983**, *37*, 461–467. Available online: http://www.ncbi.nlm.nih.gov.acces.bibl.ulaval.ca/pubmed/6829488 (accessed on 29 April 2015).

49. Muesing, R.A.; Forman, M.R.; Graubard, B.I.; Beecher, G.R.; Lanza, E.; McAdam, P.A.; Campbell, W.S.; Olson, B.R. Cyclic changes in lipoprotein and apolipoprotein levels during the menstrual cycle in healthy premenopausal women on a controlled diet. *J. Clin. Endocrinol. Metab.* **1996**, *81*, 3599–3603. Available online: http://www.ncbi.nlm.nih.gov/pubmed/8855808 (accessed on 23 March 2015). [CrossRef]

50. Friedewald, W.T.; Levy, R.I.; Fredrickson, D.S. Estimation of the concentration of low-density lipoprotein cholesterol in plasma, without use of the preparative ultracentrifuge. *Clin. Chem.* **1972**, *18*, 499–502. Available online: http://www.ncbi.nlm.nih.gov/pubmed/4337382 (accessed on 23 March 2015).

51. St Pierre, A.C.; Ruel, I.L.; Cantin, B.; Dagenais, G.R.; Bernard, P.M.; Despres, J.P.; Lamarche, B. Comparison of various electrophoretic characteristics of ldl particles and their relationship to the risk of ischemic heart disease. *Circulation* **2001**, *104*, 2295–2299. Available online: http://www.ncbi.nlm.nih.gov/pubmed/11696468 (accessed on 23 March 2015). [CrossRef]
52. Tchernof, A.; Lamarche, B.; Prud'Homme, D.; Nadeau, A.; Moorjani, S.; Labrie, F.; Lupien, P.J.; Despres, J.P. The dense LDL phenotype. Association with plasma lipoprotein levels, visceral obesity, and hyperinsulinemia in men. *Diabetes Care* **1996**, *19*, 629–637. Available online: http://www.ncbi.nlm.nih.gov/pubmed/8725863 (accessed on 23 March 2015).
53. Tzotzas, T.; Evangelou, P.; Kiortsis, D.N. Obesity, weight loss and conditional cardiovascular risk factors. *Obes Rev.* **2011**, *12*, e282–e289. Available online: http://www.ncbi.nlm.nih.gov/pubmed/21054756 (accessed on 23 March 2015). [CrossRef]
54. Reaven, P.D.; Grasse, B.J.; Tribble, D.L. Effects of linoleate-enriched and oleate-enriched diets in combination with alpha-tocopherol on the susceptibility of LDL and LDL subfractions to oxidative modification in humans. *Arterioscler. Thromb.* **1994**, *14*, 557–566. Available online: http://www.ncbi.nlm.nih.gov/pubmed/8148354 (accessed on 23 March 2015). [CrossRef]
55. Hadziabdic, M.O.; Bozikov, V.; Pavic, E.; Romic, Z. The antioxidative protecting role of the mediterranean diet. *Coll. Antropol.* **2012**, *36*, 1427–1434. Available online: http://www.ncbi.nlm.nih.gov.acces.bibl.ulaval.ca/pubmed/23390845 (accessed on 23 March 2015).

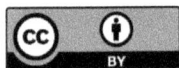

nutrients

MDPI

Article

Feasibility of Recruiting Families into a Heart Disease Prevention Program Based on Dietary Patterns

Tracy L. Schumacher [1,2,3], Tracy L. Burrows [1,2,3], Deborah I. Thompson [4], Neil J. Spratt [1,3,5,6], Robin Callister [1,2,3] and Clare E. Collins [1,2,3,*]

[1] Faculty of Health and Medicine, University of Newcastle, Callaghan, NSW 2308, Australia;
E-Mails: Tracy.Schumacher@uon.edu.au (T.L.S.); Tracy.Burrows@newcastle.edu.au (T.L.B.);
Neil.Spratt@newcastle.edu.au (N.J.S.); Robin.Callister@newcastle.edu.au (R.C.)

[2] Priority Research Centre in Physical Activity and Nutrition, University of Newcastle,
Callaghan, NSW 2308, Australia

[3] Hunter Medical Research Institute, New Lambton, NSW 2005, Australia

[4] USDA/ARS Children's Nutrition Research Centre, Baylor College of Medicine, Houston, TX 77030, USA;
E-Mail: dit@bcm.edu

[5] Priority Research Centre for Translational Neuroscience and Mental Health, University of Newcastle,
Callaghan, NSW 2308, Australia

[6] Hunter New England Local Health District, New Lambton, NSW 2305, Australia

* Author to whom correspondence should be addressed; E-Mail: Clare.Collins@newcastle.edu.au;
Tel.: +61-2491-5646; Fax: +61-24921-7053.

Received: 10 June 2015 / Accepted: 12 August 2015 / Published: 21 August 2015

Abstract: Offspring of parents with a history of cardiovascular disease (CVD) inherit a similar genetic profile and share diet and lifestyle behaviors. This study aimed to evaluate the feasibility of recruiting families at risk of CVD to a dietary prevention program, determine the changes in diet achieved, and program acceptability. Families were recruited into a pilot parallel group randomized controlled trial consisting of a three month evidence-based dietary intervention, based on the Mediterranean and Portfolio diets. Feasibility was assessed by recruitment and retention rates, change in diet by food frequency questionnaire, and program acceptability by qualitative interviews and program evaluation. Twenty one families were enrolled over 16 months, with fourteen families ($n = 42$ individuals) completing the study. Post-program dietary changes in the intervention group included small daily increases in vegetable serves (0.8 ± 1.3) and reduced usage of full-fat milk (-21%), cheese (-12%) and meat products (-17%). Qualitative interviews highlighted beneficial changes in food purchasing habits. Future studies need more effective methods of recruitment to engage families in the intervention. Once engaged, families made small incremental improvements in their diets. Evaluation indicated that feedback on diet and CVD risk factors, dietetic counselling and the resources provided were appropriate for a program of this type.

Keywords: cardiovascular diseases; diet; health education; prevention

1. Introduction

The World Health Organization reported that 17.5 million deaths were attributed to cardiovascular disease (CVD) in 2012 [1]. CVD risk factors include non-modifiable and modifiable factors, including genetic predisposition, metabolic conditions and lifestyle behaviors [2]. Offspring of parents with CVD are at increased risk due to shared genetic profiles and lifestyle behaviors [3]. In the Framingham Study, offspring with at least one parent with premature CVD had an increased age-adjusted risk of 2.3–2.6 (odds ratio) of developing CVD [4]. The Bogalusa study found that children with at least one parent with coronary artery disease (CAD) had a higher mean body mass index

(1.22 kg/m^2), total and LDL cholesterol (0.11 mmol/L, 0.14 mmol/L) and higher systolic blood pressure (1.63 mmHg) compared than children with no parental CAD [5].

Dietary patterns are an important lifestyle factor influencing the development of CVD [6,7]. Dietary patterns and eating habits are fostered within families, with younger family members modelling consumption patterns of older family members [3,8]. The Mediterranean diet is an eating pattern associated with lower risk of CVD [6], and the Portfolio diet has been shown to be efficacious in lowering CVD risk factors such as the ratio of total cholesterol to HDL cholesterol and serum triglycerides [9,10]. The Mediterranean diet is high in vegetables, fruit, nuts and olive oil with moderate intakes of fish [6]; the Portfolio diet combines foods with lipid-lowering efficacy such as soluble fibers, plant sterols and nuts [7]. Both these food-group based dietary patterns have been shown to be more effective in improving lipid profiles than diets that emphasize specific nutrient intakes such as low fat or cholesterol diets [11,12] and these food based approaches form the basis of current dietary guidelines for CVD prevention [13].

Families recruited into a dietary intervention study on the basis of one member having had an adverse CVD event, or being assessed as at high risk of CVD, may be more receptive to changing their diet. To test this hypothesis, the current study investigated: (1) the feasibility of recruiting and retaining families at increased risk of CVD into a dietary intervention program targeting alignment of existing eating patterns with heart health recommendations; (2) the dietary changes made; and (3) the acceptability of the dietary CVD prevention program.

2. Experimental Section

Families were eligible to participate in the "Love your Food, Love your Heart, Love your Family" (FHF) study if at least one member (index recruit aged 18–70 years) had experienced an adverse CVD event or was classified as being at moderate-to-high risk using Australian cardiovascular risk charts (aged 18–80 years) [14], had no other medical conditions affecting dietary intake, and had internet access. Written informed consent was obtained from all family members, with those < 18 years giving assent and having parental consent. Ethics approval was obtained from University of Newcastle Human Research Ethics Committee (H-2012-0246) and the Hunter New England Human Research Ethics Committee (HREC/12/HNE/140).

2.1. Study Design

The Protection Motivation Theory [15] proposes that health behaviors are the result of coping responses to perceived threats of vulnerability and severity. The theory posits that individuals look at the perceived benefits and usefulness of performing adaptive (helpful), and their confidence to perform them. Therefore, the intervention sought to capitalize on the awareness of personal risk, incorporate strategies to build self-efficacy for helpful tasks, and give meaningful feedback on performing the recommended strategies.

The study was a pilot parallel group randomized controlled trial. Participating families were stratified by sex of the index member, CVD event (stroke/ischemic heart condition) and time of event (≤6 months, >6 months) and randomized in blocks of six using QuickCalcs Software [16] to either the three-month intervention or feedback only control group, with assessors blinded to group allocation. Subjects received group assignment via the next available sealed envelope within their stratification.

Recruitment, baseline and follow-up assessments took place from December 2012 to May 2014. The intervention flow is summarized in Figure 1. After providing consent, families completed online questionnaires on demographics, medical history, smoking, and usual eating patterns. Fasting blood samples were analyzed for blood lipids prior to anthropometric assessments, and all individuals received a personalized feedback booklet containing lipid test results, anthropometric measures, and dietary intake analysis including macronutrient and micronutrient intakes and the percentage energy contributed by core (nutrient dense) and discretionary (energy-dense, nutrient-poor) foods. Randomization into intervention or control groups (feedback only) followed provision of the feedback booklet with those in the control group wait-listed for three months. Intervention group participants each received one 45-min dietary counselling session with an accredited practicing dietitian (APD). To ensure consistency of the intervention delivery, a resource booklet specific to the intervention and a semi-structured education session for the counselling were used, which allowed for modification of strategies to cater for families' unique needs. Participants were asked to increase their intake of specific foods to more closely align with targets. The dietary intake targets used in the current intervention included: up to two serves (60 g) of nuts per day; 2–3 daily serves (2–3 g) of plant sterols; up to five daily serves (15 g) of soluble fibers; up to seven daily (42 g) serves of soy proteins; 2–3 serves of fish per week (170–450 g, dependent on fish type); up to seven serves (approximately 650 g) of legumes/pulses/lentils per week. Unsaturated fats were promoted whilst reducing saturated fats, as well as low-sodium food choices and general healthy eating guidelines [17].

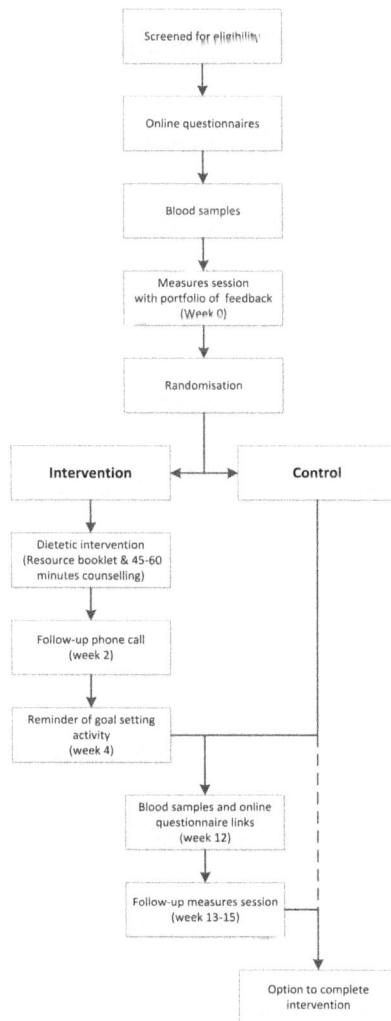

Figure 1. Intervention flow chart for study participants. Families randomized to the control group had the option of undergoing the intervention once the control period was completed.

2.2. Dietary Change Measures

Dietary intake was assessed as frequency of usual intake over the past six months using the validated Australian Eating Survey ($\geq$18 years) (AES) and Australian Child and Adolescent Eating Survey (ACAES), 120 item semi-quantitative food frequency questionnaires (FFQs) [18,19]. Nutrient intakes were computed using FoodWorks version 4.00.1158 [20] and the Australian AusNut 1999 nutrient database (All Foods, Revision 17) and AusFoods (Brands, Revision 5). Foods specific to the Mediterranean [6] and Portfolio diets [7] not included within the AES and ACAES were measured using a 72 question semi-quantitative FFQ that was specifically developed to assess intake of plant sterols, viscous fibers, soy proteins and provide specific details about fat type, sodium, legumes, nuts and fish intakes. The study-specific FFQ was comprised of 18 food habit questions and 35 intake questions with stated serve sizes aligned to the Australian Dietary Guidelines [21], Heart Foundation recommendations [22], or as natural portion sizes and 19 questions with portion size stated as "1 serving".

2.3. Qualitative Measures to Assess Feasibility, Dietary Changes and Program Acceptability

All adult family members completing the intervention were invited by post to participate in a semi-structured telephone interview. Areas of enquiry explored by interview included motivation to participate, barriers to healthy eating and dietary changes made. Individuals were interviewed by a female research team member (TS) 1–6 months (mean 1.5 months) post completion using a semi-structured discussion framework developed by the researchers. Probes and prompts were used to expand and clarify responses. The interviews were digitally recorded with the participants' consent and transcribed verbatim. A computer program (NVIVO 10) was used to assist with the organizational aspects of data analysis. Qualitative analyses were conducted by an independent experienced qualitative researcher who was not part of the research team to reduce bias and ensure accuracy of themes identified. All index participants were asked to complete a process evaluation questionnaire after completing the three-month intervention. Questions were in regards to the suggested foods and eating patterns, resources provided, changes in behavior and general feedback.

2.4. Other CVD Related Health Measures

Participants' height and weight were measured in light clothing to 0.1 cm and 0.1 kg, respectively using the Biospace BSM370 Automatic BMI Scale Stadiometer (Biospace Co. Ltd., Seoul, Korea). Waist circumference was measured at the narrowest point between the lower costal (10th rib) border and the top of the iliac crest using a non-extensible steel tape (KDFS10-02, KDS Corporation, Osaka, Japan). Brachial and central blood pressure and arterial stiffness measures (augmentation index) were obtained with the Pulsecor Cardioscope II (Pulsecor Ltd., Auckland, New Zealand) using WelchAllyn FlexiPort reusable blood pressure cuffs. Participants were seated for five minutes before the first measurement occurred, and repeat measures were taken at two-minute intervals. Participants under the age of 18 years were also provided with a familiarization trial measure to reduce potential anxiety associated with this measurement. Physical activity in adults was assessed using the International Physical Activity Questionnaire long form (IPAQ) for the previous seven days.

Blood samples were assayed for markers of insulin resistance, inflammation and blood lipid concentrations (see Table 1) from adult family members after an overnight fast by trained phlebotomists and analyzed at a single accredited (National Association of Testing Authorities) pathology service.

Table 1. Baseline characteristics of the Love your food, Love your heart, Love your family study participants, inclusive of 15 families, presented as mean ± standard deviation, except where indicated.

	Children (<18 years)	Adults		All adults
	100% Female (*n* = 3)	Males (*n* = 20)	Females (*n* = 21)	(*n* = 41, 100%)
Age (years) median (p25–p75)	12.9 (7.9–16.7)	59.4 (46.0–67.8)	56.6 (42.7–64.0)	59.0 (42.7–66.5)
Height (cm)	151.1 ± 22.0	174.8 ± 6.1	162.8 ± 6.2	168.6 + 8.6
Weight (kg)	41.9 ± 15.1	87.7 ± 15.6	75.9 ± 18.9	81.6 ± 18.2
BMI (kg/m^2)	17.8 ± 2.1	28.7 + 5.1	28.6 ± 7.2	28.7 ± 6.2
Waist (cm)	60.7 ± 6.5	99.5 ± 15.1	86.9 ± 12.2	93.1 ± 14.9
	Brachial BP (mmHg)			
systolic	100.3 ± 7.4 [a]	121.3 ± 15.6	114.3 ± 15.0	117.7 ± 15.5
diastolic	63.5 ± 7.1 [a]	71.8 ± 6.7	71.7 ± 7.8	71.7 ± 7.2
	Central BP (mmHg)			
systolic	91.8 ± 7.4 [a]	114.1 ± 16.2	109.0 ± 14.7	111.5 ± 15.5
diastolic	65.0 ± 6.0 [a]	73.5 ± 7.0	72.8 ± 7.9	73.1 ± 7.4
Arterial stiffness	43 ± 11 [a]	75 ± 34	86 ± 35	81 ± 35
	Level of physical activity [b]			
Low	N/A	10% (*n* = 2)	19% (*n* = 4)	15% (*n* = 6)
Moderate	N/A	60% (*n* = 12)	62% (*n* = 13)	61% (*n* = 25)
High	N/A	30% (*n* = 6)	19% (*n* = 4)	24% (*n* = 10)
	Smoking status			
Current	N/A	*n* = 2 (10%)	*n* = 0 (0%)	*n* = 2 (5%)
Previous	N/A	*n* = 4 (20%)	*n* = 7 (33%)	*n* = 11 (27%)
	Blood biomarkers			
Triglycerides (mmol/L)	N/A	1.3 ± 0.6	1.4 ± 0.9	1.3 ± 0.8
TC (mmol/L)	N/A	4.5 ± 1.1	5.3 ± 1.1	4.9 ± 1.2
LDL (mmol/L)	N/A	2.7 ± 1.1	3.3 ± 1.1	3.0 ± 1.1
HDL (mmol/L)	N/A	1.2 ± 0.3	1.5 ± 0.3	1.3 ± 0.4
Total: HDL ratio	N/A	3.9 ± 1.5	3.8 ± 1.0	3.9 ± 1.2
BGL (mmol/L)	N/A	5.0 ± 0.5	5.2 ± 0.8	5.1 ± 0.6
Insulin (IU/L)	N/A	8.8 ± 4.6	7.0 ± 3.4	7.9 ± 4.1
hsCRP (mg/L)	N/A	3.0 ± 3.4	2.4 ± 2.4	2.7 ± 2.9
ALT (U/L)	N/A	32.6 ± 10.8	22.5 ± 16.1	27.4 ± 14.5
AST (U/L)	N/A	30.0 ± 8.4	27.4 ± 25.8	28.7 ± 19.2
GGT (U/L)	N/A	28.0 ± 16.4	25.7 ± 25.6	26.8 ± 21.4

Abbreviations: BMI—Body mass index; Waist—waist circumference; BP—blood pressure; TC—total cholesterol; LDL—LDL cholesterol; HDL—HDL cholesterol; BGL—blood glucose level; hsCRP—high sensitivity C-Reactive Protein; [a] *n* = 2; [b] As categorized by the International Physical Activity Questionnaire.

Recruitment and retention data were measured as those enrolling and completing the intervention and by qualitative interview. Changes in dietary intakes, as measured by FFQ, are presented as mean ± standard deviation for normally distributed data and median (p25–p75) for non-normal data. An intention-to-treat analysis was used with last observation carried forward for missing data. As this was a feasibility trial, power calculations were not performed. Dietary intake themes from qualitative interviews were reported. Results for acceptability of the prevention program are summarized from program evaluation questionnaires.

3. Results

3.1. Study Participants

Twenty-one index participants enrolled with their families, totaling 59 participants across three generations. Fifteen families were retained until randomization, consisting of 41 adults and three children (Figure 2). Of the 39 adults who completed the main study, 16 adults from eight families (41%) plus one child who turned 18 during the study participated in qualitative interviews (age range 18–70 years, 47% male). Five index participants were interviewed and one other had a diagnosed CVD condition. The interviews indicated participant motivations to join the study included a long-term interest in improving diet, a desire to make positive changes in eating habits and health for self and extended family, and having existing heart health issues. Individual participants identified a key family member who drove their family's involvement, who was not necessarily the person with a CVD diagnosis.

Characteristics of the participants are summarized in Table 1. Sixteen participants (39%) reported knowing they had elevated serum cholesterol levels, with 18 (44%) taking lipid lowering medication. Twelve reported having high blood pressure (29%), with 17 (41%) on medication for this condition. Twelve (29%) had arthritis, with six taking medication (15%) and one had type 2 diabetes (medicated). Eleven of the 15 index recruits had experienced a prior CVD event; nine had been advised to attend cardiac rehabilitation, with seven having attending.

3.2. Feasibility of Recruiting and Retaining Families

Recruitment using a variety of methods (Figure 2) resulted in 51 index participants being assessed for eligibility over 16 months. Of 51 inquiries, 16 were not eligible and 14 did not return consent forms with the majority of those not returning consent forms recruited from cardiac rehabilitation and stroke units (*n* = 6) (Figure 2). Highest enrolment rates came from word-of-mouth (50%). Retention rates were highest (nine eligible, nine consented, seven completions) among those recruited from the Hunter Medical Research Institute volunteer register and media releases, and lowest among those recruited from cardiac rehabilitation classes or stroke units (11 eligible, five consents, two completions).

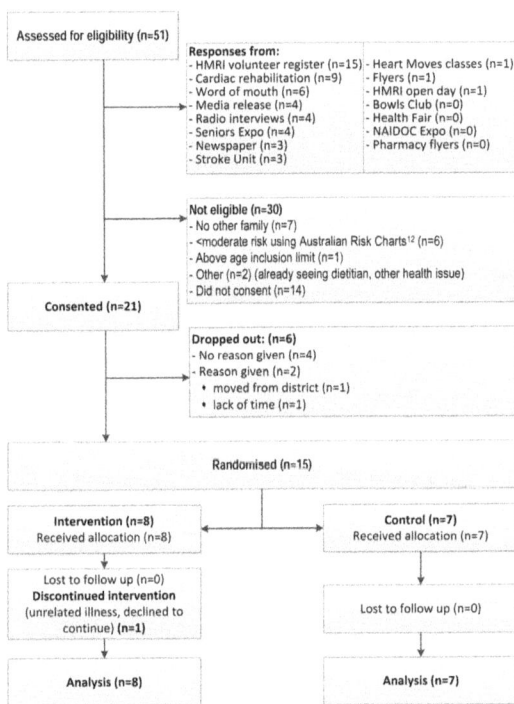

Figure 2. Flow chart showing the recruitment strategies used and number of participants assessed for eligibility and study retention.

Nutrients **2015**, *7*, 7042–7057

3.3. Nature and Extent of Dietary Changes Made

Baseline dietary intakes indicate that 63 ± 10% of energy came from nutritious, low energy-density (core) foods and 37 ± 10% from energy-dense, nutrient-poor (discretionary) foods. There was no difference in reported total energy intake at baseline between the adults or children completing the study and those who did not ($p = 0.34$ and $p = 0.32$ respectively). Analysis of dietary intakes and key components of the Mediterranean and Portfolio Diets are summarized in Table 2. Mean time between baseline and follow up was 4.5 months (±1.1). Table 3 summarizes foods habits relating to CVD health and highlights reductions in full-fat types of dairy and meat products usually eaten in the intervention group. Results at three-month follow up indicate that both groups made changes to their dietary intakes. The proportion of energy from core food groups showed improvement, as did daily vegetable intakes (Table 2).

Table 2. Baseline and follow-up dietary intakes as assessed by the Australian Eating Survey (AES), Australian Child and Adolescent Eating Survey (ACAES) and additional food frequency questionnaire assessing foods specific to the Mediterranean and Portfolio diets. Data presented as mean ± standard deviation for 15 families.

	Baseline				Follow up			
	Children	Adults			Children	Adults		
	(n = 3)	Adults (n = 41)	C (n = 18)	I (n = 23)	(n = 3)	Adults (n = 41)	C (n = 18)	I (n = 23)
Energy (kJ)	9967 ± 1619	10108 ± 2873	9582 ± 3197	10520 ± 2589	9565 ± 1942	9604 ± 261	9253 ± 2878	9878 ± 2509
PE core foods (%)	57 ± 23	63 ± 10	66 ± 14	61 ± 6	63 ± 7	66 ± 11	68 ± 13	64 ± 9
PE discretionary foods (%)	43 ± 23	37 ± 10	34 ± 14	39 ± 6	37 ± 7	34 ± 11	32 ± 13	36 ± 9
PE protein (%)	20 ± 8	19 ± 4	21 ± 5	18 ± 2	20 ± 3	19 ± 3	21 ± 4	18 ± 2
PE CHO (%)	43 ± 8	44 ± 8	40 ± 8	47 ± 5	46 ± 8	43 ± 7	39 ± 7	47 ± 6
PE fats (%)	38 ± 1	33 ± 4	34 ± 4	32 ± 4	35 ± 7	33 ± 5	35 ± 6	31 ± 3
PE sat. fats (%)	18 ± 2	13 ± 2	14 ± 2	13 ± 2	15 ± 4	13 ± 2	14 ± 2	13 ± 2
Fiber (g)	25 ± 8	29 ± 11	28 ± 13	30 ± 8	27 ± 9	30 ± 9	27 ± 8	32 ± 9
Sodium (mg)	2067 ± 402	2321 ± 679	2197 ± 614	2418 ± 724	2067 ± 244	2259 ± 671	2275 ± 715	2246 ± 650
Fruit/day	2.0 ± 1.1	2.0 ± 1.7	1.8 ± 2.1	2.2 ± 1.3	2.4 ± 1.6	1.9 ± 1.1	1.5 ± 0.7	2.2 ± 1.2
Vegetables/day	4.6 ± 1.2	4.9 ± 2.1	5.2 ± 2.2	4.7 ± 2.1	4.3 ± 0.4	5.5 ± 1.7	5.6 ± 1.7	5.4 ± 1.7
ARFS [a]	28 ± 8	35 ± 10	35 ± 8	35 ± 12	29 ± 6	39 ± 5	37 ± 5	39 ± 9
Frequency of foods specific to cardiovascular health (number of serves per day)								
Fat from added sources								
Saturated	N/A	0.3 ± 0.5	0.3 ± 0.7	0.2 ± 0.3	N/A	0.3 ± 0.7	0.5 ± 0.9	0.2 ± 0.3
Unsaturated	N/A	1.3 ± 0.8	1.4 ± 0.9	1.1 ± 0.8	N/A	1.2 ± 0.8	1.3 ± 0.9	1.1 ± 0.8
Nuts	0.2 ± 0.3	0.5 ± 0.6	0.5 ± 0.6	0.5 ± 0.5	1.1 ± 1.6	1.0 ± 1.1	0.9 ± 0.9	1.1 ± 1.2
Fish	0.3 ± 0.4	0.4 ± 0.5	0.5 ± 0.6	0.3 ± 0.3	0.5 ± 0.7	0.4 ± 0.3	0.5 ± 0.4	0.4 ± 0.3
Soy proteins	0.4 ± 0.7	0.1 ± 0.3	0.2 ± 0.4	0.1 ± 0.2	0.2 ± 0.3	0.2 ± 0.4	0.1 ± 0.3	0.3 ± 0.4
Legumes	0.1 ± 0.1	0.3 ± 0.4	0.3 ± 0.3	0.2 ± 0.5	1.2 ± 1.9	0.5 ± 0.7	0.7 ± 0.9	0.4 ± 0.5
Viscous fibers	0.2 ± 0.2	0.7 ± 0.7	0.7 ± 0.8	0.6 ± 0.6	0.3 ± 0.5	0.7 ± 0.7	0.4 ± 0.6	0.9 ± 0.8
Plant sterols	N/A	0.9 ± 1.1	1.2 ± 1.4	0.6 ± 0.9	N/A	0.7 ± 0.0	0.3 ± 0.7	1.0 ± 1.2

Abbreviations: C—Control group; I—Intervention group; N/A—Not assessed; PE—Percentage energy; ARFS—Australian Recommended Food Score; [a] measure of dietary variety.

Nutrients 2015, 7, 7042–7057

Table 3. Reported eating habits of foods related to cardiovascular disease (CVD) health.

	Baseline			Follow up		
	All (n = 44)	C (n = 20)	I (n = 24)	All (n = 44)	C (n = 20)	I (n = 24)
Type of milk normally consumed						
Don't drink milk	7%	0%	13%	7%	0%	13%
Normal	25%	15%	33%	14%	15%	13%
Reduced fat	32%	30%	33%	43%	40%	46%
Skim	32%	50%	17%	34%	40%	29%
Other	5%	5%	4%	2%	5%	0%
Type of cheese normally eaten						
Don't eat this	7%	5%	8%	7%	5%	8%
Normal	55%	40%	67%	45%	45%	46%
Reduced fat	34%	55%	17%	32%	30%	33%
Low fat	2%	0%	4%	14%	15%	12%
Not sure	2%	0%	4%	2%	5%	0%
Type of meat						
Don't eat this	2%	5%	0%	5%	10%	0%
Normal	55%	65%	46%	45%	65%	29%
Reduced fat	30%	10%	46%	39%	15%	58%
Low fat	11%	15%	8%	11%	10%	13%
Not sure	2%	5%	0%	0%	0%	0%
Type of chicken						
Don't eat this	7%	5%	8%	7%	5%	8%
Fried	2%	0%	4%	0%	0%	0%
Crumbed	9%	5%	13%	7%	10%	4%
With skin	32%	40%	25%	25%	25%	25%
Skin removed	45%	45%	46%	55%	55%	54%
Not sure	5%	5%	4%	7%	5%	8%
Adding of salt to food						
Never add salt	25%	25%	25%	16%	15%	17%
During cooking	32%	35%	29%	36%	45%	29%
To meals	27%	30%	25%	25%	15%	33%
Both meals & cooking	14%	5%	21%	20%	20%	21%
Not sure	2%	5%	0%	2%	5%	0%
Take away per week *						
None	9%	15%	4%	11%	15%	8%
<once per week	48%	45%	50%	57%	50%	62%
1–2 per week	36%	25%	46%	30%	30%	29%
3–4 per week	7%	15%	0%	2%	5%	0%
>4 per week	0%	0	0%	0%	0%	0%

Abbreviations: C—Control group; I—Intervention group; * Take away described as chinese, fish and chips, hamburgers and chips/fries, pizza.

223

Results from the qualitative interviews indicate that prior to program involvement 14 of 17 participants rated the healthiness of their diet subjectively as 6–7 on an alpha-numeric rating scale, where 10 represents the most healthy. Only two participants rated their pre-study diets as below average at three out of 10. Participants appeared to use a cognitive balancing of 'good' *versus* 'bad' aspects of their diet to justify their ratings of their usual intake pre-study. Dietary habits they acknowledged as reducing their 'healthiness rating' included the consumption of fatty meats, low vegetable intakes, and snacking on sugary foods between meals. Dietary habits perceived as increasing their 'healthiness rating' were cutting back on red meat by eating chicken and fish, and exercising 'dietary moderation' described as 'nothing in excess'. These habits were perceived by some as making their diet healthier relative to a subjective 'average' to which they mentally compared their intakes. Although almost a third of participants acknowledged little change to the healthiness of their diet post-study due to persistence of major barriers (e.g., partner reluctance, personal preference and taste), the majority reported having made permanent changes to their dietary intake and food habits. Some households reported a subjective rating improvement of 2–3 out of 10 post-program participation, suggesting substantial changes were made.

These improvements were attributed to increased knowledge and awareness due to program participation and appeared to inspire greater experimentation with healthier options and purchasing of foods reflecting increased variety and nutritional quality.

"I decided I would make a lovely rice dish, and I put in some slivered almonds and a couple of herbs and some garlic and it was lovely, and a little bit of soy sauce...I think the main thing is, after this study, was just variety. Like, if I was to make a rice dish before that I wouldn't have thought to add in nuts."

Further examples of dietary improvements given were less impulsive food shopping, more variety in fruit and vegetable selection, lower sugar and fat options, use of legumes, lentils and soy products, healthier meat options, and elimination of energy-dense, nutrient-poor foods. For all participants, including those reporting little or no change in their diet post-study, involvement in the project appeared to have increased awareness of the different components of their diet. Examples given included the proportion of energy from discretionary foods, foods with a healthy heart tick, the healthiness of different types of fat, an increased awareness of processed foods and the importance of small changes. Indeed, one participant who only reported slight changes in his diet following the study described the cumulative impact of these small changes as evidence of a shift in his food behaviors and preferences:

"I just cut out more of the bad stuff, like I'm sort of thinking it was only marginal changes I made. Look when I ate poorly like snacks and things like that, I'd probably eat too much. Whereas when I have a snack or a treat now, actually I find that I can't eat as much anyway of it. I think my taste buds have changed a little bit. But again from the converse side of things, previously when I probably didn't eat as much good food. I'm eating more good food now...It's just those marginal shifts."

3.4. Acceptability of Program to Align Current Eating Patterns with Recommendations

Eleven of the 15 index participants (73%) returned program evaluation forms. These participants all agreed or strongly agreed that this type of diet was relevant to them, but they had mixed responses regarding the ease of integration into their lives (55% positive, 18% negative, 27% neutral). Six (55%) felt it impacted negatively on grocery costs. Ten participants (91%) agreed or strongly agreed they would recommend this type of eating pattern to people in a similar situation ($n = 1$ neutral). Ten (91%) found the resource booklet easy to read and the information easy to understand, with the remainder ($n = 1$) answering neutral to both questions. Nine of the eleven participants (82%) read the booklet 2–3 or $\geqslant 3$ times, with two participants (18%) reading it once. The individualized feedback booklets were similarly valued with eight participants (73%) reading it 2–3 or $\geqslant 3$ times and three participants (27%) reading it once.

4. Discussion

The current study investigated whether families could be recruited and retained in a family CVD prevention program that was based on the Mediterranean and Portfolio eating patterns. Recruitment was challenging, with only 15 of 35 eligible families who initially expressed interest, engaging with the study through to the randomization stage. However, once randomized, the majority of these families completed the intervention. Those responding to media releases about the study and volunteer register invitations were more likely to be retained. Of interest is that amongst those families completing the trial, a key family member was found to drive the involvement and retention of the family. While overall dietary patterns were unaltered, participants made small, but incremental dietary changes, such as reducing discretionary foods and selecting fat-reduced versions of milk and cheese and fat-trimmed meats. Participants reported an increased awareness of their food habits and knowledge of food following the personalized dietary counselling they received from the study dietitian about their usual food and nutrient intakes. Evaluation of the program found that although participants noted some negatives, such as increases in grocery costs, these may have been offset by reductions in costs associated with takeaway foods. Evaluation of food costs in future studies is required. Participants used the resources and dietary feedback provided on multiple occasions and reported they would recommend the program to others in a similar situation.

A clear barrier to recruitment occurred between confirming eligibility of the index participant and the returning of consent forms from the family group, as shown by the limited number of returned consents ($n = 14$) at this stage. This suggests that persuading a family member to participate was a substantial barrier. An additional seven interested participants were deemed ineligible because they could not identify a family member to accompany them in the study. A larger Canadian family-based study had a similar focus, but recruited at-risk family members ($n = 126$) through in-patients from a tertiary care cardiac center [23]. While this study was able to randomize a greater proportion of their eligible participants, it had a 26% loss to follow-up. Recruiting using these methods may capitalize on a teachable moment, and lead to a change in lifestyle intentions [24], but does not necessarily imply a willingness to make permanent lifestyle changes amongst family members.

The lack of perceived CVD risk amongst those with actual increased risk is a significant barrier to program uptake as identified in the current study. The Protection Motivation Theory, on which the current study is based, identifies that a perception of risk must be present before any change in behavior can occur [15]. However, risk of CVD events is often poorly perceived by those with a confirmed family history of CVD, and may not be sufficient to change or act on intentions suggesting other motivators are required [25]. In the current study, some individuals lacked understanding of their medical risk factors, evidenced by the large proportion who were currently taking medications for lipid lowering or blood pressure control, but who did not identify when asked whether they had these conditions or any medical problems. Addressing appropriate awareness and management of risk is likely to be an important component in engaging people in CVD prevention programs. Future studies should consider identifying and engaging a key family member capable of influencing other family members. The recruitment approach for this study used the index person as the primary contact for the family in the first instance, but it may have been more advantageous to allow a key family member to engage on behalf of the high-risk participant.

The dietary components of this study were modelled on the Mediterranean and portfolio eating patterns as these have been shown to be efficacious in reducing CVD risk. Participants commencing the study reported dietary patterns that did not align well to these eating patterns and had higher than recommended intakes of discretionary food choices. Comparison of the dietary intakes of participants in the current study to data from the 2011–2012 Australian Health Survey (AHS) [26] indicates that this group were consuming higher energy intakes compared to the national average of 8672 kJ (value also obtained from 24-h recall), both before and after the intervention, while the proportion of energy from discretionary food choices was similar at 34.6% of total energy for adults. The macro-nutrient contributions appeared unchanged by the intervention and appears comparable to the national average, although small differences can be seen between the control and intervention groups. There was no apparent change in saturated fat intakes as analyzed by the FFQ, although questions on dietary habits (Table 3) indicate that saturated fat may have been decreased through the choosing of different cuts of meats. Within both this study and in a study of 426 family members of coronary artery disease patients by Reid *et al.* [23], participants were only able to make small increases in intakes of vegetables, showing this to be an area to be addressed in future work. Individually tailored dietary counselling immediately after personal dietary and risk biomarker feedback in the current study resulted in favorable changes in terms of selecting lower fat dairy products and fat-trimmed meat products, which may be due to capitalizing on the teachable moment the personalized feedback helped to facilitate. A possible strategy to enhance adherence in future studies includes the provision of feedback in an educational context, based on measured anthropometrics and blood lipids at an interim stage following initial dietary modifications, instead of at the end of the study as given here which may have increased motivation. Participants were contacted by a single telephone call during the three months follow-up period to discuss any difficulties they had encountered and to encourage maintenance of dietary changes made. This level of engagement was chosen and was comparable to a longer study by Jenkins *et al.* [27], which showed that more intensive follow-up did not greatly improve adherence in this type of diet.

The limitations of the current study include the recruitment of a small non-representative sample of families who volunteered. There may have been a seasonality bias influencing the reported dietary intakes impacting on both the control and intervention groups. The dietary modifications made may not be sufficient to show clinically important and statistically significant changes in serum lipids in the short term, but may benefit the individuals if continued long term [28] and a larger study with longer follow-up would be needed to evaluate this.

5. Conclusions

While the goal of primary prevention is to avert disease in high-risk individuals, the current study highlights there is little motivation to participate in CVD prevention programs when risk is poorly perceived and therefore insufficient to prompt behavior change. The program structure in the current study demonstrated promising results, but the challenges of recruitment need to be overcome. Once engaged, families were willing and able to make small incremental change in their dietary choices associated with CVD risk reduction in the long-term. Further research is needed to identify CVD-related motivators of dietary change, particularly those that engage individuals and have the ability to engage all family members in improving health behaviors.

Acknowledgments: The project received financial support by the Hunter Medical Research Institute (Grant number: HMRI 11-10). Author N.J.S. was supported by an Australian National Health & Medical Research Council Career Development Fellowship (APP1035465). The researchers wish to acknowledge Vibeke Hanson for the analysis of qualitative data and the support of the HMRI Research Volunteer Register for their assistance in participant recruitment.

Author Contributions: Authors T.L.S., T.L.B., D.I.T., N.J.S., R.C. and C.E.C. conceived and designed the experiments, T.L.S. performed the intervention, analyzed the descriptive data and drafted the initial manuscript. All authors revised and approved the final manuscript.

Conflicts of Interest: Author C.E.C. received an honoraria as a member of the Novo Nordisk Obesity Advisory Board. All authors declare no other conflicts of interest.

References

1. World Health Organization. *Global Status Report on Noncommunicable Dieases 2014*; World Health Organization: Geneva, Switzerland, 2015.
2. World Health Organization. *Global Atlas on Cardiovascular Disease Prevention and Control*; World Health Organization: Geneva, Switzerland, 2011.
3. Kral, T.V.E.; Rauh, E.M. Eating behaviors of children in the context of their family environment. *Physiol. Behav.* **2010**, *100*, 567–573. [CrossRef] [PubMed]

4.   Lloyd-Jones, D.M.; Nam, B.H.; D'Agostino, R.B., Sr.; Levy, D.; Murabito, J.M.; Wang, T.J.; Wilson, P.W.; O'Donnell, C.J. Parental cardiovascular disease as a risk factor for cardiovascular disease in middle-aged adults: A prospective study of parents and offspring. *JAMA* **2004**, *291*, 2204–2211. [CrossRef] [PubMed]

5.   Bao, W.; Srinivasan, S.R.; Valdez, R.; Greenlund, K.J.; Wattigney, W.A.; Berenson, G.S. Longitudinal changes in cardiovascular risk from childhood to young adulthood in offspring of parents with coronary artery disease: The Bogalusa heart study. *JAMA* **1997**, *278*, 1749–1754. [CrossRef] [PubMed]

6.   Estruch, R.; Ros, E.; Salas-Salvadó, J.; Covas, M.I.; Corella, D.; Arós, F.; Gómez-Gracia, E.; Ruiz-Gutiérrez, V.; Fiol, M.; Lapetra, J.; *et al.* Primary prevention of cardiovascular disease with a mediterranean diet. *N. Engl. J. Med.* **2013**, *368*, 1279–1290. [CrossRef] [PubMed]

7.   Jenkins, D.J.A.; Josse, A.R.; Wong, J.M.W.; Nguyen, T.H.; Kendall, C.W.C. The portfolio diet for cardiovascular risk reduction. *Curr. Atheroscler. Rep.* **2007**, *9*, 501–507. [CrossRef] [PubMed]

8.   Pachucki, M.A.; Jacques, P.F.; Christakis, N.A. Social network concordance in food choice among spouses, friends, and siblings. *Am. J. Public Health* **2011**, *101*, 2170–2177. [CrossRef] [PubMed]

9.   Jenkins, D.J.A.; Chiavaroli, L.; Wong, J.M.W.; Kendall, C.; Lewis, G.F.; Vidgen, E.; Connelly, P.W.; Leiter, L.A.; Josse, R.G.; Lamarche, B. Adding monounsaturated fatty acids to a dietary portfolio of cholesterol-lowering foods in hypercholesterolemia. *Can. Med. Assoc. J.* **2010**, *182*, 1961–1967. [CrossRef] [PubMed]

10. Jenkins, D.J.A.; Kendall, C.W.C.; Faulkner, D.A.; Nguyen, T.; Kemp, T.; Marchie, A.; Wong, J.M.W.; de Souza, R.; Emam, A.; Vidgen, E.; *et al.* Assessment of the longer-term effects of a dietary portfolio of cholesterol-lowering foods in hypercholesterolemia. *Am. J. Clin. Nutr.* **2006**, *83*, 582–591. [PubMed]

11. Dalen, J.E.; Devries, S. Diets to prevent coronary heart disease 1957–2013: What have we learned? *Am. J. Med.* **2014**, *127*, 364–369. [CrossRef] [PubMed]

12. Huang, J.; Frohlich, J.; Ignaszewski, A.P. The impact of dietary changes and dietary supplements on lipid profile. *Can. J. Cardiol.* **2011**, *27*, 488–505. [CrossRef] [PubMed]

13. Anderson, T.J.; Grégoire, J.; Hegele, R.A.; Couture, P.; Mancini, G.B.J.; McPherson, R.; Francis, G.A.; Poirier, P.; Lau, D.C.; Grover, S.; *et al.* 2012 update of the Canadian cardiovascular society guidelines for the diagnosis and treatment of dyslipidemia for the prevention of cardiovascular disease in the adult. *Can. J. Cardiol.* **2013**, *29*, 151–167. [CrossRef] [PubMed]

14. National Heart Foundation of Australia (National Blood Pressure and Vascular Disease Advisory Committee). *Guide to Management of Hypertension 2008. Updated December 2010*; National Heart Foundation: Melbourne, Australia, 2010.

15. Armitage, C.J.; Conner, M. Social cognition models and health behaviour: A structured review. *Psychol. Health* **2000**, *15*, 173–189. [CrossRef]

16. GraphPad Software Inc. Quickcalcs. Available online: http://graphpad.com/quickcalcs/random N1.cfm (accessed on 12 December 2012).

17. NHMRC, Australian Government. Australian Guide to Healthy Eating. Available online: http://www.eatforhealth.gov.au/guidelines/australian-guide-healthy-eating (accessed on 3 November 2014).

18. Collins, C.E.; Boggess, M.M.; Watson, J.F.; Guest, M.; Duncanson, K.; Pezdirc, K.; Rollo, M.; Hutchesson, M.J.; Burrows, T.L. Reproducibility and comparative validity of a food frequency questionnaire for australian adults. *Clin. Nutr.* **2014**, *33*, 906–914. [CrossRef] [PubMed]

19. Watson, J.F.; Collins, C.E.; Sibbritt, D.W.; Dibley, M.J.; Garg, M.L. Reproducibility and comparative validity of a food frequency questionnaire for australian children and adolescents. *Int. J. Behav. Nutr. Phys. Act.* **2009**, *6*, 17. [CrossRef] [PubMed]

20. *Xyris Software, version 4.00.1158*; Xyris Software Foodworks: Kenmore Hills, WA, Australia, 2005.

21. Department of Health and Aging, National Health and Medical Research Council, Australian Government. *Australian Dietary Guidelines*; National Health and Medical Research Council: Canberra, Australia, 2013.

22. National Heart Foundation of Australia. *Fish, Fish Oils, n-3 Polyunsaturated Fatty Acids and Cardiovascular Health*; National Heart Foundation of Australia: Melbourne, Australia, 2008.

23. Reid, R.D.; McDonnell, L.A.; Riley, D.L.; Mark, A.E.; Mosca, L.; Beaton, L.; Papadakis, S.; Blanchard, C.M.; Mochari-Greenberger, H.; O'Farrell, P.; *et al.* Effect of an intervention to improve the cardiovascular health of family members of patients with coronary artery disease: A randomized trial. *Can. Med. Assoc. J.* **2014**, *186*, 23–30. [CrossRef] [PubMed]

24. Cohen, D.J.; Clark, E.C.; Lawson, P.J.; Casucci, B.A.; Flocke, S.A. Identifying teachable moments for health behavior counseling in primary care. *Patient Educ. Couns.* **2011**, *85*, e8–e15. [CrossRef] [PubMed]
25. Imes, C.C.; Lewis, F.M. Family history of cardiovascular disease, perceived cardiovascular disease risk, and health-related behavior: A review of the literature. *J. Cardiovasc. Nurs.* **2014**, *29*, 108–129. [CrossRef] [PubMed]
26. Australian Bureau of Statistics. *4364.0.55.007-Australian Health Survey: Nutrition First Results—Food and Nutrients, 2011–2012*; Commonwealth of Australia: Canberra, Australia, 2014.
27. Jenkins, D.A.; Jones, P.H.; Lamarche, B.; Kendall, C.W.C.; Faulkner, D.; Cermakova, L.; Gigleux, I.; Ramprasath, V.; de Souza, R.; Ireland, C.; *et al.* Effect of a dietary portfolio of cholesterol-lowering foods given at 2 levels of intensity of dietary advice on serum lipids in hyperlipidemia: A randomized controlled trial. *JAMA* **2011**, *306*, 831–839. [CrossRef] [PubMed]
28. Mozaffarian, D.; Hao, T.; Rimm, E.B.; Willett, W.C.; Hu, F.B. Changes in diet and lifestyle and long-term weight gain in women and men. *N. Engl. J. Med.* **2011**, *364*, 2392–2404. [CrossRef] [PubMed]

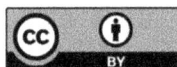

Chapter 2:
Food, Nutrients Intake and Health

nutrients

MDPI

Article

Associations between Macronutrient Intake and Obstructive Sleep Apnoea as Well as Self-Reported Sleep Symptoms: Results from a Cohort of Community Dwelling Australian Men

Yingting Cao [1,2,*], Gary Wittert [2], Anne W. Taylor [1], Robert Adams [3] and Zumin Shi [1,2]

[1] Population Research and Outcome Studies, the University of Adelaide, SAHMRI, Adelaide, SA 5005, Australia; anne.taylor@adelaide.edu.au (A.W.T.); zumin.shi@adelaide.edu.au (Z.S.)

[2] Freemasons Foundation Centre for Men's Health, the University of Adelaide, Adelaide, SA 5005, Australia; gary.wittert@adelaide.edu.au

[3] Health Observatory, Discipline of Medicine, the Queen Elizabeth Hospital Campus, the University of Adelaide, Adelaide, SA 5011, Australia; robert.adams@adelaide.edu.au

* Correspondence: yingting.cao@adelaide.edu.au; Tel./Fax: +61-8-8313-1218

Received: 25 February 2016; Accepted: 30 March 2016; Published: 8 April 2016

Abstract: *Background:* macronutrient intake has been found to affect sleep parameters including obstructive sleep apnoea (OSA) in experimental studies, but there is uncertainty at the population level in adults. *Methods:* cross-sectional analysis was conducted of participants in the Men Androgen Inflammation Lifestyle Environment and Stress cohort ($n = 784$, age 35–80 years). Dietary intake was measured by a validated food frequency questionnaire. Self-reported poor sleep quality and daytime sleepiness were measured by questionnaires. Overnight in-home polysomnography (PSG) was conducted among participants with without previously diagnosed OSA. *Results:* after adjusting for demographic, lifestyle factors, and chronic diseases, the highest quartile of fat intake was positively associated with excessive daytime sleepiness (relative risk ratio (RRR) = 1.78, 95% CI 1.10, 2.89) and apnoea-hypopnoea index (AHI) $\geqslant 20$, (RRR = 2.98, 95% CI 1.20–7.38). Body mass index mediated the association between fat intake and AHI (30%), but not daytime sleepiness. There were no associations between other intake of macronutrient and sleep outcomes. *Conclusion:* high fat is associated with daytime sleepiness and AHI. Sleep outcomes are generally not assessed in studies investigating the effects of varying macronutrient diets on weight loss. The current result highlights the potential public health significance of doing so.

Keywords: macronutrient intake; fat intake; apnoea hypopnea index; polysomnography; daytime sleepiness

1. Introduction

A body of evidence has shown the associations between macronutrient intake and sleep parameters, however, with inconsistency. Carbohydrate, particularly with high glycaemic index (GI) was associated with faster sleep onset in healthy young men [1] but was associated with increased total arousal in children compared with low GI [2]. Low intake of protein (<16% *vs.* $\geqslant$16%) has been shown to be associated with difficulty in initiating sleep, but high intake of protein ($\geqslant$19% *vs.* <19%) has been shown to be associated with difficulty maintaining sleep in middle-aged Japanese workers [3]. A fatty meal was found to aggravate apnoea in patients (overweight or obese) with obstructive sleep apnoea (OSA) [4]. A newly published randomized-crossover study by St-Onge's group found that low fibre and high saturated fat and sugar intake was associated with lighter sleep with more arousals in young and middle-aged healthy adults [5]. However, other studies suggested no association between fat intake and sleep quality [6] or insomnia symptoms [3]. Although the inconsistent results may be attributed to a variety of study designs, uncertainty remains regarding the association between macronutrient intake and sleep in the current literature.

Studies that investigate the associations between macronutrient intakes and sleep parameters (objective measurements) at the population level in the community setting are desired. One study in Caucasian and Hispanic adolescents (*n* = 319) found that total fat intake was negatively associated in girls but positively associated in boys with rapid eye movement sleep [7]. However, there are no similar studies in adults. In this study, we aimed to assess whether macronutrient intake was associated with Apnoea-hypopnea Index (AHI) and self-reported sleep symptoms in community-dwelling middle-aged men at the population level under non-experimental conditions.

2. Methods

2.1. Study Population

The Men Androgen Inflammation Lifestyle Environment and Stress (MAILES) cohort study was established in 2009, to investigate cardio metabolic disease risk factors in relation to sex steroids, inflammation, environmental and psychosocial factors in men. A detailed cohort profile has been published previously [8]. Briefly, the study population consists of 2563 community dwelling men aged 35–80 years at baseline (MAILES stage 1) from the harmonisation of two population cohort studies: all participants from the Florey Adelaide Male Ageing Study (FAMAS) (2002–2005) [9] and eligible male participants from the North West Adelaide Health Study (NWHAS) (2004–2006) [10]. The MAILES stage 2 (2007–2010) was an approximate five-year follow-up consisting of a Computer Assisted Telephone Interview (CATI), questionnaires and biomedical examinations. In total, 1815 men completed the dietary intake during stage 2.

MAILES stage 3, conducted in August 2010, consisted of a CATI including sleep related questions (*n* = 1629). The 184 who answered "yes" to the question "Have you ever been diagnosed with OSA with a sleep study" were excluded from participating in the sleep sub-study, and the 1445 men who answered "no" to the question were further asked if they were willing to participate in the sleep study (75.2% agreed). Of these, a random sample of 1087 was chosen for inclusion. A total of 857 had home based PSG (Figure 1 [11]), and 837 of them had final valid measurements and became the study population in this paper aimed at examining the association between macronutrient and AHI. Self-selection bias was examined by comparing those who underwent a sleep study with those men in the MAILES cohort who did not. Sleep study participants did not differ from non-participants in daytime sleepiness, waking frequency and obesity level but they were younger, and more likely to report frequent snoring and better general health [11]. Ethics approval was obtained from the Queens Elizabeth Hospital Human Ethics Committee for the NWHAS study (number 2010054) and the Royal Adelaide Hospital Human Research Ethics Committee for the FAMAS study (number 020305h).

2.2. Macronutrient Intake Assessment

Dietary intake was measured by the Cancer Council Victoria Diet Questionnaire for Epidemiological Studies (DQES-V3.1 (FFQ)). The FFQ has been validated in an Australian population and is widely used in epidemiological studies [12]. The questionnaire asks the participant's habitual consumption of 167 foods and six alcohol beverages over the previous 12-month on a 10-point frequency scale. Additional questions were asked about the type of breads, dairy products and fat spreads used. Macronutrient intakes were computed from the dietary data by the means of the nutrient composition tables in the NUTTAB95 database (Food Standards Australia New Zealand, Canberra, Australia, 1995).

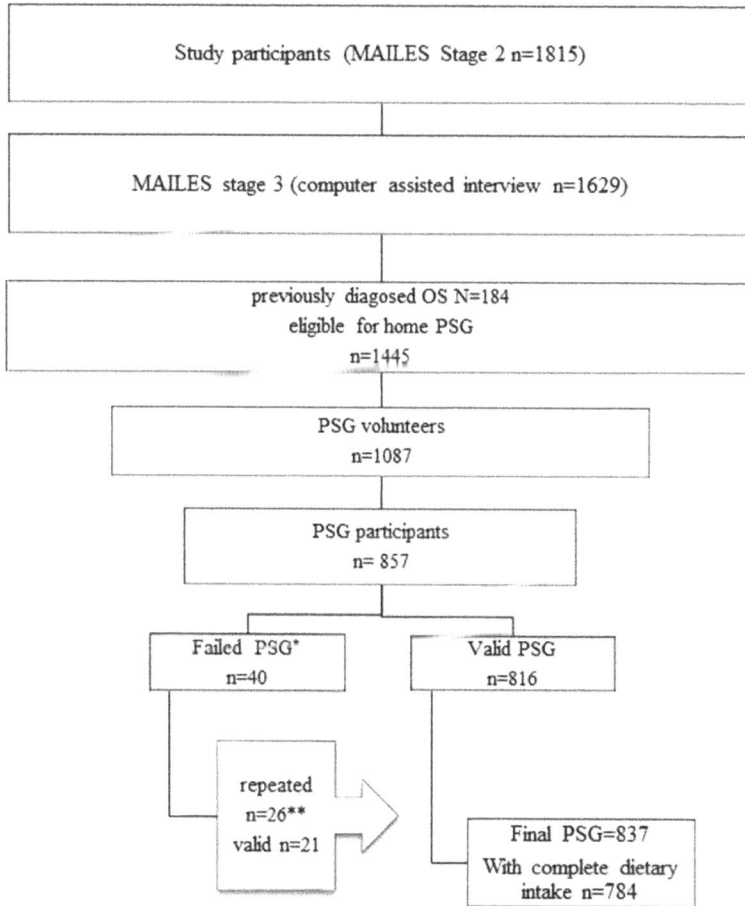

Figure 1. The flow chart of study participants with dietary intake (MAILES stage 2) and MAILES stage 3 with PSG recruitment * $n = 21$ total sleep time (TST) not $\geqslant 3.5$ h from $\geqslant 5$ h recording; $n = 3$ poor respiratory signals; $n = 2$ poor EEG; $n = 14$ no oxygen saturation (SaO$_2$); $n = 3$ all traces/recording failed. ** Includes 20 successful and 3 failed second PSG of which one was successfully reperated at a third time (this flow chart with instructions for PSG recruitment has been published previously [11]).

2.3. Sleep Assessments

Sleep measurements consisted of subjective (CATI and self-reported questionnaires) and objective (in-home PSG) approaches. Self-reported data included: (1) the STOP (snore, tiredness during daytime, observed apnoea and high blood pressure) questions [13]; (2) the Pittsburgh Sleep Quality Index (total score ranged from 0 to 21, a score >5 indicates poor sleep quality) [14]; and (3) sleepiness asked by the question "Do you feel sleepy when sitting quietly during the day or early evening? (1) yes (2) no (3) sometimes".

AHI was measured by a single overnight in-home PSG with Emblettas X100 portable sleep device [15]) and manually scored by an experienced sleep technician according to the 2007 American Academy of Sleep Medicine criteria (alternative) [16].

2.4. Other Measurements

Information on education, marital status, income, work status, physical activity, smoking, shift-work, and chronic diseases were collected by questionnaires [8]. Medication use was obtained from Medicare Australia by confidential unit record linkage, classified according to the Anatomical Therapeutic Chemical (ATC) Classification. The number of distinct medication classes (at the ATC third level) six months before clinical examination were treated as covariates.

Body weight was measured in light indoor clothing without shoes to the nearest 100 g. Height was measured without shoes to the nearest mm using a stadiometer. Waist circumference was measured to the nearest mm, midway between the inferior margin of the last rib and the crest of the ilium, in the mid-axillary line in a horizontal plane. Blood pressure was measured twice using a mercury sphygmomanometer on the right upper arm of the subject, who was seated for five minutes before the measurement.

2.5. Statistical Analysis

Macronutrient (carbohydrate, protein and fat) intakes (g) were recoded into quartiles (Q1–Q4). Chi square test was used to compare difference between categorical variables, and ANOVA was used to compare differences in continuous variables between groups. The association between quartiles of macronutrient intake and self-reported sleep (snoring and poor sleep quality) was assessed using Poisson regression. Multinomial logistic regression analysis was used to test the association between macronutrient intake and self-reported sleepiness ("yes", "sometimes" and "no"), as well as the association between macronutrient intake and AHI. AHI was divided into three categories: low (<5), medium (5–19) and high ($\geqslant$20). Using low level and the lowest quartile (Q1) of each macronutrient intake as the reference group, multivariate-adjusted associations were performed: (1) model 1 adjusted for age; (2) model 2 further adjustments for education, smoking, alcohol intake, physical activity and shift-work; (3) model 3 further adjustments for waist circumference, diabetes, depression and medication. We did a sensitivity analysis by further adjusting for energy intake in model 4. Structural equation modelling (SEM) was used to test whether body mass index (BMI) mediates the association between macronutrient intake and AHI (treated as continuous variable) and daytime sleepiness ("yes" was assigned with value 2, "no" was assigned with value 0, "sometimes" was assigned with value 1, and treated as continuous variables). Direct and indirect effects were estimated using command "estimate teffects". Linear trend across quartiles of each macronutrient intake was tested using the median value of each macronutrient intake (g) at each quartile and treating it as a continuous variable in the model. All statistical procedures were performed using STATA 13.0 (Stata Corporation, College Station, TX, USA).

3. Results

Overall, 1815 participants with dietary intake were analysed, of whom 837 without a prior diagnosis of OSA underwent successful sleep studies and 784 completed the dietary intake. Demographic characteristics by quartiles of each macronutrient intake of the participants are presented in Table 1. The mean age of the participants was 59.7 (SD 11.4) years. Characteristics of PSG participants with dietary intake are presented in Table S1.

Table 1. Characteristics of subjects according to quartiles of each macronutrient intake ($n = 1815$) [1].

Factors	Carbohydrate Intake (g)			Protein Intake (g)			Fat Intake (g)		
	Q1 (n = 454)	Q4 (n = 453)	p-Value	Q1 (n = 454)	Q4 (n = 453)	p-Value	Q1 (n = 454)	Q4 (n = 453)	p-Value
Age (years), mean (SD)	60.5 (11.7)	58.5 (11.4)	0.07	61.5 (12.1)	58.4 (10.9)	<0.001	59.9 (11.6)	59.5 (11.1)	0.47
Energy intake (kcal), mean (SD)	1539.1 (342.1)	2930.5 (606.7)	<0.001	1548.3 (348.4)	2900.5 (618.8)	<0.001	1535.1 (328.4)	2934.2 (596.9)	<0.001
Carbohydrates (g/day), mean (SD)	132.9 (26.0)	320.1 (91.5)	<0.001	157.5 (49.8)	283.1 (97.1)	<0.001	162.2 (51.2)	276.1 (93.0)	<0.001
Fat (g/day), mean (SD)	71.3 (22.2)	119.0 (34.7)	<0.001	66.5 (19.4)	123.4 (32.0)	<0.001	58.4 (10.9)	135.2 (25.8)	<0.001
Protein (g/day), mean (SD)	74.5 (23.1)	126.8 (37.1)	<0.001	64.1 (12.0)	141.5 (32.9)	<0.001	71.9 (19.0)	131.0 (39.0)	<0.001
Fibre (g/day), mean (SD)	18.4 (5.9)	37.7 (11.5)	<0.001	19.6 (7.3)	35.6 (11.0)	<0.001	21.2 (8.3)	34.3 (10.9)	<0.001
Body mass index (BMI), n (%)			0.71			0.003			0.49
<25	81 (18.7)	79 (18.2)		102 (23.4)	71 (16.3)		79 (18.2)	81 (18.6)	
25–30	214 (49.3)	207 (47.6)		211 (48.4)	201 (46.1)		214 (49.2)	152 (44.1)	
≥30	139 (32.0)	149 (34.3)		123 (28.2)	164 (37.6)		142 (32.6)	162 (37.2)	
Income, n (%)			0.08			<0.001			0.16
Low income	171 (39.1)	153 (34.2)		193 (44.3)	153 (34.3)		163 (37.1)	164 (36.5)	
Middle income	113 (25.9)	156 (34.9)		113 (25.9)	165 (37.0)		120 (27.3)	164 (36.5)	
High income	130 (29.7)	114 (25.5)		105 (24.1)	104 (23.3)		134 (30.5)	102 (22.7)	
Not stated	23 (5.3)	24 (5.4)		25 (5.7)	24 (5.4)		22 (5.0)	19 (4.2)	
Marriage status, n (%)			0.003			0.014			0.07
Married or living with a partner	323 (74.1)	342 (77.0)		316 (72.6)	343 (77.1)		351 (80.1)	324 (72.5)	
Separated/divorced	70 (16.1)	50 (11.3)		65 (14.9)	53 (11.9)		46 (10.5)	74 (16.6)	
Widowed	19 (4.4)	11 (2.5)		24 (5.5)	13 (2.9)		16 (3.7)	18 (4.0)	
Never married	22 (5.0)	40 (9.0)		28 (6.4)	33 (7.4)		24 (5.5)	30 (6.7)	
Not stated/refused	2 (0.5)	1 (0.2)		2 (0.5)	3 (0.7)		1 (0.2)	1 (0.2)	
Education, n (%)			0.07			0.18			0.10
≤High school	96 (25.3)	93 (23.3)		100 (27.0)	96 (24.2)		95 (25.1)	112 (28.1)	
Certificate	228 (60.2)	219 (54.9)		214 (57.8)	229 (57.8)		226 (59.6)	208 (52.1)	
Bachelor	52 (13.7)	83 (20.8)		50 (13.5)	69 (17.4)		53 (14.0)	75 (18.8)	
Not stated	3 (0.8)	4 (1.0)		6 (1.6)	2 (0.5)		5 (1.3)	4 (1.0)	
Current smoker, n (%)	71 (15.8)	51 (11.3)	0.22	62 (13.7)	66 (14.7)	0.35	48 (10.6)	61 (13.6)	0.36
Physical activity, n (%)			0.09			0.39			0.18
Sedentary	126 (30.6)	102 (24.2)		122 (29.4)	101 (24.0)		120 (28.7)	105 (24.9)	
Low exercise level	140 (34.0)	136 (32.2)		141 (34.0)	135 (32.1)		158 (35.4)	136 (32.3)	
Moderate exercise level	103 (25.0)	131 (31.0)		109 (26.3)	134 (31.8)		109 (26.1)	136 (32.3)	
High exercise level	43 (10.4)	53 (12.6)		43 (10.4)	51 (12.1)		41 (9.8)	44 (10.5)	
Depression, n (%)	37 (8.6)	56 (12.8)	0.17	33 (7.7)	61 (14.0)	0.016	33 (8.7)	64 (14.6)	0.029

[1] Macronutrient intake was divided into quartiles. Q1 and Q4 stand for the lowest and highest quartile. The results presented are unadjusted

Univariate analysis results between macronutrient intake and AHI and self-reported sleep parameters are presented in Table 2. No association was found between carbohydrate or protein intake and AHI. High intake of fat was positively associated with high AHI and self-reported daytime sleepiness. The prevalence of sleepiness was 46.4% and 37.0% among those with highest and lowest quartiles of fat intake. The distribution of AHI was significantly different across quartiles of fat intake with high fat intake associated with high AHI.

The prevalence ratio of self-reported sleep parameters (relative risk ratio for sleepiness) across quartiles of macronutrient intake is presented in Table 3 and Figure S1. After adjusting for age, waist circumference, education, lifestyle factors (smoking, alcohol intake, physical activity and shift work), chronic diseases and medication, the highest quartile of fat intake was positively associated with daytime sleepiness. Compared with the lowest quartile, the highest quartile of fat intake had a relative risk ratio (RRR) of 1.78 (95% CI 1.10–2.89) for daytime sleepiness (*p* for trend across quartiles was 0.305). When further adjusted for total energy intake, the association was no longer significant. There were no associations between macronutrient intakes and other self-reported sleep parameters. The RRR for AHI using multinominal logistic regression are presented in Table 4 and Figure S2. After adjusting for age, waist circumference, lifestyle factors, chronic diseases and medication, fat intake was positively associated with high AHI ($\geq$20/h) (Q4 *vs.* Q1, RRR 2.98 (95% CI 1.20–7.38) (*p* for trend across quartiles was 0.046 across quartiles). Similarly, the association was not significant after further adjusting for total energy intake. BMI mediated 30% of the association between fat intake and AHI (direct effect 0.07, indirect effect 0.03, *p* < 0.05) (Table S2 and Figure S3). However, BMI did not mediate the association between fat intake and daytime sleepiness (Table S3).

Table 2. Polysomnography and self-reported sleep measures by quartiles of macronutrient intake in grams [1].

Sleep Parameters	Quartiles of Macronutrient Intake (g)				p-Value
	Q1 (n = 196)	Q2 (n = 196)	Q3 (n = 196)	Q4 (n = 196)	
	Carbohydrate Intake (g)				
Polysomnography measures (n = 784)					
Apnoea-Hypopnea Index (/h), n (%)					0.220
<5	48 (24.5)	40 (20.4)	49 (25.0)	32 (16.3)	
5–19	108 (55.1)	108 (55.1)	95 (48.5)	110 (56.1)	
>20	40 (20.4)	48 (24.5)	52 (26.5)	54 (27.6)	
Total sleep duration (min), mean (SD)	376.8 (57.5)	376.7 (54.6)	369.1 (59.2)	365.7 (62.3)	0.380
Self-reported measures	Q1 (n = 372)	Q2 (n = 372)	Q3 (n = 372)	Q4 (n = 372)	
Daytime sleepiness (n = 1487), n (%)	133 (35.7)	160 (43.1)	159 (43.0)	157 (40.8)	0.320
Poor sleep quality (n = 773)[2], n (%)	89 (48.4)	80 (42.6)	88 (46.1)	95 (50.5)	0.450
	Protein Intake (g)				
Polysomnography measures (n = 784)					
Apnoea-Hypopnea Index (/h), n (%)					0.230
<5	48 (24.5)	43 (21.9)	46 (23.5)	32 (16.3)	
5–19	104 (53.1)	109 (55.6)	105 (53.6)	103 (52.6)	
>20	44 (22.4)	44 (22.4)	45 (23.0)	61 (31.1)	
TST (min), mean (SD)	374.6 (55.8)	375.8 (57.3)	365.4 (55.8)	376.5 (64.2)	0.200
Self-reported measures	Q1 (n = 372)	Q2 (n = 372)	Q3 (n = 372)	Q4 (n = 372)	
Daytime sleepiness (n = 1487), n (%)	131 (36.1)	164 (43.6)	152 (39.9)	157 (42.8)	0.490
Poor sleep quality (n = 773), n (%)	95 (51.4)	76 (40.0)	93 (49.7)	88 (45.6)	0.130
	Fat Intake (g)				
Polysomnography measures (n = 784)					
Apnoea-Hypopnea Index (/h), n (%)					0.004
<5	45 (23.0)	45 (23.0)	51 (26.0)	28 (14.3)	
5–19	117 (59.7)	100 (51.0)	101 (51.5)	103 (52.6)	
>20	34 (17.3)	51 (26.0)	44 (22.4)	65 (33.2)	
TST (min), mean (SD)	374.4 (54.7)	373.2 (54.1)	375.8 (61.8)	368.8 (62.9)	0.660
Self-reported measures	Q1 (n = 372)	Q2 (n = 372)	Q3 (n = 372)	Q4 (n = 372)	
Daytime sleepiness (n = 1487), n (%)	137 (37.0)	151 (41.0)	144 (38.1)	172 (46.4)	0.051
Poor sleep quality (n = 773), n (%)	86 (45.5)	89 (46.8)	85 (46.4)	92 (48.7)	0.940

[1] Data are presented by macronutrient intake in quartiles of grams (unadjusted). Q1–Q4 = quartiles of each macronutrient intake in grams. Macronutrient intake for polysomnography measurements presented are from those with polysomnography measurements (n = 784). Macronutrient intake for self-reported sleep parameters are from those with self-reported day time sleepiness data (n = 1487); [2] poor sleep quality was measured among those who had polysomnography measurements (n = 784), macronutrient intake refers to polysomnography measured.

Table 3. The prevalence ratio (95% CI) for self-reported sleep parameters across quartiles of macronutrient intakes [1].

Self-reported Sleep Symptoms	Quartiles of Macronutrient Intake (g)				n
	Q1 (n = 372) ref	Q2 (n = 372)	Q3 (n = 372)	Q4 (n = 372)	
Daytime sleepiness [2]					
Carbohydrate					
Model 1	1.00	1.60 (1.08–2.37) *	1.69 (1.10–2.58) *	1.48 (0.89–2.46)	1487
Model 2	1.00	1.58 (1.02–2.46) *	1.40 (0.87–2.26)	1.33 (0.75–2.35)	1195
Model 3	1.00	1.46 (0.92–2.31)	1.25 (0.77–2.04)	1.19 (0.66–2.13)	1147
Model 4	1.00	1.31 (0.81–2.12)	1.05 (0.61–1.81)	0.85 (0.41–1.78)	1147
Protein					
Model 1	1.00	1.62 (1.09–2.40) *	1.29 (0.86–1.94)	1.59 (1.01–2.51) *	1487
Model 2	1.00	1.75 (1.13–2.74) *	1.32 (0.84–2.08)	1.74 (1.04–2.89) *	1195
Model 3	1.00	1.51 (0.96–2.40)	1.29 (0.81–2.06)	1.62 (0.96–2.74)	1147
Model 4	1.00	1.47 (0.91–2.36)	1.21 (0.71–2.05)	1.44 (0.73–2.86)	1147
Fat					
Model 1	1.00	1.53 (1.04–2.24) *	1.23 (0.83–1.80)	1.95 (1.28–2.99) **	1487
Model 2	1.00	1.59 (1.03–2.46) *	1.23 (0.80–1.87)	1.85 (1.15–2.96) *	1195
Model 3	1.00	1.53 (0.98–2.40)	1.12 (0.72–1.72)	1.78 (1.10–2.89) *	1147
Model 4	1.00	1.56 (0.97–2.53)	1.16 (0.69–1.95)	1.90 (0.93–3.91)	1147
Poor sleep quality					
Carbohydrate					
Model 1	1.00	0.89 (0.65–1.21)	0.97 (0.69–1.36)	1.08 (0.73–1.59)	751
Model 2	1.00	0.88 (0.61–1.27)	0.96 (0.66–1.40)	0.98 (0.62–1.54)	590
Model 3	1.00	0.90 (0.62–1.31)	0.94 (0.64–1.39)	0.95 (0.60–1.53)	569
Model 4	1.00	0.86 (0.58–1.28)	0.88 (0.57–1.36)	0.84 (0.47–1.51)	569
Protein					
Model 1	1.00	0.76 (0.56–1.04)	0.94 (0.69–1.28)	0.86 (0.60–1.23)	751
Model 2	1.00	0.77 (0.54–1.12)	0.92 (0.65–1.32)	0.89 (0.59–1.34)	590
Model 3	1.00	0.77 (0.53–1.13)	0.87 (0.60–1.26)	0.83 (0.55–1.27)	569
Model 4	1.00	0.74 (0.50–1.08)	0.79 (0.52–1.19)	0.69 (0.40–1.19)	569
Fat					
Model 1	1.00	1.03 (0.76–1.39)	1.02 (0.75–1.39)	1.07 (0.77–1.49)	751
Model 2	1.00	1.12 (0.79–1.60)	1.08 (0.76–1.55)	1.11 (0.75–1.63)	590
Model 3	1.00	1.06 (0.74–1.53)	0.98 (0.68–1.42)	1.01 (0.68–1.51)	569
Model 4	1.00	1.01 (0.69–1.48)	0.90 (0.59–1.38)	0.86 (0.49–1.51)	569

[1] Poisson regression was performed for self-reported poor sleep quality and incidence rate ratio is presented; [2] multinomial logistic regression was performed for daytime sleepiness as it has three levels: "yes", "sometimes", and "no", and the results were showing those who answered "yes" compared with "no". Four models adjusted for different covariates are presented. Model 1: adjusted for age. Model 2: further adjusted for education (high school, certificate and bachelor), smoking (yes/no), alcohol intake (standard drinks 0, 1, 3), physical activity (sedentary, low, moderate and high), shift work (yes/no). Model 3: further adjusted for waist circumference (continuous), depression (yes/no), diabetes (yes/no), and medication (continuous). Model 4: further adjusted for energy intake. * $p < 0.05$, ** $p < 0.01$.

Table 4. The associations between macronutrient intake and Apnoea hypopnea index (AHI) [1].

AHI Categories	Models	Q1 (ref)	Q2	Q3	Q4	n
			Quartiles of Macronutrient Intake (g)			
AHI (/h)						
			Carbohydrate			
<5 (ref)	Model 1	1.00	1.00	1.00	1.00	169
5–19	Model 1	1.00	1.22 (0.72–2.06)	0.80 (0.45–1.41)	1.36 (0.67–2.74)	421
≥20	Model 1	1.00	1.36 (0.72–2.54)	0.96 (0.49–1.89)	1.27 (0.55–2.89)	194
						Subtotal: 784
<5 (ref)	Model 2	1.00	1.00	1.00	1.00	127
5–19	Model 2	1.00	1.79 (0.96–3.33)	1.21 (0.63–2.33)	1.77 (0.78–3.99)	338
≥20	Model 2	1.00	1.60 (0.76–3.38)	1.17 (0.54–2.54)	1.55 (0.60–4.02)	155
						Subtotal: 620
<5 (ref)	Model 3	1.00	1.00	1.00	1.00	123
5–19	Model 3	1.00	1.82 (0.94–3.52)	1.12 (0.57–2.21)	1.70 (0.73–3.95)	324
≥20	Model 3	1.00	1.44 (0.64–3.25)	1.07 (0.46–2.46)	1.47 (0.53–4.11)	149
						Subtotal: 596
<5 (ref)	Model 4	1.00	1.00	1.00	1.00	123
5–19	Model 4	1.00	1.59 (0.79–3.20)	0.87 (0.39–1.93)	1.15 (0.40–3.34)	324
≥20	Model 4	1.00	1.06 (0.45–2.49)	0.62 (0.24–1.60)	0.55 (0.16–2.05)	149
						Subtotal: 596
			Protein			
<5 (ref)	Model 1	1.00	1.00	1.00	1.00	169
5–19	Model 1	1.00	1.20 (0.72–2.01)	1.09 (0.64–1.85)	1.51 (0.79–2.87)	421
≥20	Model 1	1.00	1.09 (0.59–2.03)	1.04 (0.55–1.97)	1.80 (0.86–3.78)	194
						Subtotal: 784
<5 (ref)	Model 2	1.00	1.00	1.00	1.00	127
5–19	Model 2	1.00	1.44 (0.78–2.67)	1.18 (0.63–2.20)	1.96 (0.92–4.18)	338
≥20	Model 3	1.00	1.21 (0.57–2.54)	1.00 (0.48–2.12)	2.40 1.00–5.76) *	155
						Subtotal: 620
<5 (ref)	Model 3	1.00	1.00	1.00	1.00	123
5–19	Model 3	1.00	1.22 (0.64–2.32)	0.99 (0.51–1.89)	1.63 (0.74–3.56)	324
≥20	Model 3	1.00	1.03 (0.46–2.32)	0.83 (0.36–1.87)	2.03 (0.79–5.22)	149
						Subtotal: 596
<5 (ref)	Model 4	1.00	1.00	1.00	1.00	123
5–19	Model 4	1.00	1.09 (0.55–2.14)	0.79 (0.37–1.69)	1.13 (0.41–3.10)	324
≥20	Model 4	1.00	0.83 (0.36–1.93)	0.54 (0.21–1.38)	0.99 (0.29–3.32)	149
						Subtotal: 596

Table 4. Cont.

		Fat			
<5 (ref)	Model 1	1.00	1.00	1.00	169
5–19	Model 1	0.85 (0.51–1.40)	0.74 (0.45–1.23)	1.25 (0.68–2.30)	421
>20	Model 1	1.49 (0.80–2.77)	1.09 (0.58–2.06)	2.46 (1.21–5.00) *	194
					Subtotal: 784
<5 (ref)	Model 2	1.00	1.00	1.00	127
5–19	Model 2	0.84 (0.46–1.55)	0.67 (0.37–1.21)	1.33 (0.65–2.73)	338
>20	Model 3	1.61 (0.77–3.40)	1.10 (0.52–2.30)	2.67 (1.15–6.20) *	155
					Subtotal: 620
<5 (ref)	Model 3	1.00	1.00	1.00	123
5–19	Model 3	0.83 (0.44–1.55)	0.66 (0.36–1.22)	1.40 (0.66–2.96)	324
>20	Model 3	1.54 (0.69–3.46)	1.20 (0.54–2.67)	2.98 (1.20–7.38) *	149
					Subtotal: 596
<5 (ref)	Model 4	1.00	1.00	1.00	127
5–19	Model 4	0.67 (0.34–1.33)	0.46 (0.21–1.00) *	0.76 (0.26–2.23)	334
>20	Model 4	1.25 (0.53–2.97)	0.84 (0.32–2.21)	1.63 (0.45–5.90)	154
					Subtotal:596

[1] The results were from multinomial logistic regression. It presents comparing with the lowest level of sleep outcome, the relative risk ratio for medium or high level of having higher quartile of each macronutrient intake comparing with the lowest quartile of intake (Q2–4 vs. Q1). Four models adjusted for different covariates are presented. Model 1: adjust for age. Model 2: further adjusted for education (high school, certificate and bachelor), smoking (yes/no), alcohol intake (standard drinks 0, 1, 3), physical activity (sedentary, low, moderate and high), shift work (yes/no). Model 3: further adjusted for waist circumference (continuous), depression (yes/no), diabetes (yes/no), and medication (continuous). Model 4: further adjusted for energy intake. * $p < 0.05$.

Nutrients **2016**, 8, 207

238

4. Discussion

To the best of our knowledge, this is the first study to assess the association between macronutrient intake and sleep in a large population based cross-sectional study using objectively measured polysomnography. We found that high intake of fat was associated with daytime sleepiness and high AHI. The associations between fat intake and AHI was mediated by BMI.

Although the mechanism of the associations between macronutrient intake and sleep parameters is yet to be clear, some possibilities have been suggested by previously published work. Sleep can be regulated by various hormones that is induced by food intake through communications between hypothalamus and the brain [17]. Both dietary carbohydrates and protein can affect tryptophan metabolism through the availability tryptophan uptake into the brain via the blood brain barrier [18]. Regarding the mechanism of fat intake and sleep parameters, it is suggested that fat may affect sleep by altering circadian regulation of hormonal, central nervous and metabolic systems [19].

We found a positive association between high fat intake and daytime sleepiness. Early experimental studies showed that both infusion of lipid into the small intestine and isoenergetic meals may cause a decline in alertness and concentration [20]. Wells et.al have shown that healthy young subjects felt sleepier and less awake 2–3 h after a high-fat-low-carbohydrate meal [21]. Although carbohydrate rich meals have been demonstrated to be associated with postprandial lassitude [22], a greater decline was seen in high fat intake [20]. Other laboratory evidences suggested the potential role of gut neuro hormones in promoting hypnogenesis through vagal activation which essentially triggers fatigue [23–27]. However, we did not have data on the timing of fat intake, and dietary data collection was prior to sleep measurements, so the immediate effect of sleepiness of high-fat diet was not able to be assessed. Long-term high fat intake may lead to elevated levels of leptin and decreased levels of ghrelin [28], which could regulate arousal and wakefulness via orexin [29]. Increased sleepiness was observed in mice with high-diet fed induced obesity [30]. In large scale studies, positive associations between obesity and excessive daytime sleepiness has been reported [31,32]. This is consistent with our data that participants in the obese group had a higher risk of daytime sleepiness after adjusting for lifestyle factors (Table S4). However, obesity does not seem to be a mediator of the association between fat intake and daytime sleepiness (Table S3).High fat intake was also found to be associated with a high level of AHI ($\geqslant$20/h) in this study, after adjusting for age, waist, lifestyle factors, chronic diseases and medication. Similarly, previous experimental studies found a fatty meal the night before bed would increase AHI in OSA patients [4]. Long-term effect of high-fat diet on AHI is not clear. In non-obese rats, high-fat fed diet increases apnoea, and this could be reversed and prevented by a low dose injection of metformin (a drug for insulin resistance) [33]. This may suggest that insulin resistance induced by high fat diet may be one of the mechanisms leading to increased AHI, but was dependent on body weight. In patients with type 2 diabetes, AHI ($\geqslant$30/h) was associated with higher BMI [34]. Obesity has been suggested as one of the main risk factors of sleep apnoea [35] in the literature. In our study, being obese was strongly associated with higher AHI compared with non-obese participants (Table S5). Our mediation modelling suggests that the direct effect of BMI on AHI was about five times stronger than the effect from fat intake, and about 30% of the effect on AHI comes from BMI (Table S2 and Figure S3).

Regarding energy intake, higher energy intake was associated with high level of AHI in our study (Table S5), and our sensitivity analysis suggested that it was a confounder in the association between fat intake and AHI and daytime sleepiness. However, energy intake estimated from self-reported dietary intake has been suggested to be less accurate [36]. Moreover, soft drink and alcohol were not included in the energy intake calculation in our study.

The main merits of this study are: (1) it is the first investigation of the association between macronutrient intake and PSG measured sleep parameters as well as self-reported sleep problems in a relatively large sample; (2) we were able to adjust for a wide range of covariates including age, waist circumference, energy intake, education, smoking, alcohol intake, physical activity, shift work, depression, diabetes and medication.

Several limitations in our study need to be acknowledged. Firstly, asynchronous exploration between macronutrient and sleep were performed due to the mismatch of time of the PSG study and dietary survey. Secondly, due to the nature of the cross-sectional study, causation cannot be made. Thirdly, because the study only involved men, the findings may not be generalised to women. In addition, we only conducted one overnight PSG assessment as it is not practical to have multiple night PSG assessments in large epidemiological studies. Despite objective sleep measurement, dietary intake was estimated by FFQ, rather than 24-h food recall or actual weighing. 24-h food recall provides meal specific food intake information, which has been suggested to be associated with circadian adaption [37]. However, it is impractical to conduct 24-h food recall in studies with large sample size, and 24-h recall does not capture a long term dietary habit as FFQ does.

In conclusion, high fat intake was associated with daytime sleepiness and high AHI. BMI mediates the association between fat and AHI but not daytime sleepiness. Although a public health benefit is suggested, future studies are needed to confirm the findings at the population level.

Supplementary Materials: The following are available online at http://www.mdpi.com/2072-6643/8/4/207s1.

Acknowledgments: The present study was supported by the National Health and Medical Research Council of Australia (NHMRC Project Grant 627227).

Author Contributions: Y.C., A.W.T., G.W., R.A. and Z.S. conceived and designed the study; Y.C. analyzed the data; G.W., A.W.T., R.A. and Z.S. contributed materials/analysis tools; Y.C. wrote the paper.

Conflicts of Interest: The authors declared that there are no conflicts of interest.

References

1. Afaghi, A.; O'Connor, H.; Chow, C.M. High-glycemic-index carbohydrate meals shorten sleep onset. *Am. J. Clin. Nutr.* **2007**, *85*, 426–430. [PubMed]
2. Jalilolghadr, S.; Afaghi, A.; O'Connor, H.; Chow, C.M. Effect of low and high glycaemic index drink on sleep pattern in children. *J. Pak. Med. Assoc.* **2011**, *61*, 533–536. [PubMed]
3. Tanaka, E.; Yatsuya, H.; Uemura, M.; Murata, C.; Otsuka, R.; Toyoshima, H.; Tamakoshi, K.; Sasaki, S.; Kawaguchi, L.; Aoyama, A. Associations of protein, fat, and carbohydrate intakes with insomnia symptoms among middle-aged Japanese workers. *J. Epidemiol.* **2013**, *23*, 132–138. [CrossRef] [PubMed]
4. Trakada, G.; Steiropoulos, P.; Zarogoulidis, P.; Nena, E.; Papanas, N.; Maltezos, E.; Bouros, D. A fatty meal aggravates apnea and increases sleep in patients with obstructive sleep apnea. *Sleep Breath* **2014**, *18*, 53–58. [CrossRef] [PubMed]
5. St-Onge, M.P.; Roberts, A.; Shechter, A.; Choudhury, A.R. Fiber and saturated fat are associated with sleep arousals and slow wave sleep. *J. Clin. Sleep Med.* **2016**, *12*, 19–24. [CrossRef] [PubMed]
6. Yamaguchi, M.; Uemura, H.; Katsuura-Kamano, S.; Nakamoto, M.; Hiyoshi, M.; Takami, H.; Sawachika, F.; Juta, T.; Arisawa, K. Relationship of dietary factors and habits with sleep-wake regularity. *Asia Pac. J. Clin. Nutr.* **2013**, *22*, 457–465. [PubMed]
7. Awad, K.M.; Drescher, A.A.; Malhotra, A.; Quan, S.F. Effects of exercise and nutritional intake on sleep architecture in adolescents. *Sleep Breath* **2013**, *17*, 117–124. [CrossRef] [PubMed]
8. Grant, J.F.; Martin, S.A.; Taylor, A.W.; Wilson, D.H.; Araujo, A.; Adams, R.J.; Jenkins, A.; Milne, R.W.; Hugo, G.J.; Atlantis, E.; *et al.* Cohort profile: The men androgen inflammation lifestyle environment and stress (MAILES) study. *Int. J. Epidemiol.* **2014**, *43*, 1040–1053. [CrossRef] [PubMed]
9. Martin, S.; Haren, M.; Taylor, A.; Middleton, S.; Wittert, G. Cohort profile: The florey adelaide male ageing study (FAMAS). *Int. J. Epidemiol.* **2007**, *36*, 302–306. [CrossRef] [PubMed]
10. Grant, J.F.; Taylor, A.W.; Ruffin, R.E.; Wilson, D.H.; Phillips, P.J.; Adams, R.J.; Price, K. Cohort profile: The north west adelaide health study (NWAHS). *Int. J. Epidemiol.* **2009**, *38*, 1479–1486. [CrossRef] [PubMed]
11. Appleton, S.L.; Vakulin, A.; McEvoy, R.D.; Wittert, G.A.; Martin, S.A.; Grant, J.F.; Taylor, A.W.; Antic, N.A.; Catcheside, P.G.; Adams, R.J. Nocturnal hypoxemia and severe obstructive sleep apnea are associated with incident type 2 diabetes in a population cohort of men. *J. Clin. Sleep Med.* **2015**, *11*, 609–614. [CrossRef] [PubMed]

12. Hodge, A.; Patterson, A.J.; Brown, W.J.; Ireland, P.; Giles, G. The anti cancer council of victoria FFQ: Relative validity of nutrient intakes compared with weighed food records in young to middle-aged women in a study of iron supplementation. *Aust. N. Z. J. Public Health* **2000**, *24*, 576–583. [CrossRef] [PubMed]

13. Chung, F.; Yegneswaran, B.; Liao, P.; Chung, S.A.; Vairavanathan, S.; Islam, S.; Khajehdehi, A.; Shapiro, C.M. Stop questionnaire: A tool to screen patients for obstructive sleep apnea. *Anesthesiology* **2008**, *108*, 812–821. [CrossRef] [PubMed]

14. Buysse, D.J.; Reynolds, C.F., 3rd; Monk, T.H.; Berman, S.R.; Kupfer, D.J. The Pittsburgh sleep quality index: A new instrument for psychiatric practice and research. *Psychiatry Res.* **1989**, *28*, 193–213. [CrossRef]

15. Natus Medical Incoportaed-Sleep. Available online: http://www.embla.com/index.cfm/id/57/Embletta-X100/ (accessed on 6 April 2016).

16. Iber, C.; Ancoli-Israel, S.; Chesson, A.L.; Quan, S.F. *The AASM Manual for the Scoring of Sleep and Associated Events: Rules, Terminology and Technical Specifications*, 1st ed.; American Academy of Sleep Medicine: Westchester, IL, USA, 2007.

17. Peuhkuri, K.; Sihvola, N.; Korpela, R. Diet promotes sleep duration and quality. *Nutr. Res.* **2012**, *32*, 309–319. [CrossRef] [PubMed]

18. Brezinova, V.; Loudon, J.; Oswald, I. Tryptophan and sleep. *Lancet* **1972**, *2*, 1086–1087. [CrossRef]

19. Kohsaka, A.; Laposky, A.D.; Ramsey, K.M.; Estrada, C.; Joshu, C.; Kobayashi, Y.; Turek, F.W.; Bass, J. High-fat diet disrupts behavioral and molecular circadian rhythms in mice. *Cell Metab.* **2007**, *6*, 414–421. [CrossRef] [PubMed]

20. Wells, A.S.; Read, N.W.; Craig, A. Influences of dietary and intraduodenal lipid on alertness, mood, and sustained concentration. *Br. J. Nutr.* **1995**, *74*, 115–123. [CrossRef] [PubMed]

21. Wells, A.S.; Read, N.W.; Uvnas-Moberg, K.; Alster, P. Influences of fat and carbohydrate on postprandial sleepiness, mood, and hormones. *Physiol. Behav.* **1997**, *61*, 679–686. [CrossRef]

22. Spring, B.; Maller, O.; Wurtman, J.; Digman, L.; Cozolino, L. Effects of protein and carbohydrate meals on mood and performance: Interactions with sex and age. *J. Psychiatr. Res.* **1982**, *17*, 155–167. [CrossRef]

23. Flachenecker, P.; Rufer, A.; Bihler, I.; Hippel, C.; Reiners, K.; Toyka, K.V.; Kesselring, J. Fatigue in MS is related to sympathetic vasomotor dysfunction. *Neurology* **2003**, *61*, 851–853. [CrossRef] [PubMed]

24. Valdes-Cruz, A.; Magdaleno-Madrigal, V.M.; Martinez-Vargas, D.; Fernandez-Mas, R.; Almazan-Alvarado, S.; Martinez, A.; Fernandez-Guardiola, A. Chronic stimulation of the cat vagus nerve: Effect on sleep and behavior. *Prog. Neuropsychopharmacol. Biol. Psychiatry* **2002**, *26*, 113–118. [CrossRef]

25. Juhasz, G.; Detari, L.; Kukorelli, T. Effects of hypnogenic vagal stimulation on thalamic neuronal activity in cats. *Brain Res. Bull.* **1985**, *15*, 437–441. [CrossRef]

26. Bazar, K.A.; Yun, A.J.; Lee, P.Y. Debunking a myth: Neurohormonal and vagal modulation of sleep centers, not redistribution of blood flow, may account for postprandial somnolence. *Med. Hypotheses* **2004**, *63*, 778–782. [CrossRef] [PubMed]

27. Kirchgessner, A.L. Orexins in the brain-gut axis. *Endocr. Rev.* **2002**, *23*, 1–15. [CrossRef] [PubMed]

28. Handjieva-Darlenska, T.; Boyadjieva, N. The effect of high-fat diet on plasma ghrelin and leptin levels in rats. *J. Physiol. Biochem.* **2009**, *65*, 157–164. [CrossRef] [PubMed]

29. Sakurai, T. Roles of orexin/hypocretin in regulation of sleep/wakefulness and energy homeostasis. *Sleep Med. Rev.* **2005**, *9*, 231–241. [CrossRef] [PubMed]

30. Jenkins, J.B.; Omori, T.; Guan, Z.; Vgontzas, A.N.; Bixler, E.O.; Fang, J. Sleep is increased in mice with obesity induced by high-fat food. *Physiol. Behav.* **2006**, *87*, 255–262. [CrossRef] [PubMed]

31. Bixler, E.O.; Vgontzas, A.N.; Lin, H.M.; Calhoun, S.L.; Vela-Bueno, A.; Kales, A. Excessive daytime sleepiness in a general population sample: The role of sleep apnea, age, obesity, diabetes, and depression. *J. Clin. Endocrinol. Metab.* **2005**, *90*, 4510–4515. [CrossRef] [PubMed]

32. Resnick, H.E.; Carter, E.A.; Aloia, M.; Phillips, B. Cross-sectional relationship of reported fatigue to obesity, diet, and physical activity: Results from the third national health and nutrition examination survey. *J. Clin. Sleep Med.* **2006**, *2*, 163–169. [PubMed]

33. Ramadan, W.; Dewasmes, G.; Petitjean, M.; Wiernsperger, N.; Delanaud, S.; Geloen, A.; Libert, J.P. Sleep apnea is induced by a high-fat diet and reversed and prevented by metformin in non-obese rats. *Obesity* **2007**, *15*, 1409–1418. [CrossRef] [PubMed]

34. Foster, G.D.; Sanders, M.H.; Millman, R.; Zammit, G.; Borradaile, K.E.; Newman, A.B.; Wadden, T.A.; Kelley, D.; Wing, R.R.; Sunyer, F.X.; *et al.* Obstructive sleep apnea among obese patients with type 2 diabetes. *Diabetes Care* **2009**, *32*, 1017–1019. [CrossRef] [PubMed]

35. Kohler, M. Risk factors and treatment for obstructive sleep apnea amongst obese children and adults. *Curr. Opin. Allergy Clin. Immunol.* **2009**, *9*, 4–9. [CrossRef] [PubMed]

36. Jakes, R.W.; Day, N.E.; Luben, R.; Welch, A.; Bingham, S.; Mitchell, J.; Hennings, S.; Rennie, K.; Wareham, N.J. Adjusting for energy intake—What measure to use in nutritional epidemiological studies? *Int. J. Epidemiol.* **2004**, *33*, 1382–1386. [CrossRef] [PubMed]

37. Patton, D.F.; Mistlberger, R.E. Circadian adaptations to meal timing: Neuroendocrine mechanisms. *Front. Neurosci.* **2013**, *7*, 185. [CrossRef] [PubMed]

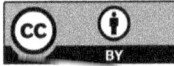

    MDPI

Article

Dietary Carbohydrate and Nocturnal Sleep Duration in Relation to Children's BMI: Findings from the IDEFICS Study in Eight European Countries

Monica Hunsberger [1,*], Kirsten Mehlig [1], Claudia Börnhorst [2], Antje Hebestreit [2], Luis Moreno [3], Toomas Veidebaum [4], Yiannis Kourides [5], Alfonso Siani [6], Dénes Molnar [7], Isabelle Sioen [8,9] and Lauren Lissner [1]

[1] Section for Epidemiology and Social Medicine, University of Gothenburg, P.O. Box 453, 40530 Gothenburg, Sweden; kirsten.mehlig@gu.se (K.M.); lauren.lissner@gu.se (L.L.)

[2] Leibniz Institute for Prevention Research and Epidemiology-BIPS GmbH, Achterstrasse 30, D-28359 Bremen, Germany; boern@bips.uni-bremen.de (C.B.); hebestr@bips.uni-bremen.de (A.H.)

[3] Growth, Exercise, Nutrition, and Development (GENUD) research group, University of Zaragoza, Domingo Miral, 50009 Zaragoza, Spain; lmoreno@unizar.es

[4] National Institute for Health Development, P.O. Box 3012, 10504 Tallinn, Estonia; toomas.veidebaum@tai.ee

[5] Research and Education Institute of Child Health, 138 Limassol Ave, #205, 2015, Strovolos 510903, Cyprus; kourides@cytanet.com.cy

[6] Institute for Food Sciences, Unit of Epidemiology and Population Genetics, National Research Council, Via Roma 64, 83100 Avellino, Italy; asiani@isa.cnr.it

[7] Department of Paediatrics, Medical Faculty, University of Pécs, Jozsef A.u., 7 H-1062 Budapest, Hungary; molnar.denes@pte.hu

[8] Department of Public Health, Ghent University, 4K3, De Pintelaan 185, 9000 Ghent, Belgium; isabelle.sioen@ugent.be

[9] Research Foundation—Flanders, Egmonstraat 5, B-1000 Brussels, Belgium

* Correspondence: monica.hunsberger@gu.se; Tel./Fax: +46-0-7033-82411

Received: 7 August 2015; Accepted: 1 December 2015; Published: 8 December 2015

Abstract: Previous research has found an association between being overweight and short sleep duration. We hypothesized that this association could be modified by a high carbohydrate (HC) diet and that the timing and type (starch or sugar) of intake may be an important factor in this context. Participants in the prospective, eight-country European study IDEFICS were recruited from September 2007 to June 2008, when they were aged two to nine years. Data on lifestyle, dietary intake and anthropometry were collected on two occasions. This study included 5944 children at baseline and 4301 at two-year follow-up. For each meal occasion (morning, midday, and evening), starch in grams and sugar in grams were divided by total energy intake (EI), and quartiles calculated. HC-starch and HC-sugar intake categories were defined as the highest quartile for each meal occasion. In a mutually adjusted linear regression model, short sleep duration as well as HC-starch in the morning were positively associated with body mass index (BMI) z-scores at baseline. HC-starch at midday was positively associated with body mass index (BMI) z-scores in children with short sleep duration, and negatively associated with BMI z-scores in those with normal sleep. After adjustment for baseline BMI z-scores, associations between total HC from starch or sugar and high BMI z-scores at two-year follow-up did not persist. Our observations offer a perspective on optimal timing for macronutrient consumption, which is known to be influenced by circadian rhythms. Reduced carbohydrate intake, especially during morning and midday meals, and following nocturnal sleep duration recommendations are two modifiable factors that may protect children from being overweight in the future.

Keywords: proportion carbohydrate intake at main meals; starch; sugar; childhood overweight; nocturnal sleep duration; breakfast consumption

---

1. Introduction

Childhood obesity is a serious threat to public health due to long-term consequences, including chronic disease in early adulthood [1]. Overweight and obesity are believed to be preventable conditions, although the issue of effective interventions for primary prevention is not well understood [2] and increased knowledge of modifiable risk factors is needed [3].

Previous investigations have shown that reduced sleep duration is associated with overweight in children and adolescents [4–6]. Nielsen *et al.* (2011) report on eight prospective cohort studies of children, all of which confirmed a significant inverse association between hours spent sleeping and future weight gain or development of obesity [4]. Findings from a Belgian longitudinal study confirmed that short sleep duration is associated with central adiposity [7]. Additionally, findings from our own cohort, the Identification and prevention of Dietary- and lifestyle-induced health EFfects In Children and infantS (IDEFICS) study, indicated that sleep duration and overweight were associated cross-sectionally, but this association was no longer observed after adjustment for other behavioral factors and for parental education [8].

Carbohydrate, *i.e.*, digestible starch and sugar, is likely to play a significant role in energy balance since it is the major macronutrient impacting blood sugar levels. Low carbohydrate intake is generally defined as <130 g/day or <26% of total energy intake (EI), while 26%–45% of EI from carbohydrates is considered to be moderate carbohydrate intake [9]. A carbohydrate proportion exceeding 45% EI is considered to be moderately high and >60% of EI from carbohydrates is considered to be high, although there is no clear established cut-off [10].

Relatively few studies have investigated the relationship between dietary carbohydrate intake and energy balance in children. However, the Feeding Infants and Toddlers Study (FITS), conducted in the USA, found that toddlers often have low intakes of fruits and green or yellow vegetables, consuming instead a high amount of starchy foods from grains. The authors highlighted this as a potential focus area for early overweight prevention efforts [11]. A study of Malaysian children found that the percentage of total EI represented by carbohydrates was significantly higher in overweight/obese children, compared with normal-weight children [12], suggesting that the proportion of EI from carbohydrates may play a role in childhood obesity.

Breakfast is often high in carbohydrate from both starch and sugar. Furthermore, the relationship between breakfast consumption patterns and overweight is not clear. Eating breakfast has long been portrayed as important, possibly enabling control of overconsumption later in the day. Several studies of breakfast-skipping behavior across European countries have shown that children who eat breakfast have a lower BMI, compared with children who do not [13–16]. However, a 2010 systematic review reported that breakfast consumption is associated with increased body weight in European children and adolescents in observational studies but that causality was not demonstrated [17]. Brown *et al.* (2013) concurred, stating that the proposed effect of consuming breakfast on obesity is not supported by scientific findings [18].

Therefore, the aims of this study were to examine whether high intake of carbohydrate modifies the association between short sleep duration and overweight, whether intake of starch and sugar differ in this regard, whether the timing (morning, midday, and evening) of carbohydrate intake is significant, and whether breakfast consumption, regardless of macronutrient composition, minimizes the risk of overweight in a mutually adjusted model (see Figure 1). The study was conducted on a geographically dispersed European sample participating in IDEFICS [19,20].

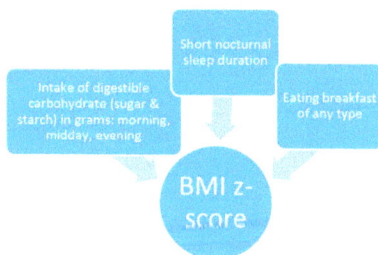

Figure 1. Factors investigated with body mass index (BMI) z-scores. Eating breakfast has a negligible relationship with carbohydrate (sugar and starch) intake during meals. Correlations range from −0.11 (evening sugar) to 0.13 (morning sugar).

2. Methods

2.1. Participants

IDEFICS is a prospective cohort study with an embedded intervention, including eight centers in Europe (Belgium, Cyprus, Estonia, Germany, Hungary, Italy, Spain and Sweden). From September 2007 to June 2008, 16,228 children aged two to nine years underwent the baseline investigation, providing lifestyle and dietary pattern information, anthropometrics and biological samples. Following recruitment, a community intervention with six key health messages was undertaken, including: (1) increasing daily physical activity; (2) decreasing daily screen time; (3) increasing fruit and vegetable intake; (4) drinking more water; (5) getting adequate sleep; and (6) being together with family. From September 2009 to March 2010, the children participated in a follow-up examination.

During the baseline and follow-up examinations, parents or legal guardians provided written informed consent for all examinations and the collection of biological samples, as well for analysis and storage of personal data and collected samples. Survey centers in the eight countries collected data according to standardized operating procedures and adherence to a predefined protocol. All questionnaires were translated from English into the respective national language and then back-translated into English at the respective study centers, in order to ensure accuracy of translations. Detailed information on the study procedures is available in [19–21].

2.2. Assessment Of Main Exposures: High Carbohydrate Intake and Sleep Duration

Dietary intake was assessed by standardized 24-h dietary recalls (24-h), based on the responses of parents or guardians (hereafter called "parents") of participating children to the Self-Administered Children and Infant Nutrition Assessment (SACINA). This computer-based instrument, previously created for the Healthy Lifestyle in Europe by Nutrition in Adolescence (HELENA) study, was developed for IDEFICS based on Young Adolescents' Nutrition Assessment on Computer (YANA-C) software [22,23]. The dietary recall part of the Self Administered Children and Infant Assessment (SACINA) instrument presents, in an interactive menu, country-specific food items with photographs of different portion sizes for the most common items, as well as probing questions regarding usual combinations of foods such as cereal and milk. The information collected through the SACINA was linked to Food Composition Tables (FCT) in order to calculate nutrient intake. The respective national FCT was used in each country except Hungary, where the German FCT was used. Nutrients are presented in standard units, grams and kilocalories (kcal), based on a standard FCT [24].

Data on diet and sleep were collected on all days of the week, including weekends. Most parents completed one 24-h recall for their child, while a subset completed more than one recall. As parents were not able to report on meals consumed at schools or kindergartens, an on-site school meal assessment, using a predefined observation-recording template with standard portions, was carried out by a teacher or school employee. A complete 24-h recall included everything the children ate or drank during their waking hours during one day. The 24-h recall allows for the calculation of energy intake, the proportion of intake from each of the macronutrients, the proportion of carbohydrate kcal from sugar and starch and hours of nocturnal sleep, hereby referred to as sleep. We defined short sleep duration as less than 10 h, based on sleep recommendations for children [25].

We restricted the present sample to interviews recalling intake Monday through Thursday, as a previous investigation on the same sample indicated that dietary intake on Friday lies between weekday and weekend intake [8,26]. Therefore, to minimize heterogencity we classified Friday as a weekend day and excluded them. In cases with more than one dietary recall, only the first complete weekday record of dietary intake was included in the analysis.

The SACINA instrument is structured around six meals without time parameters: breakfast, mid-morning snack, lunch, afternoon snack, evening meal and evening snack. If an additional snack was indicated in the interview, it was added to a previous snack in order to account for all EI. However, five was the median number of meals consumed and only 20% of children exceeded this number of meals. Eating breakfast was recorded as yes or no, based on the 24-h recall.

Importantly, as under- and over-reporting of dietary intake is a common problem, we examined total daily EI by comparing EI to the basal metabolic rate estimated by the age- and gender-specific Schofield equation [27]. Using the widely-acknowledged Goldberg cut-offs, we classified 254 (3.43%) as over-reporters and 701 (9.45%) as under-reporters and removed these 955 subjects from the analysis [28]. The prevalence of under- and over-reporting is not equally distributed across the countries. Under-reporting ranged from 1.1% in Spain to 18.44% in Cyprus, while over-reporting was most prevalent in Italy (5.6%) and lowest in Sweden (1.1%). When the under- and over-reporting subjects were excluded, Cyprus lost 19.6%, Hungary 19.4%, Germany 14.5%, Belgium 13.0%, Italy 11.5%, Estonia 11.2%, Spain 5.2% and Sweden 4.8%. An additional 107 cases were excluded because macronutrient components did not equal total EI, a result of missing data in the national FCTs.

For each meal occasion (morning, midday, and evening), starch in grams and sugar in grams were divided by total energy intake (e.g., the sum of sugar in grams for breakfast and morning snack/total daily EI). Then, HC intake for starch and sugar on each occasion was defined by assigning those in the highest quartile to the HC-starch and HC-sugar intake categories. Average intakes of starch during morning, midday, and evening meals were 50, 115, and 61 g, respectively. Similarly, average intakes of sugar were 64, 70, and 53 g, for the three meal periods. When describing total carbohydrate intake for the day, percentage of total energy from both carbohydrate sources was used.

2.3. Anthropometry and Body Mass Index (BMI)

Anthropometric data were collected at each participating survey center, according to a standard protocol. Body height was measured without shoes by trained research staff using a portable stadiometer (SECA 225). Body weight was measured with an electronic scale (TANITA BC 420 SMA), with subjects wearing light clothing. BMI-z-scores and BMI categories were calculated according to the criteria of the International Obesity Task Force (IOTF) [29]. The same procedure was followed at both examinations (baseline 2007/2008 and follow-up 2009/2010) and inter-observer reliability was assessed at each survey center [30].

2.4. Other Factors

Age, sex, highest household parental education level and survey country were included in the multivariable model. Data on parental factors were collected by a standardized parental questionnaire. Age was examined as a continuous variable. Household parental education level was categorized according to the International Standard Classification of Education (ISCED) and the original six ISCED levels were then combined into two levels [31]. ISCED levels 0–4 constitute "not high" education while levels 5 and 6 are defined as high. Moreover, we controlled for intervention when examining

BMI z-scores at follow-up, as children in the intervention had been exposed to instructions to get adequate sleep.

After limiting our sample to the first weekday recall, excluding cases with missing information about school meals or other meals outside of parental control and incomplete recalls, data from 7416 children were available. After excluding over- and under-reporters and children with incomplete sleep data, the baseline sample size was reduced to 5944. The longitudinal sample was further reduced to 4301 as some children were lost to follow-up (see Figure 2).

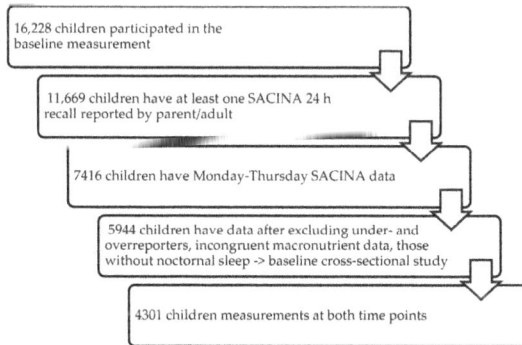

Figure 2. Study participants.

2.5. Statistical Analysis

BMI z-scores and dietary exposures are presented by short sleep duration at baseline. T-tests and regression equations controlling for country and age were used to make comparisons between short sleepers and "not-short" sleepers, presented with group means, regression coefficients and 95% confidence intervals. Linear regression was used for analysis of continuous variables (BMI-z-score, energy kcals/day, starch in grams, sugar in grams and macronutrient proportions) and logistic regression for binary outcomes (high starch and high sugar) at each time-point, eating breakfast (yes or no), high household parental education level); the respective regression coefficients are reported.

At baseline, we used a multivariable regression model to assess the association between BMI z-scores and short sleep duration (<10 h) and high intake of carbohydrate from starch and sugar at three different time-points (morning, midday, evening), while controlling for age, sex and parental education, and including country as a random intercept.

The same baseline variables were included in our prediction of BMI z-scores at two-year follow-up, in which we further controlled for BMI z-scores at baseline and exposure to the IDEFICS intervention, as mentioned above. Cross-sectionally at baseline, we assessed how being in the highest quartile of carbohydrate for starch or sugar modified the association between short sleep duration and BMI z-scores by introducing six product terms, *i.e.*, the dichotomized sleep variable multiplied by high starch and sugar intake at three time-points (morning, midday, evening). We further controlled for age, sex and parental education and included country as a random intercept.

We checked for multicollinearity between predictors and confounders included in the model by estimating the variance inflation factor (VIF), finding that none exceeded 2.0.

The significance level was set at $\alpha = 0.05$ for all analyses (2-sided tests). Statistical analyses were carried out with Stata Intercool 11.2, StataCorp LP, 4905 Lakeway Drive, College Station, TX, USA.

2.6. Ethics Statement

We certify that all applicable institutional and governmental regulations concerning the ethical use of human volunteers were followed during this research and that the IDEFICS study passed the Ethics Review process of the Sixth Framework Programme (FP6) of the European Commission. Ethical approval was obtained from the relevant local or national ethics committees by each of the eight study centers: the Ethics Committee of the University Hospital Ghent (Belgium); the National Bioethics Committee of Cyprus (Cyprus); the Tallinn Medical Research Ethics Committee of the National Institutes for Health Development (Estonia); the Ethics Committee of the University of Bremen (Germany); the Scientific and Research Ethics Committee of the Medical Research Council, Budapest (Hungary); the Ethics Committee of the Health Office, Avellino (Italy); the Ethics Committee for Clinical Research Aragon (Spain); and the Regional Ethical Review Board of Gothenburg (Sweden). All parents of the participating children gave written informed consent to data collection, examinations, collection of samples, subsequent analysis and storage of personal data and collected samples. Additionally, each child gave verbal consent after being verbally informed in simple terms, due their young age, about the study by a study nurse. This consent process was not further documented, but it was subject to central and local training and quality control procedures. Study participants and their parents could consent to single components of the study, while abstaining from others. All procedures were approved by the above-mentioned Ethics Committees.

3. Results

The study population at baseline is shown in Table 1. This study has an almost equal distribution of boys and girls in all countries and a mean age of 6.1 years at baseline. There was large inter-country variability in the proportion of children with a high intake of carbohydrate from starch and sugar respectively: generally low in Spain and high in Hungary and Italy. Short sleep duration also varied by survey country, with the lowest proportion of children categorized as short sleepers in Belgium (2.5%) and the highest in Estonia (69.6%).

Subjects who reportedly consumed breakfast consumed more morning sugar (33 g *vs.* 25 g), morning starch (26 g *vs.* 20 g), midday starch (56 g *vs.* 52 g) and evening starch (28 g *vs.* 26 g) than those reporting no breakfast. Breakfast-eaters reported consuming less midday sugar (34 g *vs.* 37 g) and less evening sugar (22 g *vs.* 29 g) than those reporting no breakfast (results not shown in tables).

In Table 2, we show cross-sectional differences in a range of baseline variables by sleep duration, adjusted for age and country at baseline. Short sleepers had significantly higher BMI z-scores than those sleeping 10 h or more. Raw numbers indicated that short sleep duration was associated with lower probability of high starch intake in the morning but the association was reversed when adjusted for age and survey country, as indicated by a positive beta-coefficient. Furthermore, regression analyses showed that short sleep was associated with less sugar intake at midday but more sugar intake in the evening. The cross-sectional analysis conducted at baseline was repeated cross-sectionally at follow-up without notable difference and is therefore not shown.

Table 3 shows mutually adjusted multivariable linear regression of BMI z-scores at baseline as a function of exposure to high starch and sugar intake at three time-points (morning, midday, and evening) and short sleep duration (referent group "normal to long sleep"), with adjustment for age, sex, high parental education level and survey country. At baseline, a significant positive association was observed between higher BMI z-scores and short sleep duration, HC intake from morning starch and higher values of total EI. A significant inverse association with BMI z-scores was observed for eating breakfast, high parental education level and HC evening starch. When it came to prediction of two-year BMI z-scores, protective associations with both breakfast consumption and high household parental education level were found. Characteristics associated with increased BMI z-scores included high intake of carbohydrate from morning starch and high intake of overall energy in a model mutually adjusted for age, sex, parental education, survey country and intervention *vs.* control study region but unadjusted for baseline BMI z-scores. When baseline BMI z-scores were included in the model, only high parental education was inversely associated with increasing BMI z-scores. HC from starch in the morning approaches significance (Regression coefficient = 0.05, p = 0.060; 95% CI = −0.001; 0.095).

Table 1. Characteristics of the study sample and distribution of covariates by country at baseline 2007/2008.

Variable	Belgium	Cyprus	Estonia	Germany	Hungary	Italy	Spain	Sweden	All
	n = 277	*n* = 699	*n* = 621	*n* = 1181	*n* = 519	*n* = 1367	*n* = 411	*n* = 869	*n* = 5944
Intervention area, *n* (%) *vs.* control	164 (59.2)	268 (38.3)	241 (38.8)	652 (55.2)	272 (52.4)	794 (58.)	368 (89.5)	394 (45.3)	3153 (53.1)
Mean age (SD)	5.5 (1.6)	6.2 (1.4)	6.5 (1.9)	6.1 (1.8)	6.5 (1.7)	6.1 (1.8)	5.5 (1.9)	5.9 (2.0)	6.1 (1.8)
Boys, *n* (%)	150 (54.2)	350 (50.1)	292 (47.0)	603 (51.1)	265 (51.1)	708 (51.8)	220 (53.5)	451 (51.9)	3039 (51.1)
Overweight, including obese, *n* (%), Cole 2012	17 (6.1)	152 (21.8)	102 (16.4)	170 (14.4)	75 (14.5)	543 (39.7)	75 (18.3)	77 (8.9)	1211 (20.4)
Mean BMI-z score at baseline (SD), Cole 2012	−0.09 (0.9)	0.40 (1.2)	0.24 (1.1)	0.18 (1.1)	0.11 (1.1)	0.97 (1.2	0.37 (1.0)	0.08 (0.9)	0.37 (1.2)
Short sleep (<10 h/night), *n* (%)	7 (2.5)	272 (38.9)	432 (69.6)	76 (6.4)	219 (42.2)	815 (59.6	128 (31.1)	112 (12.9)	2061 (34.7)
High parental education, *n* (%)	134 (48.9)	319 (52.7)	83 (13.7)	186 (16.5)	263 (51.1)	258 (19.0	226 (55.5)	593 (69.5)	2062 (35.9)
Breakfast on weekdays, *n* (%)	271 (98.2)	667 (95.4)	483 (81.3)	913 (77.3)	234 (46.6)	1221 (89.6	317 (77.1)	705 (94.5)	4811 (83.4)
Energy kcal/day on weekdays, mean (SD)	1383 (366)	1421 (362)	1718 (442)	1524 (439)	1517 (442)	1697 (404	1540 (385)	1545 (401)	1569 (424)
Mean sugar (g), morning (SD)	39 (22)	23 (13)	23 (18)	48 (32)	33 (30)	26 (17)	34 (17)	28 (17)	32 (24)
Mean starch (g), morning (SD)	25 (15)	38 (23)	17 (15)	28 (17)	27 (27)	19 (15)	18 (13)	26 (16)	25 (19)
Mean sugar (g), midday (SD)	33 (23)	20 (15)	49 (30)	43 (30)	31 (29)	34 (22)	36 (20)	30 (19)	35 (26)
Mean starch (g), midday (SD)	35 (18)	39 (23)	46 (27)	32 (26)	51 (33)	101 (55)	41 (20)	47 (23)	55 (43)
Mean sugar (g), evening (SD)	23 (19)	12 (12)	39 (26)	24 (22)	37 (26)	17 (16)	20 (14)	26 (19)	24 (21)
Mean starch (g), evening (SD)	27 (19)	25 (20)	28 (20)	22 (16)	23 (19)	37 (36)	12 (12)	36 (19)	28 (25)
HC sugar, morning, *n* (%)	99 (36)	55 (8)	73 (11)	596 (50)	178 (34)	239 (17)	110 (27)	135 (16)	1485 (25)
HC starch, morning, *n* (%)	60 (22)	334 (48)	77 (12)	403 (34)	172 (33)	186 (14)	42 (10)	212 (24)	1486 (25)
HC sugar midday, *n* (%)	64 (23)	43 (6)	271 (44)	446 (38)	108 (21)	314 (23)	104 (25)	136 (15)	1486 (25)
HC starch midday, *n* (%)	18 (7)	67 (10)	100 (16)	69 (6)	136 (26)	917 (67)	31 (8)	148 (17)	1486 (25)
HC sugar evening, *n* (%)	79 (29)	42 (6)	322 (52)	307 (26)	261 (50)	193 (14)	363 (48)	234 (27)	1486 (25)
HC starch evening, *n* (%)	55 (20)	163 (23)	157 (25)	152 (13)	83 (16)	495 (36)	20 (5)	361 (42)	1486 (25)

Footnote: household parental education level was categorized according to the International Standard Classification of Education (ISCED) and the original six ISCED levels [31] were then combined into two levels (not high *versus* high). ISCED levels 0–4 constitute "not high" education while levels 5 and 6 are defined as high education. Breakfast on weekdays was categorized as yes or no, based on the weekday 24-h recalls included in this study. High carbohydrate (HC-starch and HC-sugar categories) were calculated for starch and sugar at three time-points (morning, midday and evening) by assigning those in the highest quartile for grams of sugar/total energy intake (EI) and grams of starch/total EI to the HC groups. The number and percentage of children in each HC sub-category are given in the lower half of the table.

Table 2. Cross-sectional baseline characteristics of short sleepers (<10 h). The right-hand columns present the regression coefficients, with 95% CI (Confidence Interval).

Outcome	Not Short Sleeper *n* = 3883	Short Sleeper *n* = 2061	Regression Coefficient	95% CI
BMI score, Cole 2012	0.25	0.61	0.12	0.05; −0.18
Dietary factors modeled in multivariable model shown in Table 3				
HC morning sugar, n (%)	1080 (27.8)	405 (19.7)	0.03	−0.13; 0.19
HC morning starch, n (%)	997 (25.7)	489 (23)	0.21	0.05; 0.37
HC midday sugar, n (%)	987 (25)	499 (24)	−0.16	−0.31; −0.00
HC midday starch, n (%)	754 (19)	732 (36)	−0.08	−0.24; 0.08
HC evening sugar, n (%)	916 (24)	570 (28)	0.21	0.05; 0.36
HC evening starch, n (%)	887 (23)	599 (29)	0.07	−0.08; 0.22
Energy, kcal/day, mean	1522.8	1655.6	31.74	7.69; 55.79
Eats breakfast, %	84.17	81.82	−0.03	−0.047; −0.00
Other factor modeled in multivariable model shown in Table 3				
High parent education %	39.5	29.1	−0.029	−0.06; 0.00
Descriptive dietary factors, not in multivariable model shown in Table 3				
Starch, g/day	99.8	122.4	3.92	1.29; 6.55
Sugar, g/day	91.8	87.9	0.52	−1.88; 2.92
Carbohydrate, energy-%, day	52.3%	52.2%	0.01	−0.64; 0.65
Fat, energy-%, day	31.5%	31.0%	0.09	−0.43; 0.61
Protein, energy-%, day	15.8%	16.0%	−0.29	−0.55; 0.03

Footnote: High carbohydrate (HC-starch and HC-sugar categories) were calculated for starch and sugar at three time-points (morning, midday and evening) by assigning those in the highest quartile for grams of sugar/total energy intake (EI) and grams of starch/total EI to the HC groups.

Table 3. High carbohydrate intake from sugar and starch at three times of day and short sleep duration and association with BMI z-scores at baseline, adjusted for age, sex and country.

Exposures Measured at Baseline (*n* = 5750) [†]	Regression Coefficient	95% CI
Short sleep < 10 h *versus* ≥ 10 h	0.09	0.02; 0.16
Breakfast (yes v. no)	−0.28	−0.36; 0.19
HC morning sugar	−0.02	−0.09; 0.05
HC morning starch	0.12	0.05; 0.20
HC midday sugar	0.03	−0.04; 0.10
HC midday starch	0.02	−0.07; 0.10
HC evening sugar	−0.04	−0.12; 0.03
HC evening starch	−0.08	−0.15; −0.00
Total energy intake in kcal	0.03	0.02; 0.04
Parental education (high v. "not high")	−0.09	−0.16; 0.24

[†] *n* reduced from 5944 at baseline due to non-response on two variables: breakfast (*n* = 5772) and Parental Education (*n* = 5750). High carbohydrate (HC-starch and HC-sugar categories) were calculated for starch and sugar at three time-points (morning, midday and evening) by assigning those in the highest quartile for grams of sugar/total energy intake (EI) and grams of starch/total EI to the HC groups. CI: Confidence Interval.

In Figure 3, the effect of short sleep duration on the relationship between HC from sugar and starch at each meal occasion and BMI z-scores is shown in a mutually adjusted model including age, sex, parental education, total EI, eating breakfast and survey country. Six interaction terms were introduced to the main effects, one of which was significant, *i.e.*, the interaction between high starch at midday and short sleep. In children with short sleep duration, the risk posed by HC intake from starch at midday had a stronger effect in those with short sleep duration. We also observed that HC from starch in the evening among the children without short nocturnal sleep duration is inversely associated with BMI z-scores but the respective interaction term was not significant.

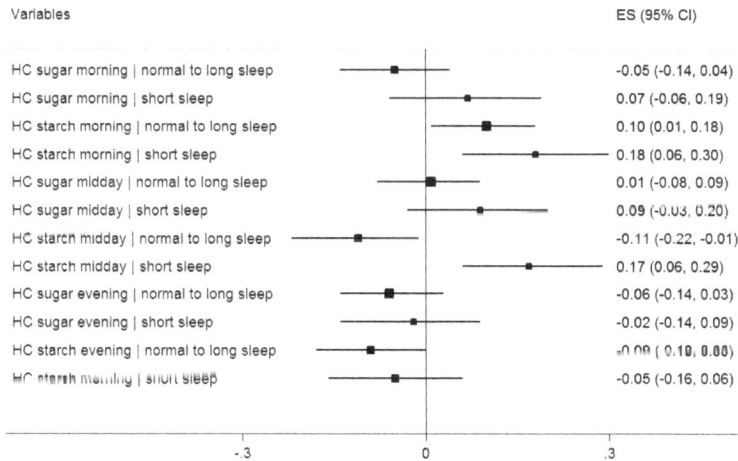

Figure 3. Effect of HC intake (sugar and starch) at 3 meal occasions on BMI z-scores at baseline by sleep duration. ES = effect size (regression coefficient). *n* reduced from 5944 at baseline due to non-response on two variables: breakfast and parental education level (*n* = 5750); Linear regression of BMI z-scores on sleep duration, HC intake variables, and their respective product terms, further adjusted for eating breakfast, parental education, age, sex, and survey country. Long sleep represents normal and long sleep ≥10 hours. CI: Confidence Interval.

There was a positive interaction between high midday sugar and short sleep duration with respect to BMI z-scores at two-year follow-up, but it was no longer observed after adjustment for baseline BMI z-scores (not shown). After adjustment for baseline BMI z-scores, only high parental education level remained significantly protective, (Regression coefficient = −0.08, *p* = 0.001, 95% CI = −0.12; −0.03; results not shown in tables).

4. Discussion

Our findings demonstrate that a high proportion of carbohydrate from starch in the morning is associated with an increased risk of a higher BMI z-scores at baseline in children participating in the IDEFICS study. Moreover, we found that high intake from starch at midday, in combination with short sleep duration, poses a risk for overweight. We also showed that eating breakfast is associated with lower BMI z-scores cross-sectionally at baseline, concurring with previous research [13,16] However, at the cross-sectional two-year follow-up analysis, eating breakfast offered no protection from increasing BMI z-scores, as has also been reported [17,18].

There is limited research on macronutrient distribution in children's diets. However, a systematic review of intervention studies published in 2014 examined the impact of dietary macronutrients on BMI and cardio-metabolic outcomes in overweight and obese children and adolescents [32]. From 14 eligible studies, five examined low carbohydrate intake related to BMI [32]. A meta-analysis of these low-carbohydrate studies in children and adolescents indicated a greater reduction in BMI in the low-carbohydrate group immediately after dietary intervention, but the authors noted that the quality of the studies was limited [32]. While our study was observational, our findings are in line with those of the systematic review of intervention studies, as we observed an association between HC intake from starch and higher BMI z-scores.

In adults, de Castro has reported that the time of day is an important factor influencing overall intake [33]. In the same cohort of adults, de Castro demonstrated that when the proportion of daily carbohydrate ingested in the morning was high, less total food energy and carbohydrate were consumed over the entire day [34]. In contrast, we found that high morning starch intake is associated with higher BMI z-scores and that breakfast-eaters consumed more total energy than those not reporting breakfast, which indicates that those skipping breakfast do not make up for skipped breakfast energy later in the day. Although de Castro did not report specifically on midday HC intake or on associations with overweight, his work may help to explain our finding that high starch intake at midday, interacting with short sleep duration, was associated with higher BMI z-scores, compared with morning carbohydrate intake. A study conducted on adults consuming a low-calorie diet studied the effects of carbohydrates consumed mostly at dinner and reported that subjects on the experimental diet underwent positive hormonal changes (leptin and adiponectin concentrations) and reported less hunger [35]. Similarly, we observed that high starch intake in the evening was inversely associated with BMI z-scores cross-sectionally at baseline. Sofer *et al.* [35] reported that simple dietary manipulation of carbohydrate distribution appears to yield additional benefits beyond calorie reduction. The hormone leptin regulates hunger, satiety and EI. Previous studies have reported that leptin secretion falls between 8:00 a.m. and 4:00 p.m., reaching the lowest point at 1:00 p.m., increasing at 4:00 p.m. and typically peaking at 1.00 p.m. [36,37]. This indicates that leptin levels are lowest at midday, which may be related to our findings that HC intake from starch in the morning and HC intake from starch at midday, interacting with short sleep duration, are positively associated with higher BMI z-scores.

It may be of particular interest that our cross-sectional findings are attributable to starch rather than sugar intake; there are plausible explanations for this. Most importantly, we report on all sugars, rather than added sugars, as a component of carbohydrate. The United States Department of Agriculture (USDA) recommends that children consume the following daily: two cups or approximately 350 g of fruit, 2.5 cups or approximately 475 g of vegetables, 6 oz. or approximately 168 g of whole grains and three cups or approximately 720 mL of dairy products. Following the USDA recommendations, a child exceeds 80 g of sugar intake when consuming just 1530 kcal per day [38]. The mean sugar intake in our study sample was 90.5 g, while the mean EI was 1569 kcal. This might indicate that added sugars do not contribute significantly to the dietary intake in our study population, *i.e.*, the sugars consumed occur naturally in foods considered to be healthy. However, it is also possible that added sugars or "bad" sugars may be under-reported by parents and therefore deflate the estimate of overall sugar intake. While we have eliminated energy over- and under-reporters from our sample based on total caloric intake, we cannot exclude the existence of a "good" food–"bad" food reporting bias.

Similar to our sleep findings, previous research has demonstrated a relationship between adiposity and short sleep duration [39,40]. Recently, a Belgian study confirmed that short sleep duration is associated with central adiposity in children [7]. We found that those with short sleep duration (<10 h) had higher BMI z-scores than those with 10 or more hours of sleep. Previous research has demonstrated that acute sleep deprivation increases snack portions [41] and that lack of sleep is associated with increased snacking, an increased number of daily meals and a preference for energy-rich foods [42]. The previously-mentioned study of Malaysian children demonstrated that children who sleep less than the recommended number of hours consumed more carbohydrates and were at higher risk of overweight/obesity [10]. Our findings indicate that children with shorter sleep duration are more at risk of overweight and that inadequate sleep potentiates the association between increased BMI z-scores and HC intake. It may be speculated that a HC diet combined with inadequate sleep may represent part of the explanation for high rates of obesity in children from a lower socioeconomic position (SEP). A number of previous studies, including the IDEFICS study, have reported that children from higher-income or more educated families tend to eat more healthfully [43–47]. However, in the context of the associations reported here, it should be pointed out that our findings are statistically independent of SEP, as defined by household parental education level.

Our findings on breakfast may be of interest, in light of inconsistencies in the literature. Our cross-sectional results at baseline are in line with other European studies reporting an association between breakfast intake and lower BMI, compared with children who skip breakfast [13–16]. However, our findings at two-year follow-up show no consistent association between breakfast consumption and lower BMI z-scores support those of a 2010 systematic review that concluded causality has not been demonstrated [17]. Similarly, a study of Danish children aged two and five also found no association between breakfast consumption and overweight [48]. Furthermore, it might be surprising that children with short sleep duration were less likely to eat breakfast than those who slept 10 or more hours, as it might be expected that those with more waking hours would have more time to consume breakfast. While the difference was statistically significant (82%: <10 h *versus* 84%: ⩾10 h), the absolute values were of low magnitude.

To our knowledge, this is the first study to simultaneously examine carbohydrate intake and its temporal distribution, short nocturnal sleep duration, breakfast habits and risk of overweight in a large cohort of children with diverse dietary cultures and lifestyle habits. Moreover, this study adhered to strict implementation of standardized operating procedures during fieldwork as well as plausibility checks during data entry. However, our study is not without limitations, the most important of which is including only one day of dietary recall. It is also important to note that the calculations are heterogeneous because macronutrients are calculated from a number of different FTC. For example, in Sweden, Germany and Hungary sugar was calculated as monosaccharide plus disaccharide, while in Estonia sugar consists of glucose, fructose, sucrose, maltose and lactose. These discrepancies might lead to subtle difficulties in comparing dietary carbohydrate intake. Finally, it should be kept in mind that the sample included in the IDEFICS study was not randomly selected and the related descriptive data cannot be considered to be representative at the country level.

5. Conclusions

This study showed BMI z-scores were cross-sectionally associated with high dietary carbohydrate intake from starch consumed in the morning, and in children with less than optimal sleep duration with high dietary carbohydrate intake from starch at midday. Breakfast consumption was not consistently associated with BMI z-scores. These findings suggest that childhood overweight might be reduced by limiting the proportion of dietary carbohydrates, particularly from starchy foods, in morning meals, and even more so in midday meals, and by encouraging the recommended amount of sleep each night.

Acknowledgments: Sources of financial support: This study was conducted as part of the IDEFICS study (http://www.idefics.edu), which was funded by the European Community within the Sixth RTD Framework Programme Contract No. 016181 (FOOD). The lead author also wishes to thank the Swedish Research Council for Health, Working Life and Welfare (http://www.forte.se/en/) for funding EPILIFE and the Stiftelsen Fru Mary von Sydows, född Wijk, Donationsfond (http://www.maryvonsydowstiftelsen.se/) for salary support. Isabelle Sioen is financially supported by the Research Foundation—Flanders (Grant No.: 1.2.683.14.N.00). The funders had no role in the design, data collection, data analysis or interpretation of data; in the writing of this manuscript; or in the decision to submit for publication. The authors are grateful for the support provided by school boards, headmasters and communities, and thank the IDEFICS children and their parents for participating in this extensive examination. The information in this document reflects the authors' views, based upon our analyses and the current literature, and is therefore provided as such.

Author Contributions: Monica Hunsberger, statistical analysis and manuscript writing; Kirsten Mehlig, statistical support and critical revisions of the manuscript; Claudia Börnhorst, statistical consulting and revisions of the manuscript; Antje Hebestreit, Luis Moreno, Toomas Veidebaum, Yiannis Kourides, Alfonso Siani, and Dénes Molnar, provided critical revisions of the manuscript; Isabelle Sioen, study design and critical revisions of the manuscript; and Lauren Lissner, study design and critical revisions of the manuscript.

Conflicts of Interest: The authors declare no conflict of interest.

References

1. World Health Organization. Global Strategy on Diet, Physical Activity, and Health: Childhood Overweight and Obesity. 2012. Available online: http://www.who.int/dietphysicalactivity/strategy/eb11344/strategy_english_web.pdf (accessed on 12 January 2015).
2. World Health Organization. Obesity and Overweight; Fact Sheet 311. 2014. Available online: http://www.who.int/mediacentre/factsheets/fs311/en/ (accessed on 12 January 2015).

3. Magarey, A.; Watson, J.; Golley, R.K.; Burrows, T.; Sutherland, R.; McNaughton, S.A.; Denney-Wilson, E.; Campbell, K.; Collins, C. Assessing dietary intake in children and adolescents: Considerations and recommendations for obesity research. *Int. J. Pediatr. Obes.* **2011**, *6*, 2–11. [CrossRef] [PubMed]

4. Nielsen, L.S.; Danielsen, K.V.; Sørensen, T.I. Short sleep duration as a possible cause of obesity: Critical analysis of the epidemiological evidence. *Obes. Rev.* **2011**, *12*, 78–92. [CrossRef] [PubMed]

5. Chen, X.; Beydoun, M.A.; Wang, Y. Is sleep duration associated with childhood obesity? A systematic review and meta-analysis. *Obesity* **2008**, *16*, 265–274. [CrossRef] [PubMed]

6. Hart, C.N.; Cairns, A.; Jelalian, E. Sleep and obesity in children and adolescents. *Pediatr. Clin. N. Am.* **2011**, *58*, 715–733. [CrossRef] [PubMed]

7. Michels, N.; Verbeiren, A.; Ahrens, W.; de Henauw, S.; Sioen, I. Children's sleep quality: Relation with sleep duration and adiposity. *Public Health* **2014**, *128*, 488–490. [CrossRef] [PubMed]

8. Hense, S.; Pohlabeln, H.; de Henauw, H.; Eiben, G.; Molnar, D.; Moreno, L.A.; Barba, G.; Hadjigeorgiou, C.; Veidebaum, T.; Ahrens, W. Sleep duration and overweight in European children: Is the association modified by geographic region? *Sleep* **2011**, *34*, 885–890. [CrossRef] [PubMed]

9. Accurso, A.; Bernstein, R.K.; Dahlqvist, A.; Draznin, B.; Feinman, R.D.; Fine, E.J.; Gleed, A.; Jacobs, D.B.; Larson, G.; Lustig, R.H.; *et al.* Dietary carbohydrate restriction in type 2 diabetes mellitus and metabolic syndrome: Time for a critical appraisal. *Nutr. Metab.* **2008**, *5*, 9. [CrossRef] [PubMed]

10. Martens, E.A.; Gonnissen, H.K.; Gatta-Cherifi, B.; Janssens, P.L.; Westerterp-Plantenga, M.S. Maintenance of energy expenditure on high-protein *vs.* high-carbohydrate diets at a constant body weight may prevent a positive energy balance. *Clin. Nutr.* **2014**, *34*, 968–975. [CrossRef] [PubMed]

11. Saavedra, J.M.; Deming, D.; Dattilo, A.; Reidy, K. Lessons from the Feeding Infants and Toddlers Study in North America: What Children Eat, and Implications for Obesity Prevention. *Ann. Nutr. Metab.* **2013**, *62*, S27–S36. [CrossRef] [PubMed]

12. Firouzi, S.; Poh, B.K.; Ismail, M.N.; Sadeghilar, A. Sleep habits, food intake, and physical activity levels in normal and overweight and obese Malaysian children. *Obes. Res. Clin. Pract.* **2014**, *1*, e70–e78. [CrossRef] [PubMed]

13. Fabritius, K.; Rasmussen, M. Breakfast habits and overweight in Danish schoolchildren. The role of socioeconomic positions. *Ugeskr. Laeger* **2008**, *170*, 2559–2563. [PubMed]

14. Henríquez Sánchez, P.; Doreste Alonso, J.; Laínez Sevillano, P.; Estévez González, M.D.; Iglesias Valle, M.; López Martín, G.; Sosa Iglesias, I.; Serra Majem, L. Prevalence of obesity and overweight in adolescents from Canary Islands, Spain. Relationship with breakfast and physical activity. *Med. Clin.* **2008**, *130*, 606–610. [CrossRef]

15. Dialektakou, K.D.; Vranas, P.B. Breakfast Skipping and Body Mass Index among Adolescents in Greece: Whether an Association Exists Depends on How Breakfast Skipping Is Defined. *Am. Diet. Assoc.* **2008**, *108*, 1517–1525. [CrossRef] [PubMed]

16. Mota, J.; Fidalgo, F.; Silva, R.; Ribeiro, J.C.; Santos, R.; Carvalho, J.; Santos, M.P. Relationships between physical activity, obesity and meal frequency in adolescents. *Ann. Hum. Biol.* **2008**, *35*, 1–10. [CrossRef] [PubMed]

17. Szajewska, H.; Ruszczynski, M. Systematic Review Demonstrating that Breakfast Consumption Influences Body Weight Outcomes in Children and Adolescents in Europe. *Crit. Rev. Food Sci. Nutr.* **2010**, *50*, 113–119. [CrossRef] [PubMed]

18. Brown, A.W.; Bohan-Brown, M.M.; Allison, D.B. Belief beyond the evidence: Using the proposed effect of breakfast on obesity to show 2 practices that distort scientific evidence. *Am. J. Clin. Nutr.* **2013**, *98*, 1298–1308. [CrossRef] [PubMed]

19. Ahrens, W.; Bammann, K.; de Henauw, S.; Halford, J.; Palou, A.; Pigeot, I.; Siani, A.; Sjöström, M. European Consortium of the IDEFICS Project. Understanding and preventing childhood obesity and related disorders—IDEFICS: A European multilevel epidemiological approach. *Nutr. Metab. Cardiovasc. Dis.* **2006**, *16*, 302–308. [CrossRef] [PubMed]

20. Ahrens, W.; Bammann, K.; Siani, A.; Buchecker, K.; de Henauw, S.; Iacoviello, L.; Hebestreit, A.; Krogh, V.; Lissner, L.; Mårild, S.; *et al.* IDEFICS Consortium. The IDEFICS cohort: Design, participation, socio-demographic characteristics and participation in the baseline survey. *Int. J. Obes.* **2011**, *35*, S3–S15. [CrossRef] [PubMed]

21. Bammann, K.; Peplies, J.; Sjöström, M.; Lissner, L.; de Henauw, S.; Galli, C.; Iacoviello, L.; Krogh, V.; Mårild, S.; Pigeot, I.; *et al.* Assessment of diet, physical activity and biological, social and environmental factors in a multi-centre European project on diet- and lifestyle-related disorders in children (IDEFICS). *Public Health* **2006**, *14*, 279–289. [CrossRef]

22. Vereecken, C.A.; Covents, M.; Sichert-Hellert, W.; Alvira, J.M.; le Donne, C.; de Henauw, S.; de Vriendt, T.; Phillipp, M.K.; Béghin, L.; Manios, Y.; *et al.* Development and evaluation of a self-administered computerized 24-h dietary recall method for adolescents in Europe. *Int. J. Obes.* **2008**, *32*, 26–34. [CrossRef] [PubMed]

23. Hebestreit, A.; Börnhorst, C.; Barba, G.; Siani, A.; Huybrechts, I.; Tognon, G.; Eiben, G.; Moreno, L.A.; Fernández Alvira, J.M.; Loit, H.M.; *et al.* Associations between energy intake, daily food intake and energy density of foods and BMI z-score in 2–9-year-old European children. *Eur. J. Nutr.* **2014**, *53*, 673–681. [PubMed]

24. Food Standard Agency; Public Health of England. *McCance and Widdowson's the Composition of Foods*, 5th ed.; Cambridge: Royal Society of Chemistry: Cambridge, UK, 1992.

25. National Heart Lung Blood Institute. How Much Sleep Is Enough? Available online: http://www.nhlbi.nih.gov/health/health-topics/topics/sdd/howmuch (accessed on 8 March 2015).

26. Svensson, Å.; Larsson, C.; Eiben, G.; Lanfer, A.; Pala, V.; Hebestreit, A.; Huybrechts, I.; Fernández-Alvira, J.M.; Russo, P.; Koni, A.C. European children's sugar intake on weekdays *versus* weekends: The IDEFICS study. *Eur. J. Clin. Nutr.* **2014**, *68*, 822–828. [CrossRef] [PubMed]

27. Schofield, W.N. Predicting basal metabolic rate, new standards and review of previous work. *Hum. Nutr. Clin. Nutr.* **1985**, *39*, S5–S41.

28. Goldberg, G.R.; Black, A.E.; Jebb, S.A.; Cole, T.J.; Murgatroyd, P.R.; Coward, W.A.; Prentice, A.M. Critical evaluation of energy intake data using fundamental principles of energy physiology: 1. Derivation of cut-off limits to identify under-recording. *Eur. J. Clin. Nutr.* **1991**, *45*, 569–581. [PubMed]

29. Cole, T.J.; Lobstein, T. Extended international (IOTF) body mass index cut-offs for thinness, overweight and obesity. *Pediatr. Obes.* **2012**, *7*, 284–294. [CrossRef] [PubMed]

30. Stomfai, S.; Ahrens, W.; Bammann, K.; Kovács, E.; Mårild, S.; Michels, N.; Moreno, L.A.; Pohlabeln, H.; Siani, A.; Tornaritis, M. Intra- and inter-observer reliability in anthropometric measurements in children. *Int. J. Obes.* **2011**, *35*, S45–S51. [CrossRef] [PubMed]

31. UNESCO. International Standard Classification of Education. 2010. Available online: http://www.uis.unesco.org (accessed on 14 December 2014).

32. Gow, M.L.; Ho, M.; Burrows, T.L.; Baur, L.A.; Stewart, L.; Hutchesson, M.J.; Cowell, C.T.; Collins, C.E.; Garnett, S.P. Impact of dietary macronutrient distribution on BMI and cardiometabolic outcomes in overweight and obese children and adolescents: A systematic review. *Nutr. Rev.* **2014**, *72*, 453–470. [CrossRef] [PubMed]

33. De Castro, J. The time of day of food intake influences overall intake in humans. *J. Nutr.* **2004**, *134*, 104–111. [PubMed]

34. De Castro, J. The time of day and the proportions of macronutrients eaten are related to daily food intake. *Br. J. Nutr.* **2007**, *98*, 1077–1083. [CrossRef] [PubMed]

35. Sofer, S.; Eliraz, A.; Kaplan, S.; Voet, H.; Fink, G.; Kima, T.; Madar, Z. Greater Weight Loss and Hormonal Changes After 6 Months Diet With Carbohydrates Eaten Mostly at Dinner. *Obesity* **2011**, *19*, 2006–2014. [CrossRef] [PubMed]

36. Coleman, R.A.; Herrmann, T.S. Nutritional regulation of leptin in humans. *Diabetologia* **1999**, *42*, 639–646. [CrossRef] [PubMed]

37. Yildiz, B.O.; Suchard, M.A.; Wong, M.L.; McCann, S.M.; Licinio, J. Alterations in the dynamics of circulating ghrelin, adiponectin, and leptin in human obesity. *Proc. Natl. Acad. Sci. USA* **2004**, *101*, 10434–10439. [CrossRef] [PubMed]

38. United States Department of Agriculture. Online Diet Assessment Tool. Available online: http://www.supertracker.usda.gov/foodtracker (accessed on 7 April 2015).

39. Patel, S.R.; Hu, F.B. Short sleep duration and weight gain: A systematic review. *Obesity* **2008**, *3*, 643–653. [CrossRef] [PubMed]

40. Beccuti, G.; Pannain, S. Sleep and obesity. *Curr. Opin. Clin. Nutr. Metab. Care* **2011**, *14*, 402–412. [CrossRef] [PubMed]

41. Hogenkamp, P.S.; Nilsson, E.; Nilsson, V.C.; Chapman, C.D.; Vogel, H.; Lundberg, L.S.; Zarei, S.; Cedernaes, J.; Rångtell, F.H.; Broman, J.E.; *et al.* Acute sleep deprivation increases portion size and affects food choice in young men. *Psychoneuroendocrinology* **2013**, *38*, 1668–1674. [CrossRef] [PubMed]

42. Chaput, J.P. Sleep patterns, diet quality and energy balance. *Physiol. Behav.* **2014**, *134*, 86–91. [CrossRef] [PubMed]

43. Fernández-Alvira, J.M.; Mouratidou, T.; Bammann, K.; Hebestreit, A.; Barba, G.; Sieri, S.; Reisch, L.; Eiben, G.; Hadjigeorgiou, C.; Kovacs, E. Parental education and frequency of food consumption in European children: The IDEFICS study. *Public Health Nutr.* **2012**, *16*, 487–498. [CrossRef] [PubMed]

44. Abudayya, A.H.; Stigum, H.; Shi, Z.; Abed, Y.; Holmboe-Ottesen, G. Socio-demographic correlates of food habits among school adolescents (12–15 years) in North Gaza Strip. *BMC Public Health* **2009**, *9*, 185. [CrossRef] [PubMed]

45. Sandvik, C.; Gjestad, R.; Samdal, O.; Brug, J.; Klepp, K.I. Does socioeconomic status moderate the associations between psychosocial predictors and fruit intake in schoolchildren? The Pro Children study. *Health Educ. Res.* **2010**, *25*, 121–134. [CrossRef] [PubMed]

46. Suliga, E. Parental education and living environmental influence on physical development, nutritional habits as well as level of physical activity in Polish children and adolescents. *Anthropol. Anz.* **2010**, *68*, 53–66. [CrossRef] [PubMed]

47. Blake, C.E.; Wethington, E.; Farrell, T.J.; Bisogni, C.A.; Devine, C.M. Behavioral contexts, food-choice coping strategies, and dietary quality of a multiethnic sample of employed parents. *J. Am. Diet. Assoc.* **2011**, *111*, 401–407. [CrossRef] [PubMed]

48. Küpers, L.K.; de Pijper, J.J.; Sauer, P.J.J.; Stolk, R.P.; Corpeleijn, E. Skipping breakfast and overweight in two and five year old Dutch children–GECKO Drenthe cohort. *Int. J. Obes.* **2014**, *38*, 569–571. [CrossRef] [PubMed]

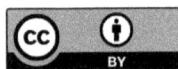

nutrients

MDPI

Article

Association of Nut Consumption with Cardiometabolic Risk Factors in the 2008/2009 New Zealand Adult Nutrition Survey

Rachel C. Brown [1,2,*], Siew Ling Tey [3], Andrew R. Gray [4], Alexandra Chisholm [1], Claire Smith [1,2], Elizabeth Fleming [1] and Winsome Parnell [1,2]

[1] Department of Human Nutrition, University of Otago, PO Box 56, Dunedin 9054 New Zealand;
E-Mails: alex.chisholm@otago.ac.nz (A.C.); claire.smith@otago.ac.nz (C.S.); liz.fleming@otago.ac.nz (E.F.);
winsome.parnell@otago.ac.nz (W.P.)
[2] Nutrition Society of New Zealand, Whanganui 4543, New Zealand
[3] Clinical Nutrition Research Centre, Singapore Institute for Clinical Sciences, A*STAR, 14 Medical Drive,
#07-02, Singapore 117599, Singapore; E-Mail: siewling_tey@sics.a-star.edu.sg
[4] Department of Preventive and Social Medicine, University of Otago, PO Box 56, Dunedin 9054, New Zealand;
E-Mail: andrew.gray@otago.ac.nz
* Author to whom correspondence should be addressed; E-Mail: rachel.brown@otago.ac.nz;
Tel.: +64-3-479-5839; Fax: +64-3-479-7958.

Received: 20 July 2015 / Accepted: 21 August 2015 / Published: 8 September 2015

Abstract: Nut consumption has been associated with improvements in risk factors for chronic disease in populations within North America, Europe and Iran. This relationship has not been investigated in New Zealand (NZ). The associations between nut consumption and cardiometabolic risk factors among New Zealanders were examined. Data from the 24-h diet recalls of 4721 participants from the NZ Adult Nutrition Survey 2008/2009 (2008/2009 NZANS) were used to determine whole and total nut intake. Anthropometric data and blood pressure were collected, as well as blood samples analysed for total cholesterol (total-C) and HDL cholesterol (HDL-C), glycated haemoglobin (HbA1c), C-reactive protein (CRP) and folate. Participants were classified according to their five-year cardiovascular disease (CVD) risk. Both whole and total nut consumers had significantly lower weight, body mass index (BMI), waist circumference and central adiposity than non-nut consumers (all $p \leqslant 0.044$). Whole blood, serum and red blood cell folate concentrations were significantly higher among whole nut consumers compared to non-whole nut consumers (all $p \leqslant 0.014$), with only serum folate higher in total nut consumers compared to non-total nut consumers ($p = 0.023$). There were no significant differences for blood pressure, total-C, HDL-C and HbA1c; however, significant negative associations between total nut consumption and CVD risk category ($p < 0.001$) and CRP ($p = 0.045$) were apparent. Nut consumption was associated with more favourable body composition and a number of risk factors, which could collectively reduce chronic disease.

Keywords: nut intake; population survey; cardiometabolic risk factors

1. Introduction

Nuts are rich in cis-unsaturated fatty acids, vitamins, minerals and a number of phytochemicals, which collectively contribute to reductions in chronic disease risk, particularly cardiovascular disease (CVD), seen in both epidemiological and intervention studies [1–6]. Typically, nut consumers have lower concentrations of total cholesterol (total-C) and low-density lipoprotein cholesterol (LDL-C), with studies showing little effect on HDL cholesterol (HDL-C) and triglyceride concentrations [6]. Although recent studies have reported significant reductions in all-cause mortality among nut consumers [1,2,7,8], the effect of nut consumption on the risk of chronic disease other than CVD is less clear.

Limited epidemiologic evidence suggests that nut consumption may have beneficial effects on blood pressure, especially among those without type 2 diabetes [9] and those with hypertension who have a Body mass index (BMI) lower than 25 kg/m^2 [10]. Two recent reviews calculated mean changes in blood pressure from over 20 intervention studies and reported significant reductions for both systolic and diastolic blood pressure following nut consumption [9,11].

Studies investigating the association between nut consumption and the risk of type 2 diabetes have produced equivocal results. Two recent meta-analyses have reported no association between nut consumption and the risk of type 2 diabetes [8,12], whereas a small, but significant reduction in the incidence of type 2 diabetes was found in another recent meta-analysis by Afshin *et al.* [13]. It has been suggested the contradictory result is likely due to the differences in study selection (e.g., one study included by Afshin *et al.* did not examine the independent effects of nuts) and a lack of adjustment for BMI in the meta-analysis by Afshin *et al.* [14]. In addition, intervention trials, which have investigated the consumption of nuts on glycaemic control, have produced mixed results [11,15].

Although nuts are energy dense, several epidemiologic studies have reported that regular nut consumers tended to be leaner than non-consumers [16–19]. In support of this finding, five clinical trials specifically designed to examine the effect of regular nut consumption on body weight have reported no weight gain or less weight gain than predicted [20–24].

Folate has attracted public health interest because the suboptimal status of this vitamin appears to be associated with an increased risk of several chronic diseases, such as CVD [25] and certain cancers [26]. Nuts, in particular peanuts, hazelnuts and walnuts, are relatively rich sources of folate [27]. Therefore, it is of interest to assess the folate status of nut consumers.

Nationally representative data from the United States of America (USA) showed that nut and tree nut consumption was associated with a lower BMI, waist circumference and systolic blood pressure [28,29]. Nut consumers also had a lower prevalence of hypertension, low HDL-C, abdominal obesity and high fasting glucose concentrations, four important risk factors for metabolic syndrome. A recent analysis of the Adventist Heart Study-2 found that there was a significant inverse association between the frequency of nut intake and metabolic syndrome [30]. Similar results were found in participants at high cardiovascular risk [31]. Further, a cross-sectional study in Iran reported a significant association between high nut consumption and reduced dyslipidemia [32].

To date, no research has examined the association of nut intake and risk factors for chronic disease in New Zealand or indeed anywhere in the Southern Hemisphere, where dietary patterns may differ from countries where relationships between nut consumption and a variety of risk factors for disease have previously been described [29,32]. This study aimed to compare known risk factors of chronic disease between nut consumers and non-nut consumers in a cross-sectional representative survey of the New Zealand population.

2. Experimental Section

2.1. Study Population

The 2008/2009 NZ Adult Nutrition Survey (2008/2009 NZANS) was a cross-sectional survey of 4721 New Zealander aged 15 years and over. A full description of the study design and methods is available elsewhere [33], and only a summary is included here. Participants were recruited using a three-stage process where 607 mesh blocks were selected using a probability-proportional-to-size design. A mesh block is defined as a small geographical area within NZ defined by Statistics NZ. Each mesh block contains approximately 110 people in urban areas and 60 in rural areas. After random selection of a household, random selection of a participant within the household occurred. Oversampling of Maori and Pacific people and age groups 15–18 years and 71 years and over was used to achieve adequate numbers for analysis by ethnicity and age.

Informed, written consent was obtained from each participant or from the guardian of participants aged less than 18 years prior to interviews. Ethical approval was gained from the NZ Health and Disability Multi-Region Ethics Committee (MEC/08/04/049). This study was conducted according to the guidelines laid down in the Declaration of Helsinki, and all procedures involving human subjects were approved by the NZ Health and Disability Multi-Region Ethics Committee (MEC/08/04/049).

2.2. Dietary Assessment

Survey data were collected at the participants' homes by trained interviewers using computer-assisted personal interview software. An interviewer-administered multiple-pass 24-h diet recall method was used to collect quantitative information on all foods and drinks the participant consumed the previous day (from midnight to midnight). It included foods and drinks consumed both at and away from home and has been previously described [33].

2.3. Determination of Nut Intake

For the purpose of this study, the term 'nuts' includes tree nuts, peanuts and mixed nuts. Tree nuts include almonds, Brazil nuts, cashews, hazelnuts, macadamias, pecans, pine nuts, pistachios and walnuts. Chestnuts, coconut and coconut products were not included in this analysis, as their nutrient profiles differ from the aforementioned 'nuts'. Nut intake was assessed using the 24-h diet recall data from the 2008/2009 NZANS, and total nut consumption was comprised of the following three categories:

(i) Whole nuts, including tree nuts, mixed nuts and peanuts eaten whole as part of a snack (e.g., mixed nut snacks) or as an addition to a food/meal (e.g., almonds sprinkled on a salad); (ii) consumed as nut butters, including those made from peanuts and tree nuts (e.g., peanut butter, hazelnut spread); and (iii) consumed as an ingredient of a recipe/dish or a commercial products (e.g., breakfast cereals, snack bars, satay sauce). Participants who reported consuming zero quantity of any nuts in their 24-h diet recall were classified as 'non-nut consumers'. 'Total nut consumers' were participants who reported consuming any of whole nuts, nut butters and/or hidden sources of nuts. 'Whole nut consumers' were participants who reported consuming any amount of whole nuts.

2.4. Blood Collection and Analysis

Non-fasting blood samples were collected from 3348 participants at local healthcare clinics. Blood was collected into three vacutainers, two containing EDTA for plasma and one additive free for serum. Vacutainers were couriered to a central processing laboratory for analysis of total-C and HDL-C, HbA1c and CRP. Further aliquots were sent to the Department of Human Nutrition, University of Otago, for analysis of whole blood, serum and red blood cell (RBC) folate concentrations.

Serum total-C was measured enzymatically and serum HDL-C using the Ultra HDL assay, on the ARCHITECT cSystem (Abbott). Serum CRP was measured using the immunoturbidimetric assay on the Abbott. HbA1c was determined in whole blood using an ion-exchange high performance liquid chromatography method (Bio-Rad Variant II). The laboratory used for these measurements subscribes to the Royal College of Pathologists Australasia Quality Assurance Program.

Whole blood and serum folate concentrations were measured using the microbiological assay with chloramphenicol-resistant Lactobacillus casei as the test micro-organism, as described by O'Broin *et al.* [34]. RBC folate concentration was calculated using the following equation:

$$RBC\,folate\ =\ whole\,blood\,folate - [serum\,folate \times (1 - haematocrit)/haematocrit] \qquad (1)$$

The accuracy of the microbiological assay was monitored using a three-level certified reference for serum folate from the National Institute of Standards Technology (NIST, USA).

2.5. Blood Pressure

Blood pressure was measured in triplicate using an Omron blood pressure monitor (Model HEM-907, Kyoto, Japan). There was a one-minute period between measurements. The first blood pressure reading is considered the most unreliable [35]; thus, the mean of the second and third measurements was calculated.

2.6. Anthropometric Measurements

Trained interviewers carried out height and weight measurements in duplicate. Standing height was measured using a stadiometer (Seca 214, Seca, Hamburg, Germany) and weight using electronic scales (Tanita HD-351, Tanita, Tokyo, Japan). BMI was calculated as weight (kg)/(height (m)^2). The World Health Organization BMI cutoffs were used to categorise BMI status in participants aged 19 years and over. The Cole age- and sex-specific BMI cutoffs were used to categorise BMI status in those aged 15–18 years [36,37].

Waist circumference (WC) was measured at the narrowest point between the lower costal border and the top of the iliac crest. Measurements were taken over light clothing using an anthropometric tape measure (Model W606PM, Lufkin, Apex Tool Group, MD, USA). Measurements were taken to the nearest 0.1 cm.

A body shape index (ABSI) was also calculated [38]. This index, based on weight, height and waist circumference, has been developed because the strong correlation between BMI and waist circumference can make it difficult to differentiate the two as epidemiological risk factors. A body shape index is relatively uncorrelated with height, weight or BMI, while remaining positively correlated with waist circumference [38]. A body shape index has been shown to be a better predictor of mortality than waist circumference [39]. A high ABSI indicates that WC is higher than expected for a given height and weight, corresponding to a more centrally-concentrated body volume. The ABSI is calculated as follows, where waist circumference and height are expressed in meters:

$$\text{ABSI} = \frac{WC}{\sqrt[3]{BMI^2}\sqrt{height}} \tag{2}$$

2.7. Cardiovascular Disease Risk

Cardiovascular disease risk was calculated for participants aged 35–74 years ($n = 1623$) using the NZ adapted Framingham Cardiovascular Risk charts [40]. These charts categorise 5-year cardiovascular disease risk (fatal and non-fatal) into the following 8 categories: <2.5%, 2.5%–5% and 5%–10% (mild risk); 10%–15% (moderate risk); 15%–20% (high risk); 20%–25%, 25%–30%; and >30% (very high risk). Risk assessment is based on sex, age, total-C:HDL-C ratio, systolic blood pressure, smoking status and the presence/absence of diabetes. Maori, Pacific and Indo-Asian (Indian, including Fijian Indian, Sri Lankan, Afghani, Bangladeshi, Nepalese, Pakistani and Tibetan) participants are moved up one risk category as their risk of CVD may be underestimated using these charts [41].

2.8. Health Risk Factor Cutoffs

Participants were categorised based on being overweight or obese (BMI ⩾25 kg/m^2); having abdominal obesity (waist circumference ⩾102 cm for males and ⩾88 cm for females); having hypertension (SBP ⩾130 mmHg or DBP ⩾85 mmHg; or having low HDL-C (⩽1.03 mmol/L for males and ⩽1.29 mmol/L for females).

Participants with diabetes were defined as those who self-reported doctor-diagnosed diabetes or those who had an HbA1c ⩾6.5% (48 mmol/mol) [42]. Participants with pre-diabetes included those who had an HbA1c between 5.7% (39 mmol/mol) and 6.4% (46 mmol/mol) inclusive and who did not self-report doctor diagnosed diabetes.

2.9. Demographic Variables

Demographic variables were selected *a priori* after reviewing the literature. Variables included sex, age category (15–18, 19–30, 31–50, 51–70, 71+ years), prioritised ethnicity, NZ Index of Deprivation (NZDep06) and education. Information was also collected during the interview on smoking status (never smoker, ex-smoker, current smoker) and use of statins.

2.9.1. Ethnicity

Self-reported ethnicity was categorised into one of three ethnic groups based on a priority classification system using the coding prioritisation order (from highest to lowest) of Maori, Pacific and New Zealand European and other (NZEO). For example, if a participant identified as both Maori and NZ European, they were classified as Maori.

2.9.2. New Zealand Index of Deprivation (NZDep06)

NZDep06 is an area-based measure of deprivation, which uses nine variables from the NZ Census reflecting specified dimensions of both material and social deprivation. Each mesh block in NZ is given a score between 1 and 10, with a score of 1 reflecting the least deprived areas and 10 the most deprived. For the purpose of the 2008/2009 NZANS, these scores were divided into quintiles where Quintile 1 represents the 20% least deprived and Quintile 5 the 20% most deprived areas.

2.9.3. Education

Participants were asked to report their highest school level qualification and, where appropriate, their highest post-school qualification. Three groups, comprising no formal school qualification, secondary school qualification only or post-school qualification (including trade certificates and university degrees), were derived for these analyses.

2.10. Statistical Analysis

The complex survey design described above was accounted for in all analyses presented here. This included incorporating both weights and clustering. The weights used were post-stratification weights for the questionnaire component of the NZANS (when comparing reported nut consumption between demographic groups and comparing anthropometric outcomes between nut consumption groups) and post-stratification weights for the blood component of the NZANS (comparing biochemical outcomes between nut consumption groups) and are intended to reflect the NZ population aged 15 years and above. Stata's default method for calculating survey-adjusted standard errors (Taylor linearization) was used for all analyses.

Log-transformations were made where this improved residual normality and/or homoscedasticity. Variables, which were log-transformed, include weight, BMI, waist circumference, total cholesterol, HDL-cholesterol, total:HDL-C ratio, C-reactive protein, HbA1c, whole blood folate, serum folate and red blood cell folate. These variables are presented as geometric means with differences reported as the percentage difference between the geometric means. Unadjusted and adjusted differences for outcomes between nut consumers and non-nut consumers are presented. Survey regression models, including sex, age group, prioritised ethnicity, NZDep06 quintile and education (blood pressure was further adjusted for smoking status and BMI category; all blood variables were further adjusted for BMI category, and CRP was further adjusted for smoking status), were used to calculate adjusted differences in outcomes between nut consumers and non-nut consumers. Survey logistic regression was used to estimate the adjusted odds ratios (OR) and 95% confidence intervals (CIs), for overweight/obese, abdominal obesity, hypertension, low HDL-C, diabetes and pre-diabetes, with the following variables entered into the model: sex, age, NZDep06, education, ethnicity and BMI. Ordinal logistic regression, including NZDep06 quintile, education and BMI category, was used to estimate the adjusted-for

(Maori, Pacific and Indo-Asian ethnicities) CVD risk category. Proportionality was examined using generalised ordinal logistic regression without adjustment for the complex survey design to see if there was evidence against proportionality at the variable level or overall. Standard regression diagnostics were used in all cases.

Stata Statistical Software 12.1 (Statacorp LP, College Station TX, USA) was used for all statistical analyses. All statistical tests were two-sided; $p < 0.05$ was considered statistically significant, and $0.05 \leqslant p < 0.10$ is noted as a non-significant tendency, where these may suggest areas for further research or support the interpretation of other results. As this study is exploratory, no formal adjustment for multiple comparisons was made, and marginally significant results should be interpreted with caution.

3. Results

3.1. Characteristics of the Sample

Table 1 describes the characteristics of the 2008/2009 NZANS sample. A total of 4721 participants were recruited and completed a 24-h diet recall.

Table 1. Characteristics of survey participants.

	All Survey Participants	
Demographic	*n*	survey weighted %
Total population	4721	
Sex		
Male	2066	48.6
Female	2655	51.4
Age		
15–18 years	699	7.0
19–30 years	718	19.7
31–50 years	1344	36.7
51–70 years	895	27.1
71+ years	1065	9.6
Ethnicity		
NZEO [a]	2980	84.3
Maori	1040	11.1
Pacific	701	4.6
NZDep06 quintile [b]		
Q1 (least deprived)	664	20.2
Q2	829	21.4
Q3	761	21.3
Q4	1072	19.0
Q5 (most deprived)	1395	18.1

Table 1. *Cont.*

		All Survey Participants
Highest educational qualification		
No school qualification	1217	18.1
School	1413	26.5
Post-school	2057	55.4
Body mass index (kg/m^2)		
<25	1409	34.9
25–29.9	1581	37.1
⩾30	1513	28.0
Smoking status		
Never smoked	2393	50.8
Ex-smoker	1274	26.5
Current smoker	1074	22.8

[a] New Zealand European and other; [b] New Zealand Index of Deprivation.

3.2. Nut Intake

The nut intakes of New Zealanders have been described previously [43]. In brief, the percentage of the population consuming whole nuts (a subset of total nuts) and nuts from all sources (total nuts, including whole nuts, nut butters and nuts from hidden sources) on the day of their 24-h diet recall were 6.9% and 28.9%, respectively. The mean daily intake among the whole population was 2.8 g and 5.2 g for whole and total nuts, respectively. Among nut consumers only, the mean daily intake was 40.3 g for whole nuts and 17.9 g for total nuts (which included whole nuts, nut butters and nuts from hidden sources). In terms of prevalence, there were no significant differences between males and females.

3.3. Anthropometric Measurements

In the fully-adjusted model, body weight, BMI, waist circumference and ABSI were significantly lower among whole nut consumers (a subset of total nut consumers) compared to non-whole nut consumers (all $p \leqslant 0.029$) and for total nut consumers (including whole nut, nut butter and nuts from hidden source consumers) compared to non-total nut consumers (all $p \leqslant 0.044$) (Table 2).

Table 2. Mean (95% CI) body composition and blood pressure among nut and non-nut consumers.

	Total n	Non-Nut Consumers	n	Nut Consumers	n	Unadjusted Difference	Unadjusted p-Value	Adjusted Difference *	Adjusted p-Value
Whole nuts									
Weight (kg)	4519	77.0 (76.2, 77.8)	4288	73.5 (70.7, 76.5)	231	−4.5 (−8.2, −0.5)	0.026	−4.0 (−7.1, −07)	0.017
Body mass index (kg/m²)	4503	27.1 (26.8, 27.3)	4272	26.1 (25.3, 26.9)	231	−3.6 (−6.6, −0.6)	0.019	−3.9 (−6.7, −1.0)	0.008
Waist circumference (cm)	4519	90.5 (89.8, 91.2)	4288	87.3 (84.9, 89.8)	231	−3.5 (−6.3, −0.6)	0.018	−3.7 (−6.1, −1.3)	0.003
ABSI	4459	0.0766 (0.0763, 0.0768)	4229	0.0759 (0.0750, 0.0768)	230	−0.0007 (−0.0016, 0.0028)	0.165	−0.0009 (−0.0017, <−0.0001)	0.029
Systolic blood pressure (mmHg)	4632	120.3 (118.9, 121.7)	4396	120.3 (115.9, 124.6)	236	<0.1 (−4.5, 4.5)	1.000	−1.4 (−5.4, 2.6)	0.497
Diastolic blood pressure (mmHg)	4632	70.7 (69.9, 71.6)	4396	70.7 (68.0, 73.5)	236	<0.1 (−2.9, 2.9)	1.000	−0.8 (−3.4, 1.8)	0.553
Total nuts									
Weight (kg)	4519	77.5 (76.6, 78.4)	3383	75.0 (73.6, 76.3)	1136	−3.3 (−5.4, −1.1)	0.003	−2.0 (−4.0, −0.1)	0.044
Body mass index (kg/m²)	4503	27.3 (27.0, 27.6)	3370	26.4 (26.0, 26.8)	1133	−3.1 (−4.9, −1.3)	0.001	−2.3 (−4.0, −0.5)	0.012
Waist circumference (cm)	4519	91.2 (90.4, 92.0)	3383	88.1 (86.8, 89.3)	1136	−3.4 (−5.0, −1.8)	<0.001	−2.5 (−3.9, −1.0)	0.001
ABSI	4459	0.0768 (0.0766, 0.0772)	3338	0.0757 (0.0752, 0.0761)	1121	−0.0012 (−0.0017, −0.0007)	<0.001	−0.0009 (−0.0013, −0.0005)	<0.001
Systolic blood pressure (mmHg)	4632	122.3 (120.8, 123.8)	3479	120.5 (118.6, 122.4)	1153	−1.4 (−3.9, 1.2)	0.289	−1.3 (−3.5, 1.0)	0.263
Diastolic blood pressure (mmHg)	4632	72.0 (71.0, 73.0)	3479	70.8 (69.6, 72.0)	1153	−0.9 (−2.5, 0.6)	0.237	−1.1 (−2.6, 0.3)	0.132

* All variables adjusted for sex, age, NZDep, education level and ethnicity; blood pressure further adjusted for smoking status and BMI; blood pressure and ABSI are presented as arithmetic means; weight, BMI and waist circumference were log transformed, and geometric means are presented, with differences reported as the percentage difference between geometric means; ABSI = a body shape index; the ABSI is calculated as follows, where waist circumference (WC) and height are expressed in metres: $ABSI = WC/BMI^{2/3}height^{1/2}$.

3.4. Blood Pressure

Neither systolic nor diastolic blood pressure differed significantly between whole nut consumers (a subset of total nut consumers) and non-whole nut consumers (both $p \geqslant 0.497$) (Table 2), nor did they differ between total nut consumers (including whole nut, nut butter and nuts from hidden source consumers) and non-total nut consumers (both $p \geqslant 0.132$).

3.5. Biochemical Outcomes

There was a non-significant tendency for a lower total-C:HDL-C ratio in whole nut consumers (a subset of total nut consumers) compared to non-whole nut consumers ($p = 0.090$), with significantly higher HDL-C ($p = 0.024$) and lower total-C:HDL-C ratio ($p = 0.036$) among total nut consumers (including whole nut, nut butter and nuts from hidden source consumers) compared to non-total nut consumers before adjustment of potential confounders. However, after adjustment, total cholesterol, HDL-C and total-C:HDL-C ratio did not differ significantly between whole nut consumers and non-whole nut consumers (all $p \geqslant 0.147$) nor between total nut consumers and non-total nut consumers (all $p \geqslant 0.310$) (Table 3).

There was a non-significant tendency for lower CRP among whole nut consumers ($p = 0.078$), but this was no longer evident after adjustment for potential confounders ($p = 0.451$); whereas among total nut consumers, CRP was significantly lower than non-total nut consumers for both the unadjusted ($p < 0.001$) and the adjusted model ($p = 0.045$).

There was no significant difference for HbA1c between whole nut consumers and non-whole nut consumers ($p = 0.646$). Glycated haemoglobin was significantly lower for total nut consumers compared to non-total nut consumer ($p = 0.021$), but this difference was no longer evident after adjusting for potential confounders ($p = 0.475$).

After adjustment for potential confounders, whole blood folate ($p = 0.004$), serum blood folate ($p = 0.001$) and red blood cell folate ($p = 0.014$) were statistically significantly higher among whole nut consumers compared to non-whole nut consumers. In contrast, for total nut consumers, only serum folate concentration was significantly higher compared to non-total nut consumers ($p = 0.023$).

Table 3. Mean (95% CI) for biochemical indices for nut consumers and non-nut consumers.

Biochemical Indices	Total n	Non-consumers	n	Nut Consumers	n	Unadjusted Difference	Unadjusted p-Value	Adjusted Difference *	Adjusted p-Value *
Whole nuts									
Total cholesterol (mmol/L)	3309	5.02 (4.97, 5.08)	3108	4.99 (4.77, 5.02)	201	−0.8 (−5.1, 3.8)	0.740	−3.2 (−7.5, 1.2)	0.147
HDL-cholesterol (mmol/L)	3309	1.33 (1.31, 1.34)	3108	1.38 (1.31, 1.44)	201	3.8 (−1.1, 9.0)	0.131	−1.0 (−4.9, 3.0)	0.611
Total-C:HDL-C ratio	3309	3.79 (3.73, 3.85)	3108	3.62 (3.44, 3.81)	201	−4.4 (−9.3, 0.7)	0.090	−2.2 (−6.4, −2.2)	0.318
C-reactive protein (mg/L)	3310	1.60 (1.53, 1.68)	3109	1.39 (120, 1.61)	201	−13.0 (−25.6, 1.6)	0.078	−5.5 (−18.5, 9.5)	0.451
HbA1c (%)	3348	5.53 (5.50, 5.56)	3147	5.49 (5.39, 5.60)	201	−0.7 (−2.6, 1.3)	0.488	−0.4 (−2.1, 1.3)	0.646
Whole blood folate (nmol/L)	2929	351 (342, 360)	2749	409 (377, 444)	180	16.6 (7.0, 27.0)	<0.001	13.0 (4.0, 22.8)	0.004
Serum folate (nmol/L)	3277	22.9 (22.1, 23.6)	3076	28.8 (25.9, 32.1)	201	26.2 (12.9, 41.1)	<0.001	19.7 (7.6, 33.1)	0.001
Red blood cell folate (nmol/L)	2821	800 (780, 821)	2646	928 (853, 1,009)	175	15.9 (6.4, 26.3)	0.001	11.6 (2.6, 21.7)	0.014
Total nuts									
Total cholesterol (mmol/L)	3309	5.03 (4.96, 5.09)	2426	5.01 (4.96, 5.11)	883	−0.3 (−2.6, 2.0)	0.778	−1.1 (−3.2, 1.0)	0.310
HDL-cholesterol (mmol/L)	3309	1.32 (1.30, 1.34)	2426	1.36 (1.33, 1.38)	883	3.0 (0.4, 5.7)	0.024	−0.3 (−2.5, 1.9)	0.781
Total-C:HDL-C ratio	3309	3.81 (3.75, 3.88)	2426	3.69 (3.59, 3.79)	883	−3.2 (−6.2, −0.2)	0.036	−0.8 (−3.5, 1.9)	0.553
C-reactive protein (mg/L)	3310	1.67 (1.58, 1.76)	2427	1.41 (1.30, 1.52)	883	−15.8 (−22.9, −8.0)	<0.001	−7.6 (−14.4, −0.2)	0.045
HbA1c (%)	3348	5.55 (5.51, 5.58)	2456	5.48 (5.43, 5.53)	892	−1.2 (−2.2, −0.2)	0.021	−0.3 (−1.3, 0.1)	0.475
Whole blood folate (nmol/L)	2929	354 (344, 364)	2161	359 (341, 377)	768	1.3 (−4.3, 7.4)	0.643	0.3 (−5.0, 6.0)	0.903
Serum folate (nmol/L)	3277	22.4 (21.6, 23.3)	2395	25.3 (23.8, 26.8)	882	12.7 (5.1, 20.8)	0.001	8.4 (1.1, 16.1)	0.023
Red blood cell folate (nmol/L)	2821	808 (785, 831)	2071	815 (774, 857)	750	0.9 (−4.8, 6.9)	0.773	−0.6 (−6.0, 5.1)	0.831

* All variables adjusted for sex, age, NZDep, education level and ethnicity; CRP was further adjusted for smoking status; total cholesterol HDL cholesterol and Total:HDL-C ratio were further adjusted for smoking status, cholesterol-lowering medication and percent energy from saturated fat; all variables were log-transformed, and geometric means are presented, with differences reported as the percentage difference between geometric means.

3.6. Cardiovascular Disease Risk

There was evidence of non-proportionality for some of the covariates, but not for the nut consumption variables. In particular, for the whole nut consumption (a subset of total nut consumption) model, there was evidence of non-proportionality for the highest levels of deprivation and education and for the total nut consumption (including whole nut, nut butter and nuts from hidden source consumption) model; there was evidence of non-proportionality for the highest level of deprivation. Modelling these did not materially change the odds ratios for nut consumption (non-survey adjusted odds ratios for the nut consumption variables were identical to two decimal places in both cases, and the interpretation of covariates was similar in both cases), and so, survey-adjusted ordinal logistic regression models assuming proportionality are presented below. There was no evidence of an association between whole nut consumption and CVD risk category (proportional odds ratio = 0.83; 95% CI: 0.58–1.19; $p = 0.321$). However, there was a significant negative association between total nut consumption and CVD risk category (proportional odds ratio = 0.61; 95% CI: 0.47–0.80; $p < 0.001$).

In both models, living in the most deprived areas, having a lower education level and having a higher BMI were all association with increased CVD risk (all $p \leqslant 0.005$).

3.7. Odds Ratios for Health Risk Factors

The odds of being overweight or obese were 40% lower for whole nut consumers (a subset of total nut consumers) compared to non-whole nut consumers ($p = 0.015$) and 36% lower for total nut consumers (including whole nut, nut butter and nuts from hidden source consumers) ($p = 0.020$) compared to non-total nut consumers (Table 4). Similarly, the odds of having abdominal obesity were 46% lower ($p = 0.012$) in whole nut consumers and 32% lower ($p = 0.004$) in consumers of all nuts. Consumers of whole nuts had 57% lower odds of pre-diabetes ($p = 0.004$). There was no significant difference in the odds of pre-diabetes or diabetes between consumers of all nuts and non-nut consumers (both $p \geqslant 0.346$).

There were no significant differences in the odds of having low HDL-C or hypertension for whole and total nut consumers compared to non-consumers (all $p \geqslant 0.448$).

Table 4. Odds ratio (95% CI) for diabetes and risk factors for chronic disease by nut consumption.

	Unadjusted Odds ratio	Unadjusted *p*-Value	Adjusted Odds ratio *	Adjusted *p*-Value †
Whole nuts				
Overweight or obese	0.66 (0.44, 0.99)	0.045	0.60 (0.40, 0.90)	0.015
Abdominal obesity	0.57 (0.37, 0.89)	0.012	0.54 (0.34, 0.87)	0.012
Hypertension	0.91 (0.61, 1.38)	0.682	0.85 (0.53, 1.36)	0.502
Low HDL-C	0.77 (0.49, 1.22)	0.268	0.97 (0.61, 1.55)	0.904
Diabetes	0.91 (0.45, 1.81)	0.780	1.05 (0.49, 2.26)	0.898
Pre-diabetes	0.52 (0.31, 0.88)	0.016	0.43 (0.34, 0.76)	0.004

Table 4. *Cont.*

	Unadjusted Odds ratio	Unadjusted *p*-Value	Adjusted Odds ratio *	Adjusted *p*-Value †
Total nuts				
Overweight or obese	0.72 (0.57, 0.91)	0.006	0.74 (0.58, 0.95)	0.020
Abdominal obesity	0.66 (0.52, 0.84)	0.001	0.68 (0.52, 0.88)	0.004
Hypertension	0.83 (0.65, 1.04)	0.116	0.90 (0.69, 1.19)	0.456
Low HDL-C	0.78 (0.61, 0.99)	0.042	0.90 (0.70, 1.17)	0.448
Diabetes	0.63 (0.42, 0.96)	0.031	0.80 (0.51, 1.27)	0.346
Pre-diabetes	0.80 (0.63, 1.03)	0.082	0.88 (0.67, 1.16)	0.360

* Calculated using survey multiple logistic regression and adjusted for sex, age, NZDep06, education, ethnicity and BMI (except for overweight/obesity and abdominal obesity, which were not adjusted for BMI); † overall *p*-value from regression models; overweight or obesity, BMI $\geqslant 25$ kg/m^2; abdominal obesity, waist circumference $\geqslant 102$ cm for males and $\geqslant 88$ cm for females; hypertension, systolic BP $\geqslant 130$ mmHg or diastolic BP $\geqslant 85$ mmHg; low HDL-C, $\leqslant 1.03$ mmol/L for males and $\leqslant 1.29$ mmol/L for females; pre-diabetes included those with an HbA1c result between 5.7% (39 mmol/mol) and 6.4% (46 mmol/mol) inclusive and did not self report doctor diagnosed diabetes; diabetes included those who self-reported doctor-diagnosed diabetes or those who had an HbA1c $\geqslant 6.5\%$ (48 mmol/mol).

4. Discussion

This is the first study to assess the association between nut consumption and risk factors for chronic disease, in a cross-sectional survey of a population in NZ. This study confirms the results from large cross-sectional surveys undertaken in the Northern Hemisphere [29–32], which report that nut consumption is associated with better outcomes for a number of risk factors for chronic disease. Body weight, BMI and measures of central adiposity were significantly lower among nut consumers compared to non-nut consumers, as was the risk of being overweight or obese. In addition, CRP, a marker of inflammation, was significantly lower among total nut consumers compared to non-nut consumers. Furthermore, whole blood, serum and red blood cell folate were significantly higher among whole nut consumers compared to non-whole nut consumers. Collectively, these differences are likely to confer long-term beneficial health effects among regular nut consumers.

Although there were some significant differences between total-C and the total-C:HDL-C ratio between nut consumers and non-nut consumers, these disappeared after adjustment for potential confounders. This is in contrast to the majority of epidemiologic studies and randomised controlled trials, which show better lipid profiles or improvements in blood lipids and lipoproteins with the inclusion of nuts in the regular diet. A meta-analysis of 25 clinical trials reported dose-response reductions in total-C and LDL-C, with no effect on HDL-C, and a reduction in triglycerides [6]. However, the findings of the present study in regards to blood lipoproteins are not unique. A cross-sectional analysis of the Prevencion con Dieta Mediterranea (PREDIMED) study also found no evidence of an association between nut consumption and dyslipidemia [31]. Furthermore, O'Neil *et al.* failed to show a difference in total cholesterol between 'out of hand nut' consumers and non-consumers in a representative sample from the USA [44]. Out of hand nut consumers were defined as those who ate nuts solely as nuts, not as components of other food products. This is similar to the definition for whole nut consumers used in the present study. It has been suggested that these consumers may differ from consumers of nuts from all sources in that they make a conscious decision to eat nuts. Conversely, analysis of National Health and Nutrition Examination Survey (NHANES) data 1999–2004 reported significantly higher concentrations of HDL-C among nut consumers compared to non-consumers [29]. In addition, Askari *et al.* reported that nut consumption was associated with a reduction in LDL-C, triglycerides and apoB:apoA ratio, with total-C significantly reduced among female participants only, in an Iranian cohort [32].

The blood samples collected in the present study were not collected in a fasting state; therefore, LDL-C and triglycerides were unable to be measured. A meta-analysis has suggested that reductions in total and LDL-C are blunted in those who are obese [6]. One possible explanation for the lack of association between cholesterol concentrations and nut consumption observed in this study could be the high rates of obesity in the NZ population, where over 36% are classified as overweight and 28% as obese [45].

Despite the lack of difference in these specific lipoproteins, there was a significant negative association between total nut consumption and CVD risk category. The calculation of the CVD risk category takes into account the total-C:HDL-C ratio, as well as sex, age, systolic blood pressure and smoking and diabetes status.

A more consistent finding across different populations is the significantly lower body weight, BMI and waist circumference observed among nut consumers [46,47]. In agreement with other investigators [31,44,48,49], this study found a lower risk of being overweight and obesity among nut consumers, despite the fact that nut consumers report higher energy intakes compared to non-nut consumers. This finding is consistent with other epidemiological studies [16–19], which show that nut consumers tend to be leaner than non-nut consumers, and clinical trials [20–24], which report that when nuts are added to the diet, there is no weight gain or less weight gained than predicted. There are several mechanisms that may explain this consistent finding. Firstly, the composition of nuts, which contain protein and fibre, may result in dietary compensation. Indeed, a recent review estimated that dietary compensation accounted for 65%–75% of the additional energy provided by nuts [50]. Recent studies have also suggested that a substantial proportion of the energy in nuts is lost in the faeces, suggesting that the metabolisable energy from nuts is 9%–32% less than that predicted using the Atwater factors [51–53]. A third explanation is possibly the increase in metabolic rate observed with the higher intake of unsaturated fats, although this has only been reported in studies investigating peanuts [20,54,55].

There were no significant differences in blood pressure between nut and non-nut consumers in the present study. Data from NHANES 1999–2004 revealed that nut consumers had significantly lower systolic blood pressure and prevalence of hypertension [29]. However, most clinical trials investigating the effects of nut consumption on blood pressure have small sample sizes and tend to show mixed results, with the majority reporting no effect on blood pressure [11,56].

Both epidemiological studies and clinical trials have also produced mixed results regarding the relationship between nut consumption and the risk of developing type 2 diabetes. Analysis of NHANES data showed lower prevalence of risk factors associated with metabolic syndrome among nut consumers [29]. In a cross-sectional analysis of the PREDIMED study in a group of individuals with a wide range of nut intake and at high risk of cardiovascular disease, nut consumption was associated with a significant reduction in the risk of obesity, metabolic syndrome and diabetes [31]. However, there were no significant associations for the components of metabolic syndrome, including high blood pressure, dyslipidemia and fasting hyperglycaemia. Collectively, the evidence suggests no association between diabetes risk and nut consumption, which is in agreement with the present study, where there was no difference in the risk of diabetes between nut and non-nut consumers. The risk of pre-diabetes was significantly reduced only among whole nut consumers compared to whole non-nut consumers. This may reflect the more healthful effects of nuts when consumed alone rather than as components of other foods. Given the equivocal findings on the association of nut consumption and diabetes and metabolic syndrome, more well-designed studies are required in order to draw definitive conclusions.

C-reactive protein is a marker of inflammation, which has been positively correlated with CVD [57]. In the present study, CRP was significantly lower among total nut consumers compared to non-total nut consumers. O'Neil *et al.* reported that 'out of hand' nut consumers had significantly lower CRP compared to non-nut consumers [44]. Only around one-quarter of intervention studies in this area have reported significant reductions in CRP with the regular consumption of nuts [58–60]. A limitation of the current study is that only CRP was measured, not high sensitivity CRP (hsCRP), which is a more sensitive measure.

Whole blood, serum and red blood cell folate concentrations were higher among whole nut consumers, whereas only serum folate was higher among total nut consumers. This finding is consistent with those of O'Neil *et al.*, who reported significantly higher serum and red blood cell folate among nut consumers in the NHANES 1999–2004 dataset [29]. Folate is also present in fruit and vegetables, and many breakfast cereals are fortified with folic acid. Therefore, these higher concentrations of blood folate could be due to the intake of nuts, but may also be a marker of a healthier diet.

The results of the present study should be interpreted with several limitations in mind. Firstly, the cross-sectional design of the study means causal inferences cannot be drawn. The improvements in risk factors observed among nut consumers in this study and others may be due to the addition of nutrient dense nuts to the diet. An alternative explanation is that nut consumption may be a marker of a healthier diet. Nut consumers may simply be more health conscious than non-consumers. Thus, a healthier lifestyle may explain the association of nuts with risk factors (*i.e.*, the associations observed could be the result of residual confounding by health consciousness). This explanation cannot be excluded in the present study. A further limitation was that dietary intake relied on memory and included only one 24-h diet recall for the identification of nut consumers, so it may not represent usual nut intake. Therefore, the effects of regular nut consumption on the risk factors examined here may have been under- or over-estimated. In addition, blood samples were not fasting in order to enhance compliance. Thus, LDL-C and triglycerides were unable to be measured. Furthermore, CRP was measured, which is less sensitive than hsCRP. Waist circumference was measured over light clothing, and this is known to introduce bias to the measurement [61]. Lastly, individuals with type 1 and 2 diabetes could not be differentiated; however, over 90% of people with diabetes in NZ are reported to have type 2 diabetes [62].

The strengths of this study include the rigorous coding of food items collected through a multi-stage process and the use of NZ-specific compositional data, allowing confidence in the collected estimates of the intake for nuts. Other strengths of the study are its large sample size, permitting precise estimation of the effects, and the use of a representative, after weighting, population-based sample. In addition, several unique outcomes in relation to nut consumption were investigated, including ABSI and cardiovascular risk category.

5. Conclusions

In summary, this is the first study using national data from NZ to examine the effects of nut consumption on risk factors for chronic disease. In agreement with other studies conducted in the U.S., Europe and Iran, nut consumers were leaner with reduced central adiposity and had better outcomes for a variety of biochemical indices compared to non-consumers, which collectively may reduce the risk of chronic disease.

Acknowledgments: We thank the 4721 New Zealanders who participated in the 2008/2009 New Zealand Adult Nutrition Survey. The New Zealand Ministry of Health funded the 2008/2009 New Zealand Adult Nutrition Survey. The New Zealand Crown is the owner of the copyright for the survey data. The results presented in this paper are the work of the authors.

Author Contributions: The authors' contributions were as follows: R.B., W.P., A.G. and L.F. designed and/or conducted the research; R.B. performed the statistical analyses with assistance from A.G.; C.S. and L.F. managed the dietary analysis; W.P. was the principal investigator of the 2008/2009 Zealand Adult Nutrition Survey; R.B., S.L.T., A.G. and A.C. wrote the manuscript; R.B. has primary responsibility for the final content; all authors reviewed and approved the final manuscript.

Conflicts of Interest: The authors declare no conflict of interest.

References

1. Grosso, G.; Yang, J.; Marventano, S.; Micek, A.; Galvano, F.; Kales, S. Nut consumption and all-cause, cardiovascular, and cancer mortality risk: A systematic review and meta-analysis of epidemiologic studies. *Am. J. Clin. Nutr.* **2015**, *101*, 783–793. [CrossRef] [PubMed]
2. Hshieh, T.T.; Petrone, A.B.; Gaziano, J.M.; Djousse, L. Nut consumption and risk of mortality in the Physicians' Health Study. *Am. J. Clin. Nutr.* **2015**, *101*, 407–412. [CrossRef] [PubMed]

3. Kris-Etherton, P.M.; Yu-Poth, S.; Sabate, J.; Ratcliffe, H.E.; Zhao, G.; Etherton, T.D. Nuts and their bioactive constituents: Effects on serum lipids and other factors that affect disease risk. *Am. J. Clin. Nutr.* **1999**, *70*, S504–S511.

4. Nash, S.D.; Nash, D.T. Nuts as part of a healthy cardiovascular diet. *Curr. Atheroscler. Rep.* **2008**, *10*, 529–535. [CrossRef] [PubMed]

5. Ros, E. Health benefits of nut consumption. *Nutrients* **2010**, *2*, 652–682. [CrossRef] [PubMed]

6. Sabate, J.; Oda, K.; Ros, E. Nut consumption and blood lipid levels: A pooled analysis of 25 intervention trials. *Arch. Intern. Med.* **2010**, *170*, 821–827. [CrossRef] [PubMed]

7. Bao, Y.; Han, J.; Hu, F.B.; Giovannucci, E.L.; Stampfer, M.J.; Willett, W.C.; Fuchs, C.S. Association of nut consumption with total and cause-specific mortality. *N. Engl. J. Med.* **2013**, *369*, 2001–2011. [CrossRef] [PubMed]

8. Luo, C.; Zhang, Y.; Ding, Y.S.; Shan, Z.L.; Chen, S.J.; Yu, M.; Hu, F.B.; Liu, L.G. Nut consumption and risk of type 2 diabetes, cardiovascular disease, and all-cause mortality: A systematic review and meta-analysis. *Am. J. Clin. Nutr.* **2014**, *100*, 256–269. [CrossRef] [PubMed]

9. Mohammadifard, N.; Salehi-Abarghouei, A.; Salas-Salvado, J.; Guasch-Ferre, M.; Humphries, K.; Sarrafzadegan, N. The effect of tree nut, peanut, and soy nut consumption on blood pressure: A systematic review and meta-analysis of randomized controlled clinical trials. *Am. J. Clin. Nutr.* **2015**, *101*, 966–982. [CrossRef] [PubMed]

10. Djousse, L.; Rudich, T.; Gaziano, J.M. Nut consumption and risk of hypertension in US male physicians. *Clin. Nutr.* **2009**, *28*, 10–14. [CrossRef] [PubMed]

11. Barbour, J.A.; Howe, P.R.; Buckley, J.D.; Bryan, J.; Coates, A.M. Nut consumption for vascular health and cognitive function. *Nutr. Res. Rev.* **2014**, *27*, 131–158. [CrossRef] [PubMed]

12. Zhou, D.H.; Yu, H.B.; He, F.; Reilly, K.H.; Zhang, J.Y.; Li, S.S.; Zhang, T.; Wang, B.Z.; Ding, Y.L.; Xi, B. Nut consumption in relation to cardiovascular disease risk and type 2 diabetes: A systematic review and meta-analysis of prospective studies. *Am. J. Clin. Nutr.* **2014**, *100*, 270–277. [CrossRef] [PubMed]

13. Afshin, A.; Micha, R.; Khatibzadeh, S.; Mozaffarian, D. Consumption of nuts and legumes and risk of incident ischemic heart disease, stroke, and diabetes: A systematic review and meta-analysis. *Am. J. Clin. Nutr.* **2014**, *100*, 278–288. [CrossRef] [PubMed]

14. Liu, Z.; Wei, P.; Li, X. Is nut consumption associated with decreased risk of type 2 diabetes? *Am. J. Clin. Nutr.* **2014**, *100*, 1401–1402. [CrossRef] [PubMed]

15. Viguiliouk, E.; Kendall, C.W.; Blanco Mejia, S.; Cozma, A.I.; Ha, V.; Mirrahimi, A.; Jayalath, V.H.; Augustin, L.S.; Chiavaroli, L.; Leiter, L.A.; et al. Effect of tree nuts on glycemic control in diabetes: A systematic review and meta-analysis of randomized controlled dietary trials. *PLoS ONE* **2014**, *9*, e103376. [CrossRef] [PubMed]

16. Bes-Rastrollo, M.; Sabate, J.; Gomez-Gracia, E.; Alonso, A.; Martinez, J.A.; Martinez-Gonzalez, M.A. Nut consumption and weight gain in a Mediterranean cohort. The SUN study. *Obesity* **2007**, *15*, 107–116. [CrossRef] [PubMed]

17. Bes-Rastrollo, M.; Wedick, N.M.; Martinez-Gonzalez, M.A.; Li, T.Y.; Sampson, L.; Hu, F.B. Prospective study of nut consumption, long-term weight change, and obesity risk in women. *Am. J. Clin. Nutr.* **2009**, *89*, 1913–1919. [CrossRef] [PubMed]

18. Martinez-Gonzalez, M.A.; Bes-Rastrollo, M. Nut consumption, weight gain and obesity: Epidemiological evidence. *Nutr. Metab. Cardiovasc. Dis.* **2011**, *21*, S40–S45. [CrossRef] [PubMed]

19. Mozaffarian, D.; Hao, T.; Rimm, E.B.; Willett, W.C.; Hu, F.B. Changes in diet and lifestyle and long-term weight gain in women and men. *N. Engl. J. Med.* **2011**, *364*, 2392–2404. [CrossRef] [PubMed]

20. Alper, C.M.; Mattes, R.D. Effects of chronic peanut consumption on energy balance and hedonics. *Int. J. Obes. Relat. Metab. Disord.* **2002**, *26*, 1129–1137. [CrossRef] [PubMed]

21. Fraser, G.E.; Bennett, H.W.; Jaceldo, K.B.; Sabate, J. Effect on body weight of a free 76 kilojoule (320 calorie) daily supplement of almonds for six months. *J. Am. Coll. Nutr.* **2002**, *21*, 275–283. [CrossRef] [PubMed]

22. Hollis, J.; Mattes, R. Effect of chronic consumption of almonds on body weight in healthy humans. *Br. J. Nutr.* **2007**, *98*, 651–656. [CrossRef] [PubMed]

23. Sabate, J.; Cordero-MacIntyre, Z.; Siapco, G.; Torabian, S.; Haddad, E. Does regular walnut consumption lead to weight gain? *Br. J. Nutr.* **2005**, *94*, 859–864. [CrossRef] [PubMed]

24. Tey, S.L.; Brown, R.; Gray, A.; Chisholm, A.; Delahunty, C. Nuts improve diet quality compared to other energy-dense snacks while maintaining body weight. *J. Nutr. Metab.* **2011**. [CrossRef] [PubMed]
25. Strain, J.J.; Dowey, L.; Ward, M.; Pentieva, K.; McNulty, H. B-vitamins, homocysteine metabolism and CVD. *Proc. Nutr. Soc.* **2004**, *63*, 597–603. [CrossRef] [PubMed]
26. Kim, Y.I. Folate and carcinogenesis: Evidence, mechanisms, and implications. *J. Nutr. Biochem.* **1999**, *10*, 66–88. [CrossRef]
27. Segura, R.; Javierre, C.; Lizarraga, M.A.; Ros, E. Other relevant components of nuts: Phytosterols, folate and minerals. *Br. J. Nutr.* **2006**, *96*, S36–S44. [CrossRef] [PubMed]
28. O'Neil, C.E.; Fulgoni, V.L., III; Nicklas, T.A. Tree Nut consumption is associated with better adiposity measures and cardiovascular and metabolic syndrome health risk factors in U.S. Adults: NHANES 2005–2010. *Nutr. J.* **2015**, *14*, 64. [CrossRef] [PubMed]
29. O'Neil, C.E.; Keast, D.R.; Nicklas, T.A.; Fulgoni, V.L. Nut consumption is associated with decreased health risk factors for cardiovascular disease and metabolic syndrome in U.S. adults: NHANES 1999–2004. *J. Am. Coll. Nutr.* **2011**, *30*, 502–510. [CrossRef] [PubMed]
30. Jaceldo-Siegl, K.; Haddad, E.; Oda, K.; Fraser, G.E.; Sabate, J. Tree nuts are inversely associated with metabolic syndrome and obesity: The Adventist health study-2. *PLoS ONE* **2014**, *9*, e85133. [CrossRef] [PubMed]
31. Ibarrola-Jurado, N.; Bullo, M.; Guasch-Ferre, M.; Ros, E.; Martinez-Gonzalez, M.A.; Corella, D.; Fiol, M.; Warnberg, J.; Estruch, R.; Roman, P.; *et al.* Cross-sectional assessment of nut consumption and obesity, metabolic syndrome and other cardiometabolic risk factors: The PREDIMED study. *PLoS ONE* **2013**, *8*, e57367. [CrossRef] [PubMed]
32. Askari, G.; Yazdekhasti, N.; Mohammadifard, N.; Sarrafzadegan, N.; Bahonar, A.; Badiei, M.; Sajjadi, F.; Taheri, M. The relationship between nut consumption and lipid profile among the Iranian adult population; Isfahan Healthy Heart Program. *Eur. J. Clin. Nutr.* **2013**, *67*, 385–389. [CrossRef] [PubMed]
33. University of Otago; Ministry of Health. *Methodology Report for the 2008/09 New Zealand Adult Nutrition Survey*; Ministry of Health: Wellington, New Zealand, 2011.
34. O'Broin, S.; Kelleher, B. Microbiological assay on microtitre plates of folate in serum and red cells. *J. Clin. Pathol.* **1992**, *45*, 344–347. [CrossRef] [PubMed]
35. Egan, B.M.; Zhao, Y.; Axon, R.N. US trends in prevalence, awareness, treatment, and control of hypertension, 1988–2008. *JAMA* **2010**, *303*, 2043–2050. [CrossRef] [PubMed]
36. Cole, T.J.; Bellizzi, M.C.; Flegal, K.M.; Dietz, W.H. Establishing a standard definition for child overweight and obesity worldwide: International survey. *BMJ* **2000**, *320*, 1240–1243. [CrossRef] [PubMed]
37. Cole, T.J.; Flegal, K.M.; Nicholls, D.; Jackson, A.A. Body mass index cut offs to define thinness in children and adolescents: International survey. *BMJ* **2007**, *335*, 194–197. [CrossRef] [PubMed]
38. Krakauer, N.Y.; Krakauer, J.C. A new body shape index predicts mortality hazard independently of body mass index. *PLoS ONE* **2012**, *7*, e39504. [CrossRef] [PubMed]
39. Krakauer, N.Y.; Krakauer, J.C. Dynamic association of mortality hazard with body shape. *PLoS ONE* **2014**, *9*, e88793. [CrossRef] [PubMed]
40. Jackson, R. Updated New Zealand cardiovascular disease risk-benefit prediction guide. *BMJ* **2000**, *320*, 709–710. [CrossRef] [PubMed]
41. New Zealand Guidelines Group. *New Zealand Primary Care Handbook 2012*, 3rd ed.; New Zealand Guidelines Group: Wellington, New Zealand, 2012.
42. American Diabetes Association. Diagnosis and classification of diabetes classification. *Diabetes Care* **2010**, *33*, S62–S69.
43. Brown, R.C.; Tey, S.L.; Gray, A.R.; Chisholm, A.; Smith, C.; Fleming, E.; Blakey, C.; Parnell, W. Patterns and predictors of nut consumption: Results from the 2008/09 New Zealand Adult Nutrition Survey. *Br. J. Nutr.* **2014**, *112*, 2028–2040. [CrossRef] [PubMed]
44. O'Neil, C.E.; Keast, D.R.; Nicklas, T.A.; Fulgoni, V.L. Out-of-hand nut consumption is associated with improved nutrient intake and health risk markers in US children and adults: National Health and Nutrition Examination Survey 1999–2004. *Nutr. Res.* **2012**, *32*, 185–194. [CrossRef] [PubMed]
45. University of Otago; Ministry of Health. *A Focus on Nutrition: Key Findings of the 2008/09 New Zealand Adult Nutrition Survey*; Ministry of Health: Wellington, New Zealand, 2011.
46. Jackson, C.L.; Hu, F.B. Long-term associations of nut consumption with body weight and obesity. *Am. J. Clin. Nutr.* **2014**, *100*, 408S–411S. [CrossRef] [PubMed]

47. Tan, S.Y.; Dhillon, J.; Mattes, R.D. A review of the effects of nuts on appetite, food intake, metabolism, and body weight. *Am. J. Clin. Nutr.* **2014**, *100*, 412S–422S. [CrossRef] [PubMed]
48. Jaceldo-Siegl, K.; Joan, S.; Rajaram, S.; Fraser, G.E. Long-term almond supplementation without advice on food replacement induces favourable nutrient modifications to the habitual diets of free-living individuals. *Br. J. Nutr.* **2004**, *92*, 533–540. [CrossRef] [PubMed]
49. O'Neil, C.E.; Keast, D.R.; Fulgoni, V.L.; Nicklas, T.A. Tree nut consumption improves nutrient intake and diet quality in US adults: An analysis of National Health and Nutrition Examination Survey (NHANES) 1999–2004. *Asia Pac. J. Clin. Nutr.* **2010**, *19*, 142–150. [PubMed]
50. Mattes, R.D. The energetics of nut consumption. *Asia Pac. J. Clin. Nutr.* **2008**, *17*, 337–339. [PubMed]
51. Ellis, P.R.; Kendall, C.W.C.; Ren, Y.; Parker, C.; Pacy, J.F.; Waldron, K.W.; Jenkins, D.J.A. Role of cell walls in the bioaccessibility of lipids in almond seeds. *Am. J. Clin. Nutr.* **2004**, *80*, 604–613. [PubMed]
52. Grundy, M.; Grassby, T.; Mandalari, G.; Waldron, K.; Butterworth, P.J.; Berry, S.; Ellis, P. Effect of mastication on lipid bioaccessibility of almonds in a randomized human study and its implications for digestion kinetics, metabolizable energy, and postprandial lipemia. *Am. J. Clin. Nutr.* **2015**, *101*, 25–33. [CrossRef] [PubMed]
53. Novotny, J.A.; Gebauer, S.K.; Baer, D.J. Discrepancy between the Atwater factor predicted and empirically measured energy values of almonds in human diets. *Am. J. Clin. Nutr.* **2012**, *96*, 296–301. [CrossRef] [PubMed]
54. Claesson, A.L.; Holm, G.; Ernersson, A.; Lindström, T.; Nystrom, F.H. Two weeks of overfeeding with candy, but not peanuts, increases insulin levels and body weight. *Scand. J. Clin. Lab. Investig.* **2009**, *69*, 598–605. [CrossRef] [PubMed]
55. Coelho, S.B.; de Sales, R.L.; Iyer, S.S.; Bressan, J.; Costa, N.M.B.; Lokko, P.; Mattes, R. Effects of peanut oil load on energy expenditure, body composition, lipid profile, and appetite in lean and overweight adults. *Nutrition* **2006**, *22*, 585–592. [CrossRef] [PubMed]
56. Blanco Mejia, S.; Kendall, C.W.; Viguiliouk, E.; Augustin, L.S.; Ha, V.; Cozma, A.I.; Mirrahimi, A.; Maroleanu, A.; Chiavaroli, L.; Leiter, L.A.; et al. Effect of tree nuts on metabolic syndrome criteria: A systematic review and meta-analysis of randomised controlled trials. *BMJ Open* **2014**, *4*, e004660. [CrossRef] [PubMed]
57. Bartunek, J.; Vanderheyden, M. Inflammation and related biomarkers in cardiovascular disease. *Biomark. Med.* **2012**, *6*, 1–3. [CrossRef] [PubMed]
58. Jenkins, D.J.A.; Kendall, C.W.C.; Banach, M.S.; Srichaikul, K.; Vidgen, E.; Mitchell, S.; Parker, T.; Nishi, S.; Bashyam, B.; de Souza, R.; et al. Nuts as a replacement for carbohydrates in the diabetic diet. *Diabetes Care* **2011**, *34*, 1706–1711. [CrossRef] [PubMed]
59. Rajaram, S.; Connell, K.M.; Sabate, J. Effect of almond-enriched high-monounsaturated fat diet on selected markers of inflammation: A randomised, controlled, crossover study. *Br. J. Nutr.* **2010**, *103*, 907–912. [CrossRef] [PubMed]
60. Zhao, G.; Etherton, T.D.; Martin, K.R.; West, S.G.; Gillies, P.J.; Kris-Etherton, P.M. Dietary alpha-linolenic acid reduces inflammatory and lipid cardiovascular risk factors in hypercholesterolemic men and women. *J. Nutr.* **2004**, *134*, 2991–2997. [PubMed]
61. Wills, S.D.; Bhopal, R.S. The challenges of accurate waist and hip measurement over clothing: Pilot data. *Obes. Res. Clin. Pract.* **2010**, *4*, e163–e246. [CrossRef] [PubMed]
62. Coppell, K.J.; Anderson, K.; Williams, S.; Manning, P.; Mann, J. Evaluation of diabetes care in the Otago region using a diabetes register, 1998–2003. *Diabetes Res. Clin. Pract.* **2006**, *71*, 345–352. [CrossRef] [PubMed]

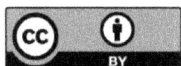

nutrients

MDPI

Article

Double Burden of Malnutrition in Rural West Java: Household-Level Analysis for Father-Child and Mother-Child Pairs and the Association with Dietary Intake

Makiko Sekiyama [1,*], Hong Wei Jiang [2], Budhi Gunawan [3], Linda Dewanti [4], Ryo Honda [5], Hana Shimizu-Furusawa [6], Oekan S. Abdoellah [3] and Chiho Watanabe [6]

[1] Graduate Program in Sustainability Science-Global Leadership Initiative (GPSS-GLI), Graduate School of Frontier Science, The University of Tokyo, 5-1-5 Kashiwanoha, Kashiwa City 277-8563, Japan

[2] Research Institute for Humanity and Nature, 457 4 Motoyama, Kamigamo, Kita-ku, Kyot 603-8047, Japan; jiang@chikyu.ac.jp

[3] Institute of Ecology, Research Institute, Padjadjaran University, Jl. Sekeloa Selatan I, Bandung 40132, Indonesia; budhi_gunawan@unpad.ac.id (B.G.); oekan.abdoellah54@gmail.com (O.S.A.)

[4] Faculty of Medicine, Airlangga University, Jl. Mayjen. Prof. Dr. Moestopo 47, Surabaya 60132, Indonesia; lindaperisdiono@yahoo.com

[5] RSET, Institute of Science and Engineering, Kanazawa University, Kakuma-machi, Kanazawa 920-1192, Japan; rhonda@se.kanazawa-u.ac.jp

[6] Department of Human Ecology, School of International Health, The University of Tokyo, 7-3-1 Hongo, Bunkyo-ku, Tokyo 113-0033, Japan; hana-shimizu@umin.ac.jp (H.S.-F.); chiho@humeco.m.u-tokyo.ac.jp (C.W.)

* Correspondence: sekiyama@k.u-tokyo.ac.jp; Tel.: +81-4-7136-4859; Fax: +81-4-7136-4878

Received: 22 June 2015 ; Accepted: 23 September 2015 ; Published: 2 October 2015

Abstract: Indonesia is facing household-level double burden malnutrition. This study aimed at examining (1) household-level double burden for the mother-child and father-child pairs; (2) risk of adiposity of double burden households; and (3) associated dietary factors. Subjects were 5th and 6th grade elementary school children ($n = 242$), their mothers ($n = 242$), and their fathers ($n = 225$) in five communities (1 = urban, 4 = rural) in the Bandung District. Questionnaires on socioeconomic factors, blood hemoglobin measurements, and anthropometric measurements were administered. For adults, body fat percentage (BF%) was estimated by bioelectrical impedance (BF%-BI) and by converting skinfold thickness (ST) data using Durnin and Womersley's (1974) formula (BF%-ST). Food frequency questionnaires were also completed. Double burden was defined as coexistence of maternal or paternal overweight (Body mass index (BMI) $\geqslant$ 23) and child stunting (height-for-age z-score <-2) within households. Maternal-child double burden occurred in 30.6% of total households, whereas paternal-child double burden was only in 8.4%. Mothers from double burden households showed high adiposity; 87.3% with BF%-BI and 66.2% with BF%-ST had BF% >35%, and 60.6% had waists >80 cm. The major dietary patterns identified were "Modern" and "High-animal products". After controlling for confounding factors, children in the highest quartile of the "High-animal products" dietary pattern had a lower risk of maternal-child double burden (Adjusted OR: 0.46, 95% CI: 0.21–1.04) than those in the lowest quartile. Given that the "High-animal products" dietary pattern was associated with the decreased risk of maternal-child double burden through a strong negative correlation with child stunting, improving child stunting through adequate intake of animal products is critical to solve the problem of maternal-child double burden in Indonesia.

Keywords: double burden; malnutrition; adiposity; food frequency questionnaire; Indonesia

1. Introduction

Nutrition transition comprises food consumption and physical activity changes caused by lifestyle transformations resulting from rapid urbanization and modernization [1]. Whereas this process occurred gradually in developed countries, in many developing countries it has been proceeding at a faster rate [2]. Consequently, many developing countries are facing increasing rates of overweight and obesity [3,4], though undernutrition is still prevalent in these countries. This coexistence of overnutrition and undernutrition is often referred as the double burden of malnutrition [2,5,6]. Researchers have revealed that double burden occurs not only at the country level [5,7], but also at the household level [8,9].

As for household-level double burden, most literature has examined the relationship between mother and child. These studies revealed that in several countries mothers are overweight whereas their children are stunted in the same household [9,10]. However, the relationship between father and child at the household level has scarcely been investigated.

Body mass index (BMI) has been commonly used to define maternal overweight in double burden households [2,6,9,10], despite the fact that it does not directly measure adiposity. Excess adiposity is associated with increased risk of non-communicable diseases (NCDs) such as type 2 diabetes and cardiovascular disease [11,12]. NCDs are the leading cause of global disease burden [13], with 80% of mortality from NCDs occurring in low- and middle-income countries [14]. However, the actual risk of adiposity among mothers in double burden households has not been studied.

Identification of risk factors of the double burden household has been investigated from the perspective of socioeconomic characteristics of these households [10,15,16]. Several studies have revealed that double burden is associated with older maternal age [6,10], maternal short stature [15,16], larger family size [15,17], and higher levels of maternal education [6,10]. However, food consumption patterns of household members, which mediate socioeconomic characteristics of the household, and physical characteristics of household members, have scarcely been studied as associated factors of double burden. For example, higher risk of double burden in urban residents was interpreted to be associated with a rapid shift to inactivity and an energy-dense diet [10], but empirical data for explaining such an association are limited. One such example of the limited literature is that of a study in Malaysia, which concluded that the variety of food available to children decreases the risk of double burden [17].

Until recently, three studies have reported double burden of malnutrition at the household level in Indonesia [2,6,18] using secondary data analysis with a large sample size. The first study analyzed data from the Indonesian Nutrition Surveillance System (INSS) in 2000–2003 and found that overweight mother and stunted child pairs were found among 11% of rural households in Indonesia [6]. The latter two studies used the same dataset, the Indonesian Family Life Survey (IFLS), from different years. Roemling and Qaim [2] analyzed 1993 (IFLS1), 1997 (IFLS2), 2000 (IFLS3), and 2007 (IFLS4) data as a panel and found the proportion of double burden households increased between 1993 and 1997, but remained relatively stable since that time. Vaezghasemi analyzed 2007 (IFLS4) data and found that 19% of households had at least one underweight and one overweight member of the household [18]. These studies have investigated determinants of double burden households using socioeconomic characteristics of the households, whereas the relationship between double burden and food intake patterns has not been analyzed.

The objectives of this study were (1) to examine double burden structure at the household level, not only for the mother-child pair but also for the father-child pair; (2) to compare the adiposity related physical characteristics of double burden household members and non-double burden household members; and (3) to explore the association of dietary patterns of the household members with the occurrence of double burden. The targets for this study were five communities (1 urban and 4 rural) in the Bandung District in West Java, Indonesia.

2. Methods

2.1. Study Area and Subjects

The present study was conducted as a part of the Environmental Research in Rural Asia (ENVRERA) project that aimed to examine the effects of subsistence change (*i.e.*, from self-subsistence to commercial cash cropping) on chemical exposures and on the well-being of people [19]. The study communities were selected so that they varied in terms of their subsistence patterns. The study sites included five communities within the Citarum Watershed, West Java, Indonesia: Bongas (B), an agricultural village facing the Saguling dam with a fish culture and rice cropping; Cihawuk (C), an agricultural village with vegetable cropping; Taruma Jaya (T), an agricultural village with dairy husbandry and vegetable cropping; Pasir Pogor (P), an agricultural village with rice cropping; and Sekeloa (S), an urban community in Bandung city (Figure 1).

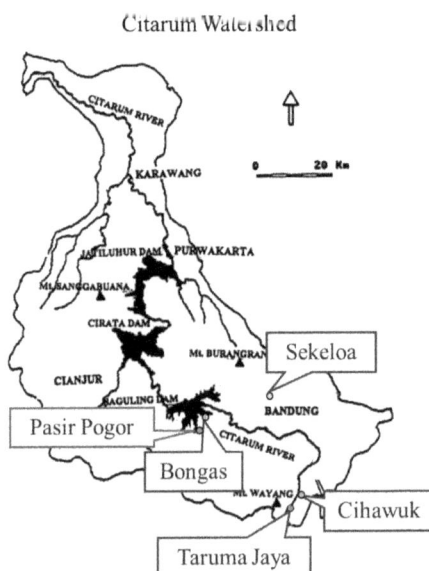

Figure 1. Map of the study sites.

Data collection was conducted from August to September 2006 in communities B, C, and T, and in March 2007 in communities P and S. One of the authors (Budhi Gunawan) selected two elementary schools from each community and obtained the permission from the school head to collaborate on this project. Then, school teachers selected 50 students in the 5th and 6th grades of each elementary school who met the inclusion criteria. The inclusion criteria for a student were that his/her mother, father, and sister/brother could participate in the study. In case we could not obtain 50 students from the 5th and 6th grades of each elementary school, students whose mothers or fathers were not available but another adult (aged 20 years or above) was available were recruited for the study. These selection criteria were used to enable us to examine within (siblings or husband and wife) and between household variation in terms of chemical exposures and their related health effects. In each household that fulfilled the selection criteria, four members (two adults and two children) were invited to participate in the study. A total of 929 people participated in the ENVRERA project in the five communities. Because the ages of the sisters/brothers of 5th or 6th grade school children were diverse, this paper only targeted 5th or 6th grade school children. Furthermore, as our interest was to analyze double burden for mother-child and father-child pairs and it was difficult to recruit fathers to a survey conducted during the daytime, this paper only targets 242 children in 5th or 6th grade whose mothers were also available. Thus, the final sample for this paper was 242 children and their mothers (*n* = 242) and fathers (*n* = 225). Breakdown of the number of participants by community was as follows; 242 children (communities B = 51, C = 52, T = 4 8, P = 50, S = 41), 242 mothers (communities B = 51, C = 52, T = 48, P = 50, S = 41), and 225 fathers (communities B = 47, C = 52, T = 48, P = 49, S = 29).

2.2. Physical Check-up

A health camp was set up at each elementary school where questionnaire surveys on socioeconomic characteristics, anthropometric measurements, urine and blood sampling and testing, and questionnaire surveys on their food consumption habits using food frequency questionnaires (FFQ) were conducted.

2.3. Questionnaire Survey on Socioeconomic Characteristics

Names, ages, genders, occupations, and education history of all household members, as well as possession of goods of the household, water source and sanitation, and land ownership were asked using a structured questionnaire. Possession of goods was asked for five items including a radio, TV, refrigerator, telephone, and mobile phone. Possession of each item was scored as 1, and a total score was used as a "possession of goods" score.

2.4. Anthropometric Measurements

Anthropometric measurements were taken by one of the authors (Makiko Sekiyama) following standard methods [20]. Body weight was measured to the nearest 0.1 kg and the percentage of body fat (BF%) was estimated using bioelectrical impedance with a body composition analyzer (DC-320, Tanita Co., Ltd., Tokyo, Japan). Height was measured to the nearest 0.1 cm using a portable stadiometer. Skinfold thicknesses at the biceps, triceps, subscapular, and suprailiac were measured three times with GPM skinfold calipers (Siber Hegner & Co., Ltd., Zurich, Switzerland) that can measure up to 40 mm with a precision of 0.2 mm. The three measurements at each site were averaged for the statistical analyses. For an adult, using skinfold thickness data, BF% was calculated according to Durnin and Womersley [21]. Waist and hip circumference was measured with a plastic tape with a precision of 1 mm and waist-to-hip ratio (WHR) was calculated for adults. Mid-upper arm circumference (MUAC) was also measured with a plastic tape with a precision of 1 mm. For children, z-scores for height-for-age (HAZ) were calculated as nutritional indicators based on the WHO growth references published in 2007 for children older than 5 years [22] using EPI-INFO (Version 7, Centers for Disease Control and Prevention, Atlanta, GA, USA).

2.5. Hemoglobin (Hb)

Capillary whole blood was collected via finger prick from each participant by one of the authors (Linda Dewanti; an Indonesian physician), with Hb concentrations measured on site using a battery operated photometric analyzer (Test-mate; EQM Research, Cincinnati, OH, USA).

2.6. FFQ (Food Frequency Questionnaire)

A FFQ including 22 food items was developed based on the results of one of the author's (Makiko Sekiyama) preliminary surveys [23,24]. The 22 food items were rice, potato, tofu/tempeh, fresh vegetable, cooked vegetable, indigenous fruit, non-native fruit, egg, salted fish, freshwater fish, sea fish, chicken, beef, goat meat, duck meat, noodle, tea/coffee, milk, meatball, fried sweets, bread, and snack. The consumption frequency was asked using 9 alternatives and converted into weighing factors for statistical analysis: (1) almost never = 0; (2) one to three times per month = 0.07; (3) once per week = 0.1; (4) two to four times per week = 0.4; (5) five to six times per week = 0.8; (6) once per day = 1; (7) two to three times per day = 2.5; (8) four to six times per day = 5; and (9) more than six times per day = 6. Indigenous fruits are those planted locally such as papayas and guavas, whereas non-native fruits are those not planted locally but available in the market or local shop such as apple, orange, and grape.

2.7. Ethics

Ethical approval for the study was obtained from the Research Ethics Committee at Graduate School of Medicine, the University of Tokyo (Approval No. 1505) and Padjadjaran University. The purpose and procedures of the study were explained to the participants and written informed consent was obtained from all study subjects.

2.8. Statistical Analysis

Stunting was defined as a height-for-age z-score (HAZ) <-2 according to the World Health Organization (WHO) growth standards [22]. BMI was calculated as a ratio of weight (kg)/height (m)^2. Concerning the overweight cutoff, Asian populations were found to have a higher level of BF% at lower levels of BMI than other ethnic groups [25]. Thus, adult overweight was classified as a BMI (in kg/m^2) $\geqslant 23$ to capture the increased risk of NCDs [26]. Double burden was defined as coexistence of maternal or paternal overweight and child stunting within the same household. Namely, paternal-child double burden was coexistence of paternal overweight and child stunting within the same household, and maternal-child double burden was coexistence of maternal overweight and child stunting within the same household.

A principal component analysis based on the 22 food items was conducted to assess the major dietary patterns among the subjects. In determining the number of factors to retain, we considered the results of the Scree test, eigenvalues greater than 1, and interpretability of the factors [27]. Factors were then rotated with an orthogonal rotation procedure (varimax rotation). Labeling of dietary patterns was based on the interpretation of foods with high factor loadings for each dietary pattern [28]. Only foods with a factor loading $\geqslant |0.25|$ were included in this study. Factor scores for each dietary pattern were categorized into quartiles (quartile 1 represented a low intake of the food pattern; quartile 4 represented a high intake of the food pattern), separately for child, mother, and father. Association between dietary patterns with child stunting, with maternal overweight, and with paternal overweight was analyzed using logistic regression analysis, adjusted for potential confounders.

Age, gender, and physical characteristics were compared between maternal-child double burden and non-double burden households. Comparisons between double burden and non-double burden households were conducted using a t-test for maternal height, which was the only variable to fit a normal distribution. For other parameters that did not fit a normal distribution, comparisons were made using the Mann-Whitney U-test. Relevant socioeconomic factors associated with maternal-child double burden were analyzed using logistic regression analyses. Descriptive statistics were used to examine the full distribution of variables. Using appropriate cutoffs, categorical variables were created for maternal age (<30, 30–39.9, or $\geqslant 40$ year), maternal education (no schooling, elementary or secondary school, or >secondary school), maternal height (<145, 145–149.9, or $\geqslant 150$ cm), and parity (1–2, 3–5, or $\geqslant 6$). Each socioeconomic factor was firstly put in the univariate logistic regression analysis to examine its association with maternal-child double burden, then only those associated at the $p < 0.1$ level were included in the multiple logistic regression models. Associations between dietary patterns of mother and child and the maternal-child double burden were also analyzed using logistic regression analysis, adjusted for potential confounders. For all analyses using logistic regression models, odds ratios (ORs) and corresponding 95% confidence intervals (CIs) were calculated with statistical significance defined as $p < 0.1$. All analyses were performed using the Statistical Package for Social Science (SPSS) software package (Version 10.0, SPSS Inc., Chicago, IL, USA).

3. Results

3.1. Characteristics of the Subjects

Table 1 shows the ages and physical characteristics of the study subjects. For the children, the mean age was 11.1 years, mean HAZ was −2.15, and the stunting ratio was 57.9%. For the fathers, the mean age was 41.6 years, mean BMI was 21.1 kg/m², and the proportion of overweight (BMI ⩾ 23) was 18.7%. For the mothers, the mean age was 36.9 years, mean BMI was 23.8 kg/m², and the proportion of overweight (BMI ⩾ 23) was 53.7%.

Table 1. Characteristics of child, father, and mother subjects.

	n	Age	Height (cm)	HAZ [a]	Stunting (HAZ < −2)	Weight (kg)	BMI [b] (kg/m²)	Overweight (BMI ⩾ 23)
		Mean ± SD	Mean ± SD	Mean ± SD	%	Mean ± SD	Mean ± SD	%
Child	242	11.1 ± 0.95	132.0 ± 7.08	−2.15 ± 1.01	57.9	27.9 ± 5.33	15.7 ± 1.73	
Father	225	41.6 ± 9.06	160.1 ± 6.35			54.1 ± 8.43	21.1 ± 2.68	18.7
Mother	242	36.9 ± 6.83	149.1 ± 4.97			53.1 ± 9.15	23.8 ± 3.67	53.7

[a] Height-for-age z-score; [b] Body mass index; SD: Standard deviation.

Socioeconomic characteristics of the subject households were also obtained from the questionnaire survey. Regarding the land ownership, only 13.2% of the households owned paddy fields and 22.4% of the households owned vegetable fields. Consequently, though the main occupation of the subject father was agricultural work (30.2%), 60.2% of them were agricultural wage laborers. The main water source of the subject households were spring (60.8%) and well (37.3%), while some of the households in community B used lake water especially in dry season due to the scarcity of well water. 57.2% of the subject households owned their private toilet facilities, whereas 49.7% of them used the shared or public toilet facilities.

With regard to the birth-related factors, the mean parity of the subject mothers was 3.28 ± 1.63. Information of birth weight, which is the important birth-related factors affecting future nutritional status, was not obtained from the study subjects, because the bulk of child deliveries were made at home without measurement of birth weight.

3.2. Paternal-Child and Maternal-Child Double Burden

Table 2 shows that paternal-child double burden (coexistence of paternal overweight and child stunting) was found only in 8.4% of the targeted households, whereas maternal-child double burden (coexistence of maternal overweight and child stunting) was observed in 30.6% of the targeted households.

Table 2. Maternal-child and paternal-child pair double burden.

		Non-Obese (%)		Obese (%)	
		Father	Mother	Father	Mother
Child	Non-Stunting (%)	29.8	19.0	10.2	23.1
	Stunting (%)	51.6	27.3	8.4	30.6

3.3. Dietary Patterns of the Subjects

Two major dietary patterns, explaining 25.7% of the total variance in the consumption of the 22 food items, were identified in the principal component analysis. For each of the two major dietary patterns, foods with a high factor loading (set at 0.25 or greater) are shown in Table 3. The first dietary pattern was named as the "Modern" dietary pattern, which was characterized by a high consumption of flesh foods such as egg (factor loading = 0.559), freshwater fish (0.557), and milk (0.524), and of instant snack foods such as meatball (0.541), fried sweets (0.483), noodle (0.473), and snack (0.462). The second dietary pattern was named as the "High-animal products" dietary pattern because it was characterized by high consumption of animal products such as beef (0.556), goat (0.487), chicken (0.349), and duck (0.258), but low consumption of salted fish (−0.465). One example of the salted fish available in this area is the small fish of the *Engraulidae* family (called *ikan teri* in the Indonesian language). Because of its salty taste, local people consume very small portions of salted fish with large amounts of rice.

Table 3. Factor loading matrix for the major factors (dietary patterns) identified by using food consumption data.

	Factor 1 ("Modern" Dietary Pattern)	Factor 2 ("High-Animal Products" Dietary Pattern)
Rice		
Potato	0.322	
Tofu/tempeh	0.543	
Fresh vegetable		−0.406
Cooked vegetable		−0.340
Indigenous fruit	0.624	
Non-native fruit	0.420	0.593
Egg	0.559	
Salted fish		−0.465
Freshwater fish	0.557	
Sea fish	0.387	
Chicken	0.475	0.349
Beef	0.333	0.556
Goat		0.487
Duck		0.258
Noodle	0.473	
Tea/coffee		−0.397
Milk	0.524	0.261
Meatball	0.541	
Fried sweets	0.483	−0.296
Bread	0.429	
Snack	0.462	

Absolute values < 0.25 were not listed in the table; the first factor explained 16.7% of the total variance and the second factor explained 8.96% of the total variance.

3.4. Dietary Patterns and Child Stunting, Paternal Overweight, and Maternal Overweight

Table 4 shows associations between dietary patterns of children and child stunting, dietary patterns of fathers and paternal overweight, and dietary patterns of mothers and maternal overweight. After controlling for potential confounding factors, mothers in the middle (Q2–Q3) and highest quartile (Q4) of the "Modern" dietary pattern had higher risk of overweight (Adjusted OR = 2.34, 95% CI = 1.20–4.57 for Q2–Q3; Adjusted OR = 2.63, 95% CI = 1.12–6.17 for Q4) compared with the lowest quartile (Q1 = reference). Children in the highest quartile (Q4) of the "High-animal products" dietary pattern had a lower risk of stunting (Adjusted OR = 0.36, 95% CI = 0.16–0.80) than those in the lowest quartile (Q1). Fathers in the highest quartile (Q4) of the "High-animal products" dietary pattern had a higher risk of overweight (Adjusted OR = 3.92, 95% CI = 1.13–13.6) than those in the lowest quartile (Q1). Confounding factors considered in this analysis were age, gender, and possession of goods for children, and age, possession of goods, and occupation for fathers and mothers. Possession of goods was used as a proxy for household socioeconomic status and occupation was used as a proxy for physical activity level.

Nutrients 2015, 7, 8376–8391

Table 4. Association of the two identified dietary patterns with child stunting, maternal overweight, and paternal overweight.

			Child Stunting OR (95% CI)	p	Maternal Overweight OR (95% CI)	p	Paternal Overweight OR (95% CI)	p
Model 1 [a,c]	Modern	Q1	1.00	–	1.00		1.00	–
		Q2–Q3	0.85 (0.45–1.61)	0.623	2.60 (1.36–4.98)	0.004	1.81 (0.68–4.80)	0.232
		Q4	0.76 (0.37–1.57)	0.459	3.53 (1.65–7.53)	0.001	3.33 (1.19–9.30)	0.021
	High-animal products	Q1	1.00	–	1.00	–	1.00	–
		Q2–Q3	0.59 (0.30–1.14)	0.115	0.89 (0.48–1.66)	0.708	2.83 (0.92–8.71)	0.071
		Q4	0.38 (0.18–0.79)	0.010	1.07 (0.52–2.21)	0.853	6.16 (1.93–19.7)	0.002
Model 2 [b,c]	Modern	Q1	1.00	–	1.00	–	1.00	–
		Q2–Q3	1.03 (0.53–2.00)	0.929	2.34 (1.20–4.57)	0.013	1.28 (0.45–3.60)	0.647
		Q4	1.01 (0.46–2.21)	0.980	2.63 (1.12–6.17)	0.026	1.00 (0.30–3.26)	0.994
	High-animal products	Q1	1.00	–	1.00	–	1.00	–
		Q2–Q3	0.60 (0.30–1.19)	0.143	0.92 (0.48–1.76)	0.802	2.59 (0.78–8.54)	0.119
		Q4	0.36 (0.16–0.80)	0.012	0.95 (0.44–2.04)	0.892	3.92 (1.13–13.6)	0.032

[a] Unadjusted; [b] Adjusted for age, gender, and possession of goods for children; adjusted for age, possession of goods, and occupation for fathers and mothers; [c] For each dietary pattern, quartile values were separately calculated for child, mother, and father; associations between child dietary patterns and child stunting, between maternal dietary patterns and maternal overweight, and between paternal dietary patterns and paternal overweight were examined. OR: odds ratio; CI: confidence interval.

3.5. Age, Gender, and Physical Characteristics of Maternal-Child Double Burden Households

Age, gender, and physical characteristics were compared between maternal-child double burden and maternal-child non-double burden households (Table 5). For the children, age and gender were not different between double burden and non-double burden groups. As for physical characteristics of the children, height, weight, HAZ, BMI, waist, hip, MUAC, sum of skinfold thickness, and Hb were compared between double burden and non-double burden groups. In terms of physical characteristics of the mothers, height, weight, BMI, waist, hip, WHR, MUAC, sum of skinfold thickness, BF% measured by bioelectrical impedance (BF%-BI), BF% calculated using skinfold thickness based on Durnin and Womersley's (1974) formula (BF%-ST), and Hb were compared between double burden and non-double burden groups. The results show that for the children, height ($p < 0.001$) and HAZ ($p < 0.001$) were significantly lower in the double burden group. For mothers, weight ($p < 0.001$), BMI ($p < 0.001$), waist ($p < 0.001$), hip ($p < 0.001$), WHR ($p < 0.05$), MUAC ($p < 0.001$), sum of skinfold thickness ($p < 0.001$), BF%-BI ($p < 0.001$), BF%-ST ($p < 0.001$), and Hb ($p < 0.01$) were significantly higher in the double burden group. Mothers from double burden households showed high adiposity: BF%-BI = 39.0% ± 5.51%, BF%-ST = 35.1% ± 6.90%, waist = 82.1 ± 9.38 cm.

3.6. Association of Maternal-Child Double Burden with Sociodemographic Variables

Table 6 shows sociodemographic characteristics of maternal-child double burden and maternal-child non-double burden households and the association with maternal-child double burden. Sociodemographic factors that were significantly associated with maternal-child double burden included age of the child (OR = 1.34, 95% CI = 0.96–1.88), maternal education higher than secondary school level (OR = 0.33, 95% CI = 0.09–1.15), and maternal occupation as housewife (OR = 0.49, 95% CI = 0.22–1.12) in the univariate analysis. Then, the variables that were significantly associated with maternal-child double burden in the univariate analysis ($p < 0.1$) were entered into a multivariate analysis. The results show that age of the child (Adjusted OR = 1.44, 95% CI = 1.00–2.08) and maternal occupation as housewife (Adjusted OR = 0.45, 95% CI = 0.19–1.05) remained as significant factors for maternal-child double burden.

3.7. Association of Maternal-Child Double Burden with Dietary Patterns of Mother and Child

Table 7 shows associations between dietary patterns of child and mother, and maternal-child double burden from the logistic regression analysis. After controlling for the confounding factors detected in Table 6, children in the highest quartile of the "High-animal products" dietary pattern had a lower risk of maternal-child double burden (Adjusted OR = 0.46, 95% CI = 0.21–1.04) than those in the lowest quartile.

Table 5. Age, gender, and physical characteristics of children and mothers from maternal-child double burden and maternal-child non-double burden households.

	Double Burden Mean ± SD (N = 73)	n	Non-Double Burden Mean ± SD (N = 169)	n	p [a]
Child characteristics					
Age in months	140.5 ± 8.94		138.0 ± 10.8		0.154
Gender					
Male		32		83	0.834
Female		41		86	
Height (cm)	129.8 ± 4.64		134.2 ± 7.54		0.000
Weight (kg)	26.7 ± 3.40		28.5 ± 5.90		0.055
HAZ [b]	−2.72 ± 0.53		−1.90 ± 1.06		0.000
BMI	15.8 ± 1.40		15.7 ± 1.86		0.217
Waist (cm)	56.6 ± 3.91		57.5 ± 5.74		0.364
Hip (cm)	69.1 ± 6.18		69.8 ± 5.96		0.264
MUAC (mm)	18.4 ± 1.44		19.0 ± 4.84		0.771
Sum of skinfold thickness (mm)	31.5 ± 7.34		31.8 ± 11.7		0.321
Hb (g/dL)	12.7 ± 1.55		13.1 ± 1.00		0.184
Maternal characteristics					
Age	35.7 ± 6.20		37.4 ± 7.03		0.074
Height (cm)	148.7 ± 5.25		149.3 ± 4.85		0.620
Weight (kg)	58.2 ± 6.87		50.9 ± 9.14		0.000
BMI [c] (kg/m^2)	26.3 ± 2.29		22.8 ± 3.66		0.000
Waist (cm)	82.1 ± 9.38		75.5 ± 13.0		0.000
Hip (cm)	97.9 ± 10.4		91.8 ± 13.5		0.000
WHR [d]	0.86 ± 0.23		0.82 ± 0.16		0.016
MUAC [e] (mm)	28.2 ± 2.06		26.2 ± 5.87		0.000
Sum of skinfold thickness (mm)	86.5 ± 23.9		64.0 ± 28.6		0.000
BF%-BI [f] (%)	39.0 ± 5.51		32.9 ± 6.61		0.000
BF%-ST [g] (%)	35.1 ± 6.90		31.7 ± 6.80		0.000
Hb [h] (g/dL)	13.4 ± 1.30		12.6 ± 1.84		0.001

[a] Comparisons between double burden and non-double burden households were conducted using a *t*-test for maternal height, which was the only variable to fit a normal distribution; for other parameters, which did not fit a normal distribution, comparisons were made using the Mann-Whitney U-test; [b] Height-for-age z-score; [c] Body mass index; [d] Waist to hip ratio; [e] Mid-upper arm circumference; [f] Body fat percentage measured by bioelectrical impedance; [g] Body fat percentage calculated using skinfold thickness based on Durnin and Womersley's (1974) formula [21]; [h] hemoglobin. SD: Standard deviation.

Table 6. Socioeconomic characteristics and associations with maternal-child double burden.

	Double Burden		Non-Double Burden		Univariate		Multivariate [a]	
	%	Mean ± SD	%	Mean ± SD	OR (95% CI)	p	Adjusted OR (95% CI)	p
Child characteristics								
Age		11.2 ± 0.74		11.0 ± 0.90	1.34 (0.96–1.88)	0.089	1.44 (1.00–2.08)	0.051
Gender								
Male	43.8		49.1		1.00 (Reference)	–		
Female	56.2		50.9		1.24 (0.71–2.15)	0.451		
Maternal characteristics								
Age								
<30 year	15.5		12.7		1.00 (Reference)	–		
30–40 year	54.9		44.6		1.01 (0.44–2.30)	0.988		
≥40 year	29.6		42.8		0.57 (0.24–1.36)	0.202		
Education								
No schooling/Elementary school	23.6		51.9		1.00 (Reference)	–	1.00 (Reference)	–
Secondary school	5.1		9.7		1.15 (0.53–2.47)	0.727	1.29 (0.59–2.82)	0.526
>Secondary school	1.3		8.4		0.33 (0.09–1.15)	0.083	0.35 (0.10–1.27)	0.111
Height								
<145 cm	22.5		15		1.00 (Reference)	–		
145–149.9 cm	32.4		38.9		0.55 (0.25–1.22)	0.14		
≥150 cm	45.1		46.1		0.65 (0.31–1.38)	0.26		
Parity								
1–2	9		27.8		1.00 (Reference)	–		
3–5	18.4		35		1.62 (0.88–3.00)	0.123		
>6	3		6.8		1.35 (0.49–3.74)	0.558		
Occupation								
Farmer	5.1		6.3		1.00 (Reference)	–	1.00 (Reference)	–
Merchant, services	2.1		5.1		0.52 (0.14–1.89)	0.322	0.59 (0.15–2.24)	0.435
Other wage labor	0		0.8		0.00 (0.00–0.00)	0.999	0.00 (0.00–0.00)	0.999
Housewife	22.8		57.8		0.49 (0.22–1.12)	0.091	0.45 (0.19–1.05)	0.064
Household characteristics								
Possession of goods		3.53 ± 1.74		3.59 ± 1.82	0.98 (0.84–1.15)	0.819		

[a] The variables that were associated with maternal-child double burden in the univariate analysis ($p < 0.1$) were entered into multivariate analysis; SD: Standard deviation; OR: odds ratio; CI: confidence interval.

Table 7. Association of double burden with dietary patterns.

			Child Diet		Maternal Diet	
			OR (95% CI)	*p*	OR (95% CI)	*p*
Model 1 [a]	Modern	Q1	1.00	–	1.00	–
		Q2–Q3	1.07 (0.55–2.09)	0.847	0.99 (0.50–1.95)	0.972
		Q4	0.92 (0.42–2.03)	0.841	0.92 (0.42–2.03)	0.840
	High-animal products	Q1	1.00	–	1.00	–
		Q2–Q3	0.79 (0.41–1.51)	0.479	1.36 (0.68–2.71)	0.381
		Q4	0.48 (0.21–1.07)	0.073	0.92 (0.40–2.08)	0.834
Model 2 [b]	Modern	Q1	1.00	–	1.00	–
		Q2–Q3	1.12 (0.57–2.21)	0.740	1.01 (0.51–2.02)	0.972
		Q4	0.98 (0.44–2.16)	0.949	0.92 (0.40–2.11)	0.839
	High-animal products	Q1	1.00	–	1.00	–
		Q2–Q3	0.81 (0.42–1.57)	0.786	1.45 (0.72–2.95)	0.300
		Q4	0.46 (0.21–1.04)	0.064	1.01 (0.43–2.33)	0.991

[a] Unadjusted; [b] Adjusted for child's age and mother's occupation, which were significantly associated with maternal-child double burden (Table 6); OR: odds ratio; CI: confidence interval.

4. Discussion

4.1. Double Burden Structure at the Household Level

To the best of our knowledge, this is the first study that examined double burden structure at the household level for both mother-child and father-child pairs in the same household using primary data in Indonesia. We found that double burden in mother-child pairs exist in 30.6% of the subject households, whereas that of father-child pairs exists in only 8.4% of the subject households.

The percentage of double burden in mother-child pairs observed in this study was higher than that of the previous study conducted in rural Indonesia [6]. Those authors reported that maternal overweight and child stunting coexisted in 11% of the rural population throughout Indonesia. As pointed out by Vaezghasemi [18], the prevalence of double burden largely differs across the provinces in Indonesia. Among 13 provinces analyzed in Vaezghasemi's study, the prevalence of double burden in West Java was 4th highest. Thus, the higher prevalence of double burden observed in maternal-child pairs in our study would be partly attributable to this regional difference.

Our study revealed that the risk of double burden within the same household was larger among mother-child pairs than for father-child pairs. Among households whose mothers were overweight, only 24.0% had an overweight father and the rest (76.0%) had a non-overweight father. This gender difference in the prevalence of overweight has been reported in several studies in Indonesia [2,29], and is more pronounced than other countries in Asia such as China, Vietnam, and Nepal [30].

4.2. Adiposity Related Physical Characteristics of Double Burden Household Members

A novel aspect of our study is that the data include physical measurements related to adiposity. Among children, physical characteristics were not different between double burden and non-double burden groups except for height and HAZ. Among mothers, however, almost all physical characteristics differed between the double burden and non-double burden groups. Mothers in the double burden group had higher BF%, waist and hip circumference, WHR, MUAC, and the sum of skinfold thickness than those in the non-double burden group.

It is frequently stated in the literature that in the case of obesity or adiposity the BF% exceeds 25% in males and 35% in females [12,31]. In our analyses, we used two methods, BF%-BI and BF%-ST, for estimating BF%. The percentage of mothers whose BF% exceeded 35% was 87.3% using the BF%-BI method and was 66.2% using the BF%-ST method. A Tanita bioelectrical impedance with a body composition analyzer is often reported to underestimate BF% especially for fat individuals [32]. Durnin and Womersley's [21] formula has been used to estimate BF% in Indonesian adults [33–35] and has been reported to underestimate BF% by 1% compared with the deuterium dilution technique [35].

Considering these technical biases, it was judged that at least 66% of mothers from double burden households have obesity or adiposity based on BF% criteria. Moreover, 60.6% of mothers from double burden households had a waist larger than 80 cm, which is frequently used as an Asian threshold of waist circumference for metabolic syndrome [36]. It has been noted for a given BMI that Asians have a higher body fat percentage compared with Caucasians [25], and thus we determined overweight as a BMI (in kg/m^2) $\geqslant$23 to capture the increased risk of NCDs [26]. Even with this strict definition of overweight, more than 60% of mothers from double burden households were categorized either with adiposity or metabolic syndrome.

4.3. Dietary Patterns Relevant to Double Burden

Studies on the double burden problem in Indonesia scarcely mentioned the association between double burden and dietary patterns. In this study, to identify the dietary patterns of the study subjects, we administered a FFQ not at the household level but at the individual level, though we recruited father, mother and child pairs from the same household. In the subject area, frequent snacking outside the house is commonly observed not only for adults but also for children [23]. Also, family members do not always take their meals together. Thus, it was judged to be necessary to obtain FFQ data from each individual. Using the FFQ data, dietary patterns of the study subjects were identified by means of principal component analysis and two major dietary patterns, "Modern" and "High-animal products", were identified.

The "Modern" dietary pattern was predominantly characterized by higher consumption of flesh foods and instant snack foods. In this study area, instant snack foods such as meatball (called *bakso* in the Indonesian language), noodle, and fried sweets are sold in retailers in the village (called *Warung* in the Indonesian language) and peddlers. People often consume these snack foods instead of taking their meals and the extent of the contribution of these foods to overall nutrition is relatively high fat but low micronutrients [23]. A considerable body of literature has reported that traditional population groups throughout the world are replacing their traditional food patterns rich in complex carbohydrates, micronutrients, and fiber with diets high in refined sugars, animal products, and highly processed foods [37]. Considering the contents and the greatest preference in the principal component analysis, this dietary pattern likely reflects the nutrition transition phenomenon in this subject area. With regards to the relationships with nutritional status, after controlling for confounding factors, mothers in the middle quartiles and the highest quartile of the "Modern" dietary pattern had a higher risk of overweight. This finding is in agreement with other studies that reported that modified dietary patterns after the initiation of nutrition transition, frequently called a "Western diet", have a positive association with overweight among women [38,39].

The second dietary pattern identified by principal component analysis was the "High-animal products" dietary pattern, which was characterized by high consumption of animal products such as beef, goat, chicken, and duck but low consumption of salted fish. With regards to its association with nutritional status, after controlling for confounding factors, children in the highest quartile had a lower risk of stunting than those in the lowest, and fathers in the highest quartile had a higher risk of overweight than those in the lowest. In developing countries, consumption of animal products such as meat is often low in rural areas because of economic constrains [40]. Our data show that the median intake frequency of meat was mostly less than once per week among the subjects in the lowest quartile of the "High-animal products" dietary pattern; for example, among children, median intakes of chicken: one to three times per month; beef: almost never; goat: almost never; and duck: almost never. Animal products such as meat are not only the source of the animal proteins but also readily available sources of iron, zinc, and preformed vitamin A [40]. It has been reported in many studies that deficient intake of iron, zinc, and vitamin A, which are serious problems in some places in the world, impairs linear growth in children [41,42].

In our analysis, the "High-animal products" dietary pattern was associated with decreased risk of maternal-child double burden; after controlling for confounding factors, children in the highest quartile had a lower risk than those in the lowest. This association was highly related to the strong negative correlation of the "High-animal products" dietary pattern with child stunting. There was no association between the "High-animal products" dietary pattern and maternal overweight. For example, quartiles of the "High-animal products" dietary pattern were not different between overweight and non-overweight mothers (by χ^2 test), but quartiles of the "High-animal products" dietary pattern among overweight mothers were significantly different between those with stunted children and those with non-stunted children ($p < 0.1$ by χ^2 test). Thus, it was judged that it is critical to improve the issue of child stunting through adequate intake of animal products.

4.4. Limitations

Our study has a few limitations that should be considered. First, the sample size is small compared with previous studies discussing double burden issues in Indonesia. However, it is difficult to recruit father- and mother-child pairs from the same household to understand double burden structure in the household. Further, adiposity related physical characteristics and detailed information of food consumption frequencies are not easy to assess when targeting a large sample. Second, we adapted cutoff points for Asian populations for the classification of overweight, taking into account that Asians tend to have higher risk of NCDs at lower BMIs. This means that caution is warranted in terms of comparing our results with previous studies. Third, our food consumption data do not offer quantitative data and, thus, principal components analysis was conducted based on the consumption frequency. Even with this limitation, we adapted the principal components analysis considering the increasing interest in nutritional epidemiology to capture the association between diet and its health effects through dietary patterns, not through a single nutrient or food, because combined effects and interactions of multiple nutrients cannot be captured by analyzing a single nutrient or food [27,38,43]. Despite these limitations, we believe the present study provides useful information for understanding the degree of emerging household-level double burden of malnutrition in Indonesia.

5. Conclusions

The prevalence of double burden of malnutrition within the same household was three to four times higher for mother-child pairs than for father-child pairs in West Java, Indonesia. Furthermore, mothers from double burden households showed high levels of adiposity. Thus, further studies and policies should address overweight and the risk of NCDs among overweight mothers in double burden households as a rising health threat in Indonesia. This study also demonstrated the significance of dietary pattern, which has been scarcely examined before in studies on double burden of malnutrition. Dietary pattern characterized by high consumption of animal products but low consumption of salted fish, as identified by a principal component analysis, was associated with the decreased risk of maternal-child double burden through a strong negative correlation with child stunting. Therefore, improving child stunting through adequate intake of animal products is critical to solve the problem of maternal-child double burden in Indonesia.

Acknowledgments: This study was financially supported by the Ministry of Environment, Japan (H-063). The authors greatly appreciate the kind cooperation of the people in the study communities. We are also grateful to Dede Tresna, Ade Sudrajat, Ibnu Hurri, Iwan Setiawan, Ivan Apun Rahadian and Shanty Permanasari for their assistance in data collection. Also, thanks are due to John Freeman, The University of Tokyo, for editing the entire manuscript and providing useful advice.

Author Contributions: Makiko Sekiyama carried out data collection, data analysis, and was responsible for manuscript writing. Linda Dewanti carried out blood collection and analysis. Budhi Gunawan and Oekan S. Abdoellah were responsible for community liaison. Ryo Honda and Hana Shimizu-Furusawa collaborated on data collection. Chiho Watanabe and Hong Wei Jiang were responsible for manuscript editing and management of the study.

Conflicts of Interest: The authors declare no conflicts of interest.

References

1. Belahsen, R. Nutrition transition and food sustainability. *Proc. Nutr. Soc.* **2014**, *73*, 385–388. [CrossRef] [PubMed]
2. Roemling, C.; Qaim, M. Obesity trends and determinants in Indonesia. *Appetite* **2012**, *58*, 1005–1013. [CrossRef] [PubMed]
3. Malik, V.S.; Willett, W.C.; Hu, F.B. Global obesity: Trends, risk factors and policy implications. *Nat. Rev. Endocrinol.* **2013**, *9*, 13–27. [CrossRef] [PubMed]
4. Popkin, B.M., Adair, L.S.; Ng, S.W. Global nutrition transition and the pandemic of obesity in developing countries. *Nutr. Rev.* **2012**, *70*, 3–21. [CrossRef] [PubMed]
5. Khan, S.H.; Talukder, S.H. Nutrition transition in Bangladesh: Is the country ready for this double burden. *Obes. Rev.* **2013**, *14*, 126–133. [CrossRef] [PubMed]
6. Oddo, V.M.; Rah, J.H.; Semba, R.D.; Sun, K.; Akhter, N.; Sari, M.; de Pee, S.; Moench Pfanner, R., Bloem, M.; Kraemer K Predictors of maternal and child double burden of malnutrition in rural Indonesia and Bangladesh. *Am. J. Clin. Nutr.* **2012**, *95*, 951–958. [CrossRef] [PubMed]
7. Sengupta, A.; Angeli, F.; Syamala, T.S.; Van Schayck, C.P.; Dagnelie, P. State-wise dynamics of the double burden of malnutrition among 15–49 year-old women in India: How much does the scenario change considering Asian population-specific BMI cut-off values? *Ecol. Food Nutr.* **2014**, *53*, 618–638. [CrossRef] [PubMed]
8. Wong, C.Y.; Zalilah, M.S.; Chua, E.Y.; Norhasmah, S.; Chin, Y.S.; Siti Nur'Asyura, A. Double-burden of malnutrition among the indigenous peoples (Orang Asli) of Peninsular Malaysia. *BMC Public Health* **2015**, *15*, 680. [CrossRef] [PubMed]
9. Garrett, J.L.; Ruel, M.T. Stunted child-overweight mother pairs: Prevalence and association with economic development and urbanization. *Food Nutr. Bull.* **2005**, *26*, 209–221. [PubMed]
10. Jehn, M.; Brewis, A. Paradoxical malnutrition in mother-child pairs: Untangling the phenomenon of over- and under-nutrition in underdeveloped economies. *Econ. Hum. Biol.* **2009**, *7*, 28–35. [CrossRef] [PubMed]
11. Hawley, N.L.; Minster, R.L.; Weeks, D.E.; Viali, S.; Reupena, M.S.; Sun, G.; Cheng, H.; Deka, R.; Mcgarvey, S.T. Prevalence of adiposity and associated cardiometabolic risk factors in the Samoan genome-wide association study. *Am. J. Hum. Biol.* **2014**, *26*, 491–501. [CrossRef] [PubMed]
12. Phillips, C.M.; Tierney, A.C.; Perez-Martinez, P.; Defoort, C.; Blaak, E.E.; Gjelstad, I.M.; Lopez-Miranda, J.; Kiec-Klimczak, M.; Malczewska-Malec, M.; Drevon, C.A.; *et al.* Obesity and body fat classification in the metabolic syndrome: Impact on cardiometabolic risk metabotype. *Obesity* **2013**, *21*, E154–E161. [CrossRef] [PubMed]
13. Murray, C.J.; Vos, T.; Lozano, R.; Naghavi, M.; Flaxman, A.D.; Michaud, C.; Ezzati, M.; Shibuya, K.; Salomon, J.A.; Abdalla, S.; *et al.* Disability-adjusted life years (DALYs) for 291 diseases and injuries in 21 regions, 1990–2010: A systematic analysis for the Global Burden of Disease Study 2010. *Lancet* **2012**, *380*, 2197–2223. [CrossRef]
14. Lozano, R.; Naghavi, M.; Foreman, K.; Lim, S.; Shibuya, K.; Aboyans, V.; Aggarwal, R.; Ahn, S.Y.; AlMazroa, M.A.; Alvarado, M.; *et al.* Global and regional mortality from 235 causes of death for 20 age groups in 1990 and 2010: A systematic analysis for the Global Burden of Disease Study 2010. *Lancet* **2012**, *380*, 2095–2128. [CrossRef]
15. Fernald, L.C.; Neufeld, L.M. Overweight with concurrent stunting in very young children from rural Mexico: Prevalence and associated factors. *Eur. J. Clin. Nutr.* **2007**, *61*, 623–632. [CrossRef] [PubMed]
16. Lee, J.; Houser, R.F.; Must, A.; de Fulladolsa, P.P.; Bermudez, O.I. Disentangling nutritional factors and household characteristics related to child stunting and maternal overweight in Guatemala. *Econ. Hum. Biol.* **2010**, *8*, 188–196. [CrossRef] [PubMed]
17. Saibul, N.; Shariff, Z.M.; Lin, K.G.; Kandiah, M.; Ghani, N.A.; Rahman, HA. Food variety score is associated with dual burden of malnutrition in Orang Asli (Malaysian indigenous peoples) households: Implications for health promotion. *Asia Pac. J. Clin. Nutr.* **2009**, *18*, 412–422. [PubMed]
18. Vaezghasemi, M.; Öhman, A.; Eriksson, M.; Hakimi, M.; Weinehall, L.; Kusnanto, H.; Ng, N. The effect of gender and social capital on the dual burden of malnutrition: A multilevel study in Indonesia. *PLoS ONE* **2014**, *9*, e103849. [CrossRef] [PubMed]

19. Konishi, S.; Parajuli, R.P.; Takane, E.; Maharjan, M.; Tachibana, K.; Jiang, H.W.; Pahari, K.; Inoue, Y.; Umezaki, M.; Watanabe, C. Significant sex difference in the association between C-reactive protein concentration and anthropometry among 13- to 19-year olds, but not 6- to 12-year olds in Nepal. *Am. J. Phys. Anthropol.* **2014**, *154*, 42–51. [PubMed]

20. Weiner, J.S.; Lourie, J.A. *Practical Human Biology*; Academic Press: London, UK, 1981.

21. Durnin, J.V.G.A.; Womersley, J. Body fat assessed from total body density and its estimation from skinfold thickness: Measurements on 481 men and women aged from 17 to 72 years. *Br. J. Nutr.* **1974**, *32*, 77–97. [CrossRef] [PubMed]

22. De Onis, M.; Onyango, A.W.; Borghi, E.; Siyam, A.; Nishida, C.; Siekmann, J. Development of a WHO growth reference for school-aged children and adolescents. *Bull. World Health Organ.* **2007**, *85*, 660–667. [CrossRef] [PubMed]

23. Sekiyama, M.; Roosita, K.; Ohtsuka, R. Snack foods consumption contributes to poor nutrition of rural children in West Java, Indonesia. *Asia Pac. J. Clin. Nutr.* **2012**, *21*, 558–567. [PubMed]

24. Sekiyama, M.; Roosita, K.; Ohtsuka, R. Developmental stage-dependent influence of environmental factors on growth of rural Sundanese children in West Java, Indonesia. *Am. J. Phys. Anthropol.* **2015**, *157*, 94–106. [CrossRef] [PubMed]

25. Ramachandran, A.; Snehalatha, C. Rising burden of obesity in Asia. *J. Obes.* **2010**. [CrossRef] [PubMed]

26. WHO Expert Consultation. Appropriate body-mass index for Asian populations and its implications for policy and intervention strategies. *Lancet* **2004**, *363*, 157–163.

27. Zazpe, I.; Sánchez-Tainta, A.; Toledo, E.; Sánchez-Villegas, A.; Martínez-González, M.Á. Dietary patterns and total mortality in a Mediterranean cohort: The SUN project. *J. Acad. Nutr. Diet.* **2014**, *114*, 37–47. [CrossRef] [PubMed]

28. Newby, P.K.; Tucker, K.L. Empirically derived eating patterns using factor or cluster analysis: A review. *Nutr. Rev.* **2004**, *62*, 177–203. [CrossRef] [PubMed]

29. Usfar, A.A.; Fahmida, U. Do Indonesians follow its Dietary Guidelines? Evidence related to food consumption, healthy lifestyle, and nutritional status within the period 2000-2010. *Asia Pac. J. Clin. Nutr.* **2011**, *20*, 484–494. [PubMed]

30. Watanabe, C.; Umezaki, M.; Sekiyama, M.; Shimizu, H.; Konishi, S.; Jiang, H.W.; Arizono, K.; Inaoka, T.; Gunawan, B.; Abdoellah, O. Subsistence transition and its effects on local natural and chemical environments in rural and urban communities of Asian-pacific countries. Available online: https://eco.con fex.com/eco/2009/techprogram/P20225.HTM (accessed on 6 June 2015).

31. WHO. Physical Status: The Use and Interpretation of Anthropometry. WHO: Geneva, Switzerland, 1995.

32. Sluyter, J.D.; Schaaf, D.; Scragg, R.K.; Plank, L.D. Prediction of fatness by standing 8-electrode bioimpedance: A multiethnic adolescent population. *Obesity* **2010**, *18*, 183–189. [CrossRef] [PubMed]

33. Guricci, S.; Hartriyanti, Y.; Hautvast, J.G.A.J.; Deurenberg, P. Relationship between body fat and body mass index: Differences between Indonesians and Dutch Caucasians. *Eur. J. Clin. Nutr.* **1998**, *52*, 779–783.

34. Küpper, J.; Bartz, M.; Schultink, J.W.E.; Lutiko, W.; Deurenberg, P. Measurements of body fat in Indonesian adults: Comparison between a three compartment model and widely used methods. *Asia Pac. J. Clin. Nutr.* **1998**, *7*, 49–54. [PubMed]

35. Hastuti, J.; Kagawa, M.; Byrne, N.M.; Hills, A.P. Development and validation of anthropometric prediction equations for estimation of body fat in Indonesian men. *Asia Pac. J. Clin. Nutr.* **2013**, *22*, 522–529. [PubMed]

36. Alberti, K.G.; Zimmet, P.; Shaw, J. Metabolic syndrome—A new world-wide definition. A consensus statement from the international diabetes federation. *Diabet. Med.* **2006**, *23*, 469–480. [CrossRef] [PubMed]

37. Romaguera, D.; Samman, N.; Rossi, A.; Miranda, C.; Pons, A.; Tur, J.A. Dietary patterns of the Andean population of Puna and Quebrada of Humahuaca, Jujuy, Argentina. *Br. J. Nutr.* **2008**, *99*, 390–397. [CrossRef] [PubMed]

38. Cunha, D.B.; de Almeida, R.M.; Sichieri, R.; Pereira, R.A. Association of dietary patterns with BMI and waist circumference in a low-income neighbourhood in Brazil. *Br. J. Nutr.* **2010**, *104*, 908–913. [CrossRef] [PubMed]

39. Flores, M.; Macias, N.; Rivera, M.; Lozada, A.; Barquera, S.; Rivera-Dommarco, J.; Tucker, K.L. Dietary patterns in Mexican adults are associated with risk of being overweight or obese. *J. Nutr.* **2010**, *140*, 1869–1873. [CrossRef] [PubMed]

40. Gibson, R.S.; Hotz, C. Dietary diversification/modification strategies to enhance micronutrient content and bioavailability of diets in developing countries. *Br. J. Nutr.* **2001**, *85*, S159–S166. [CrossRef] [PubMed]

Nutrients **2015**, *7*, 8376–8391

41. Hadi, H.; Stoltzfus, R.J.; Dibley, M.J.; Moulton, L.H.; West, K.P., Jr.; Kjolhede, C.L.; Sadjimin, T. Vitamin A supplementation selectively improves the linear growth of Indonesian preschool children: Results from a randomized controlled trial. *Am. J. Clin. Nutr.* **2000**, *71*, 507–513. [PubMed]

42. Norgan, N.G.; Bogin, B.; Cameron, N. Nutrition and growth. In *Human Growth and Development*, 2nd ed.; Cameron, N., Bogin, B., Eds.; Elseviser: New York, NY, USA, 2012; pp. 123–152.

43. Denova-Gutiérrez, E.; Castañón, S.; Talavera, J.O.; Gallegos-Carrillo, K.; Flores, M.; Dosamantes-Carrasco, D.; Willett, W.C.; Salmerón, J. Dietary patterns are associated with metabolic syndrome in an urban Mexican population. *J. Nutr.* **2010**, *140*, 1855–1863. [CrossRef]

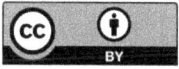

nutrients

MDPI

Article

Dietary Changes over 25 Years in Tianjin Residents: Findings from the 1986–1988, 2000–2004, and 2008–2011 Nutrition Surveys

Xuan Wang, Yuntang Wu, Xumei Zhang, Meilin Zhang and Guowei Huang *

Department of Nutrition and Food Science, School of Public Health, Tianjin Medical University,
22 Qixiangtai Road, Heping District, 300070 Tianjin, China; wangxuan@tmu.edu.cn (X.W.);
wuyuntang@tmu.edu.cn (Y.W.); zhangxumei@tmu.edu.cn (X.Z.); defjmmm@163.com (M.Z.)
* Correspondence: huangguowei@tmu.edu.cn; Tel.: +86-22-8333-6606; Fax: +86-22-8333-6603

Received: 13 October 2015; Accepted: 14 January 2016; Published: 22 January 2016

Abstract: In China, the rates of chronic diseases characteristic of countries in nutritional transition have been increasing. However, few studies have examined diet changes in recent decades. We analyzed dietary changes in Tianjin, China. The data in this descriptive, population-based study in ⩾18-year-old adults were collected from three surveys from 1986 to 2011. Food consumption and nutrient intake were compared among the three surveys separately for urban and rural areas. Differences in food consumption between urban and rural areas in different periods were also shown. The consumption of cereals, vegetables, and oils decreased, and that of fruits and beans increased in both urban and rural areas. Moreover, the total consumption of animal foods, especially milk, increased (0.01% in 1986–1988; 1.72% in 2008–2011) in rural areas. Although milk consumption also increased in urban areas, consumption of other animal foods decreased (19.33% in 1986–1988; 13.74% in 2008–2011). Meanwhile, cereals consumption rebounded from 22.63% in 2000–2004 to 29.75% in 2008–2011. Moreover, the lack of dairy products and some nutrients, e.g., retinol, calcium, and dietary fiber (<80% of recommended nutrient intake), in the diet persisted in both urban and rural areas. In conclusion, differences in diet between urban and rural areas decreased over time.

Keywords: nutrition survey; dietary pattern; urban area; rural area

1. Introduction

Human survival has always been based on foods and nutrients, which are also important factors affecting the population's quality and are closely related to economic and social development. Meanwhile, economic progress and high levels of education can also change people's dietary patterns. Technological changes have reduced physical activity for work, travel, home production, and leisure. Chinese consumption patterns have been transformed by changes in food technology, import controls, food pricing, and mass media. China has undergone many marked dietary pattern shifts since 1949. These include: (1) a period (1949–1957) when food production was inadequate and cereal consumption was low; (2) the famine (1957–1962), which was linked with the Great Leap Forward; (3) a strong recovery (1962–1979); (4) the subsequent reform period (1979–1985) after the liberalization of food production, when the annual economic growth rate was greater than 10%; and (5) the current period (since 1985), in which continued rapid economic growth and a remarkable shift in diet structure has occurred [1–4]. Rapid economic and social change has transformed urban China and much of its rural sector as well [5].

The classic Chinese diet includes cereals and vegetables with few animal foods. It is a diet that many scholars consider to be the healthiest when adequate intake is achieved. An earlier study showed rapid changes in diet [6]. As the classic dietary pattern shifts, intakes of cereals and many lower-fat, mixed dishes are being replaced, animal foods are becoming popular, and the consumption of edible oils is increasing quickly. This shift in diet composition and corresponding body composition has been accompanied by many positive and some negative changes [2]. Although infectious diseases and hunger, the important causes of death in the 1950s, no longer affect most of the population, the mortality burden has shifted to diet-related, non-communicable diseases (DR-NCDs), with a rapid increase in the prevalence of obesity. Obesity and non-communicable diseases are the major causes of morbidity, disability, and mortality in China, and the health system has to develop in order to care for people with these conditions [7–9].

In 1985, China entered the fifth dietary pattern period (*i.e.*, the current period), during which the economy has further improved. China has been undergoing a fast shift towards a stage of nutrition transition dominated by a high intake of fat and animal foods by 2004, as well as a high prevalence of DR-NCDs [10]. Because of these, the Ministry of Health consigned the Chinese Nutrition Society constituting the "Chinese Dietary Guidelines" (2007) and the "Food Guide Pagoda (FGP) for Chinese Residents" (2007) which were published after two years of hardships [11]. To our knowledge, no study based on the changes after that has been carried out in China to date. The present study added some new information after 2007, which had not been assessed before, and explored a nutritional shift in different time periods by using a sample from urban and rural Tianjin, one of four large cities in China. We used data on individual diets from three independent representative samples of the Tianjin population to examine the differences in food and nutrient intake and in the source of energy, protein and fat for the periods of 1986–1988, 2000–2004, and 2008–2011(contained several key time points of dietary changes during these periods). Moreover, we compared the latest data with FGP (2007) to reveal the changes in 2008–2011. The full implications of these changes are then discussed.

2. Experimental Section

2.1. Data Sources and Subjects

Data from urban and rural areas were analyzed respectively in this study because of the imbalance in economic development between urban and rural areas in China. Data for this study were primarily obtained from three sources. First, the nutrition survey data from 1986 to 1988 in urban and rural Tianjin (S1); second, annual household consumption surveys data from 2000 to 2004 (S2); and the third, nutrition survey data from 2008 to 2011 in urban and rural Tianjin (S3). The three surveys covered all six districts from urban areas and all five counties from rural areas in Tianjin. Data from 1986 to 1988 and from 2000 to 2004 were partially available [12–14]. The use of the data for 2008–2011 survey was approved by the ethics committee of Tianjin Medical University.

A multistage, random cluster sample was used to draw the sample in three surveys. The surveys collected information on all individuals, including all age groups, living in the household. Our study included adults aged at least 18 years ($\geqslant$18 years) in three surveys to comprise the study population (Table 1). Moreover, the data for further comparison were converted to the level of reference person (an 18-year-old man with light physical activity weighing 60 kg) so that the results are consistent and comparable.

Table 1. Composition of study population in Tianjin by three surveys (*n*, %)

Population Group	1986–1988		2000–2004		2008–2011	
	Urban (%)	Rural (%)	Urban (%)	Rural (%)	Urban (%)	Rural (%)
Sex						
Male	7061 (48.5)	1603 (49.3)	8076 (49.1)	5426 (49.4)	4674 (47.2)	3737 (49.0)
Female	7488 (51.5)	1649 (50.7)	8385 (50.9)	5555 (50.6)	5222 (52.8)	3891 (51.0)
Total	14,549	3252	16,461	10,981	9896	7628
Age (years)						
18–29	3577 (24.6)	826 (25.3)	2316 (14.1)	2888 (26.3)	1017 (10.3)	1985 (26.0)
30–39	3334 (22.9)	760 (23.4)	4111 (25.0)	2712 (24.7)	2723 (27.5)	1840 (24.1)
40–49	2990 (20.6)	659 (20.3)	3137 (19.0)	2559 (23.3)	2672 (27.0)	1755 (23.0)
50–59	2464 (16.9)	650 (20.0)	3979 (24.2)	1787 (16.3)	1898 (19.2)	1419 (18.6)
60–	2184 (15.0)	357 (11.0)	2918 (17.7)	1035 (9.4)	1586 (16.0)	629 (8.3)
Total	14,549	3252	16,461	10,981	9896	7628

2.2. Dietary Analysis

Dietary data were collected via in-home interviews by a combination of the weighting method and a seven-day consecutive record method. A food-weighted record method was used for S1 and S2. The method was determined by weighing all food consumed by the household over seven consecutive randomly selected days. All remaining food was weighed and recorded at the beginning and the end of the survey. Household food consumption was determined by examining changes in every kind of food from the beginning to the end of each day. All the newly brought foods were recorded. Food eating outside was estimated when weighing was not possible. A seven-day consecutive record method was used in S3; every household member was asked to record all food consumed over the previous 24 h for each of the seven days, no matter where it was eaten. Individuals were asked to record the name and amounts of food consumed for every meal. The amount of food in each dish was estimated according to some food pictures which showed different amounts of food on a 20 cm paper plate (e.g., Figure 1). Compared to the food-weighted record method, food intakes assessed by 24 h recall were similar, and the relative differences were less than 10% of most food items [15]. Data obtained by these methods correlated well with respect to individual food items and calculated nutrients.

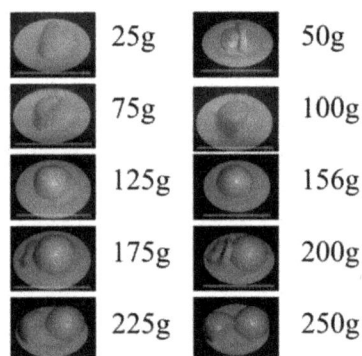

Figure 1. Example of selection pictures for aiding estimatation of the amount of steamed buns eaten.

The food groups included were based on Chinese Food Composition Table [16]. The following twenty food groups were included: cereals and grain products; potatoes and starches; beans and their products; vegetables; mushrooms; fruits; nuts and seeds; red meat and their products; poultry and their products; fish and shellfish; milk and dairy products; egg and egg products; snack and cakes;

fast food; drinks; alcohol; sugar; flavors; fats and oils. However, S3 for 2008–2011 did not include sugar, flavors, drinks and alcohol. In order to ensure the consistency of the food category and the readability of the information, we removed these four groups. According to the results of three surveys, food items with similar nutritional profiles were merged, and food items people ate less were put together into new group which was called others. In total, 12 sub-categories were summarized to compare the average food consumption. Moreover, 10 main food groups were used to compare the food proportion according to the Food Guide Pagoda [17].

Food and nutrient intakes were assessed by calculating the amount for each reference person per day according to the constitution of the population. A quantitative assessment of dietary intake was analyzed using a computer dietary analysis. We determined total calories; percentage of calories from total carbohydrate, protein, and fat; percentage of proteins from different kinds of foods; and the following nutrients: cholesterol, fiber, vitamin A (retinol), vitamin B1 (thiamine), vitamin B2 (riboflavin), niacin, vitamin C (ascorbic acid), calcium, iron, zinc, and selenium using the Chinese Food Composition Table [16]. The total retinol value of the diet was evaluated by the retinol equivalent (RE). Food intakes were compared with the levels in the 2002 Chinese National Nutrition and Health Survey (NNHS) [18,19] and the recommended intakes in the food guide pagoda (2007) [17], including intake of cereals (250–400 g/day), vegetables (300–500 g/day), fruits (200–400 g/day), meats and poultry (50–75 g/day), fish and seafood (50–100 g/day), eggs and egg products (25–50 g/day), milk and dairy products (300 g/day), beans (30–50 g/day), and oil (25–30 g/day). We also determined the percentage of selected recommended nutrient intakes (RNIs) and adequate intakes (AIs) [17]. The intake of vitamin A was compared using AI; total fat ($\leqslant$30% kcal/day), cholesterol ($\leqslant$300 mg/day), vitamin B1, vitamin B2, niacin, vitamin C, calcium, iron, zinc, and selenium were compared using RNI.

2.3. Statistical Analysis

The food and nutrient intake were calculated using Microsoft Office Excel 2003 (Microsoft Corp., Redmond, WA, USA). All analyses were performed separately for urban and rural areas. Mean daily nutrient intake was derived for descriptive purposes. Values were expressed as means $\pm$ SD. Nutrient intake and food consumption among the periods of 1986 to 1988, 2000 to 2004, and 2008 to 2011 were compared using an analysis of variance. The statistical analysis was performed with SPSS 13.0 for Windows (Chicago, IL, USA).

3. Results

3.1. Food Consumption Patterns

3.1.1. Proportions for Different Food Groups

A reduction of proportions for cereals, vegetables, and oil and an increase of proportions for fruits, beans, milk and dairy products were found in both urban and rural areas for the periods of 1986–1988, 2000–2004, and 2008–2011 (Supplementary Table S1). Especially the proportions for fruits and milk and dairy products increased sharply (*i.e.*, from 1.01% for 1986–1988 to 16.29% for 2008–2011 and from 0.01% for 1986–1988 to 1.72% for 2008–2011, respectively) in rural areas, while the proportion for cereals decreased significantly. Whereas the proportions for cereals increased to 29.75% for 2008–2011 after falling to the lowest 22.63% for 2000–2004 in urban areas. Moreover, it also showed that the total proportion for animal foods except milk and dairy products decreased in urban areas and increased in rural areas.

3.1.2. Average Intakes for Different Food Groups

The mean food consumption levels from 2002 NNHS and FDP (2007) were used as reference. The average intakes for different food groups for the periods of 1986–1988, 2000–2004, and 2008–2011 were compared to each other (Table 2). Furthermore, a comparison of differences between urban and rural areas in three periods was carried out for each food group (Figure S1).

Cereals

In urban areas, cereal intake decreased considerably from 1986–1988 to 2000–2004, but increased during the period of 2008–2011 ($p < 0.001$) (Table 2). In rural areas, the mean intake of cereals decreased gradually, from 483.03 g/reference person/day to 442.26 g/reference person/day ($p = 0.807$) (Table 2). Therefore, the shift in cereal intake for rural areas was not obvious among the three discrete stages from 1986 to 2011. The difference between urban and rural residents' intakes increased from 88.36 g/reference person/day for 1986–1988 to 222.43 g/reference person/day for 2000–2004, and then decreased to 51.04 g/reference person/day for 2008–2011(Figure S1). Both urban and rural residents' cereal and tubers products intakes became slightly higher than the levels of FGP (Table 2).

Vegetables and Fruits

Intake of vegetables increased significantly in both urban and rural areas from 1986–1988 to 2000–2004, but decreased slightly for 2008–2011(Table 2). Urban residents' intake was higher than rural residents'. The difference between urban and rural residents' intakes decreased from 68.84 g/reference person/day for 1986–1988 to 53.86 g/reference person/day for 2000–2004 and then to 9.73 g/reference person/day for 2008–2011 (Figure S1). Moreover, both urban and rural residents' vegetable intake in 2008–2011 was just a little lower than the recommended level of FGP (Table 2). However, the mean intake of fruits increased considerably across all three time periods in both urban and rural areas (Table 2). The intake of fruits for 2008–2011 was 4.57-fold and 25.28-fold higher than that for 1986–1988 in urban and rural areas, respectively. The difference between urban and rural residents' intake decreased to 1.31 g/reference person/day (Figure S1). Furthermore, both urban and rural residents' fruit intake in 2008–2011 was in the recommended range of FGP (Table 2).

Animal Foods

The mean intake of total animal foods increased over time in both urban and rural areas. Rural residents' intake showed a more significant shift (the mean intake of total animal foods increased by 106.77 g/reference person/day during the study period), especially with regard to the intake of milk and dairy products (Table 2). Although the intake of milk was still less than the level of FGP recommended, the intake for 2008–2011 was 176.31-fold higher than that for 1986–1988. Although the overall increase (6.85 g/reference person/day) in intake for urban residents was less than that for rural residents, urban residents' daily intake of total animal foods was higher than that for rural residents across all periods from 1986 to 2011. However, the intake of total animal foods except milk and dairy products decreased in urban areas and increased in rural areas (Table 2). Urban residents' intake of meat and eggs was higher than the level of FGP recommended, while intake of milk was lower than that level. Rural residents' intake of egg in 2008–2011 was higher than the level of FGP recommended, while intake of fish and milk was far lower than that (Table 2).

Beans and Bean Products

The intake of beans decreased from 1986–1988 to 2000–2004, but then increased considerably for 2008–2011 in both urban and rural areas, and was even higher than the level of FGP (Table 2). The mean intake of beans decreased by 5.72 g/reference person/day for urban residents and by 2.09 g/reference person/day for rural residents, and then increased by 82.77 g/reference person/day and 55.30 g/reference person/day in urban and rural areas, respectively.

Table 2. Average food consumption of different dietary food groups for urban and rural residents in Tianjin in three different periods ($\bar{x} \pm s$, g/reference person/day).

Food Category	Urban				Rural				2002 NNHS		Food Guide [a] in 2007
	1986–1988	2000–2004	2008–2011	p Value	1986–1988	2000–2004	2008–2011	p Value	Urban	Rural	
Plant foods											
Cereals and grain products	391.67 ± 41.97	242.06 ± 10.12 **	391.22 ± 40.77 ##	0.000	483.03 ± 34.95	464.49 ± 84.28	442.26 ± 31.41	0.807	366.1	415.3	250–400 [b]
Potatoes and starches	39.03 ± 16.27	36.00 ± 2.29	29.92 ± 4.04	0.565	31.30 ± 6.9	35.33 ± 11.80	42.67 ± 13.72	0.523	31.9	56.2	—
Beans and their products	21.23 ± 5.49	15.51 ± 10.52	98.28 ± 24.80 ***##	0.000	12.23 ± 2.56	10.14 ± 6.67	65.44 ± 20.60 ***##	0.001	15.5	16.2	30–50
Vegetables	272.67 ± 58.52	374.62 ± 19.62 *	289.07 ± 82.72	0.011	203.83 ± 46.98	321.76 ± 66.8	279.34 ± 58.96	0.069	251.9	284.1	300–500
Fruits	48.27 ± 6.90	208.82 ± 14.10 **	220.49 ± 58.23 **	0.000	8.67 ± 6.40	89.45 ± 5.57 **	219.18 ± 56.38 ***##	0.000	69.3	36.6	200–400
Vegetable oils	37.63 ± 7.50	24.10 ± 2.61 **	27.23 ± 4.63 *	0.018	17.00 ± 3.84	25.11 ± 2.60	29.76 ± 5.43 *	0.012	40.2	29.9	25–30 [c]
others	56.90 ± 28.40	66.20 ± 11.39	89.15 ± 35.11	0.323	20.97 ± 6.73	10.61 ± 0.61	76.00 ± 20.23 ***##	0.000	—	—	—
Animal foods											
Meats and poultry and their products	83.30 ± 2.34	96.21 ± 3.65	80.34 ± 14.04 #	0.024	19.93 ± 4.84	32.11 ± 0.69 *	64.40 ± 8.51 ***##	0.000	104.4	69.9	50–75
Fish and shellfish	62.50 ± 8.34	49.62 ± 12.67	48.58 ± 7.88	0.206	26.73 ± 8.36	23.13 ± 3.34	37.93 ± 7.18 #	0.043	44.9	24.4	50–100
Egg and egg products	72.43 ± 11.96	54.43 ± 3.65 *	65.53 ± 20.51 *	0.018	29.87 ± 5.76	38.53 ± 8.14	60.72 ± 23.70	0.062	33.2	19.9	25–50
Milk and dairy products	44.00 ± 6.71	61.32 ± 13.39	74.19 ± 2.78 #	0.045	0.13 ± 0.06	7.20 ± 9.32	22.92 ± 10.02 *	0.046	65.8	11.2	300
Animal oils and fats	0.77 ± 0.17	0.08 ± 0.05 **	1.34 ± 0.84 ##	0.007	6.47 ± 2.27	2.31 ± 0.73 *	3.93 ± 0.97*	0.013	3.8	10.5	—
Total	1133.53 ± 62.02	1228.97 ± 70.48	1415.34 ± 44.18 **	0.006	860.16 ± 12.17	1057.20 ± 39.56 *	1344.55 ± 60.54 *##	0.000	—	—	—

[a]: from the Chinese food guide pagoda in 2007; [b]: both from cereals and tubers products; [c]: total oil(both from animal and vegetable); * $p < 0.05$; ** $p < 0.01$: vs. 1986–1988; # $p < 0.05$: vs. 2000–2004; ## $p < 0.01$: vs. 2000–2004; Abbreviation: 2002 NNHS: 2002 Chinese National Nutrition and Health Survey.

Oils

The shift in oil intake in both urban and rural residents is very interesting. Urban residents' mean intake of oils was higher than that for rural residents for 1986–1988. Urban residents' mean intake of oils decreased by 14.15 g/reference person/day for 2000–2004, while rural residents' mean intake of oils increased by 3.95 g/reference person/day. Then, both urban and rural residents' intake increased for 2008–2011. Overall, rural residents' mean intake of oils came from behind and was higher than that for urban residents, and was even higher than the level of FGP recommended (Table 2).

3.2. Caloric and Nutrient Intakes

3.2.1. Caloric Intakes

Urban residents' mean caloric intakes decreased over time, while there were no big changes in rural areas (Table 3). Urban residents' mean caloric intakes were higher than rural residents' intakes for 1986–1988. During the five-year period from 2000 to 2004, urban residents' mean caloric intakes decreased by 671.46 kcal/reference person/day, while rural residents' increased by 131.13 kcal/reference person/day. The difference between urban and rural residents' caloric intakes increased to 444.29 kcal/reference person/day by 2000–2004. Then, urban residents' intakes increased (by 164.84 kcal/reference person/day) and rural residents' decreased (by 141.41 kcal/reference person/day) for 2008–2011. Finally, rural residents' intakes were slightly higher than those of urban residents. The difference between urban and rural residents' caloric intakes decreased to 138.04 kcal/reference person/day by 2008–2011(Table 3).

3.2.2. Nutrients Intakes and Selected Nutrients Intakes as Percent of RNI or AI

Urban residents' protein, fat, and carbohydrate intakes all decreased over time. Both protein and fat intakes increased in rural areas, but carbohydrate intake slightly decreased (Table 3). The intake of dietary fiber increased for both urban and rural residents. And it had increased by 185.24% in urban areas and by 249.34% in rural areas by 2008–2011 (Table 3). Rural residents' mean intake of cholesterol increased more quickly than did urban residents' (135.61% *vs.* 4.82%, respectively), and the cholesterol intake for rural residents was closer to that of urban residents for 2008–2011 (Table 3). Additionally, retinol significantly decreased among urban residents for both 2000–2004 and 2008–2011 ($p < 0.01$), riboflavin and niacin significantly increased among rural residents for 2008–2011, and thiamine significantly decreased for all residents and calcium and selenium significantly increased among rural residents for both 2000–2004 and 2008–2011 (Table 3).

3.3. Composition of Energy, Protein and Fat

Regarding the food sources for energy, energy from cereals and grain products decreased remarkably and that from animal foods and others increased significantly in rural areas in this study period (Table 4). In urban areas, after an increased proportion of animal foods, the proportion fell to 20.73% for 2008–2011 from 24.54% for 2000–2004. Furthermore, an increasing trend in energy from beans and their products and a decreasing trend in that from pure energy foods were found in both urban and rural areas (Table 4). Nutrient sources of energy changed remarkably: energy from carbohydrates decreased from 54.10% to 51.00% (lower than the RNI) in urban areas and from 67.9% to 55.26% (similar to the RNI) in rural areas, whereas energy from both protein and fat increased both in urban and rural areas (Figure 2). And these changes were more obvious in rural areas.

Among the energy components, there was little change in the proportion of energy from protein, but the proportion of protein from animals increased while protein from cereals decreased considerably. This change was especially remarkable for rural residents; only 16.32% of their protein came from animal foods for 1986–1988, but that increased to 17.3% for 2000–2004 and to 34.48% for 2008–2011, while protein from cereals decreased from 69.88% to 40.17% (Figure 2).

Table 3. Average energy and nutrients intake (percentage of RNI/AI) for urban and rural residents in Tianjin in three different periods ($\bar{x} \pm s$, /reference person/day)

Energy/Nutrients	Urban				Rural				RNI/AI
	1986–1988 (%)	2000–2004 (%)	2008–2011 (%)	p Value	1986–1988 (%)	2000–2004 (%)	008–2011 (%)	p Value	
Energy (kcal)	2649.07 ± 272.18 (110.38)	1977.61 ± 92.86 ** (82.40)	2142.45 ± 156.31 * (89.25)	0.003	2290.77 ± 71.12 (95.45)	2421.90 ± 96.30 (100.91)	2223.49 ± 38.91 (95.02)	0.098	2400
Protein (g)	83.63 ± 7.07 (111.51)	73.81 ± 4.97 (98.41)	78.08 ± 1.05 (104.11)	0.104	64.60 ± 2.31 (86.13)	70.26 ± 4.29 (93.68)	78.11 ± 0.58 ** (104.55)	0.010	75
Fat (g)	98.20 ± 13.95	75.91 ± 4.85 *	81.21 ± 5.16	0.025	52.83 ± 4.25	52.47 ± 2.34	78.48 ± 9.09 **##	0.001	
Carbohydrate (g)	357.57 ± 33.42	250.19 ± 10.37 **	275.02 ± 26.11 *	0.001	389.87 ± 25.54	417.45 ± 20.00	315.24 ± 30.77 *##	0.004	
Dietary fiber (g)	6.03 ± 0.55 (24.12)	10.13 ± 0.50 (40.52)	17.20 ± 7.95 **# (68.80)	0.015	5.27 ± 0.32 (21.08)	16.24 ± 2.58 ** (64.96)	18.41 ± 7.82 **## (73.64)	0.006	25
Retinol Equiv. (µg)	1377.00 ± 136.54 (172.13)	444.38 ± 122.22 ** (55.55)	624.15 ± 27.10 ** (78.02)	0.000	590.20 ± 73.72 (73.78)	426.469 ± 153.89 (53.31)	576.24 ± 94.85 (72.03)	0.217	800
Thiamine (mg)	1.93 ± 0.40 (137.86)	1.01 ± 0.08 (72.14)	1.10 ± 0.10 (78.57)	0.002	2.40 ± 0.17 (171.43)	1.44 ± 0.14 ** (102.86)	1.11 ± 0.07 ** (80.00)	0.300	1.4
Riboflavin (mg)	1.13 ± 0.12 (80.71)	1.10 ± 0.08 ** (78.57)	1.16 ± 0.17 * (82.86)	0.744	0.73 ± 0.06 (52.14)	0.75 ± 0.04 (53.57)	1.14 ± 0.20 **## (81.43)	0.002	1.4
Niacin (mg)	15.33 ± 0.85 (109.5)	18.05 ± 0.72 ** (128.93)	17.03 ± 0.22 (121.64)	0.004	14.40 ± 0.46 (102.86)	15.09 ± 0.76 (107.79)	16.9 ± 0.39 **# (120.78)	0.010	14
Ascorbic acid (mg)	94.00 ± 21.17 (94.00)	165.43 ± 45.41 (165.43)	101.33 ± 0.03 (101.33)	0.055	58.13 ± 11.02 (58.13)	85.20 ± 24.19 (85.2)	95.29 ± 8.57 (95.29)	0.37	100
Calcium (mg)	475.1 ± 67.05 (59.39)	611.25 ± 92.44 (76.41)	625.15 ± 57.97 (78.14)	0.936	406.83 ± 30.03 (50.85)	482.40 ± 34.29 * (60.3)	504.86 ± 97.01 **## (63.11)	0.000	800
Iron (mg)	28.03 ± 2.80 (186.87)	24.20 ± 1.24 (161.33)	24.02 ± 2.88 (160.13)	0.081	25.90 ± 1.21 (172.57)	20.76 ± 1.36 (138.4)	25.26 ± 1.12 **# (168.4)	0.002	15
Zinc (mg)	11.51 ± 1.07 (76.73)	12.09 ± 1.41 (80.60)	12.90 ± 1.43 (86.00)	0.546	10.12 ± 0.36 (67.47)	13.22 ± 0.43 * (88.13)	12.87 ± 1.47 * (85.8)	0.001	15
Selenium (µg)	46.93 ± 3.67 (93.86)	60.51 ± 8.93 (121.02)	64.28 ± 3.52 (128.56)	0.053	25.31 ± 0.49 (50.62)	40.52 ± 2.06 * (81.04)	61.70 ± 7.17 **# (123.4)	0.000	50
Cholesterol (mg)	486.26 ± 58.29 (162.09)	498.69 ± 45.93 (166.23)	509.72 ± 107.69 (169.91)	0.916	191.53 ± 29.71 (63.84)	247.82 ± 54.93 (82.61)	451.27 ± 25.03 **## (150.42)	0.001	300

* $p < 0.05$: vs. 1986–1988; ** $p < 0.01$: vs. 1986–1988; # $p < 0.05$: vs. 2000–2004; ## $p < 0.01$: vs. 2000–2004. Abbreviation: RNI: recommended nutrient intake; AI: adequate intake.

Energy from fat also slightly increased among urban residents to higher than the RNI. However, the proportion of fat from animals showed a decreasing trend (from 48.12% for 2000–2004 to 37.85% for 2008–2011) (Figure 2). For rural residents, there was an obvious increase of the proportion of energy from fat overall and fat from animals specifically (Figure 2). Thus, the energy and food composition patterns are now more similar between urban and rural areas.

Table 4. The proportion of energy from different dietary food groups for urban and rural residents in Tianjin in three different periods (%).

Food Category	Urban			Rural		
	1986–1988	2000–2004	2008–2011	1986–1988	2000–2004	2008–2011
Cereals and grain products	48.61	37.54	41.90	68.68	74.53	48.73
Beans and their products	2.21	2.02	3.35	1.12	1.48	3.28
Potatoes and starches	1.16	1.45	1.59	1.05	0.10	1.48
Animal foods	16.79	24.54	20.73	5.18	7.74	16.56
Pure energy foods	16.51	16.19	15.24	17.27	12.04	15.92
Others	14.68	18.26	17.19	6.70	4.10	14.03
Total	100.00	100.00	100.00	100.00	100.00	100.00

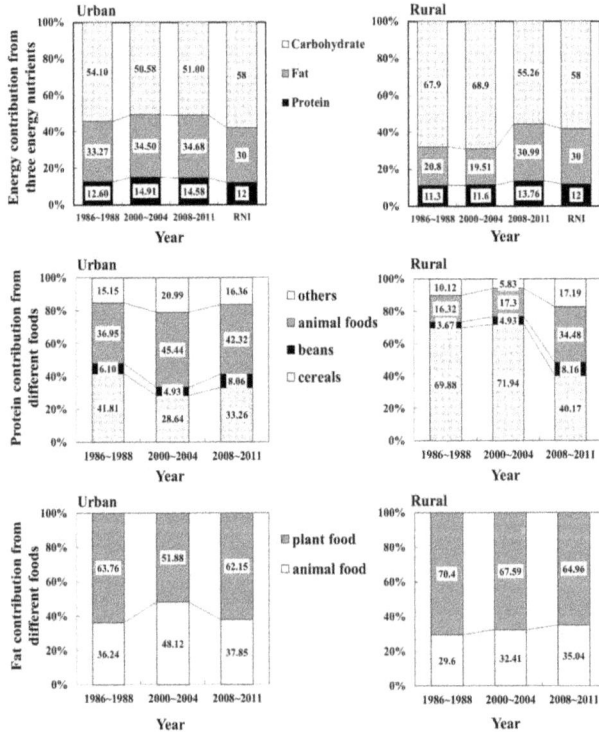

Figure 2. Composition of energy from three energy nutrients and compositions of protein and fat from different foods for urban and rural residents in three different periods.

4. Discussion

After the fourth, or reform period, from 1979 to 1985, China experienced remarkable economic progress [4]. There was a significant increase in food production capacity and food yield. Living standards and food accessibility per capita increased rapidly. The current period (since 1985) is the fifth period. Our study included data only from the fifth period, in which there was further economic improvement. The total gross domestic product (GDP) increased from 201.7 billion USD in 1980 (the fourth period) to 354.6 in 1990, 1079.9 in 2000 and 5685.5 in 2010 (the fifth period). The per capita GDP was 309, 343, 945 and 4387 USD respectively in these years [20]. The three periods (1986–1988, 2000–2004 and 2008–2011) in this study are just around these years. Fortunately, we observed many dietary changes which indicated a slight and significant improvement in the pattern of food intake in both urban and rural areas.

During the period of 1986 to 1988, food intake of key food types (cereals, vegetables, animal foods) in urban areas was abundant except for fruits, beans, milk, and the oil. In particular, animal food was very popular. However, the intake of most key food types (fruits, animal foods) in rural areas was extremely rare except for cereals. Lack of calcium (due to a lack of milk and beans) and dietary fiber (due to choice of cereals and inadequate vegetables and fruits) became a problem for both urban and rural residents. Moreover, lack of riboflavin (due to choices in vegetable types or a lack of animal foods), ascorbic acid (due to a lack of fresh fruits) and selenium (due to a lack of animal foods) were found particularly in rural areas. After this period, the first food-based dietary guideline (FBDG) was established in China in 1989, and a FGP was established in association with a revision of the FBDG in 1997 [11].

To solve the problem in the first period, the recommendation in 1997 to consume "appropriate amounts" of animal food, "plenty" of vegetables and fruits, and consume milk, beans or dairy- or bean-products "everyday" were hoped to benefit both ends of the population [11]. During the period of 2000 to 2004, although rural residents consumed a little more animal food, urban residents did not change their total amount of animal foods. There was just a slight change in the proportion of animal food (an increase in meat, poultry, milk and their products, a decrease in seafood, egg and their products). In addition, an evident decrease in cereal intake and an increase in the intake of vegetables and fruits were observed in urban areas. Cereals were no longer the main source of energy. About 50% of the energy came from protein and fat, and most of this was from animal foods. Meanwhile, there was also an obvious change in rural areas, especially the consumption of fruit (9.32-fold increase) and milk (54.38-fold increase). However, lack of calcium and dietary fiber was still a major problem. In addition, lack of retinol (due to choices in vegetable or animal foods types) became a new problem for both urban and rural residents. Furthermore, lack of energy (due to low in cereals intake) and thiamine (due to choice of refined grains) in urban areas and lack of riboflavin (due to low in animal foods intake) in rural areas were found. These changes indicated that the guide partly affected consumption. Moreover, a study showed the awareness rate of the FBDG among Chinese adults increased from 31.9% to 99.2% after education [21]. Therefore, secular and regular education should be effective to increase the awareness and provide people a scientific and reasonable guidance.

During the second period, consumption of large amounts of meat, poultry, and oils and small amount of cereals resulted in a rapid increase in the prevalence of non-communicable disease. By 2004, nearly one-fourth of all Chinese adults were overweight. Moreover, the rate of change in the Chinese overweight status was one of the most rapid in the world, far larger than that in the United States [22,23], and these changes are accelerating [24]. There is in China a large increase in nutrition-related causes of death, such as cancer and cardiovascular disease [25,26]. These causes are directly linked to diet, activity, and obesity [27,28]. Therefore, basic, scientific guideline on a balanced diet is needed for the Chinese population.

Before the third period in this study, a further revision of the FBDGs and the FGP took place in 2007. In China, most of the studies on dietary changes were before the third period [2,10,19]. They found a shift toward a high-fat, high-energy-density and low-fiber diet in the Chinese nutrition transition. In this study, we added some new findings after 2007. We found an increase in the consumption of cereals and in the intake of dietary fiber and thiamine during the period of 2008 to 2011, although the energy intake from carbohydrates was only 51%. This might related to the guidelines which added "including appropriate amount of coarse grains" and the improved awareness of healthy diet among Chinese adults. We also found an increase in bean consumption and a decrease in meat consumption in urban areas. In the meantime, a sharp increase in the consumption of fruits and beans products was found in rural areas. Nevertheless, intake of cholesterol for both urban and rural residents remarkably exceeded 300 mg/day. Furthermore, intakes of every kind of animal food and edible oil also increased significantly for rural residents. One of the reasons for the consumption of a large amount of edible oils may be that both the importation of soybean oil and that domestic production skyrocketed [29,30].

Additionally, the intake of energy and various nutrients for both urban and rural areas can reach 80% RNI/AI or above, but the intake of calcium, retinol and dietary fiber was still not up to the 80% RNI/AI though they increased more than the previous period. A higher intake of iron was also found in this study. This might be partially due to a higher intake of animal food and can explain the lower prevalence (4.6%) of anemia in Tianjin [31]. However, the iron intake was much higher than RNI (over 160%). The result was similar with that of the 2002 NNHS [18]. Moreover, epidemiological studies provide evidence that elevated iron stores are a risk factor for developing cardiovascular and metabolic abnormalities, such as atherosclerosis, diabetes and metabolic syndrome [32,33]. Therefore, a high iron intake in the population is of concern and needs further research. In a word, scientific and reasonable dietary guideline are very important and useful for residents.

The classic Chinese diet includes cereals and vegetables with few animal foods [34]. Many studies indicate that diets largely based on plant foods offer a number of nutritional benefits [35–37]. Lower consumption of meats and higher consumption of grains have long been considered to be part of a healthy diet to help reduce risks for cardiovascular disease [37–40]. However, increased meat consumption and decreased cereal consumption over time is a worldwide phenomenon, especially during recent years, among developing countries that have enjoyed rapid economic development. This dietary pattern is related to increased chronic morbidity, while a greater intake of vegetables, fruits, cereals, nuts, and beans has been independently associated with a lower risk for several chronic diseases, such as cardiovascular disease and many cancers [36,37,41]. Recent findings related to global climate change suggest that high-meat diets are less sustainable [42,43]. Although the nutritional status significantly improved, Chinese will still face the simultaneous challenges of undernutrition and overnutrition for a certain period of time.

This study had several limitations. First, the study population was only from Tianjin, China. Therefore, caution should be used when generalizing the findings from this study to broader populations with different socioeconomic status. Secondly, the third survey used 24 h recall, and the other two used weighted-food records (a gold standard method to assess dietary intakes). Because the relative differences of food and nutrients intakes were less than 10% by two methods [15], we considered data from the three surveys as comparable. Finally, dietary patterns may be affected by many other factors, such as psychosocial–behavioral, educational levels and healthy status [44]. Thus, further study is needed to improve our observation.

5. Conclusions

From this study, we found that there are signs of decline of meat intake in the third period, and meat consumption had peaked and began to decrease in urban areas. Although the contribution of fat to total energy intake did not decrease, fats from plant sources increased. Furthermore, after a very large decrease in cereal consumption, it began to show an increasing trend. Consumption of both beans and milk products showed a stable increase. Although the nutrition transition of rural areas was usually a period slower than urban areas, the dietary structure of rural residents was more and more close to urban residents'. During the important stage of nutrition transition, both the people's efforts and the national efforts are necessary to improve human health.

Nutrients **2016**, *8*, 62

Acknowledgments: The authors would like to thank the Statistical Bureau of Tianjin for their assistance. We also thank the Food and Nutrition Advisory Steering Committee of Tianjin for supporting the project. This work was supported by grants from the National Science and Technology Support Program (No. 2012BAI02B02) and from the National Natural Science Foundation of China (No. 81302422).

Author Contributions: X.W. and G.H. conceived and designed the experiments; X.W., Y.W., X.Z. and M.Z. performed the study; X.W., X.Z., and M.Z. performed statistical analysis; X.W., and G.H. wrote the paper; and X.W. and G.H. had primary responsibility for the final content. All authors read and approved the final manuscript.

Conflicts of Interest: The authors declare no conflict of interest.

References

1. Popkin, B.M. Will China's Nutrition Transition Overwhelm Its Health Care System and Slow Economic Growth? *Health Aff.* **2008**, *27*, 1064–1076. [CrossRef] [PubMed]

2. Du, S.; Lu, B.; Zhai, F.; Popkin, B.M. A New Stage of the Nutrition Transition in China. *Public Health Nutr.* **2002**, *5*, 169–174. [CrossRef] [PubMed]

3. Piazza, A. Food Consumption and Nutritional Status in the P.R.C. In *Westview Special Studies on East Asia*; Westview Press: Boulder, CO, USA, 1986.

4. Popkin, B.M.; Keyou, G.; Zhai, F.; Guo, X.; Ma, H.; Zohoori, N. The nutrition transition in China: A cross-sectional analysis. *Eur. J. Clin. Nutr.* **1993**, *47*, 333–346. [PubMed]

5. World Bank. *World Development Indicators*; World Bank: Washington, DC, USA, 2009.

6. Campbell, T.C.; Parpia, B.; Chen, J. Diet, lifestyle, and the etiology of coronary artery disease: The Cornell China study. *Am. J. Cardiol.* **1998**, *82*, 18T–21T. [CrossRef]

7. Popkin, B.M.; Horton, S.; Kim, S.; Mahal, A.; Shuigao, J. Trends in diet, nutritional status, and diet-related noncommunicable diseases in China and India: The economic costs of the nutrition transition. *Nutr. Rev.* **2001**, *59*, 379–390. [CrossRef] [PubMed]

8. Popkin, B.M.; Horton, S.; Kim, S. The Nutrition Transition and Prevention of Diet-Related Chronic Diseases in Asia and the Pacific. *Food Nutr. Bull.* **2001**, *22*, s1–s58.

9. Popkin, B.M.; Kim, S.; Rusev, E.R.; Du, S.; Zizza, C. Measuring the full economic costs of diet, physical activity and obesity-related chronic diseases. *Obes. Rev.* **2006**, *7*, 271–293. [CrossRef] [PubMed]

10. Zhai, F.; Wang, H.; Du, S.; He, Y.; Wang, Z.; Ge, K.; Popkin, B.M. Prospective study on nutrition transition in China. *Nutr. Rev.* **2009**, *67*, S56–S61. [CrossRef] [PubMed]

11. Ge, K. The transition of Chinese dietary guidelines and food guide pagoda. *Asia Pac. J. Clin. Nutr.* **2011**, *20*, 439–446. [PubMed]

12. Wang, D.S.; Xu, G.C.; Wang, Z.L.; Che, S.P.; Mo, J.X.; Ren, D.L.; Jin, J.M.; Zhang, W.Q. Nutritional problems and improvement measures of Tianjin urban and rural residents dietary. *Tianjin Yi Xue Yuan Xue Bao* **1991**, *15*, 1–6.

13. Wang, X.; Huang, G.W.; Tian, H.G.; Dong, S.R.; Yin, H.G.; Cao, X.H. Investigation on dietary nutrition of urban residents in Tianjin from 2000 to 2004. *Chin. J. Public Health* **2007**, *23*, 1245–1247.

14. Huang, G.W.; Tian, H.G.; Wang, X.; Dong, S.R.; Yin, H.G.; Cao, X.H. Dietary survey of urban and rural residents in tianjin from 2000 to 2004. *Acta Nutr. Sin.* **2007**, *29*, 435–437.

15. Li, Y.; He, Y.; Zhai, F.; Yang, X.; Hu, X.; Zhao, W.; Ma, G.S. Comparison of assessment of food intakes by using 3 dietary survey methods. *Clin. J. Prev. Med.* **2006**, *40*, 273–280.

16. Yang, Y.X.; Wang, G.Y.; Pan, X.C. Chinese Center for Disease Control and Prevention nutrition and food security. In *China Food Composition*; Peking University Medical Press: Peking, China, 2009.

17. Wang, L.D. *Comprehensive Report of Chinese National Nutrition and Health Survey in 2002*; People's Medical Publishing House: Peking, China, 2005.

18. Zhai, F.Y.; He, Y.N.; Ma, G.S.; Li, Y.P.; Wang, Z.H.; Hu, Y.S.; Zhao, L.Y.; Cui, Z.H.; Li, Y.; Yang, X.G. Study on the current status and trend of food consumption among Chinese population. *Zhonghua Liu Xing Bing Xue Za Zhi* **2005**, *26*, 485–488. [PubMed]

19. Chinese Nutrition Society. *Dietary Guidelines for Chinese Residents*; The Tibet People's Publishing House: Tibet, China, 2010.

20. National Bureau of Statistics of China. Indices for Total Amount and Rapidity of Socioeconomic Development. *Part 1–2, China Statistical yearbook 2010*; China Statistical Publisher: Beijing. Available online: http://www.stats.gov.cn/tjsj/ndsj/ (accessed on 14 January 2016).

21. Liang, H.; Huang, W.; Wang, J.Y. Shenzhen citizens' cognitive level on "Guidance on Chinese people's Meal Nutrition". *Occup. Health* **2005**, *21*, 10–13.

22. Popkin, B.M. An overview on the nutrition transition and its health implications: The Bellagio meeting. *Public Health Nutr.* **2002**, *5*, 93–103. [PubMed]

23. Popkin, B.M. The Nutrition Transition in the Developing World. *Dev. Policy Rev.* **2003**, *21*, 581–597. [CrossRef]

24. Wang, H.; Du, S.; Zhai, F.; Popkin, B.M. Trends in the distribution of body mass index among Chinese adults, aged 20–45 years (1989–2000). *Int. J. Obes. (Lond.)* **2007**, *31*, 272–278. [CrossRef] [PubMed]

25. Beaglehole, R. Global cardiovascular disease prevention: Time to get serious. *Lancet* **2001**, *358*, 661–663. [CrossRef]

26. Ezzati, M.; Lopez, A.D.; Rodgers, A.; Vander Hoorn, S.; Murray, C.J.; Comparative Risk Assessment Collaborating Group. Selected major risk factors and global and regional burden of disease. *Lancet* **2002**, *360*, 1347–1360. [CrossRef]

27. Popkin, B.M. Understanding global nutrition dynamics as a step towards controlling cancer incidence. *Nat. Rev. Cancer* **2007**, *7*, 61–67. [CrossRef] [PubMed]

28. Critchley, J.; Liu, J.; Zhao, D.; Wei, W.; Capewell, S. Explaining the increase in coronary heart disease mortality in Beijing between 1984 and 1999. *Circulation* **2004**, *110*, 1236–1244. [CrossRef] [PubMed]

29. Wallingford, J.C.; Yuhas, R.; Du, S.; Zhai, F.; Popkin, B.M. Fatty acids in Chinese edible oils: Value of direct analysis as a basis for labeling. *Food Nutr. Bull.* **2004**, *25*, 330–336. [CrossRef] [PubMed]

30. Popkin, B.M.; Du, S. Dynamics of the nutrition transition toward the animal foods sector in China and its implications: A worried perspective. *J. Nutr.* **2003**, *133*, S3898–S3906.

31. Jing, Y.; Lu, G.S.; Wang, L.; Zhou, Y.J.; Sun, J.; Bai, Y. Epidemiological study of anemia in 18 to 60 years old population in Tianjin area. *J. Prev. Med. Clin. PLA* **2012**, *30*, 406–408.

32. Basuli, D.; Stevens, R.G.; Torti, F.M.; Torti, S.V. Epidemiological associations between iron and cardiovascular disease and diabetes. *Front. Pharmacol.* **2014**, *5*, 117. [PubMed]

33. Felipe, A.; Guadalupe, E.; Druso, P.; Carlos, M.; Pablo, S.; Oscar, C.; Luis, V.; Diego, M.; Jaime, R.; Inés, U.; Federico, L. Serum Ferritin Is Associated with Metabolic Syndrome and Red Meat Consumption. *Oxid. Med. Cell. Longev.* **2015**, *2015*, 769739. [CrossRef] [PubMed]

34. Du, S.; Mroz, TA.; Zhai, F.; Popkin, B.M. Rapid income growth adversely affects diet quality in China–particularly for the poor! *Soc. Sci. Med.* **2004**, *59*, 1505–1515. [CrossRef] [PubMed]

35. Foster, G.D.; Wyatt, H.R.; Hill, J.O.; McGuckin, B.G.; Brill, C.; Mohammed, B.S.; Szapary, P.O.; Rader, D.J.; Edman, J.S.; Klein, S. A randomized trial of a low-carbohydrate diet for obesity. *N. Engl. J. Med.* **2003**, *348*, 2082–2090. [CrossRef] [PubMed]

36. Leitzmann, C. Vegetarian diets: What are the advantages? *Forum Nutr.* **2005**, *57*, 147–156. [PubMed]

37. Sabaté, J. The contribution of vegetarian diets to human health. *Forum Nutr.* **2003**, *56*, 218–220. [PubMed]

38. Dietary Guidelines for Americans 2010. Available online: http://health.gov/dietaryguidelines/dga2010/DietaryGuidelines2010.png (accessed on 14 January 2016).

39. Astrup, A.; Meinert Larsen, T.; Harper, A. Atkins and other low-carbohydrate diets: Hoax or an effective tool for weight loss? *Lancet* **2004**, *364*, 897–899. [CrossRef]

40. Dansinger, M.L.; Gleason, J.A.; Griffith, J.L.; Selker, H.P.; Schaefer, E.J. Comparison of the Atkins, Ornish, Weight Watchers, and Zone diets for weight loss and heart disease risk reduction: A randomized trial. *JAMA* **2005**, *293*, 43–53. [CrossRef] [PubMed]

41. Grosso, G.; Yang, J.; Marventano, S.; Micek, A.; Galvano, F.; Kales, S.N. Nut consumption on all-cause, cardiovascular, and cancer mortality risk: A systematic review and meta-analysis of epidemiologic studies. *Am. J. Clin. Nutr.* **2015**, *101*, 783–793. [CrossRef] [PubMed]

42. Gerber, P.J.; Vellinga, T.V.; Steinfeld, H. Issues and options in addressing the environmental consequences of livestock sector's growth. *Meat Sci.* **2010**, *84*, 244–247. [CrossRef] [PubMed]

43. Horrigan, L.; Lawrence, R.S.; Walker, P. How sustainable agriculture can address the environmental and human health harms of industrial agriculture. *Environ. Health Perspect.* **2002**, *110*, 445–456. [CrossRef] [PubMed]

44. Wang, Y.; Beydoun, M.A.; Caballero, B.; Gary, T.L.; Lawrence, R. Trends and correlates in meat consumption patterns in the US adult population. *Public Health Nutr.* **2010**, *13*, 1333–1345. [CrossRef] [PubMed]

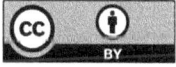

MDPI AG

St. Alban-Anlage 66

4052 Basel, Switzerland

Tel. +41 61 683 77 34

Fax +41 61 302 89 18

http://www.mdpi.com

Nutrients Editorial Office

E-mail: nutrients@mdpi.com

http://www.mdpi.com/journal/nutrients